THE ROUTLEDGE HANDBOOK OF DIET AND NUTRITION IN THE ROMAN WORLD

The Routledge Handbook of Diet and Nutrition in the Roman World presents a comprehensive overview of the sources, issues and methodologies involved in the study of the Roman diet. The focus of the book is on the Mediterranean heartland from the second century BC to the third and fourth centuries AD.

Life is impossible without food, but what people eat is not determined by biology alone, and this makes it a vital subject of social and historical study. The Handbook takes a multi-disciplinary approach in which all kinds of sources and disciplines are combined to study the diet and nutrition of men, women and children in city and countryside in the Roman world. The chapters in this book are structured in five parts. Part I introduces the reader to the wide range of textual, material and bioarchaeological evidence concerning food and nutrition. Part II offers an overview of various kinds of food and drink, including cereals, pulses, olive oil, meat and fish, and the social setting of their consumption. Part III goes beyond the perspective of the Roman adult male by concentrating on women and children, on the cultures of Roman Egypt and Central Europe, as well as the Jews in Palestine and the impact of Christianity. Part IV provides a forum to three scholars to offer their thoughts on what physical anthropology contributes to our understanding of health, diet and (mal)nutrition. The final section puts food supply and its failure in the context of community and empire.

Paul Erdkamp is Professor of Ancient History at the Vrije Universiteit Brussel, Belgium. His research interests focus on the demography and economy of the Roman world, including living standards and food supply. In addition he has published on Republican historiography and Roman warfare. He is author of *Hunger and the Sword. Warfare and Food Supply in Roman Republican Wars* (1998) and *The Grain Market in the Roman Empire* (2005) and edited *A Companion to the Roman Army* (2007), *The Cambridge Companion to Ancient Rome* (2013) and, with Koen Verboven and Arjan Zuiderhoek, *Ownership and Exploitation of Land and Natural Resources in the Roman World* (2015).

Claire Holleran is Senior Lecturer in Classics and Ancient History at the University of Exeter, UK. Her research interests focus on Roman social and economic history, particularly the city of Rome, urban economies, the retail trade and demography. She is the author of *Shopping in Ancient Rome: The Retail Trade in the Late Republic and the Principate* (2012), and co-editor with April Pudsey of *Demography and the Greco-Roman World* (2011), and with Amanda Claridge of *A Companion to the City of Rome* (2018).

THE ROUTLEDGE HANDBOOK OF DIET AND NUTRITION IN THE ROMAN WORLD

Edited by
Paul Erdkamp and Claire Holleran

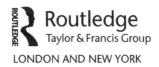

Routledge
Taylor & Francis Group

LONDON AND NEW YORK

First published 2019
by Routledge
2 Park Square, Milton Park, Abingdon, Oxon OX14 4RN

and by Routledge
605 Third Avenue, New York, NY 10017

First issued in paperback 2021

Routledge is an imprint of the Taylor & Francis Group, an informa business

British Library Cataloguing-in-Publication Data
A catalogue record for this book is available from the British Library

Library of Congress Cataloging-in-Publication Data
A catalog record has been requested for this book

ISBN 13: 978-1-03-209456-4 (pbk)
ISBN 13: 978-0-8153-6434-4 (hbk)

Typeset in Bembo
by Florence Production Ltd, Stoodleigh, Devon, UK

CONTENTS

FIGURES

TABLES

NOTES ON CONTRIBUTORS

L.M. Banducci is an Assistant Professor of Greek and Roman Studies at Carleton University, Canada. Her research centres on the archaeology of pre-Roman and Roman Italy, particularly with regards to foodways, domestic technology, and material economy. She specializes in artefact analysis: examining how everyday objects were made, used, and re-purposed. Her current research includes studying the petrology of Roman cooking vessels, and 3D scanning serving vessels from the Capitoline Museums as part of the *Capturing the Life Cycle of Ceramics in Rome* project. She also serves as the Director of Finds at the excavations of the city of Gabii, overseeing the study and publication of the artefacts from this vast site.

Kim Beerden is a Lecturer in Ancient History at Leiden University. Her research explores the history of ancient mentalities, especially the topic of religious dealings with uncertainty. She is the author of a comparative study on ancient divination titled *Worlds Full of Signs: Ancient Greek Divination in Context* (Brill, 2013) but has also published in the field of food and foodways and is currently interested in notions of fat and fattening.

Chryssi Bourbou is a Bioarchaeologist at the Ephorate of Antiquities at Chania (Hellenic Ministry of Culture). She currently holds a senior postdoctoral position at the University of Fribourg (Switzerland), investigating aspects of Roman childhood and weaning patterns. She is the author of various scientific papers and monographs, such as *Health and Disease in Byzantine Crete (7th–12th centuries AD)* (Ashgate, 2010) and co-editor (with L. Schepartz and S. Fox) of the volume *New Directions in the Skeletal Biology of Greece* (American School of Classical Studies at Athens, 2009). Her main research interests include the bioarchaeological analysis of Greek populations, with special emphasis on non-adults, and the application of stable isotope analysis for detecting dietary and weaning patterns.

Wim Broekaert was a postdoctoral researcher in Ancient History at Ghent University. He has published widely on many aspects of Roman trade. He published *Navicularii et negotiantes*, a prosopographical study of Roman merchants and shippers, in 2013.

Willy Clarysse is emeritus professor of Greek and Ancient History at the KULeuven and a member of the Royal Flemish Academy of Belgium. His research is focused on the multicultural and multilingual society of Greco-Roman Egypt, with a special interest for onomastics and prosopography. He is the editor of Greek and demotic papyri, including *Les ostraca grecs d'Elkab* (1990) and *Counting the People in Hellenistic Egypt* (with D.J. Thompson; Cambridge University Press 2006) and the editor of the Leuven Database of Ancient Books (LDAB) online.

John Donahue is Professor of Classical Studies at the College of William and Mary in Virginia. His books, articles and reviews focus on Latin epigraphy and Roman social history, especially ancient health, diet and dining practices. His most recent book is entitled, *Food and Drink in Antiquity: A Sourcebook of Readings from the Greco-Roman World* (2015).

Paul Erdkamp is Professor of Ancient History at the Vrije Universiteit Brussel. His research interest focus on the demography and economy of the Roman world, including living standards and food supply. In addition he has published on Republican historiography and Roman warfare. He is author of *Hunger and the Sword. Warfare and Food Supply in Roman Republican Wars* (Brill 1998) and *The Grain Market in the Roman Empire* (Cambridge University Press 2005) and edited the *Blackwell Companion to the Roman Army* (Wiley-Blackwell 2007), *Cambridge Companion to Ancient Rome* (Cambridge University Press 2013) and, with Koen Verboven and Arjan Zuiderhoek, *Ownership and Exploitation of Land and Natural Resources in the Roman World* (Oxford University Press 2015).

Miko Flohr is Lecturer in Ancient History at Leiden University. His research focuses on the material remains of cities in Roman Italy, and takes a particular interest in the history of everyday economic life in urban shops and workshops. He authored *The World of the Fullo: Work, Economy and Society in Roman Italy* (Oxford University Press, 2013), and co-edited, with Andrew Wilson, *Urban Craftsmen and Traders in the Roman World* (Oxford University Press, 2016) and *The Economy of Pompeii* (Oxford University Press, 2017).

Paul Halstead is Professor of Archaeology at the University of Sheffield. His research explores farming, food and society in late prehistoric–early historic Greece, drawing especially on zoo-archaeological analysis of animal remains and on ethnographic study of 'traditional' rural economies in the Mediterranean. The latter is the focus of his *Two Oxen Ahead: Pre-Mechanized Farming in the Mediterranean* (Wiley Blackwell, 2014).

Annette M. Hansen (MSc) studied Classical and Near Eastern Archaeology (BA, 2010) and Arabic Studies (BA, 2010) at Bryn Mawr College and obtained an MSc in Archaeological Science at the University of Oxford (Keble College, 2012). She is currently completing her PhD project: *The Agricultural Economy of Islamic Jordan, from the Arab Conquest until the Early Ottoman Period* through an NWO Sustainable Humanities fellowship. In addition, she is senior archaeobotanist at archaeological projects in Jordan and Israel. Hansen's main interests are the agricultural and food economies of the Near East from the Late Roman to Islamic periods. She uses an interdisciplinary approach in her research, integrating evidence from (ethno-)archaeo-botany, Arabic written sources and economic history.

F.B.J. (Frits) Heinrich (MA, MSc) studied History (BA, 2009) and Classical and Mediterranean Archaeology (BA, 2010, Research MA, 2011) at the University of Groningen and obtained an MSc in Archaeological Science at the University of Oxford (Brasenose College, 2012). He is currently completing his PhD. In 2017 he was also an Adam Smith Fellow in Political Economy at the Mercatus Center at George Mason University. In addition, he is senior archaeobotanist at archaeological projects in Egypt and Sudan. His main interests are the Roman agricultural economy and premodern agricultural economics, topics which he primarily approaches through (ethno-)archaeobotany, biochemistry, economics and papyrology.

Claire Holleran is Senior Lecturer in Classics and Ancient History at the University of Exeter. Her research interests focus on Roman social and economic history, particularly the city of Rome, urban economies, the retail trade and demography. She is the author of *Shopping in Ancient Rome; the Retail Trade in the Late Republic and the Principate* (Oxford University Press, 2012), and co-editor with April Pudsey of *Demography and the Greco-Roman World* (Cambridge University Press, 2011), and with Amanda Claridge of *A Companion to the City of Rome* (Wiley-Blackwell, 2018).

Tünde Kaszab-Olschewski is an Archaeologist and Lecturer in Archeology of the Roman Provinces at the University of Cologne. Her research interests focus on Roman civil life in the provinces, particularly the rural and small settlements with agricultural and craftsman production. She is the author of *Siedlungsgenese im Bereich des Hambacher Forstes* (Archaeopress, 2006), co-editor and author with Jutta Meurers-Balke of *Grenzenlose Gaumenfreuden. Römische Küche in einer germanischen Provinz* (Philipp von Zabern Verlag, 2010), and with Ingrid Tamerl of *Wald- und Holznutzung in der römischen Antike* (DGUF-Verlag 2017).

Kristina Killgrove is Teaching Assistant Professor at the University of North Carolina. She earned degrees in both Anthropology (PhD) and Classical Archaeology (MA) from the University of North Carolina at Chapel Hill. Her research interests focus on bioarchaeology in the Roman world, including ways to reconstruct diet, disease and migration from human skeletal remains. Her current research is based at the sites of Gabii and Oplontis. She is the author of numerous journal articles and book chapters, and she writes about archaeology, anthropology, and classics for the general public at *Forbes* and *Mental Floss*.

David Kraemer is Professor of Talmud and Rabbinics at the Jewish Theological Seminary He has published eight books on topics as varied as Rabbinic understandings of human suffering, beliefs concerning death and the afterlife in Rabbinic Judaism, and the Jewish family. His publications include *Jewish Eating and Identity Through the Ages* (2007).

Educated at the University of Toronto, **Geoffrey Kron** teaches Greek history at the University of Victoria (Canada). His research focuses on Greco-Roman social and economic history, including agriculture, particularly animal husbandry, social equality and living standards, including nutrition, housing, and public health in the ancient world.

Christian Laes is Professor of Latin and Ancient History at the University of Antwerp and Senior Lecturer in Ancient History at the University of Manchester. He has published five monographs and more than 80 international contributions on the sociocultural history of Roman and Late Antiquity. Human life course (childhood, youth, sexuality, disabilities) has been one of the focuses of his research. The research for this chapter was carried out when he was a Senior Research Fellow at the Institute of Advanced Social Research, University of Tampere.

Alexandra Livarda is an Assistant Professor at the Department of Classics and Archaeology of the University of Nottingham (UK). Much of her work has focused on the archaeology of food and the social role of plants in Roman and medieval societies of Northwestern Europe. She has also worked extensively in the Aegean, where she has co-directed the excavation research project at the Bronze Age town of Palaikastro, Crete, and contributed as an archaeobotanist to several other projects. Her research interests also include ancient sensory studies, the archaeology of rituals and ancient trade networks.

Michael MacKinnon is Professor of Classics at the University of Winnipeg. He specializes in the exploration of the role of animals in Greek and Roman antiquity, with a concentration on the integration of the zooarchaeological, ancient textual and iconographic databases that provide evidence to this effect. As a zooarchaeologist, he has been involved in more than 60 different archaeological projects, chiefly in the Mediterranean region. He is the author of *Production and Consumption of Animals in Roman Italy: Integrating the Zooarchaeological and Textual Evidence* (2004: Journal of Roman Archaeology Supplement 54).

Annalisa Marzano is Professor of Ancient History at the University of Reading, and a Fellow of both the Royal Historical Society and the Society of Antiquaries of London. She has participated in a number of archaeological projects in Italy, Libya and Egypt and published widely on a range of topics related to the social and economic history of the Roman world. Her research is characterized by an interdisciplinary approach combining archaeological, documentary and literary sources. She is the author of *Roman Villas in Central Italy: A Social and Economic History* (2007) and *Harvesting the Sea: The Exploitation of Marine Resource in the Roman Mediterranean* (2013). She is also co-editor, with Guy Métraux, of *The Roman Villa in the Mediterranean Basin: Late Republic to Late Antiquity* (2018).

Shana D. O'Connell is a Lecturer in Classics at Howard University in Washington, DC. In 2015, she received her PhD in the History of Art from Johns Hopkins University. Her research interests include the depiction of still life, materiality and perspective in Campanian wall painting, and artistic technique and ornament as diachronic phenomena in ancient Greco-Roman art. She is also the specialist of painted plaster for the Huqoq Excavation Project in Israel.

Emmanuelle Raga is scientific collaborator at the Université Libre de Bruxelles. Her research focuses on the normative discourse about food in Western Late Antiquity as a heuristic tool for the understanding of the 'Transformation of the Roman World'.

Erica Rowan is a lecturer in Classical Archaeology at Royal Holloway (UK). Her research focuses on ancient diet and consumption practices, the formation and evolution of ancient cultural identities, routes of connectivity and economic developments, particularly in Roman Italy. She has articles in the *American Journal of Archaeology* and *Environmental Archaeology* and she is currently working on a monograph, *Food and Diet in Republican and Imperial Roman Italy* (Bloomsbury) and co-editing a volume with Daniel King entitled *Greek Diet and Medicine in the Roman World*. She is the senior archaeobotanist on projects in Italy, Tunisia and Turkey, looking at material from the Bronze Age to Late Antiquity.

1

INTRODUCTION

Paul Erdkamp and Claire Holleran

Life is impossible without food, but what people eat is not determined by biology alone, and this makes it a vital subject of social and historical study. Food is as complex as society itself, as variations in diet reflect differences in gender and age, social and economic position, cultural and ideological attitudes, technical and agricultural know-how, and climatic and geographic background. What one eats is not a question of choice alone, but also of social conditioning and limited possibilities. At the same time, food is a means of expressing the place of oneself or another in society, and a symbol of one's ideas and beliefs, which becomes even more complex if manners of preparation and consumption of food are taken into account, and with whom food and drink are enjoyed or not. Hence, it is not surprising that food and commensality are such popular areas of research in history, anthropology and other social studies. Rituals and ceremonies of festive meals, symbolic and metaphoric uses of food, religious and philosophic attitudes, and the material context of banquets are excellently discussed in recent publications, and these topics occur in this volume as well, but primarily when directly related to the nature and quality of the food and drink consumed in the Roman world. To be sure, diet and nutrition can only be understood in relation to their social, political, economic and cultural aspects, if only because the images emerging from our written and material sources are very much determined by them. As we have seen, food reflects the complexity of society itself, and hence we cannot discuss food without touching upon its social, cultural, economic and material contexts. However, this is not the main perspective of this book. In general, the aim of this book is to analyse the evidence for the nutrition of various segments of society, trying to offer as much nuance and differentiation as the imperfect sources for the Roman world allow.

The volume covers the entire Roman world, and while this includes those lands beyond the Mediterranean that were gradually subjected to Roman influence and political domination, the focus will be on the Mediterranean heartland. Much of the evidence derives from the late Republic and Principate, and hence, in practice the focus is on the period from the second century BC to the third century AD, but earlier and later times are discussed as well. Treating such a long period in thematic chapters might give the impression of a static approach, but it is clear that very much changed between mid-Republican Rome and the days of high empire, when previously unknown plants had been introduced in the Mediterranean world and central Europe and some exotic foodstuffs, such as pepper, became surprisingly widespread. One of the main questions of this volume is whether we also see a change in living standards and nutrition.

The introduction continues with, first, a brief overview of the past perspectives and debates in the literature on food in classical antiquity; second, a discussion of the need for multi-disciplinarity due to the limitations of the various kinds of sources and related disciplines; third, a brief explanation of the structure of the book.

Ancient Food Studies

The history of food is a flourishing subject.[1] Numerous journals are devoted to food and foodways in historical perspective.[2] Regular conferences are dedicated to food history, such as the annual meetings of the Oxford Symposium on Food and Cookery, the European Institute for Food Culture and History, the Association for the Study of Food and Society (ASFS) in North America, and the Asian Food Study Conference, as well as the biennial symposium of the International Committee for Research into European Food History. In 2013, the 82nd Anglo-American Conference of Historians in London reflected the zeitgeist by choosing Food in History as its conference theme. Landmark publications include *The Oxford Companion to Food* (1999), *The Cambridge World History of Food* (2000), and more recently, the ambitious six-volume *Cultural History of Food* (2012), spanning antiquity to the modern age. *The Food Bibliography*, a bibliographic database jointly compiled by the Harvard University Centre for Italian Renaissance Studies and the European Institute for Food Culture and History currently contains some 20,880 records in eight different languages.[3] Dedicated research centres include Social and Cultural Food Studies (FOST) at the Vrije Univeristeit Brussel (Belgium), the Institut Européen de l'Histoire de l'Alimentation in Tours (France), the SOAS Food Studies Centre in London (UK), and the Centre for the History of Food and Drink at the University of Adelaide (Australia). There are also now numerous undergraduate and graduate programmes on food history in European and North American universities.[4]

Antiquity is at the forefront of this trend, although ancient food studies have a long history. Research goes back to at least the mid-nineteenth century, when studies were predictably antiquarian in their approach.[5] Soyer (1853), for example, drew primarily on literary evidence to compile a comprehensive catalogue of ancient foodstuffs. Food and dining was also very often a part of the 'daily life' works of the first half of the twentieth century, such as Friedländer (English trans. [1908]–1913) and Carcopino (1939; 1941). By the mid-twentieth century, more detailed studies of specific foodstuffs had also begun to appear, focusing in particular on the so-called 'Mediterranean triad' of grain, wine and olive oil, and especially on the staple of grain.[6] In the early 1960s, André (1961) was still relying principally on literary sources, albeit supplemented by pictorial evidence, mainly from Pompeii and other Campanian sites. By the end of that decade, however, Brothwell and Brothwell (1969) were making much greater use of archaeology, including zooarchaeology and archaeobotany, although they still relied chiefly on literature for their broad study of food in antiquity, particularly for the Graeco-Roman period.[7]

The basic listing or cataloguing of literary references to foodstuffs can, of course, only take us so far, not least because the identification of cereals, beans and plants mentioned in ancient literature with their modern counterparts is not always straightforward (André, 1985; Wilkins, 2012, 15).[8] Moreover, the listing of foodstuffs tells us little about the frequency of consumption of particular foods, or their availability to the population as a whole, and inevitably leads to a focus on the elites. It tells us nothing about the nutritional value of food. It does not take account of taboos or religious or cultural restrictions that limit the access of certain population groups to specific foodstuffs. Nor does it include considerations of the role that food played in social relations and in the creation and preservation of particular identities. In short, while it might tell us something about Roman food, it says little about Roman diet. In fact, the study of foodstuffs and the study of diet and nutrition may overlap and intersect, but they are by no means synonymous (Rowan, 2014b, 1.3.2).

White's (1976) article on food requirements and food supplies in classical times was one of the first studies to consider ancient food as it related to diet and nutrition more fully. While his analysis is still heavily dependent on ancient literature, he makes use of archaeological material, which he divides into four categories: the remains of food and food debris; skeletal remains and teeth; surviving artefacts; and painted or sculpted representations of food-related activities (White, 1976, 145). The focus is primarily on cereals and bread, but the (albeit limited) consideration of diet across different social groups and the important research questions that this article posed about the relationship between diet, nutrition and health, famines and food shortages, and the food supply of large urban populations and of armies marked an important step forward in approach. The inclusion of a chart in Appendix E listing the calorific, protein, fat and carbohydrate values of common ancient foodstuffs, such as chestnuts, walnuts, figs, grapes, raisins and olives is also noteworthy. This was followed soon afterwards by Foxhall and Forbes' pivotal article (1982) on grain as a staple food, considering the role of cereals in the diet of various segments of society and applying modern nutritional information to ancient populations to establish the amount of grain required to support an individual based on their age and sex.

In the 1980s and 1990s the field was dominated by Peter Garnsey, who produced a series of groundbreaking publications, focusing in particular on famine and food supply and (mal)nutrition (Garnsey, 1983; 1988; 1991; 1998; 1999). Drawing on a combination of ancient literature (most notably the medical writer Galen), biological science, anthropology, sociology, comparative evidence, skeletal data and archaeological material, he argued that much of the population of the Graeco-Roman world suffered from endemic undernourishment (*contra* Waterlow, 1989).[9] He emphasised that there was no single Mediterranean diet, and that access to food and vulnerability to food crises was determined by factors such as social status, age, gender and geographical location. This included not only regional variations in diet and susceptibility to famine and food shortages, but also differences in food supply between urban and rural populations. While rural populations had a direct connection to the food supply, urban populations were primarily dependent on the market. However, urban populations had something of an advantage in that the urban food supply was a matter of political importance, and elites very often intervened in the market to ensure an adequate food supply, while distributions of food, particularly grain, and the provision of public banquets were part of the world of euergetism. Consequently the urban grain supply, particularly that of Rome, and the relationship between food and politics have been the focus of a number of other important studies (e.g., Rickman, 1980a; Sirks, 1991; Virlouvet, 1995; 2009; Aldrete and Mattingly, 1999; Mattingly and Aldrete, 2000; Erdkamp, 2002; 2005; 2008; Broekaert and Zuiderhoek, 2012b).

In *Food and Society in Classical Antiquity* in particular (1999), Garnsey expanded his focus to consider the cultural and social aspects of food and commensality in more depth. As he emphasises in the preface, 'food is a biocultural phenomenon . . . at once nutrition, needed by the body for survival, and cultural object, with various non-food uses and associations' (Garnsey, 1999, xi). This reflects a longer-term trend in ancient food studies to consider the cultural, social, and religious factors that determined access to food. As Bradley noted (2001, 36), for example, while the consumption of food is essential, 'the *manner* in which food is consumed and shared is a matter of cultural construction', and in the Roman world, communal meals were important markers of status and one's role within a community.[10] Social hierarchies were reinforced by carefully considered seating plans and, very often, by the serving of different food and wine to diners as a reflection of their standing within the social hierarchy.

Commensality and the social context of meals have, therefore, received much attention, encouraged in part by a renewed interest in the Greek *symposium* from the 1980s onwards (Murray, 1990; Slater, 1991; Nielsen and Nielsen, 2001; Nadeau, 2010; Smith and Taussig, 2012). Given the nature of the ancient literary evidence, much of this work has focused on banquets taking place within elite households (*cenae* and *convivia*), which were crucial events in acquiring and maintaining the social and political status of Roman elites, including that of the emperor himself (e.g., Vössing, 2004). D'Arms (1990; 1991), for example, explored the social world of the Roman *convivium*, while Dunbabin (1991; 2003) considered the physical spaces in which such meals took place, as well as providing a detailed analysis of artistic representations of Roman banquets and the role of the formal meal in Roman political and civic life (see also Stein-Hölkeskamp, 2005). The collection of essays edited by Nielsen and Nielsen expanded the focus to consider the experience of formal meals among the elite family more broadly, including children (Bradley, 2001; Nielsen, 2001), while a 2003 special edition of *The American Journal of Philology* focused on dining in the Roman world and included an exploration of the complexities of female posture at the *convivium* (Roller, 2003).[11] Petronius' much-studied Cena of Trimalchio in the *Satyricon* provides a satirical account of a wealthy freedman imitating the dining culture of the elite, although much of the humour for a contemporary audience must have been found in his misreading of the carefully constructed language of the aristocratic banquet (Wallace-Hadrill, 1994, 6; see also Dupont, 1977 on the *cena Trimalchionis*).

Scholarship has also noted the sharing of food among those outside of the upper echelons of society, where communal meals took place in a variety of ritual, religious and social settings. Public feasting (the *cena* and the *epulum*) was, for example, a central part of civic life in the Roman world, whether it was banquets sponsored by the emperor in Rome or by local elites in Italy and the provinces, or meals linked to religious festivals or to the lifecycle, such as marriages and funerals (Donahue, 2003; 2004a). At a family and community level, the communal meal was also commonplace, be it an everyday family meal or people meeting together for a social, political or religious purpose. Meals accompanied funerals (Graham, 2005, 58–63; Lindsay, 2001), and were a central part of the life of *collegia*; the well-known inscription from Lanuvium detailing the laws of the *collegium* of Diana and Antinous includes many rules regulating the behaviour of members at banquets (AD 136; *CIL* 14.2112).[12] Urban inhabitants also ate together in commercialised settings, such as bars and inns (Ellis, 2012). Commensality was equally important among particular religious groups, including (but by no means limited to) Jews, Christians and the Qumran-Essene communities (Bilde, 2001; Hallbäck, 2001; Noy, 2001; White, 2001; Smith, 2003; 2015). For certain groups, such as Jews, and to a lesser extent philosophers and early Christians, regulations restricting the type of food that could be eaten, and with whom, became part of the construction of their identity (Feely-Harnick, 1981; Garnsey, 1999, 82–99; Kraemer, 2009; Rosenblum, 2010; Erdkamp, 2011; Freidenreich, 2011; Nadeau, 2012; see also Beer, 2010). Furthermore, for Roman writers, changes in diet were a reflection of wider social, economic and cultural developments and shifting identities (Purcell, 2003).

Research into Roman diet has, therefore, moved beyond the initial focus on adult male elites in Rome and Italy. This trend can also be seen in the broadening geographical scope, which has moved beyond the 'core' Mediterranean regions to consider other areas. Eating and drinking in Roman Britain, for example, has been the subject of several specialised studies, relying by necessity almost entirely on archaeological material (e.g. Meadows, 1997; 1999; Alcock, 2001; Cool, 2006). Developments in osteoarchaeology and archaeobotany in particular have made such studies possible; from the 1970s onwards, for example, the collection, identification and interpretation of plant remains became commonplace in archaeological excavations, a trend facilitated by the introduction of machine-assisted flotation techniques, the increased frequency of pollen analysis, and developments in techniques of phytolith analysis.[13] The food supply of the Roman army has been considered in some depth (e.g. Davies, 1971; Erdkamp, 1998; Roth, 1999; Kehne, 2011). The relationship between diet and health in ancient medical writers – most notably Galen, whose treatises *On the Powers of Food* and *On Barley Soup* in particular, and to a lesser extent *On Hygiene*, explored the health-giving properties of foods (Grant, 2000) – and the role of food as medicine, have been explored (e.g. Garnsey, 1999; Mazzini, 1999; Wilkins and Hill, 2006, 213–244; Nadeau, 2012). Numerous cookbooks of ancient recipes have been published, inspired in large part by the ancient 'cookbook' attributed to Apicius, which was most likely compiled around the fourth to fifth century AD.[14] Such cookbooks are mainly aimed at a popular audience but give some sense of how Roman food might actually have tasted (e.g., Giacosa, 1992; Dalby and Grainger, 1996; Grant, 1999; Renfrew, 2004; Segan, 2004; Grainger, 2006). The recent publication of *A Companion to Food in the Ancient World* (Wilkins and Nadeau, 2015), with chapters by almost 40 different authors covering all of these topics and more, and a new sourcebook on food and drink in antiquity (Donahue, 2015b), both intended to introduce a new audience to ancient food studies, are testimony to the thriving nature of the discipline.

The need for multidisciplinarity

Diet and nutrition are important topics in themselves, but they are also crucial aspects of demographic and economic history. It is often held that, if living standards and nutrition improved, population rose, and vice versa. Studies of past societies have shown, however, that there is no simple correlation between nutrition on the one hand and mortality and fertility on the other, but it does seem that below a certain level of nutrition, further decrease resulted in higher levels of mortality and lower levels of fertility.[15] In particular, infant mortality is related to the nutritional status of women. The food supply may also be linked to mortality more indirectly, as in the rise in deaths that is observable in premodern Europe even after minor harvest failures, which was due to the spread of infectious diseases rather than the direct consequences of hunger. In times of dearth the number of deaths increased among all classes more or less evenly, but with a time lag among the higher classes, indicating that price rises caused rising mortality primarily through diseases, and that nutritional status offered little protection against the latter. At some point in early-modern Europe, the correlation between harvest failure and mortality disappeared, which is not so much related to rises in productivity as to changes in government and society, which protected the most vulnerable and prevented the disastrous cycle of disease and death from happening. The Roman world does not offer us the demographic data that are required to study the link between nutrition and mortality in the same way as for later premodern societies, but two interesting observations may result from the comparison: first, the link between nutrition, fertility and mortality was undoubtedly as complex in Roman times as in later premodern societies; second, social, political and economic conditions were as important in determining these links as the physical environment of agriculture, climate and biology.[16]

Equally complex is the correlation between nutrition and economy. Nobel Prize winner Robert Fogel argued that most people in premodern societies were simply not adequately fed and healthy enough to be very productive and that progress in productivity in modern society was made possible by recent developments in health and nutrition.[17] The economic historian Gregory Clark maintained that thousands of years of economic development made little progress in living standards. The technological advance and rising labour input between the Neolithic Revolution and the Industrial Revolution did not mean that the individuals involved were fed any better. People in premodern Europe worked harder not in order to fulfil their nutritional needs with better foods – on the contrary, Clark argues – but to feed more of them. There is no trend in improving living conditions up to the Industrial Revolution, but that does not mean that there are no differences in living standards between premodern societies. However, these differences are not linked to technology or economic progress, but to demography. The main point of Clark is that under Malthusian constraints, living standards and nutrition are determined by the balance between mortality and fertility. Clark points to Polynesians, who lived well-nourished lives, not because they spend so many hours working or because their environment was so very productive, but because high mortality resulting from infanticide, human sacrifice and endemic warfare kept population low.[18] Malthusian models have rightly come under severe criticism and so has Clark's, because the links between population, living standards, fertility and demography are not as rigid as Malthusians suppose, but the provocative way in which Clark poses his extreme statements offer food for thought: to what extent is food and nutrition a function of productivity and technology, of agriculture and climate, and to what extent is access to food determined by social and political factors? Basically, the question is to what extent was there scope for improvement in diet and nutrition in the Roman world? Did they actually improve?

Answering these questions requires a multidisciplinary approach in which all kinds of sources are combined. Written and visual sources, which offer a wealth of details on diet, food and dishes, have a long tradition in the exploration of ancient food and foodways. Literary sources, including fiction, biographies, letters and philosophical discourses, mention rations offered to soldiers, citizens or slaves, and meals eaten by various classes of society, sometimes going into considerable detail.[19] Agricultural writers inform us how to produce, process and store a wide range of foodstuffs. Medical treaties provide us with their authors' insights into nutritional aspects of health and food. Inscriptions mention the involvement of magistrates and benefactors in the market supply and provisioning of various foodstuffs on different occasions and in different contexts, including bread, wine, olive oil, meat and fish. In particular the papyri may be supposed to offer particularly valuable information regarding the daily lives of common people in Roman Egypt. On a much smaller scale we have similar evidence in the wooden Vindolanda tablets, which contain official and private documents of a cohort stationed at Hadrian's Wall. However, even regarding the papyri or the Vindolanda tablets, it turns out to be not so very easy to combine the available data into a reconstruction of diet and nutrition of individual people, as it is difficult to generalize the fragmented data into a coherent and comprehensive picture. The literary and epigraphic sources are subject to social and gender bias, as the authors are generally male members of elite urban classes, or at least closely connected to the upper layers of society. Hence, literary accounts provide details concerning the more or less luxurious meals of the richest members of society, but there is a tendency to mention the exceptional and remarkable rather than narrating the mundane *minutiae* of upper-class everyday life. It is also not the case that these urban writers do not pay attention to the food of poor inhabitants of the countryside. Ovid (*Metamorphoses* 8.630–678) is quite specific in his narration of the meal that an elderly couple of smallholders offers to Jupiter and Mercury in the guise of common travellers, while the poem Moretum famously describes in much detail the morning meal of a farmer before he ploughs his fields. However, these narratives primarily reflect the author's desire to depict these characters as sober-living and content rustics and the prejudices of both writers and their well-to-do urban audience. This is even true of medical writers, who might be thought to be trustworthy witnesses of the realities of rural foodways or the differences in the diet and food habits of men and women, but their prescriptive accounts are partly based on their ideas of what should be, and not what is.

When discussing the diet of the common people in the city and in the countryside, we need to differentiate among those social and economic classes that are too easily lumped together as 'the masses' or 'the common people'. There is no reason to doubt the literary sources, such as Columella or Galen, that describe poor dwellers of the countryside as largely living on porridges of coarse grains, or some of them as surviving the winter on dried apples and vetches (normally considered fodder rather than food). But what part of the populace is actually described in these passages? How large is this segment of society, and how common was it for the urban and rural poor to survive on the most frugal of diets? Between the unemployed and homeless beggars who literally starved in the streets of the cities and the highest echelons of society, i.e., the senators, urban councillors and large-landowners, there are many levels of poverty and prosperity, and hence we need to differentiate between various social and economic layers of society. The most vulnerable groups in society are likely to have been the unemployed in the cities, the landless rural proletariat, and in particular the women and children of these classes. The social and gender bias of the written sources and their fragmented, one-sided and incomplete nature makes it nearly impossible to describe on the basis of this kind of evidence only the diet and nutrition of the inhabitants of town and countryside in the Roman world in sufficient shades of grey.

It is often said that archaeology lacks the geographical and social bias of the written sources, but that does not mean that the data unearthed by paleobotanists, archaeozoologists and other specialists are straightforward and uncomplicated, even apart from the fact that archaeological research into food and diet is not evenly spread among the countries that once formed the Roman Empire. The fact that most finds of pepper are located in Britain is, for example, due to the excellent state of archaeological research in this far corner of the Roman Empire rather than its greater presence there. Nevertheless, archaeology is less determined by an urban, upper-class and male perspective than the written sources.

We may distinguish three kinds of archaeological evidence on food and foodways: first, the food itself and the waste associated with it; second, the material environment of consumption, providing insight into the social context of meals of various social groups; and third, the tools and equipment of the processing, preparation, storage and consumption of food and drink.[20] Most valuable are the insights offered by food remains that are found in the physical context of their processing or consumption, i.e. primary deposits, but much of the evidence derives from secondary deposits, i.e. remains that have been moved and disposed elsewhere. The list of foodstuffs represented by the botanical and faunal material found in a wide variety of contexts, going from kitchen and dinner room floors to waste-pits and sewers, is endless.[21] The context of these finds, broadly defined, is crucial for their interpretation. For example, the presence or absence of waste and by-products sheds light on processing activities, whether animals were slaughtered at a different location than their meat was consumed, or whether foodstuffs were cooked at the same location as they were eaten. Hence, written sources on everyday practices are vital for our understanding of the context of archaeological findings. Also the comparison with practices of later times – for example, on storage, processing and preparation of food – is very important, as this informs us about practices that may be lacking from the written evidence and the archaeological remains.

Crucially, the botanical and faunal remains are not a random representation of the diet and hence there is no simple correlation between what is found and what was eaten. The bias in the remains of plants and animals is due to their physical characteristics and the ways of storage and preparation that partly determine their chance of survival. Not only the food itself, but also the containers in which it was stored and distributed, are subject to unequal degradation. For example, stone fruit such as peaches, cherries and apricot will more likely be found than fruit or vegetables that have no robust parts, while dairy products leave far fewer traces than wine or olive oil, which were processed, stored and transported in almost indestructible presses and amphorae. Soil conditions are important too, as bones decompose in acid soils much faster than in others. Finally, ways of preparation determine survival rates of particular foodstuffs, as the charred remains of food that came close to fire during its preparation had a vastly greater chance of survival into modern days than foodstuffs that were prepared without fire. In short, what is mostly found is not necessarily what was mainly eaten.

The consumption of meat and fish is a particularly valuable indicator of changes in living standards, as a rise in spending power will not result in more consumption of the same, but in a gradual shift of consumption towards more luxurious items. As Willem Jongman pointed out, Engel's Law predicts that the spending on basic necessities at first rises with income, but as income increases further, people will generally spend more on expensive sources of calories, such as meat or fish. In other words, a rise in meat consumption reflects a general rise in income.[22] There is a tendency to associate meat consumption in Greek society with animal sacrifices, with little meat consumption outside a context of religious feasts.[23] It is commonly assumed that this was much less the case in Roman times and that many people, including the urban and rural poor, had regular access to meat.[24] However, it is not unproblematic to prove a general rise in meat consumption in Roman times on the basis of the archaeological data.

The analysis of animal bones at various sites throughout the Roman Empire does point to a widespread shift in meat consumption and meat processing. We see relative changes in the proportion of the main meat-providing animals, with a shift towards pigs in some places, cattle in others.[25] These changes not only reflect regional ecological and cultural variances, but also differences between urban and rural sites and between civil and military contexts.[26] Pork was the favoured meat of the Romans, and in the provinces it is particularly associated with high-status, Romanized and military sites.[27] The age distribution of slaughtered animals sheds light on the animal husbandry at various sites, while the composition of bone-finds informs us about slaughtering practices. Cut-marks on bones indicate increasing professionalism of butchering practices in urban contexts. The predominance of older animals shows that livestock was often held particularly for the secondary products, i.e., traction in the case of oxen, wool and milk in the case of sheep and goats. Only pigs were held primarily for their meat. Unequal preservation of animal remains leads to some bias in the remains, as smaller animals are less well preserved and therefore underrepresented. Nevertheless, recent studies confirm the increasing consumption of, for example, chicken. Also dairy products are generally underrepresented in the evidence, as both the products (milk, cheese) and the equipment – generally made of wood – are perishable. Recent studies have also shed light on the widespread consumption of fish. The written evidence seemed to suggest that this was a relatively expensive product, while fishing techniques in the ancient Mediterranean world used to be seen as underdeveloped and unproductive. Careful analysis of faunal remains has indicated a greater role of marine foods and pointed out the vital importance of coastal lagoons and wetlands for the consumption of marine foods in a wider area.[28] All in all, the archaeological data indicate a widespread increase in the role of meat and fish in the everyday food consumption of large segments of society, but it remains unclear to what extent this trend affected the poorer classes.

The statistical analysis of data from different sites requires standardly applied methods and practices, as it would be difficult otherwise to compare results and to draw more general conclusions from separate case studies. Archaeologists distinguish various contexts, such as urban or rural, civil or military, villa or smallholding, local or Roman, and deduce patterns based on the variations between these contexts and the changes over time. Scholars need to apply standard measures and measurements in order to prevent distortions stemming from inter-observer differences or variations in recording practices.[29] However, the main limitation is that it remains very difficult to translate data of finds spread over time and space into reconstructions of individual consumption among the various segments of society. For example, we find a wide variety of foodstuffs in the sewers of one particular insula-building in Herculaneum, including common items such as figs, grapes, olives, eggs and shell-fish, but also small birds, coastal fish and crustaceans, some of which are regarded as expensive and luxurious.[30] Nevertheless, conclusions regarding the diet of the inhabitants of the apartments above are not straightforward, as it is not easy to distinguish the common from the exceptional, to determine the social make-up of these *insulae* and to distinguish the diet of the various households and their members. Zooming in on the diet of particular groups of different age, gender and social class requires a multidisciplinary approach that takes into account all kinds of written, visual and archaeological sources. In view of the unequal entitlement to food and the cultural views on what was appropriate food for men, women and children of different ages, the challenge is to go beyond the statistics of findings at particular sites and to answer the question of which foodstuffs in what quantities and at which frequencies were consumed by individual men, women and children of different social classes.

It is precisely in the bioarchaeological research into the health and nutrition of individuals from the past that giant steps forward have been made in recent decades. We may distinguish the study of health, which is mainly the field of paleopathology and postcranial morphology, and the investigation of diet by means of the biochemical analysis of human remains and the investigation of teeth. Dental evidence has been used to reconstruct individual diets by linking rates of caries and calculus to differences in the composition of the diet.[31] Paleopathology investigates patterns of disease on the basis on skeletal remains, while an important aspect of postcranial morphology is the study of differences in stature, in particular the length of the femur, and developments over time thereof, as an indication of changes in health and nutrition.[32]

Deficiencies in the intake of nutrients leave traces in human skeletons, which offers insight into the health and/or diet of individuals. In particular since the last quarter of the twentieth century, studies of human remains from antiquity have, for instance, explored the presence of *enamel hypoplasia* (stress lines in tooth enamel) as possible indicators of food deprivation and *cribra orbitalia* (the porous condition of eye-sockets) as possibly showing chronic anaemia.[33] In the light of the emphasis on malnutrition and deprivation in premodern societies in food studies at the time, one could even say that many researchers expected to find indicators of poor diets. As important as such research is, one has to realize the complexities of the correlation between stress markers in human bones, disease and nutrition in order to avoid *a priori* assumptions and distorted results. Specialists are now careful in their conclusions, pointing out that skeletal lesions or other features of human bones can be caused by various conditions and thus are not specific for one particular disease or disorder. Insufficient intake of nutrients may have been caused by an inadequate diet, but also by diseases or disorders that hampered the body's ability to absorb nutrients. Rickets and similar conditions are often diagnosed, but may possibly have been caused more often by gastro-intestinal diseases than by deficiencies of the diet. Similarly, anaemia can be related to several causes, one of which may be iron-deficiency in the diet, but the symptoms may just as likely have been caused by a genetic condition of the blood-cells, lead-poisoning or parasites. In short, diagnosis is difficult on the basis of osteological data alone.[34] On the other hand, not all effects of a deficient intake of minerals and vitamins can be deduced from the skeleton, while there are many diseases or disorders that leave no marks on the bones (or at least not marks that are specific for that disease).

Stature is used as a proxy for health and nutrition in past populations and even as an indicator of economic performance.[35] Koepke and Baten (2005) investigated the long-term development of bodily length within Europe from the start of the common era into the early-modern period (see also Flohr in this volume). Their graphs show that stature increased after the fall of the Roman Empire in the West and again when the Black Death struck in the fourteenth century. Hence, while carefully considering the possible determinants of changes in average stature, they conclude that the changes over time reflect a Malthusian scenario, in which average nutrition declined when population rose and improved when population fell. Potential height within a population is genetically determined and whether this potential is reached in individuals can be related to many interconnected determinants, including changes in diet, diseases, urbanization and employment, and hence it is difficult to link long-term trends to one cause. Short-term effects of temporary shortages were probably compensated afterwards, which can be related to variations in timing and duration of the physical development of children over time. The long-term effects of deprivation on the mental health of survivors are far beyond the potential of our sources.

Apart from the investigation of dental remains, individual diet is examined in the biochemical analysis of bone and dental remains. Stable isotope analysis is based on the fact that the biochemical characteristics of tissue reflect the properties of the food consumed when that tissue was formed. Carbon isotopes differ according to the photosynthetic pathways of terrestrial and marine plants, and animals consuming these plants, while nitrogen levels are linked to the consumer's position in the food chain. A 'higher' position in the food chain results in higher $\delta^{15}N$ levels (the so-called trophic level effect). As various foodstuffs have different carbon and nitrogen characteristics, the biochemical analysis of human tissue broadly reveals the composition of an individual's diet. However, isotope analysis cannot distinguish specific foodstuffs; an individual's diet is only revealed in broad categories, such as wheat and/or barley as opposed to millet, marine or terrestrial food, etc.[36] Moreover, more should be known about the impact of biochemical processes on stable isotope values and the possible distortion of reconstructions of diets.[37] Nevertheless, even if only in broad terms, individual results can be taken as the basis for comparative analysis of specific features of particular social, cultural and geographical communities and gender and age-groups.[38]

As dental tissue is formed at different ages and retains its biochemical characteristics, in particular the isotope analysis of deciduous teeth in comparison to the teeth and bones of adults reflects changes in diet at different ages. Change over time in the biochemical characteristics within the dental tissue of an individual is interpreted as indicating a change in physical surroundings, which in turn may indicate migration.[39] The problem here is that little is known of the impact of local variations in physical conditions on isotope values, so that 'migration' may be very local.

The distinction between boys and girls at relatively young ages is difficult to make on the basis of skeletons, so it is not possible to study differences in gender at young ages. It would have been particularly interesting to compare the ideas expressed in medical treatises on the appropriate nourishment of male and female children with the picture emerging from isotope analysis. However, the written and bioarchaeological evidence can be combined in the study of weaning ages in the Roman world. The trophic level effect applies to breastfeeding as well, so that breastfed children have higher nitrogen properties than their mothers. Comparing nitrogen isotopes of infants and children with those of adult women in the same community reveals the age at which the isotope values of infants lower to the same level as that of their mother, in other words the age at which infants are weaned onto foods similar to those eaten by adults. Variations within the Roman world can be linked to cultural differences.[40]

We may conclude with the observation that, in contrast to bioarchaeological evidence, which reveals diet and nutrition at the individual level, but in broad terms, written evidence, paleobotany and zooarchaeology offer very detailed information, which, however, is not easily broken down into the individual level. Archaeological research avoids the urban, upper-class and male biases of the written sources, but the written evidence is vital for shedding light on the contexts of the archaeological finds of food, waste and physical settings of consumption in the Roman world, and it offers insights to cultural and ideological aspects of food that are not always visible in the material evidence. The context of material evidence is crucial for interpretations that avoid the biases inherent in archaeological data. In sum, a multidisciplinary approach will not only reveal the geographical, cultural and social variations in diet and nutrition in the Roman world, but also the changes over time that ultimately can be linked to demographic and economic developments.

What follows

This book is structured in five parts. The first part introduces the reader to the wide range of evidence concerning food and nutrition, the nature of the various sources, and their methodological implications. Kim Beerden sets out to deconstruct the idea that literary and documentary textual evidence allows us to draw an objective image of diet and nutrition, but she also points out that the sources offer a wealth of information on attitudes, norms and values related to food. Shana O'Connell explains the functions and motives of the various genres of pictorial sources, which determine the image emerging from the visual evidence. For those readers who are unfamiliar with the way archaeobotanists, zooarchaeologists, physical anthropologists and other specialists in these fields generate and interpret their data, the next chapters in this section clarify the key concepts and methodological tools in each field of expertise. Laura Banducci explains the methods archaeologists use to answer questions regarding diet from the artefacts involved in the preservation, processing and cooking of food. Alexandra Livarda and Paul Halstead explore the methods employed in the study of plant and animal evidence respectively, and the limitations and the possibilities in this line of inquiry, with the aim of shedding light on the potential of archaeobotanical and archaeozoological research. Chryssi Bourbou deals with the contribution of osteoarchaeology to the reconstruction of Roman dietary patterns, through the study of specific pathological conditions and stable isotope analysis.

The overview of the various items of food and drink in Part II focuses on variation and diversity. John Donahue places the various meals in a social context, which shaped their character and influenced the food that was consumed. There was, for example, a distinction between the meals that were eaten by different members of a household in and outside of a domestic setting, particularly in cities, where the largest part of the population did not have the opportunity to prepare large meals in their private dwellings. The other chapters discuss particular kinds of food, stressing the variety within each category. Variation, for example, in the sense of different kinds of cereals and pulses and the food items made from them, ranging from gruel to white bread, which are discussed by Frits Heinrich and Annette Hansen. Such variation characterizes all the categories that are distinguished in this section: Erica Rowan outlines the evidence for the trade and consumption of table olives and olive oil, elucidating the dietary and nutritional role of this staple food. In his chapter on beverages, Wim Broekaert discusses among others wine and wine-related drinks, which vary from the famous Falernian wine to the pulp that remains after pressing, which was given to the servile workforce to drink. Michael MacKinnon emphasizes the need for a nuanced reconstruction of the consumption of meat and other animal products across time and space by integrating textual and visual evidence with faunal remains from Roman archaeological sites. Annalisa Marzano discusses the entire range of seafood, from common saltwater fish to the most luxurious items on the aristocratic dinner tables, emphasizing the vital contribution of marine foods to the diet of many people. In all of these chapters, the question 'who ate what' is related to the issues of preservation, storage and transportation, with obvious implications for the availability of, on the one hand, vegetables, fruit, herbs and spices, and, on the other, meat and other animal products such as milk and cheese. In short, in this section the consumption of the broad range of items in each category by various groups in society is related to production, processing, preservation, distribution and cultural preferences regarding consumption.

The volume is concerned with the 'Roman world', but this label encompasses a wide geographical, social and cultural range. Descriptions and studies of food in the Roman world tend to be dominated by the perspective of the adult male Greek or Roman in the Mediterranean core-regions of the Roman Empire. The next section aims to go beyond this viewpoint. Christian Laes gives particular attention to women and children within urban and rural households. Other societies often show that the entitlement of women and children to food was inferior to that of adult men, and the Roman world also offers indications of their inferiority and dependency in this regard. This section furthermore aims to identify the particular views on food of peoples beyond the Graeco-Roman core. The ethnic and cultural diversity within the empire was reflected in varied diets. At the same time, acculturation and the distribution of goods through trade and army supply introduced Roman ideas and Mediterranean food items to a much wider world. Three regions and/or peoples are selected to discuss these issues: Tünde Kaszab-Olschewski exposes the diversity of diet across the provinces of central and western Europe; David Kraemer discusses the diet of Jews in Palestine and the diaspora, but he points out that the diverse attitudes to food make it impossible to speak of a 'Jewish' diet; Willy Clarysse explores the unique possibilities of the papyri and ostraca to explore the diet of various segments of the populace of Roman Egypt, although it remains difficult to draw general conclusions from the numerous scraps of information. The section ends with the impact of Christianity on food and eating culture. Emmanuelle Raga shows that, while food and diet at first played no great role in early Christian discourse, it became a central issue in the developing Christian ethos, leading to the spread of asceticism as the proper way of life of a good Christian.

New research in the field of physical anthropology has created new possibilities to shed light on the nature of the diet and quality of nourishment of various groups at different times and regions in the Roman world. However, the interpretation of the data generated by recent research is not beyond debate; opinions differ not only on diet, nourishment and the extent of malnutrition in the various parts of the Roman world, but also on what this kind of research can and cannot reveal. Part IV therefore provides a forum to three scholars to offer their thoughts on the issues of diet, malnutrition and stature. Kristina Killgrove offers a careful survey of what recent bioarchaeological investigations in Italy tell us about the diet and nutrition of various segments of society. Geoffrey Kron argues that relatively low levels of social inequality resulted in nutritious diets and high levels of living standards for most people, reflected in high stature as revealed by average femur lengths in Italy and beyond. Miko Flohr responds by drawing attention to the limits of what physical anthropology, and in particular femur length, can tell us about average levels of nutrition, arguing that at this point it is not yet possible to draw definite conclusions.

In the final section, Claire Holleran explores the urban food supply. Despite the elite ideology of autarky and the role of imperial rulers in feeding certain segments of society, a large part of the population of the Roman world depended on commercial channels for their access to food, and few were entirely separated from the market. Hence the commercial channels involved in the distribution of various foodstuffs are an important aspect of diet and nourishment. However, local authorities and imperial rules intervened regularly in the food supply, determining the margins in which the market operated. Supply systems sometimes failed, in extreme cases leading to widespread starvation and famine (which is related to but should be separated from the issue of structural malnourishment), but it is nearly impossible to quantify the impact of famines on the basis of the ancient sources alone. Paul Erdkamp attempts to assess the impact of food crises by analysing their causes and the coping strategies available to individuals and communities in the Roman world and by comparing the impressionistic accounts of ancient authors to the hard data of early-modern documentary evidence.

Notes

1 For an overview of intellectual trends in food history in 2012, see the collection of essays edited by Claflin and Scholliers (2012), especially the introduction by the editors. See also Super, 2002 for a discussion of general trends up to that date.

2 For example, *Petits Propos Culinaires* (1979–); *Food and Foodways* (1984–); *Food, Culture and Society* (1996–); *Gastronomica* (2001–); *Food and History* (2003–). See Claflin and Scholliers, 2012, 1, 7.

3 www.foodbibliography.eu/index_en.asp (accessed 27 July 2016).

4 A list of programmes is available on the *ASFS* website: www.food-culture.org/food-studies-programs (accessed 28 July 2016).

5 Lombardo 1995, 256. See Rowan, 2014b, chapter 1 for a useful overview of the development of ancient food studies.

6 For example, Jasny, 1941–1942; 1944a; 1950; Moritz, 1958.

7 Salza Prina Ricotta was still taking a literary approach in 1983, exploring Roman cooking and meals through separate chapters on authors from Cato through to Juvenal, but see Gowers, 1993 for a more sophisticated analysis of ancient literary accounts of food and dining. Also Dupont, 1977. See also Hudson, 1989 for food in satire. For a brief overview of food in literature, see also Leigh, 2015.

8 For a more modern (and very useful) take on the antiquarian encyclopaedic approach, see Dalby, 2003. See also for individual entries for specific fruits, vegetables, fish, cereals, etc. showing the difficulties of equating ancient terminology with modern foodstuffs.

9 On dietary deficiency, see also Sippel, 1987.

10 For a brief overview, with further reading, see Donahue, 2015a, 253–259.

11 On the place of women and children at banquets, see also Vössing, 2012, 138–143.

12 See also *CIL* 6.10234 for a similar focus on feasting in the *collegium* of Aesculapius and Hygia. For further examples, see Donahue, 2003, 434. See also Ascough, 2008; Harland, 2012.

13 Rowan, 2014b, 11–12; also Pearsall, 2000, 3–6. In general on archaeobotany, see Pearsall, 2000; Livarda in this volume.

14 For a recent translation of Apicius, see Grocock and Grainger, 2006; on ancient cookery books, including Apicius, see Nadeau, 2015. See also Faas, 1994, who provides a series of recipes alongside a brief culinary history of Rome and a discussion of ingredients and cooking processes, with the proviso that it is not intended as a practical cookery book, since few of the recipes are easy to prepare and are, in any case, not necessarily suitable for the modern palate.

15 Schofield, 2006.

16 On the political aspects of food supply, see in particular Garnsey, 1999; Erdkamp, 2005; Alston and Van Nijf, 2008.

17 Fogel, 1989/2012.

18 Clark, 2007, in particular chapter 3, 'Living standards', pp. 40–70.

19 For an exhaustive analysis of the evidence on grain consumption, see Foxhall and Forbes, 1982.

20 Thus, Pitts, 2015.

21 For an exhaustive study of paleobotanical remains, see Van der Veen et al., 2011.

22 Jongman, 2007a.

23 Cf. Ekroth, 2007.

24 MacKinnon, 2004. Cf. Corbier, 1989.

25 Regarding Britain, see Cool, 2006.

26 Chandezon, 2015.

27 On pig-raising, see MacKinnon, 2004.
28 Marzano, 2013b; Mylona, 2015.
29 Thus, Killgrove in this volume.
30 Robinson and Rowan, 2015.
31 Prowse, 2011. Bonsall, 2014, points out that medical writings suggest differences in diet between men and women, but that analysis of dental health of men and women in Roman Britain indicate broadly similar diets. This is an interesting example of combining different sources. However, we should take into account great cultural variations within the vast Roman Empire.
32 See also Waldron, 2006.
33 See in particular Garnsey, 1999, in particular pp. 43–61. On the history of bioarchaeology, MacKinnon, 2007.
34 E.g. recently, Redfern et al., 2015.
35 Kron, 2005a.
36 E.g. Prowse et al., 2004; Craig et al., 2009.
37 Craig et al., 2013.
38 The bibliography is rapidly growing. See for example an analysis of Christian diet: Rutgers, 2009. On the difference between urban and suburban Rome, Killgrove and Tykot, 2013.
39 Prowse et al., 2007; Killgrove, 2010a.
40 Powell et al., 2014.

PART I

Evidence and methodology

2

TEXTUAL EVIDENCE

Roman reflections of realities

Kim Beerden

Introduction

The textual sources on the topic of food and foodways in the ancient world are certainly abundant, and in many senses they are also rich and varied. There are literary sources: poetry in the shape of comedy, satire or epic; as well as prose – consider agricultural manuals, medical-philosophical treatises, 'Apicius' and Athenaeus. In addition to such literary texts, there are documentary (epigraphical and papyrological) sources. This discussion about the study of ancient food and foodways through textual sources will refer to both literary and documentary sources, except for the papyrological sources: these are extensively discussed elsewhere in this volume.[1]

Evaluation of the sources

Although the textual sources are plentiful in terms of quantity, they are both very revealing about a number of topics – and silent on others. They also have their inherent limitations. The ancient past is what has been – and the past cannot be *known* as such. All we have are the sources, which are always *reflections* of a past reality. Our interpretations of these reflections shape our vision of the past. Critical evaluation of the sources is key: three factors, then, come into play. First, the subjectivity of the author; second, the subjectivity of our interpretation of the sources; and third, the issue of representativity.

The first issue is the subjectivity of the author: we may think of a sliding scale – on the left side we find sources such as dental and bone remains, sources that the author had no intention of leaving. Moving towards the middle of the sliding scale, epigraphical sources emerge;[2] then literary sources such as ancient historiography; and furthest to the right genres such as comedy can be found, which intentionally and explicitly play with ideas about the historical context in which they are created.

For any of the textual sources discussed here, it holds that the author will have written his (usually not her) work with a particular aim; from a particular perspective; within a particular geographical and historical context; and within the context of his genre (the boundaries of which he might at the same time stretch). '[These] works belong to different cultural and social levels, they often form part of a rigidly defined literary genre, and are above all affected by the demands of the intended readership' (Gabba, 1983, 75). It follows that any textual source shows a particular reflection of a topic at a particular moment in a particular place in time.

Sources on food are based on the realities of a historical context, but are at the same time layered with perceptions, norms and values. Due to the great cultural importance of food and foodways the sources are perhaps even more normative than sources on other topics. Whether this is an issue or not, depends on the question that is being asked. When students of ancient food and foodways ask questions about perceptions, norms, symbols and values related to their topic, they will usually have at least some textual source materials to turn to in order to find possible answers. Take the important work *The Loaded Table*: its author studies Roman mentalities by investigating how food is represented in different literary genres – a perfectly viable and important approach: 'The literary medium need not be seen as an obstruction; indeed, the kinds of evasions and prejudices that seem to cloud it can be illuminating in themselves' (Gowers, 1993, 2). However, when other kinds of questions are raised – those that deal with the realities of food and foodways in the context of society – the textual (and especially the literary) sources should be used with caution.

The second issue is the subjectivity of our modern interpretation of the sources. We should be careful not to impose our own norms or morals on the ancient evidence. As historians, we try to understand the past in the best ways we can. It is, however, clear that our experiences of food differ from those in the ancient world in so many ways. As a result, we should take into account that we may have serious difficulty in considering issues related to everyday experiences of food shortages, autarky and so on.

The third issue is the representative character of the sources. It can be very hard to find supportive evidence for statements found in the literary sources because there might only be one source on an issue – ideally, there should be other sources confirming or disconfirming the first source. This brings attention to the wider issue of whether or not a source, or a group of sources, can be seen as representative. If questions deal with realities of food – for example, did the Romans eat seabass? – how may we define representativeness? Perhaps there are some literary sources attesting this, and in combination with archaeological remains it may be plausibly argued that seabass was eaten. But which segment of society ate this fish? And during which period of time did they do this? In other words: how much evidence do we need before we feel we know something definitive about Roman realities?

The existence of these three issues does not mean textual sources should not be used for the study of historical realities of food and foodways: each source should be treasured and interpreted to the fullest and to our best abilities as historians. At the same time it should not be used to construct more of an ancient historical context than can be plausibly deduced. Every source has to do with a reality about which we are eager to find out more, but we should not get carried away and jump to conclusions that might not be as 'hard' as they seem – in terms of subjectivity; interpretation; or representative character of the source.

All in all, it is necessary to consider in which ways sources reflect the perceptions, norms and values of its subjective author. Ideas about these issues will have consequences for the ways the source can be used by a subjective historian. It is one of the core tasks of any student of the ancient world to consider each textual source in the context of connections between reflections of realities and possible historical realities.

Genres and their pitfalls

This chapter discusses the contributions, biases and shortcomings of each genre of textual evidence we may use for the study of Roman food and foodways – and suggest how we may approach a variety of sources.

Poetry and fictional prose

Many sources in this category briefly refer to food – we may think of Ovid's aphrodisiacs (Ov., *Ars Am*. II.12) – and others deal with it more extensively. I will restrict myself to the latter category here: one example is the *Moretum*. In this poem, assigned to Virgil,[3] a poor farmer bakes his bread and decides to make a soft cheese paste/salad by adding ingredients such as garlic to his soft cheese:

> The [garlic] bulb, saved with the
> leaves, he dips in water, and drops into the mortar's hollow circle.
> Thereon he sprinkles grains of salt, adds cheese hardened with
> consuming salt, and heaps on top the herbs he has collected; with
> his left hand he wedges the mortar between his shaggy thighs,
> while his right first crushes with a pestle the fragrant garlic, then
> grinds all evenly in a juicy mixture.[4]

After eating his bread and this *moretum*, he is ready to face another day in the fields. Which conclusions might we draw? Should we see the way this farmer prepares his bread and *moretum* as realistic? Was this food daily fare for farmers? Or does the author aim to show us something about the poor and how they lived, using the preparation of food as a metaphor? Fortunately, there are other sources on this topic but this is not always the case.[5]

Roman satire touches upon many topics related to food: Wilkins distinguishes nostalgia, rural purity, gluttony, hierarchies, and ideas about the elite (Wilkins and Hill, 2006, 268). Food – which food was eaten as well as how it was eaten – was a prime way of distinguishing between various groups and classes in a society. Petronius' *Satyricon* 26–78 is a prime example of such satire. The freedman Trimalchio misbehaves: but how? Which topics are problematized? What does this say about norms and values, and what about realities? The same questions may be asked from the 'dinner-invitation poems' by the likes of Martial and Juvenal: which issues are satirized here?

> If the thought of a gloomy dinner at home depresses you, Toranius, you can go hungry with me. If it's your habit to take a snack beforehand, you won't lack for cheap Cappadocian lettuces and smelly leeks, chopped tunny will lurk in halves of egg. A green cabbage-sprout fresh from the chilly garden will be served on a black plate for your oily fingers to handle, and a sausage lying on snow-white porridge and pale beans with ruddy bacon. If you wish for the bounties of dessert, you will be offered withering grapes and pears that bear the name of Syrian and chestnuts roasted in a slow fire, produce of cultured Naples.[6]

While this category is an extremely useful group of sources for the study of attitudes towards food and foodways, it leaves us guessing on many other topics.

'Non-fictional prose'

Recipes and agricultural information

The most important sources of this genre are Cato's *De agri cultura* (second century BC), Varro's *De re rustica* (first century BC), Columella's *De re rustica* (first century AD), and Palladius' *Opus agriculturae* (fourth/fifth century AD) – but Pliny the Elder's *Historia Naturalis* should not be overlooked. The first four are agricultural manuals for the wealthy farmer, and contain a wealth of information. For our purposes it is most important to focus on recipes and the information on the production of foodstuffs that these texts provide. Although we call these sources 'manuals', they are certainly no dry or technical descriptive texts. The use of rhetorical strategies should not be downplayed. For example, Varro's biting wit and humor have certainly received attention (Cardauns, 2001, 25–29) and the work has been described as a 'philosophical and satirical dialogue' with an intellectual and political agenda – and not only as the technical treatise that it has often been considered to be (Nelsestuen, 2015, 2–8). Cato, Columella and Palladius, too, should be considered as authors who put a personal stamp on their work. It has been argued that there are three ways to 'read' these 'manuals': as nonfictional treatises about the theory and practice of agriculture; as literary works; and as moralistic works about self-representation of the elite within Roman society (Diederich, 2007, 2). A fourth may be added: that of agriculture in the context on views on Roman expansion (Spanier, 2010).

Pliny the Elder as well provides recipes and other agricultural information – especially in books 17 and 18, but also on related topics such as botany, zoology, and pharmacology – in his encyclopaedic *Historia naturalis*. Pliny cites many sources and is a critical author, but it is still hard for us to evaluate how far his information is correct.[7]

'Apicius'

Apicius' *De re coquinaria* is the only 'cookery book' we have from antiquity, although recipes may also be found in sources such as Cato and Columella, as discussed above. The questions regarding who has written this 'cookery book', when, and for whom have all been problematized in the literature – and these questions are a clue to its reliability. The source as we know it is normally dated to the fourth century AD and was named after a famous gourmet (Apicius) from the first century.[8] Its genesis was probably a dynamic process: 'a late compilation of a number of different works which combine medical interests, rare food, and adaptation of cheap foods to make equivalents of expensive foods' (Wilkins and Hill, 2006, 208). The following fragments give an idea of what to expect from this text:

> I Peeled cucumbers. Serve with *liquamen* or *oenogarum*: you will find this makes them more tender, and they will not cause flatulence or heaviness.
>
> II Peeled cucumbers, another method. Stew with boiled brains, cumin and a little honey, celery seed, *liquamen*, and oil. Bind with eggs, sprinkle with pepper, and serve.
>
> III Cucumbers, another method. Dressing for salad: pepper, pennyroyal, honey or *passum*, *liquamen*, and vinegar. Sometimes asafoetida is added.[9]

A cookery book is certainly no objective source – consider the values, norms and expectations of the cookery books on our own shelves. Apicius should certainly not be taken at face value: the 'recipes', discussed one by one in ten books, were not just a systematic and factual exploration of the Roman kitchen (although some recipes can be found in other sources, too[10]). So, what does Apicius convey about what Romans ate?

There are two ways of answering this question: first, to see Apicius as a source that people used to cook from (a manual), and second, as a normative source that was not used in practice (and is aspirational) (Wilkins and Hill, 2006, 246). Those arguing the first say that the cookery book was perhaps aimed at cooks working in elite households (the extensive use of spices and exotic ingredients points to this, although at the same time some recipes are very simple!). The books were in Vulgar Latin and contained many Greek loan words,[11] so there is certainly a possibility that cooks without much literacy would use them. If so, did they use these recipes in a literal sense, or should they be seen as blueprints used for inspiration? The fact that most recipes are very vague in terms of quantities of the ingredients should not be forgotten here. This would, at the same time, render the cookery book useless to the untrained.

Those arguing for the second option, of 'Apicius' as a normative source, take a different approach: 'It is deeply unlikely until recently that the cook could read [. . .]. The books on food and cookery that have survived from the period [. . .] are aimed at those at the eating end of the proceedings rather than those at the cooking end' (Wilkins and Hill, 2006, 245). They argue that perhaps 'Apicius' was not used at all in practice: was its possession a mark of status for rich Romans? This leads us to consider the following option: are the recipes not at all objective or meant to be used in practice, but normative in the sense that they show which culinary expectations or wishes rich Romans had, or should have had?

Although these questions cannot be definitively answered, the recipes should, most probably, not be used to illustrate consumption in the Roman world outside the world of the elite. Even then, it should be questioned how far they reflect the real or ideal table of the elite.

Medical-philosophical writings

Diet was an important aspect of ancient medicine because food could bring balance to, or disturb, the humors. Other foods served as drugs (Grant, 2000, 6–7). Consequently, Galen – the second-century doctor and philosopher – addressed food in a number of different ways and in different contexts in the course of his vast intellectual output, among others in his *On the Powers of Food*. Of course, Galen's writings are known to have been polemic and have certainly been written from his particular philosophical point.[12] Still, evaluations of his work for the study of food are generally positive. In Galen's work, 'medicine and food are combined with an observant eye for sociological details. There are few writings from the Roman world who allow us such a window on everyday life.'[13]

When speaking about norms and food, the works of Seneca are more explicit examples of how food is seen through a particular philosophical lens: that of Stoicism. Seneca abhorred luxury, also in terms of food, because he perceived it as decidedly un-Roman and as unrestrained behavior. However, more can be said: Seneca uses 'culinary description [. . .] [as] another "dialect" in his language of moral exposition and a penetrating means of exemplifying and exposing human irrationality, moral weakness, and philosophical shortcomings' (Richardson-Hay, 2009, 75). He tells us about the first-century gourmet Apicius (after whom the collection of recipes is presumably named) who, according to Seneca, led a life full of greed and desire – poisoning himself by means of food and drink:

> After he had squandered a hundred million sesterces upon his kitchen, after he had drunk up at every one of his revels the equivalent of the many largesses of the emperors and the huge revenue of the Capitol, then for the first time, when overwhelmed with debt and actually forced, he began to examine his accounts.[14]

When he had considered his financial situation, Seneca adds, Apicius committed suicide by means of actual poison. Food, in Seneca, 'is code for moral purpose, ethical perception, interpretation, rational capability, and personal fortitude' (Richardson-Hay, 2009, 96). Seneca is a fantastic source for those who wish to study these issues through the lens of food – but those who wish to study food practices should not take this source at face value.

'Symposium literature'

Although there are other texts from Roman times, such as Plutarch's *Dinner of the Seven Wise Men*, that could serve as examples of symposium literature ('Literature which purported to record what happened at specific symposia, real or imaginary': Mossman, 1997, 120), here we focus on Athenaeus as an illustration of the genre. The sophist Athenaeus' *Deipnosophistae* is an extremely valuable literary source for Roman perceptions of the study of food and foodways in classical and Roman Greece. The elite received special attention. In the 15 known books, probably written at the end of the second century AD (although this has been subject of debate), many subjects related to the history of food and foodways are discussed by the banqueters who have gathered for their banquet in the city of Rome:

> In response to such people we should note that drinking-styles vary by city, as Critias establishes in his *Constitution of the Spartans* (88 B 33 D–K), in the following passage: Chians and Thasians (drink) from left to right, from large cups; Athenians (drink) from left to right, from small cups; and Thessalians propose toasts with large vessels to anyone they want. The Spartans, however, drink from individual cups, and the slave who pours the wine (replaces) whatever they drink.[15]

The context of the banquet is fictionalized: a number of known philosophers, rhetoricians, and so on are mentioned by name and other names are hinted at (Bowie, 'Athenaeus [3]', Brill's New Pauly). Apart from the past, the banqueters also reflect on topics from their own present, for example, where reflections on luxury and austerity are concerned (Braund, 2000, 12; Wilkins, 2000, 37). The discussions cite, and refer to, existing sources from the Graeco-Roman world, especially from Greek comedy (which we would often not know in other ways). However, it should be noted that it has been argued that Athenaeus may have misrepresented and misquoted citations: 'taking liberties with his texts, even by our standards being a little bit naughty with them'.[16]

Athenaeus' greater aim is not to provide information about food. Rather it is to write a work that 'reflects the Platonic model' of symposiastic literature and reflects programmatic elements: 'the testing of the present against the past; competitive testing of memory as a pastime at the symposium; the consumption of drink or food once the verbal achievement is complete'; and gluttony (Wilkins, 2000, 25).[17] A. Lukinovich summarizes as follows: 'Athenaeus' true passion is not the banquet itself, but everything having to do with the theme of "the banquet" in literature and in conversation' (Lukinovich, 1990, 265).

All in all, the *Deipnosophistae* should be seen as a literary work in the context of the Second Sophistic – full of wit and play – based on learned research. Attitudes toward consumption – and especially among the elite – are clearly reflected, but how far these were widely shared is unknown.[18]

Epigraphic

Although epigraphic sources differ from the literary sources discussed above in many ways, this does not necessarily mean they are free from normative thinking or implicit aims. This is usually referred to as 'epigraphic bias' (Bodel, 2001, 46–48): 'All that is clear is that each and every public inscription is the result of a deliberate choice, whether motivated by the need to proclaim rules or privileges in permanent form or to give equally permanent expression to the highly competitive value-systems of most ancient communities' (Millar, 1983, 135). As with literary sources, it is unclear how representative the – public and private – epigraphical sources are. After all, inscriptions too are a product of a particular time and place. However, quantitative research may help to answer such questions: Louis Robert's 'mettre en série' aids us here. According to Robert, one piece of epigraphic evidence is not enough. Instead, as many sources as possible should be collected – they should be analyzed as a series or corpus. While doing so, patterns of distribution and diachronic changes should be taken into account.

One category of our epigraphic sources related to food is public inscriptions concerned with communal dining. The inscriptions on public dining show that a benefactor (whether emperor, or a citizen from one of the different *ordines* in a particular city, or someone else altogether) has the means to provide food or a feast. Also, we may gain an insight into which groups were important in a particular city, or it becomes clear that the benefactor favors the group for a different reason. One inscription may illustrate this point:

> The most devoted sisters of Caesia Sabina, the daughter of Cn. Caesius Athictus, erected this statue. She alone of all the women gave a feast to the mothers of the *centumviri* and to their sisters and daughters and to municipal women of every rank. And on the days of the games and of the feast of her own husband, she offered a bath with free oil.[19]

A woman functions as public benefactor here, and provides especially for other women of the city: although women were usually not invited, this inscription explicitly invites women of all ranks to a special public meal. But what does this mean? 'Are these banquets, then, to be understood as occasions similarly marked by limited social interaction among classes of women, [. . .] or did such gatherings represent a genuine opportunity for female solidarity [. . .]?' (Donahue, 2004a, 115) Why was the inscription written – and how did it increase the status of the woman, her husband or the family more generally?

Other epigraphic sources important for the study of food are varied: think of Diocletian's price edict (301 AD) in which maximum prices of – among others – a great many foodstuffs were imposed;[20] or epigraphic sources about the management of imperial estates, revealing the juridical structures in which agriculture took place (Lo Cascio, 2007, 642–643). 'Inscribed *instrumentum*' is another category, and extremely important for the study of the ancient economy, including those aspects related to food. Amphorae take an important place: a number of different kinds of inscriptions were produced during production, transportation and distribution of amphorae. Amphorae stamps, for example those on the terracotta in Monte Testaccio, reveal where the container was made – and as a consequence, trade patterns and the size of the economy.[21] Dipinti on amphorae may reveal the quality of contents, the place of production or the people involved in production – especially when they are studied together, as a corpus. Some examples from Roman Britain are: '(Property) of Attius Secundus, tribune: a jar of three modii';[22] 'Flavoured sauce of fish-tails, matured for the larder. . .';[23] and 'Falernian (wine from the vineyard of) Lollius'.[24]

Towards a fruitful study of food

After this critical discussion of the different genres, which has essentially deconstructed ideas about their objectivity, it has become time to ask the following constructive question: how might we move on towards a fruitful study of – real and ideal – food and foodways in the Roman world?

As for the study of ideal food and foodways: the sources are rich for those interested in images and norms and values related to food, of course taking into account that every source should still be approached in a critical manner.

As for the study of the reality of food and foodways: the answer can only be that textual and other sources – which will here be conveniently referred to as 'archaeological' sources – should be discussed in combination and as complementary. Two important methodological issues arise. First, what has been called 'epistemic independence' between archaeological and textual evidence cannot be assumed: 'they may support one another, but evidence from the textual record is not necessarily independent, in the relevant epistemic sense, from evidence from the material record' (Kosso, 1995, 178). Different independent kinds of sources may point toward the same conclusions: for example, finds of fish bones, textual sources, and human bone analysis may all point toward the idea that fish was eaten. If we are sure that the different sources were produced independently (and have not influenced one another) the conclusions gain in strength (Alberione Dos Reis, 2005, 49–50). The second methodological point is that a careful balance in terms of optimism must be maintained. On the one hand, we should take care not to fall victim to the so-called 'positivist fallacy' where we connect textual sources to archaeological ones, producing 'fallible connections'.[25]

When combining the sources, a fruitful approach may be to change the order in which we examine them.[26] Although many ancient historians and classicists first think of texts, why not start with the archaeological sources and only then look at textual sources to correct or confirm these? Of course, archaeological sources are not exempt from critical evaluation. However, so many of these sources have become – and are still becoming – available (or are re-investigated with the aid of new techniques) that this may be the right time to change our outlook. We may answer questions about Roman realities by starting our analysis with visual; material; archaeobotanical; zooarchaeological; and dental and bone evidence – and then turn to the textual sources.

Notes

1 See Clarysse, this volume.

2 Although sometimes overlooked in discussions of textual sources, these documentary sources should be treated with caution as much as literary texts – and be evaluated critically: Millar, 1983, 98.

3 However, the author was perhaps Ausonius: 'we meet with many an echo of Virgil, but nothing that is stamped as Virgilian.' Fairclough and Goold, 2000, 371, 379. Cf. the commentary by Laudani, 2004, 9–45.

4 Verg. *Moretum* 94–100: servatum gramine bulbum | tinguit aqua lapidisque cavum demittit in orbem. | his salis inspergit micas, sale durus adeso | caseus adicitur, lectas super ingerit herbas, | et laeva testam saetosa sub inguina fulcit, | dextera pistillo primum fragrantia mollit | alia, tum pariter mixto terit omnia suco. Edition and translation: Fairclough and Goold (Loeb Classical Library).

5 Ov. *Fast.* 4.367; Colum. *Rust.* 12.57. These should, however, also be critically evaluated.

6 Mart. *Epigrams* V.78.1–15. si tristi domicenio laboras, | Torani, potes esurire mecum. | non deerunt tibi, si soles προπίνειν, | viles Cappadocae gravesque porri, | divisis cybium latebit ovis. | ponetur digitis tenendus unctis | nigra coliculus virens patella, | algentem modo qui reliquit hortum, | et pultem niveam premens botellus, | et pallens faba cum rubente lardo. | mensae munera si voles secundae, | marcentes tibi porrigentur uvae | et nomen pira quae ferunt Syrorum, | et quas docta Neapolis creavit | lento castaneae vapore tostae [. . .]. Edition and translation: D.R. Shackleton Bailey (Loeb Classical Library).

7 Dalby, 2003: s.v. 'Pliny "the Elder" '.

8 Attestations to, and discussion of, the identity of M. Gavius Apicius: Bode, 1999, 6–20; but see also Lindsay, 1997, 148–153; and 144–148 of the same article for a discussion about the genesis of the work.

9 Apicius III.VI (76–78). I Cucumeres rasos: sive ex liquamine, sive ex oenogaro: sine ructu et gravitudine teneriores sentries. II Aliter cucumeres rasos: elixabis cum cerebellis elixis, cumino et melle modico, [[vel]] apii semine, liquamine et oleo. Ovis obligabis, piper asparges et inferes. III Aliter cucumeres: piper, puleium, mel vel passum, liquamen et acetum. Interdum et silfi accredit. Edition and translation: Flower and Rosenbaum, 1958.

10 E.g., Bode compares Apicius I.6 to Palladius 11.14.9.

11 Dalby, 2003: s.v. 'Apicius'.

12 Cf. the various articles in Gill et al., 2009; and Hankinson, 2008.

13 Grant, 2000, 12. See also Wilkins, 2003, 361, 371–373; Nutton, 1996, 361–363 on an evaluation of the sources Galen uses, as well as his own contribution.

14 Sen. *Ad Helv*. 10.9. Cum sestertium milliens in culinam coniecisset, cum tot congiaria principum et ingens Capitolii vectigal singulis comi-sationibus exsorpsisset, aere alieno oppressus rationes suas tunc primum coactus inspexit. Edition and translation: J.W. Basore (Loeb Classical Library).

15 Ath. *Deipnosophistae* 11.462.e–f. Πρὸς οὓς λεκτέον ὅτι τρόποι εἰσὶ πόσεων κατὰ πόλεις ἴδιοι, ὡς Κριτίας παρίστησιν ἐν τῇ Λακεδαιμονίων Πολιτείᾳ διὰ τούτων· ὁ μὲν Χῖος καὶ Θάσιος ἐκ μεγάλων κυλίκων ἐπιδέξια, ὁ δ᾽ Ἀττικὸς ἐκ μικρῶν ἐπιδέξια, ὁ δὲ Θετταλικὸς | ἐκπώματα προπίνει ὅτῳ ἂν βούλωνται μεγάλα. Λακεδαιμόνιοι δὲ τὴν παρ᾽ αὑτῷ ἕκαστος πίνει, ὁ δὲ παῖς ὁ οἰνοχόος ὅσον ἂν ἀποπίῃ. Translation and edition: S. Douglas Olson (Loeb Classical Library).

16 Pelling, 2000, 188. Cf. Wilkins and Hill, 1996, 429–438.

17 Cf. König, 2012, 90–120.

18 Braund and Wilkins, 2000, 39. On Athenaeus as a literary work see, however, also Jacob, 2013; Paulas, 2012, 403–439.

19 From Veii, second or third century, *CIL* 11.3811=*ILS* 6583. Caesiae Sabinae | Cn. Caesi Athicti. | Haec sola omnium | feminarum | matribus (centum) vir(orum) et | sororibus et filiab(us) | et omnis ordinis | mulieribus minicipib(us) | epulum dedit, diebusq(ue) | ludorum et epuli | viri sui balneum | cum oleo gratuito |dedit, | sorores pissimae. Edition and translation: Donahue, 2004a, 114.

20 There are other attestations of fixing of prices, see: Noethlichs, 'Edictum [3] Edictum Diocletiani' (visited 12 March 2016). On price-fixing more generally, see also Holleran, this volume.

21 Pucci, 2001, 145–147. For Monte Testaccio see Blázquez et al., 1994–2013.

22 Atti Secundi tr(ibuni) | lagunu(m) m(odiorum) iii. RIB 2492.7, in Collingwood and Wright, 1994, 3–4.

23 Possibly: cod(ae) ting(tae) ve(tus) | penuar(ium) [. . .] OL. RIB 2492.11, in Collingwood and Wright, 1994, 5–6.

24 Fal(ernum) (Lollianum). RIB 2492.18, in Collingwood and Wright, 1994, 7.

25 Small, 1995, 4. The term 'positivist fallacy' that Small refers to is borrowed from Anthony Snodgrass.

26 However, both kinds of evidence should be seen as equally important. On archaeology as text, and text as archaeology see the two very methodologically insightful papers by Dyson, 1995, 25–44; and Hedrick, 1995, 45–88.

3

VISUAL EVIDENCE

Picturing food and food culture in Roman art

Shana D. O'Connell

Introduction

As thematic studies of visual culture become increasingly common, the depiction of food and food culture promises new insight into patterns of actual or aspirational consumption as well as the role of quotidian subjects in ancient aesthetics and art history. Similar to the textual evidence for diet and nutrition, discussed by Kim Beerden in this volume, the visual evidence necessitates a critical evaluation of its formal characteristics, function, and representativeness. In this chapter, I present a sketch of visual sources primarily from painting and mosaic in Campania and North Africa from the first century BC through to the first century AD.[1] These regions offer a substantial quantity of visual evidence for the types of food items depicted and provide parallels to textual sources on depictions of food. Additionally, where possible, I note archaeological context in order to suggest how social space and the conditions of viewing inform the significance of visual representations.

Formal analysis of visual sources

In ancient Greco-Roman art depictions of food serve a variety of visual functions from ornament to narrative. Because most of the visual evidence for food comes from architectural surface decoration (wall paintings, floor mosaics, relief sculpture), artists had flexibility in how to use food as a subject. The style of individual examples largely depends on medium, region, and date, but the appearance of food, for example a pomegranate or loaf of bread, does not vary significantly whether it is part of a still-life or a scene with human figures. Similarly, depictions of food are consistent between domestic, commercial, and funerary spaces.

Food, particularly fruit, frequently appears as an ornament, alone, or woven into a garland along with flowers, greenery, ribbons, and cultic items (for comparison see Dunbabin, 1999, 29). As examples from ancient tombs or sacred architecture demonstrate, in these contexts it is usually symbolic. In tombs, depictions of food associated with the afterlife or fertility and rebirth, such as single pomegranates or eggs, fill in the spaces between figures (discussed further below). On the interior walls of the Ara Pacis—designed to imitate a sacred precinct—the relief sculpture portrays thick garlands weighed down by produce from all seasons of the year. The supernatural abundance asserts a message of largess and, along with suspended *paterae* and *bucrania*, echoes the solemnity of the religious procession depicted on the monument's exterior walls (Kleiner, 1992, 90–91).

Artists also depicted food as an autonomous subject, often, but not always, portrayed within an illusionistic frame or decorative border. Scholars frequently refer to such depictions as "still-life," or "*xenia*," a Greek term discussed in greater detail below. In the tradition of European painting, "still-life" refers to a work of art that eschews human figures in favor of objects, small animals, food, flowers, and so forth.[2] Some examples of still-lifes from Campanian wall painting are not only depictions of food but also depictions of panel paintings of food. These motifs feature illusionistic frames, sometimes with shutters, as if they are set upon shelves or hung on the wall (Croisille, 2015, 30–31 and *passim*). Within the frames artists depicted foods, tablewares, and other objects arranged on and around three-dimensional shelves, plinths, or windows. In later paintings of the Third and Fourth Style, the frames become increasingly flat so that they are only nondescript monochrome lines. The realism of objects and space within the frame continues for many, but not all, still-lifes.

In Second Style wall paintings, un-framed still-lifes appear fully integrated into an illusionistic scene such as a bowl of fruit sitting on a ledge or freshly killed game hanging from a wall (Croisille, 2015, 24–31).[3] In later Third and Fourth Style paintings, still-lifes are depicted on neutral backgrounds with little suggestion of a space (Croisille, 2015, 34–35, 42). Usually a decorative border appears as an organizational feature (rather than an illusionistic frame) similar to the geometric borders that separate different subjects in mosaics (Croisille, 2015, 34; Dunbabin, 1999, Pl. 47, fig. 117).[4]

Finally, food appears in scenes with human or divine figures. It might be part of a scene of distribution (De Caro, 2001, 104–105) or *convivium* (Dunbabin, 1999, 312, Pl. 46).[5] And in mythological paintings it adds to an environment and supports the story depicted. For example, in paintings from Campania, fruit-laden baskets symbolize the fertility of Arcadia (De Caro, 2001, 40–42), or serve as a wedding gift from a centaur to Pirithoös (De Caro, 2001, 44).

Common subjects of visual sources

The eruption of Mt. Vesuvius in AD 79 preserved a large corpus of visual evidence at Pompeii, Herculaneum, and the villas at Oplontis and Stabiae. The extent of preservation at these sites in Campania demonstrates the ubiquity of food in visual culture and offers an important source for the study of diet and nutrition. To date, most scholarship on depictions of food has centered on identification or the relationship between images and text (Croisille, 2015; Squire, 2009; De Caro, 2001). Much work remains to be done on the archaeological context of visual sources in this region and throughout the Roman Empire. Nonetheless, the subjects of Campanian art offer a point of departure. In his study of still-life, S. De Caro identifies "utility" as an organizing principle of objects, particularly food and tableware (2001, 21–22). Adapted for the present discussion, his summary of subjects that relate to food and dining from Campanian painting comprises the following:

1. Edible land, sea, and air animals such as poultry, goats, birds, hares, rabbits, deer, fish, crustaceans, and mollusks.
2. Edible plant life such as gourds, cucumbers, asparagus, mushrooms, nuts, grains, and fruit.
3. Bread, cheese, and eggs.
4. Tablewares and containers, including vases, plates, and cups made of metal, glass, or terracotta as well as woven baskets.

The subjects of the visual sources not only offer evidence for consumption patterns but also relative value. Peaches, for example, were considered to be a recent import in the first century AD (Jashemski and Meyer, 2002, 151–152) and they appear in Campanian painting, including two famous still-lifes from the garden cryptoporticus at the Casa dei Cervi (IV.2) in Herculaneum (Croisille, 2015, 64–66, 88). The choice to depict non-native produce is striking because textual sources suggest moral value was related to tradition and local cultivation. Another still-life from the cryptoporticus shows a mixture of fruit—apples and pomegranates—with peaches (Croisille, 2015, 66). Does this painting, along with the still-lifes of peaches alone, suggest equal symbolic value between the different types of fruit? Would an ancient viewer have reflected on the origins of the fruit depicted? As recent studies suggest, the subjects of the paintings could be a self-conscious reflection on the consumption of "everyday" foods and their pictorial illusion of sensuality.[6]

Visual sources in commercial and private contexts

Visual evidence for Roman food and foodways comes from commercial, domestic, funerary, and sacred contexts throughout the Mediterranean. The social function of a space and the audience and viewing conditions demonstrate the significance of visual sources for the study of diet and nutrition. At the same time, there is similarity in the style and subject matter of the visual sources regardless of the function of a particular space. This consistency not only demonstrates the interconnectedness of private and public display or regional trends but also food as a multivalent subject of visual representation.

While we may assume that elite tastes govern a majority of visual sources, it is important to keep in mind that viewing or making works of art was not limited to elites.[7] Little is known about artists of surviving works and yet they produced art with parallels in the descriptions of works by the most famous artists of the Greco-Roman world, including those credited with depictions of food like Sosos of Pergamon (discussed below).[8] Additionally, ancient wall painters and mosaicists had to account for the physical location of their designs and a viewer's perception. In the following examples, I discuss how artists adapted their techniques of representation in order to emphasize the sensuality of food and to make it appear present as if it was an ingredient, a cooked dish, the remnants of a luxurious banquet, or a dedicatory offering.

At Ostia and Pompeii, paintings of food and tableware decorate commercial areas, perhaps as depictions of items sold and consumed there. In a second-century painting from a tavern in Ostia comestibles are displayed in three groups (Croisille, 2015, 113). The only indication of space is the apparent three-dimensionality of the objects themselves. At the left is a plate set atop a plinth. On the plate there is a cup, some olives, a knife, and carrot or parsnip. Next there is a glass cup holding five olives and set on another plinth. At the right are two round objects—possibly wrapped meat or cheese—hanging from a nail. There is little overlap between individual objects; even the olives are painted as single dots of pigment. This composition allowed viewers to identify the subjects of the painting at a glance and perhaps see them as items for sale (Croisille, 2015, 44; Mielsch 2001, 200). Additionally, the artist's technique makes the food and tableware appear to project towards a viewer. The three-dimensional plinths elevate the plate and cups and the nail holds up the meats. The plate is depicted as if it is seen from an angle above such that its surface looks as if it is tilting forward in order to better show off its contents. Similarly, the transparency of the cup indicates its solidity while also framing a view of the olives it contains.[9] The visibility of the foods makes it seem as if they are fully available to the eye and evokes the perception of a hungry guest who purchases a meal at the establishment.

The still-lifes from the *tablinum* at the Praedia of Julia Felix (II.4.3) in Pompeii demonstrate a similar approach to space and perspective in an effort to highlight a variety of foods,[10] including fruit, grains, eggs, game, fish, and more (Croisille, 2015, 76–82).[11] The relatively large-scale (1 m × 0.72 m) still-lifes appeared in a frieze just above eye-level on the north wall of the room (Figure 3.1). A simple reddish-brown line frames each of the compositions as if they were paintings hung on the wall. Painted at a similar height, in the atrium, is a very fragmentary still-life that included a basket and fruit (Figure 3.2).

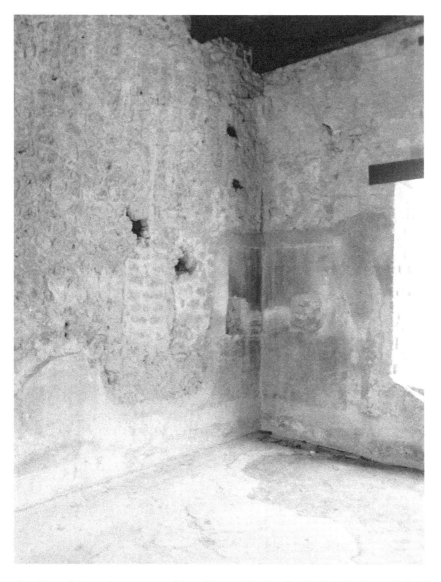

Figure 3.1 View of the northeast corner of the *tablinum* of the Praedia of Julia Felix (Pompeii, II.4.3), 2014 photograph by author, with permission of the Soprintendenza Speciale per I Beni Archeologici di Pompei, Ercolano e Stabia.

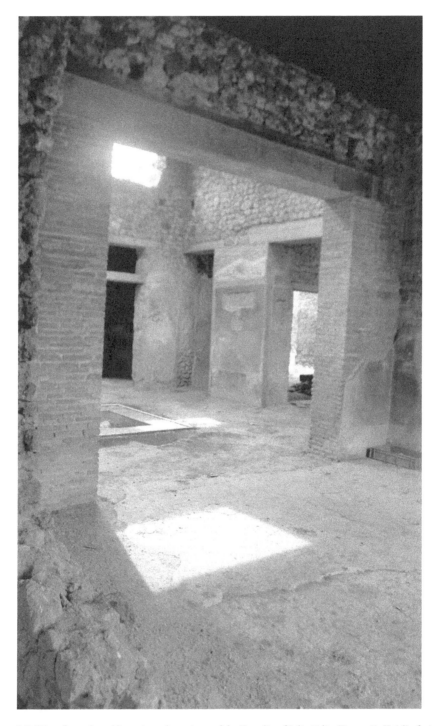

Figure 3.2 View from the *tablinum* into the atrium of the Praedia of Julia Felix (Pompeii, II.4.3), facing
northwest, 2014 photograph by author, with permission of the Soprintendenza Speciale per
I Beni Archeologici di Pompei, Ercolano e Stabia.

The paintings come from a private residence within the complex that also featured a large garden with an outdoor *triclinium*, baths, and rooms for rent; an inscription names Julia Felix as the proprietress. Appropriately the wall paintings of the *tablinum* mixed private and commercial imagery: in addition to the food and dining-related subjects, there is a depiction of writing implements and coins (Croisille, 2015, 79).

Like the painting from the tavern at Ostia, the still-lifes of the Praedia portray food and tablewares with an appearance of corporeality. One of the compositions—another of the most famous paintings of ancient Roman art—features a large glass vessel set on a plinth and packed with fruit (Croisille, 2015, 80). The vessel's transparency shows off the technical skill of its anonymous painter and draws attention to the quinces, apples, pears, pomegranates, and grapes within. Perhaps the depiction of transparent glass is as much a comment on the deceptive nature of art (Squire, 2009, 402; Naumann-Steckner, 1991, 97) as it is a virtuoso subject. Certainly it functions as a frame for the perfectly ripe fruit visible within. By contrast, the terracotta vessels in the same composition required a different approach in order to suggest or show their contents. One, a lidded amphora, leaves the viewer to imagine it contains liquid—wine or oil—based on its shape, while the other, with its lid removed, shows off a pile of small brown objects (dried plums?) piled up above its rim.

In a pendant composition to the still-life with the glass vase, there is silver tableware set on a plinth along with game, a white bottle, and fringed towel (Croisille, 2015, 78). From left to right the silver includes a vase with flared mouth and a spoon with a long handle resting obliquely over it (possibly a *cochlear* for eating escargot), a plate of eggs, and an oinochoe. Although the silver is opaque and reflective, the plate is shown from a slight angle above, like the plate from the tavern at Ostia. Thus it gives a full view of the eggs arranged on its surface. A similar approach to the depiction of a round shape is evident in the transparent glass vase as well. Although fruit conceals much of the rim, a section of it on the left is visible and suggests that the curve of the mouth is a wide oval. Thus the mouth of the vase, like the plate, indicates that it is seen at a slight angle from above. This perspective is not consistent with the side-view of the vase but it maximizes the food's visibility.

A third composition from the *tablinum* shows live fish swimming through blue water (for comparison see Croisille, 2015, 142–143). The side-view of the fish is common in painting and mosaic, regardless whether the fish are alive, in water, or freshly caught and spilling forth from a basket (Croisille, 2015, 119). This view makes each fish easily identifiable by type and it recalls the perspective of a diner who looks down on to a plate of cooked fish lying on one side.

While most Campanian paintings feature food ready-to-eat, rather than consumed, a trompe l'oeil theme of floor mosaics depicts the remnants of a feast. The Elder Pliny credits the invention of this motif—the *asarotos oikos* or unswept floor—to the fourth-century BC mosaicist, Sosos of Pergamon (Dunbabin, 1999, 26–27). One of the best-preserved examples, now in Rome, depicts chicken bones, fish skeletons, partially eaten nuts, fruit, and more. This illusionistically rendered food appears in three bands of mosaic that corresponded to the placement of dining couches in a room. Each piece of food appears to cast a shadow, as if it is something recently tossed onto the floor. Adding temporality to the mosaic is the depiction of a small mouse nibbling on a nut. Like the paintings discussed above, the *asarotos oikos* represents food as an object of consumption. Rather than a tantalizing portrayal of food ready-to-eat, however, this image is the aftermath of a luxurious meal.

The illusionistic techniques of ancient artists make it possible to identify many different types of foods in painting and mosaic. This high-quality of illusionism must remind us, however, that ancient artists were not interested in documentary evidence for the study of diet.[12] They produced works in a variety of contexts and for different patrons. Interdisciplinary study is therefore necessary to understand the significance of visual representations of food as advertisement, demonstration of wealth, and more.

Xenia: Vitruvius on visual sources

Textual sources suggest at least one interpretation of the paintings of food as symbols of hospitality. The testimony of the architect Vitruvius even seems to offer a name—*xenia*—and a social and artistic practice to associate with visual evidence. His account also illustrates the seemingly contradictory relationship between luxury and humility that is often evident in textual sources on food. In a discussion of Greek houses, he writes:

> When the Greeks were more refined and more wealthy, they outfitted dining rooms and bedrooms with well-stocked pantries for their arriving guests, and on the first day would invite them to dinner; subsequently they would send over chickens, eggs, vegetables, fruit, and other rustic produce. For this reason painters who in their pictures imitated the things that were sent to guests called such paintings "hospitalities," *xenia*.[13]

The connection between *xenia* and painting offers a useful source for the iconography and reception of surviving depictions of food.[14] It also explains why these subjects were not limited to areas used for food preparation and dining. A painting or mosaic of chickens, eggs, vegetables, fruit, and the like conveyed a message of hospitality and therefore wealth and abundance to visitors. At the Casa dei Ceii (Pompeii, I.6.15), for example, paintings from the *triclinium* and *fauces* feature similar depictions of food.[15] In the *fauces*, on the interior wall above the entrance, there is a still-life of two pairs of birds, pomegranates and quinces and a handful of nuts on a white background (Figure 3.3).

As visitors left the Casa dei Ceii the painting was a reminder of *xenia* regardless of whether or not they had dined there. Similarly, in the *tablinum* at the Casa dell'Ara Massima (Pompeii, VI. 16.15) small roundels show food (fruit, poultry) and tablewares against a monochrome background.[16] The only sign of three-dimensional space (besides the objects themselves) are "shelves" that divide the composition into registers. Did a visitor see these paintings with

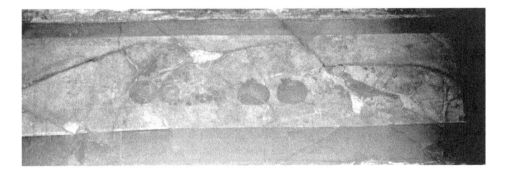

Figure 3.3 Detail of fruit and birds in a Third Style wall painting above the entrance to the Casa dei Ceii (Pompeii, I.6.15), 2014 photograph by author, with permission of the Soprintendenza Speciale per I Beni Archeologici di Pompei, Ercolano e Stabia.

shelves as visual allusions to a well-stocked pantry? Like the still-life from the *fauces*, the still-lifes in the *tablinum* were part of a well-trafficked area in the house.

At the Casa dei Vettii (Pompeii, VI.15.1), a depiction of Priapus with a basket of fruit brings the symbolism of *xenia* into a cultic scene (De Caro, 2001, 115). The painting depicts the god in Eastern attire as he holds a scale and weighs his large phallus against a bag of money. While the subjects of a *xenia* painting were humble, as Vitruvius' *reliquasque res agrestes* suggests, the ability of the host to provide food for guests was a demonstration of wealth. And, as noted above, the ability to afford such decor was also indicative of means.[17] The concept of *xenia* therefore offers a useful lens through which to understand the relationships between décor and viewers or house-owner and guest.

Visual sources in tombs and votives

The portrayal of food as an object of cult is no doubt among its oldest functions in the visual arts. In ancient Italy there is a long history of depicting food and feasting as part of tomb decoration. Lucanian tombs, dating to the fourth century BC, feature paintings with pomegranates, eggs, and grapes as offerings. Single pomegranates also function as ornament between figures (Pontrandolfo et al., 2002, 35 and *passim*; De Caro, 2001, 40–41). Similarly, Etruscan tomb paintings depict feasts that include eggs and pomegranates (Steingraber, 2006, 211 and *passim*).[18]

An unusual late fourth-century BC terracotta votive, now in Basel, features a plate on which a mouse nibbles on a leaf while surrounded by nuts, an apple, grapes, figs, and a pear (Figure 3.4).[19]

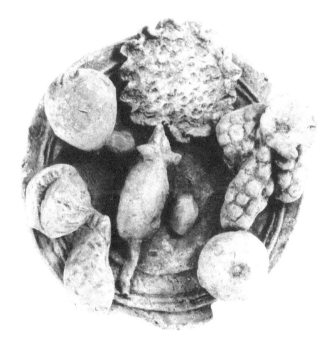

Figure 3.4 Late fourth-century BC terracotta votive of a nibbling mouse on a plate (diameter of 14.5 cm) with fruit and nuts, Antikenmuseum Basel und Sammlung Ludwig, Inv. Lu 128.

The food is dedicatory and the mouse adds a temporal element, similar to the one in mosaic of the *asarotos oikos* mentioned above. Animals often appear with food, sometimes as scavengers like the rooster, partridge, cat, or rabbit (Croisille 2015, 50, 55, 22, 77) in various paintings and mosaics. These depictions are not limited to the funerary context but rather are a ubiquitous motif.

Later in date, the wall paintings of the Tomb of Vestorius Priscus at Pompeii decorate the walls of the tomb and its enclosure with similar imagery. [20] The paintings include a banquet, and still-lifes of a silver drinking service and a peacock standing near/next to a plate of offerings (Mols and Moormann, 1993–1994, 27–32).[21] Both of the still-lifes demonstrate the same pictorial techniques discussed above. The service is set on a table that appears to "tilt" forward and the plate of offerings is depicted as if from slightly above (Mols and Moormann, 1993–1994, 30, 34). Instead of visually presenting the items and food as objects of human consumption, however, the perspective displays them as offerings in commemoration of the 22-year-old man to whom the tomb was dedicated. Similarly, a tomb painting from Rome features a lavish transparent glass vase filled with fruit (Croisille, 2015, 55). The vessel fully displays a view of its contents and casts a shadow on its supporting plinth. Two birds stand on either side, and one, a partridge, even lifts its beak to nibble some grapes spilling from the vessel's mouth.

Conclusion: Visual sources on food production and distribution

Although this chapter has emphasized depictions of food as an object of human consumption, all types of media (painting, mosaic, sculpture) depicted it as the subject of production and distribution as well. By way of a conclusion I will present several examples related to bread. Paintings at an Etruscan tomb in Orvieto not only depict butchered meat but also figures baking bread in preparation for a banquet (Steingraber, 2006, 211–213). At Rome, the monumental tomb of Eurysaces, a freedman and wealthy baker, includes a frieze that shows the production of bread from grinding grain to placing loaves in an oven (Hackworth-Peterson, 2003). Unusual cylinders built into the tomb evoke actual equipment used during the baking process (Hackworth-Peterson, 2003, 246). In a painting from the House of the Baker (Pompeii, VII.3.30), a togate citizen is shown handing a loaf of bread to a man (Roberts, 2013, 28–29). Piled around the "baker" are more yellow loaves waiting to be distributed. The painter depicted lines on each loaf that divide it into wedges. These lines appear in other depictions of bread from still-life (Croisille, 2015, 45, 96) and evoke the actual cuts visible in a carbonized loaf from Herculaneum (Roberts, 2013, 65). Scoring makes bread easier to share, a realistic detail of the paintings that underscores their significance as signs of generosity.

Visual sources for the ancient Roman diet recall the role of food in daily life if they feature human figures, like the scenes of baking bread and distribution, or focus on the foods and utensils meant for human use. Although it may be difficult to recover the degree to which they reflect historical reality, the visual sources continually remind us of the many people for whom the depictions of butchered game, round loaves of bread, or colorful fruits and fish were served forth.

Notes

1 Throughout this chapter I cite visual reproductions of paintings and mosaics in Croisille, 2015; De Caro, 2001; and Dunbabin, 1999.
2 On the problematic use of the term "still-life" to describe ancient paintings see Squire, 2009, 360–371.
3 B. Wesenberg identifies these as "integrated" still-life and argues that they transition between the viewer's reality and the fantastic illusion of the wall painting (1993). M. Squire goes further to show

how depictions of food were visual arguments that engaged viewers in a discourse on the nature of pictorial illusion (2009, 398–408).

4 This compositional strategy is not well represented in the literature on still-life. For an example see the *triclinium* paintings at the Casa dei Ceii (I.6.15) in *Pompei: pitture e mosaici* (hereafter *PPM*), vol. 1, 1990.

5 For discussion and additional reproductions see also Dunbabin, 2003, 159–161.

6 Blake, 2016; Croisille, 2015, 104–110; Squire, 2009, 412.

7 See Clarke, 2003.

8 It is still often assumed that the artists were copying now lost Greek panel paintings, e.g., De Caro, 2001, 22 and *passim*. In her seminal article, B. Bergmann convincingly argues for a more nuanced approach to the wall paintings' imagery (1995). More recently see Pearson, 2015.

9 F. Naumann-Steckner suggests it is possible that the glass is not meant to appear transparent but rather the "olives" are a depiction of surface decoration similar to actual "blobbed" glasses (1991, 97).

10 A number of still-lifes attributed to the Praedia do not survive. For additional reproductions, including eighteenth-century prints see *PPM*, vol. 3.

11 For a discussion of the relationship between the visual effects of the still-lifes—especially transparency—and perception see O'Connell, 2015, 95–137; currently, I am revising my work on this topic for publication.

12 For example, depictions of glass and metal vessels emphasize material qualities (e.g. transparency, reflectivity) and only approximate actual vessels in form and scale (Naumann-Steckner, 1991, 95–97; Riz, 1990, 4).

13 *De Architectura* 6.7.4. . . . Nam cum fuerunt Graeci delicatiores et fortuna opulentiores, hospitibus advenientibus instruebant triclinia, cubicula, cum penu cellas, primoque die ad cenam invitabant, postero mittebant pullos, ova, holera, poma reliquasque res agrestes. Ideo pictores ea, quae mittebantur hospitibus, picturis imitantes xenia appellaverunt. Translation: Rowland 1999.

14 Other sources on *xenia* include Philostratos' *Imagines*, in which two paintings are identified as *xenia*, and Martial's books of epigrams entitled *Xenia* and *Apophoreta*. For an overview of these sources see Croisille, 2015, 104–110. For further discussion of reception see Squire on Philostratos (2009, 416–427) and Blake on Martial (2016).

15 *PPM* vol. 1; Croisille, 2015, 31–33.

16 Croisille, 2015, 70–71.

17 Squire describes Campanian paintings of food as successfully fusing elegance and luxury with the moral ideal of simplicity and traditional Roman values (2009, 408–419).

18 Cf. also an Etruscan bronze statuette of a woman holding a pomegranate at the Harvard Art Museums, Inv. No. 1956.43.

19 Traces of red, yellow, and violet paint remain (Berger, 1982, 97).

20 Mols and Moormann argue that the tomb commemorates specific aspects of Priscus' life and career (1993–1994).

21 On the service see Tamm, 2005.

4

MATERIAL EVIDENCE ON DIET, COOKING AND TECHNIQUES

L.M. Banducci

Introduction

Archaeological artefacts are an important source of information for Roman diet and eating behaviours. When we consider a modern home and how many different objects we have for storing, transporting, mixing, cooking, and serving foods, it is no wonder that many of these domestic artefacts feature as the most commonly recovered items on archaeological sites. The tools for preparing and consuming food were produced, used, and discarded throughout Roman settlements. This massive amount of what is largely household waste provides indirect evidence for diet and nutrition. Archaeologists excavate cooking and dining vessels and other tools made of ceramic, metal, glass, and more rarely, bone and wood.

The manner in which archaeologists have chosen to study these artefacts has changed a great deal in recent decades. The banality of these artefacts and their similarity to the tools of the modern kitchen means that their analysis by scholars has sometimes been superficial. It has seemed obvious that an ancient vessel that looks like a modern jug must have been used to contain and pour liquid. Quite often such assumptions about object function are not incorrect. Without further examination, however, we cannot move beyond the simple conclusion that "Romans poured liquids", leaving unanswered questions like, *which* liquid did this jug contain? How much liquid? Who used it? Was it always used for the same thing? How was it cleaned? Detailed artefact analysis can explore such questions and contribute to Roman food studies by enhancing our knowledge and understanding of the methods of food and drink preparation or cooking, the quantities consumed, and the manner in which they were consumed. This chapter explains the methods archaeologists use to extrapolate these answers.

Ceramic vessels

The recognition that ceramic vessels reflect daily food behaviours has always been implicit in scholars' work; however, only recently has this become of explicit interest. Bronze Age Aegean ceramicists provide an exemplary model after which Romanists can expand their approaches to this subject area.

There are several disciplines through which to approach the study of vessels in the context of diet and nutrition: morphology and material composition, use wear, and residue analysis. The most fruitful conclusions combine these approaches to consider the foodways of ancient Romans. After explaining these approaches below, I outline the various types of vessel that we can identify.

Morphology

The starting point for the study of ceramic vessels and diet is their morphology – their physical form. The relationship between vessel function and vessel morphology has been much debated in archaeological scholarship. The term "function" has its own limitations and multiple meanings, since an object can have many overlapping functions, and may be used in ways for which it was not originally designed (Binford, 1962, 219; Schiffer, 1992, 9–12; Preston, 2000). The form of a vessel can be used to understand its ideal or perhaps intended function, rather than how it was actually used by its ancient owner. Archaeologists can measure several features of vessels in order to consider how a vessel's morphology might reflect and affect its function (see Table 4.1).

Material composition

The composition of the clay of vessels plays an important role in their use. Analysis of the clay surface magnified with a lens can reveal the basics of its composition and the examination of clay with a light polarizing microscope reveals its microscopic mineral composition. Archaeometric approaches are becoming increasingly common in Roman archaeology: this includes petrology, the study of the mineral composition through polarized light microscopy and elemental analyses like x-ray fluorescence and Neutron Activation Analysis, which are focused specifically on clay sourcing (Peña, 1990; Peña and Gallimore, 2014; Mirti and Davit, 2001; Morra et al., 2013).

For the study of vessel function and thus diet, several factors can be examined. The general chemical composition of a vessel's clay matrix, whether primarily ferrous or calcareous, can affect how the vessel will withstand different types of use. In general, ferrous clays are best for helping the vessel withstand thermal shock; that is, quick and dramatic changes in temperature (being placed on and off a fire). Calcareous clays are best for vessels to withstand mechanical shock; that is, knocking or dropping (Olcese, 2003, 19–21).

Furthermore, the inclusion of temper in this matrix affects the vessel's performance. Temper includes the minerals, stones, fossils, or fibres that appear naturally in clay or were added to the clay by the potter to create certain effects. A vessel's ability to conduct heat well throughout its walls, and thus to heat food evenly and efficiently, is also affected by the nature of its clay and tempering. Scientists have created a series of trials with experimental clay briquettes and discs to test the parameters affecting thermal conductivity in ancient vessels. The type of clay, the type of temper, the proportion of temper in the clay, and the original firing temperature of the ceramic are each important to consider. In general quartz temper, especially in angular particles, increases vessel conductivity. The porosity caused by the temper and the orientation of the pores together also has a great effect on thermal conductivity. In one experiment, granite temper comprising about 10% of the clay matrix increased conductivity in clay when it was fired at 550°C and also at 850°C. However, the same experiment conducted with temper making up 40% of the clay matrix resulted in elongated pores in the vessel wall and lower thermal conductivity, in some cases lower than in clay with no temper at all (Hein et al., 2008; Müller et al., 2015).[1]

Table 4.1 Morphological and material variables examined to consider function

Variable name	Definition
Size	Diameter and height, vessel volume
Access to contents	Open/closedness; angle/width of opening suggesting liquid/dry contents
Stability	Centre of gravity and base size and shape
Graspability/purchase	How easy is it to move empty, full, heated?
Durability and flexibility	Resistance to thermal and mechanical stresses
Surface treatment	Porosity/permeability and slippery/stickiness/friction
Wall thickness	The width of the wall

Traces of use

Observation of the traces of use on artefacts provides a vital contribution to our understanding of these artefacts for food preparation and consumption. Use wear analysis, sometimes called alteration analysis, involves the examination of artefact surfaces for abrasion and the accretion of foreign material. The most common form of abrasion is from tool use, in the repetitive stirring of a pot, for example, but abrasion can also occur because of general everyday knocking or stacking (Griffiths, 1978, fig. 8; Banducci, 2014a, fig 2). The study of this wear can determine the interaction between the vessel and the food it contained. Was the user stirring frequently or vigorously a semi-liquid food, like porridge? Was the user frequently cutting on a plate, for a meat or vegetable product?

Accretion of residues can be the result of a number of different activities. A cooking pot used over a charcoal or wood cooking fire acquires layers of soot released from the burning fuel. This soot is both absorbed into the pores of the vessel and becomes caked on its exterior such that even centuries of burial in the ground do not erase the blackened discoloration. On the interior of vessels, residues from food can be found absorbed into vessel walls and on their surface. Patches of charred food, perhaps from over-boiling or the cooking fire being too close or hot, remain on the inside of some cooking pots. The study of the patterning of these blackening residues can reveal the location of the cooking vessel relative to the cooking fire and the manner of cooking, and subsequently, the type of food being cooked (Banducci, 2014a). For example, we can observe that a flat-bottomed, low-walled pan, typically called a *tegame*, is often blackened on its exterior base, demonstrating that it was elevated above the fire. The food on its interior was likely exposed to high heat and perhaps was fried or sautéed vigorously (Banducci, Forthcoming) (see Figure 4.1).

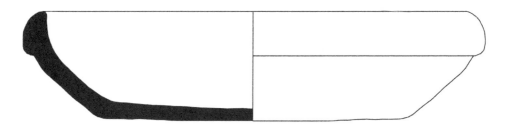

Figure 4.1 Shallow open-form pan, or *tegame*, frequently blackened with soot on its exterior (drawing by author).

Uncharred food residues on the interior of vessels and absorbed into vessel walls can also provide direct evidence for diet. An increasingly sophisticated method in archaeological sciences is the identification of these organic residues using a variety of different devices for chemical analysis. Most commonly, a gas chromatograph and mass spectrometer are used in concert to identify the chemical compounds of the residues and allow scientists to hypothesize the original food product.[2] This technique is particularly good at identifying lipids. It is difficult to identify the exact foodstuff from which these lipids originated, but rather, the category of foodstuff: mammal fats, marine animal fats, dairy fats, or plant oils (Heron and Evershed, 1993, 264–69). There are limitations to residue analysis because of the frequent mixing of plant and animal products in cooking vessels and because of the opportunities for the degradation and contamination of chemical samples over the course of their burial and excavation. Experimental testing has been undertaken in order to account for some of these variables and to try to isolate particular markers that are diagnostic of certain food products (Evershed, 2008a; 2008b).

Ceramic forms

There are few Roman texts that mention ceramic vessel types by name. Many examples in Latin literature appear in didactic or encyclopaedic texts: the works of Cato, Varro, Columella, Pliny the Elder, and Apicius. These authors mention vessels mostly for wine and oil production and, in a few instances, in the context of cooking. Later authors of recipe compilations, Vinidarius and Anthimus, who wrote in the fifth to sixth centuries AD, also explain which cooking vessels should be used for which task. Ancient texts like these are often used to determine the labels scholars apply to archaeological vessels. Scholars have associated terms like *patina*, *caccabus*, *olla*, and *clibanus* with specific artefacts (Bats, 1988; Cubberley et al., 1988). Andrew Donnelly's scrutiny of how these terms are used, and the cooking verbs associated with each vessel (e.g., "boiling", "frying") reveals that there are major inconsistencies within and among Latin authors about which vessels are used for which function (Donnelly, 2015). Thus, we should be careful about labelling different vessel types and then associating those vessels with ancient texts. Just because archaeologists agree that a certain form can be referred to as an *aula* or *olla*, this does not mean that when Cato mentions *aulae*, he intended our chosen form.

Dolia

This vessel is both for storage and large-scale food preparation. *Dolia* sunk into the ground, *dolia defossa*, were used for storing wine as it fermented. Burying the vessels would help insulate them from changes in temperature, keeping the wine at a consistent temperature of perhaps 10°C, through the winter and into the summer (Rossiter, 1981, n. 39). Throughout the area of Mount Vesuvius and at Ostia many storage magazines contain these *dolia*.[3] In the Caseggiato dei Doli at Ostia, 35 *dolia* are preserved sunken into the ground of one room. Many have their total volume inscribed on their rim or upper wall, on average 1040 litres each (Pasqui, 1906, 357–359).

For olive oil production large storage jars, perhaps of the same form as *dolia*, were not sunken into the ground but rather were moved between rooms depending on the stage of oil production. This is suggested both by instructions in the farming manuals of Cato and Columella and by the archaeological evidence for oil processing facilities. These buildings are rarely found with embedded *dolia* (Rossiter, 1981, 359).

Dolia may have also been used for the processing or storage of fish sauce, albeit less frequently. In Pompeii, a house identified as a shop for garum and other fish sauces contains several *dolia defossa* with remains of fish sauce inside. These were originally *dolia* for wine processing (one of them has the letters *VR* for *vinum rubrum*, red wine, incised on its exterior). This fish sauce was likely produced outside the facility, but was either in temporary storage before it was sold to Pompeian customers, or perhaps it was undergoing its last stages of maceration and was being flavoured with particular ingredients by the shop owner (Curtis, 1979, 10–12, 15–20; Peña, 2007, 87).

Amphorae

These are vessels with ovoid bodies, narrow necks and bases often ending in a point, double handles, and thick walls (see Figure 4.2). Amphorae were made throughout the Roman world and their form comes out of a tradition of similar vessels produced by Greeks and Phoenicians from at least the eighth century BC. Roman amphorae most often contained wine, oil or fish sauce, but also dry goods like wheat and nuts (Peña, 2007, table 5.4 and Appendix table A1). Production areas of amphorae are often closely associated with production areas of the foodstuffs they contained. Evidence for amphora production has been found within agricultural estates containing vineyards or facilities for olive oil production, and also at independent sites that seemed to serve a number of nearby estates (Peacock and Williams, 1986, 41–43).

A first method for determining the contents of amphorae is by examining labels painted on their exterior, *tituli picti* (Peacock and Williams, 1986, 17).[4] These labels were not applied to all amphorae and when they were they are not always visible because of the preservation conditions of the soil. *Tituli picti* were written in a number of different ways. In some cases,

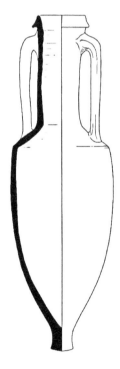

Figure 4.2 Dressel 1 amphora (drawing by author).

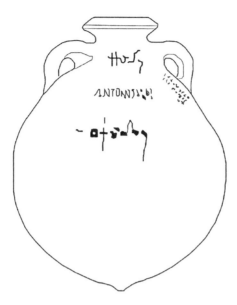

Figure 4.3 Dressel 20 amphora (after Peacock and Williams, 1986, fig. 5).

the *titulus* states the intended contents of the amphora, their quantity, the name of an individual involved in the transaction (e.g., the estate owner) and the location of the foodstuff's production.[5]

In other cases, the *titulus* has been used to extrapolate the original contents of the amphora. One spherical amphora from Baetica, Spain, produced in great quantities between the first century and third century AD, presents such a situation. This type, called Dressel 20, has *tituli* notations with a series of numbers (see Figure 4.3). One number indicates the empty weight of the amphora in Roman pounds, another number indicates the weight of the contents inside the amphora (with the weight of the amphora subtracted). Based on the mass of olive oil and the volume of this amphora type, archaeologists are able to confirm that olive oil is what Dressel 20 amphorae transported (Rodriguez-Almeida, 1972, 121–122). These amphorae comprise the majority of the hill of Monte Testaccio in Rome, thus illustrating the large quantity of Spanish olive oil imported into the city.

The remains of amphorae as part of shipwrecks also provide an opportunity to observe what they contained. In a few cases the contents are preserved in residue inside the amphorae. For example, recent work on the amphorae of the first century BC shipwreck off the coast of Albegna, Italy has confirmed that the Dressel 1A amphorae it transported were carrying wine from central-southern Italy. The amphora tested was well-sealed with lime-pozzolana paste. The liquid inside was significantly deteriorated and contaminated with seawater and clay matter; yet, it was clearly Italian wine perhaps with gypsum added for flavouring. This was determined using a combination of residue analysis (ICP-MS), isotopic analysis (with isotope ratio mass spectrometry), and analysis of the pollen residue remaining in the liquid (Arobba et al., 2014).

Vessels for food preparation and cooking

These ceramics can be divided into two groups: vessels for preparing and storing foods, and vessels for cooking foods. Cooking vessels are typically composed of ferrous clay, and have a higher proportion of temper, and are thus coarser than serving vessels. Roman cooking vessels are found in many shapes, from deep open-form vessels with rounded or flat bottoms, as well as deep closed-form vessels (see Figures 4.4a and 4.4b). These are often called *pentole* and *olle* in the Italian-language literature. Both of these forms can have handles or not. Handles would have made the vessel easier to remove from the heat, though the pronounced rim of both vessels was also probably part of their graspability. *Olle* tend to be the most common cooking vessel found in Republican Roman sites. The morphology of the vessel has specific implications for cooking. A vessel that is deeper than it is wide, like an olla, minimizes the amount of surface area of its liquid and thus the area from which liquid can vaporize and escape. This can produce faster boiling times and/or less loss of liquid. This may suggest the frequent preparation of liquid

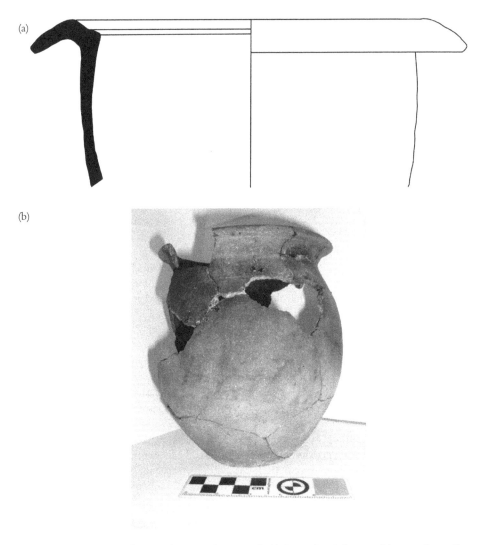

Figure 4.4 a) Deep open-form cooking vessel, or *pentola*. b) Deep closed-form cooking vessel, or *olla*, blackened by soot on its upper section (drawing and photo by author).

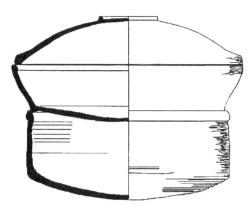

Figure 4.5 African cooking ware vessels arranged for a double-boiler or bain marie (Fentress, 2010, fig. 1).

or semi-liquid slow-stewing foods, either of starchy porridge-like quality (the *puls* of emmer grain which Cato discusses) or of a mixed pottage variety (Olcese, 2003, 37–39). The sooting patterns on *olle* suggest that they were typically seated in a charcoal bed, with their lower half surrounded by charcoal, perhaps on a masonry stove typical of Roman houses throughout Italy (see Figure 4.4b).

Creative assessments of the form and sooting patterns of ceramic vessels from the imperial period have also been used to suggest innovative cooking techniques. Three very popular cooking vessel forms (Hayes forms 23, 196, and 197) made in North Africa are often recovered together on archaeological sites in the Mediterranean region (see Figure 4.5).

Based on their sizes, the arrangement of their surface treatment, and the patterning of their soot, Elizabeth Fentress argues that they would have been used in conjunction as a double-boiler or bain marie. The bottom vessel, Hayes 197, would have contained boiling water and heated the contents of the vessel above, Hayes 23, at a constant temperature of 100°C or lower, depending on the height of the water. Form 23 rarely has soot on its base, unlike 197, which is frequently sooted, suggesting it was elevated over a fire (Fentress, 2010, 147). This arrangement of vessels may have worked well for delicate dairy or egg dishes, like those mentioned by both Cato and Apicius, as well as in the production of yoghurt.[6]

Another oft-cited vessel is the Roman *clibanus*, a ceramic cooking bell which is essentially a shallow basin turned upside down to cover bread dough. Baking bread under a vessel has its earliest attestation in Roman sources in Cato's *de agricultura* who describes the vessel being covered with charcoal (Cato, 74–76). Other ancient and medieval sources suggest that this would have been a common way to cook bread through the conduction of heat (Sparkes, 1962, 128; Cubberley et al., 1988; Cubberley, 1995). Archaeological evidence for *clibani*, however, is not as common as we might expect (Ikäheimo, 2003, 91, n. 420). The form typically identified as such in Republican sites has a large flange circling its top, but other shallow vessels of cooking ware without a flange might be equally well-suited (see Figure 4.6) (Olcese, 2003, 88–89; Zifferero, 2004; Bertoldi, 2011, 108–109). Perhaps, then there were several non-flanged vessels which were used as baking covers, but which scholars have identified as bowls or lids instead.

Traces of soot on the exterior of the flanged *clibanus* form suggest that it was not always covered directly by charcoal, but rather may have been surrounded by active fire, perhaps in

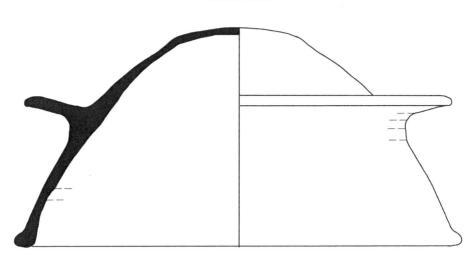

Figure 4.6 Cooking bell, or *clibanus* (drawing by author).

an oven (Banducci, Forthcoming). The cooking bell would have then created a controlled internal temperature regardless of how the fire may have diminished. Comparison with other Mediterranean cooking practices (traditional and contemporary) also suggests that the Roman ceramic cooking bell was not only used to cook bread. The Croatian *peka*, a ceramic vessel similar in scale and form to the *clibanus*, can be used in a wood-fired oven for both bread baking and to cover another shallow vessel that contains meat and vegetable stew (Randic, 2001, 325). Two to four hours of cooking serves to soften the ingredients and combine their flavours.

When compared with cooking vessels, vessels for preparing foods (for grinding or combining ingredients) can vary widely in form and composition. In general, vessels ideal for food preparation but not heating are composed of calcareous clays that allow for adequate resistance to mechanical shock.

Common vessel forms include handled jugs, *olle*, similar to those for cooking, but made of calcareous fabric, and open-form basins, sometimes called *mortaria*. *Mortaria* are generally identified based on the following characteristics: they have a thickened everted rim, they have a spout moulded into this rim, and their interior wall contains incised lines or added grit for grinding. These characteristics can be found in small as well as larger bowls; however, the canonical *mortarium* is greater than 20 cm in diameter. *Mortaria* were made in Italy beginning in the fifth century BC out of local clay with black volcanic augite particles (Merlo, 2005). The production of this form spread in the Roman period such that *mortaria* were produced throughout the provinces (Hartley, 1973; Blakely et al., 1992). The central interior portion of *mortaria* is frequently found worn: depending on the clay and grit composition of the vessel, the ceramic matrix can be worn down so that the grit remains protruding on pedestals, the grit itself can be ripped out so the interior vessel remains pock-marked, and in some case the vessel wall is worn through completely. These common wear patterns confirm that *mortaria* were actively used for abrasive grinding; the worn condition of archaeological examples may also suggest that *mortaria* were used frequently or remained in use in Roman households for generations.

Residue analysis of a series of 600 *mortaria* from Roman Britain and Germany was recently undertaken in order to clarify what might be processed in these vessels. Through gas chromatography, GC-MS, and staple isotope analysis, it was determined that these *mortaria* were used to process both plant and animal products. At one site, Stanwick, there was slightly greater evidence for the processing of dairy products, perhaps for cheese; however, in general the multi-functionality of the *mortarium* in the western provinces was the most important finding of the study (Cramp et al., 2011).

Vessels for serving food

Vessels for serving food, bowls and plates, and cups and jugs for drink, present a vast and well-studied category of material.[7] Ceramic serving vessels took their formal cues from Greek pottery and metal ware. They were typically slipped with black, red, or dark orange slip, or were burnished to a sheen depending on the period and location of production. Unslipped vessels were used with slightly less frequency. The clay of slipped and plainware serving vessels was typically fine or well-levigated; it contains few inclusions visible to the unaided eye. The study of serving vessels refers more to consumption habits and customs, rather than diet and nutrition specifically; however, several pertinent observations can be made.

Bowls and drinking cups are often difficult to distinguish since they are both open-form vessels. Cups made of thin-walled wear tend to be more cylindrical in profile than conical. Otherwise, their forms are similar and scholars usually draw a distinction between them based on their rim diameters. Use wear analysis has suggested a further insight into these vessels' interaction with foods. Wear on black gloss bowls from central Italy have shown a tendency to have worn patches and circular wear lines that illustrate stirring and scooping of foodstuffs (Banducci, 2014a, 195–196). Edward Biddulph furthermore recreated common wear marks on two *terra siglliata* bowl forms, Dragendorff 33 and 27, in order to suggest what they may have contained. Though similar in scale, these two bowls are quite different in form, Dragendorff 27 having a rounded profile and 33 being carinated. Biddulph's experiment suggested that the first bowl type was used for grinding or scooping, while the second must have contained a liquid frequently stirred, like the Roman spiced wine *mulsum* (Biddulph, 2008, 92–93) (see Figure 4.7).

Plates and platters have straight walls that are roughly parallel with the ground. Although sometimes thought of as the serving plates for bite-sized morsels, analysis of cut marks on the surface of black gloss plates from Republican central Italy has demonstrated that cutting food with a sharp tool must have been frequent (Banducci, 2014a, 197–198). This may have been meats or vegetable products – no residue analysis of appropriate samples has been undertaken.

A further avenue to understand serving vessels' reflection of diet might be to study the production and appearance of these vessels in whole ceramic assemblages. At different sites in different periods, there was a shifting prevalence of bowls over plates and vice versa, as well as a change in vessel size (for example, from plates for individual diners, to large platters). Such changes can be reflective of changing types of foods (Bats, 1988; Principal, 2006; Hudson, 2010).

Vessels of other materials

Metal

Metal vessels were used for food preparation, cooking and serving in the Roman period; however, the archaeological evidence is minimal, likely because of a tendency to reuse metal. Hundreds of bronze vessels preserved in Pompeii suggest that there was some frequency of use. Although the morphology of many of these look like they would have been used for cooking

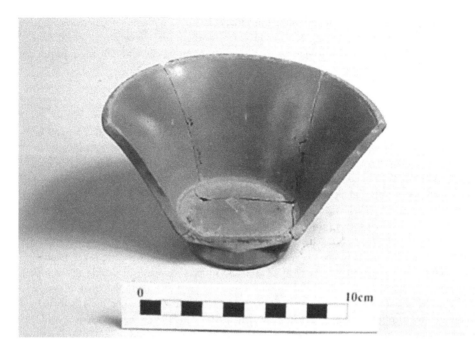

Figure 4.7 *Terra sigillata* bowl (Dragendorff 33 form) with marks from stirring (Biddulph, 2008, 92; photo by Jeff Hobson).

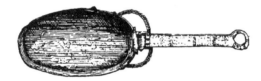

Figure 4.8 Iron "frying pan" from the Fayum, Egypt, now in the Royal Ontario Museum (Harcum, 1921, fig. 5).

(deep open-forms and shallow flat pans), they do not have exterior sooting the way we would expect for cooking vessels (Tassinari, 1993, I, 232). This may, however, be a result of extensive cleaning or conservation following their recovery from the site over the course of the eighteenth and nineteenth centuries. Extensive cleaning is recorded for four iron "frying pans" recovered from Roman Egypt in the nineteenth century and now in the Royal Ontario Museum. These have long handles that fold in over the pan prompting Cornelia Harcum to suggest that they were part of a soldier's equipment (Harcum, 1921, 45–46) (see Figure 4.8).

Hoards of silver and pewter items from the western Roman provinces demonstrate the artistic quality of serving vessels (Johns, 2010; Hobbs, 2010). Some plates, platters, and bowls are extremely ornate and must represent some manner of conspicuous consumption or elite gift-giving; yet the majority of silver platters that have been recovered have minimal decoration and seem to have actually been used for the serving of food. The cost of the metal and the control of these resources by the Roman state particularly in the Late Roman period,

however, means that these objects were only used by the most elite house
18–20).

Glass

From the third century BC, glass vessels produced in the eastern Medi....
their way throughout the expanding Roman territory. Their preservation in the archaeolog...
record is limited due to their delicacy; but they do appear as grave goods, in the Vesuvian area,
and in rare circumstances at other archaeological sites. They appear in forms for pouring,
drinking, and serving, rather than for food preparation or cooking. Blown glass pouring vessels
come in different sizes. The smallest, only a few centimetres tall, were clearly meant for
unguents, not drinks; however, jugs between 15 cm and 39 cm high must have held liquid for
drinking – perhaps wine and water to be mixed in craters or individual diners' cups (Cima and
Tomei, 2012, 118–123; Dunbabin, 1993). Blown glass and mosaic glass bowls and plates of
various scales – with diameters sometimes as wide as 30 cm – were likely used in the dining
rooms of the elite for the service of food (Cima and Tomei, 2012, 94–95, 112–113). Large
clear glass bowls are reminiscent of Roman wall paintings, which depict vessels full of fruit.[8]

Wood

There is little archaeological evidence for the use of wood for domestic vessels. While this is
certainly because of preservation conditions (most Roman wood is preserved in anaerobic soil
in Roman Britain), it is also likely that wood was not frequently used for food preparation. The
mass production of pottery was simply too economical to sustain a competitive wood vessel
industry (Pugsley, 2003, 101). These vessels were made in a variety of local woods: boxwood,
walnut, alder, oak, maple. The quality of preserved wood vessels varies; some seem to be made
roughly with little skill, while many demonstrate fine craftsmanship: thin walls, carved details,
and forms similar to both glass and ceramic vessels. Bowls, some small enough to be drinking
cups, are both turned on a lathe and hand carved. They range from the simple hemisphere with
an incurved rim, to a wider flanged form (see Figure 4.9) (Pugsley, 2003, 106–109).

Only a few examples of plates survive, several from Roman Britain and several from Italy.
Four from Herculaneum are clearly of very fine manufacture and seem to have been made to
imitate the forms of ceramic *terra sigillata* plates (Pugsley, 2003, 103–104).

Other artefacts for food preparation

Cooking stands

Ceramic cooking stands or stoves on which vessels would have been perched provide evidence
for a common cooking method. From Bronze Age Italy and into the second century BC,
cooking stands of various forms are ubiquitous, although sometimes difficult to identify when
broken into fragments. The most common early example was a portable stove designed with
a full wall and "hot plate" built in, but by about the seventh century, these were replaced by
stands of a simple U-shape that supported the cooking vessel above the heating fuel (Scheffer,
1981) (see Figure 4.10). This change in form may reflect a change in cooking fuel used (from
wood to charcoal), a change in the material qualities of the cooking vessels, or perhaps a change
in the types of food being cooked or food preferences, from foods which need to be separated
from the heat source to foods which can stand high heat (Banducci, 2015).

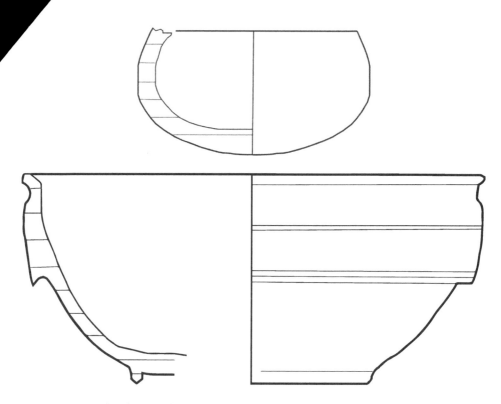

Figure 4.9 Two styles of wooden bowl from Roman Britain (Pugsley, 2003, fig. 5.1 and 5.12).

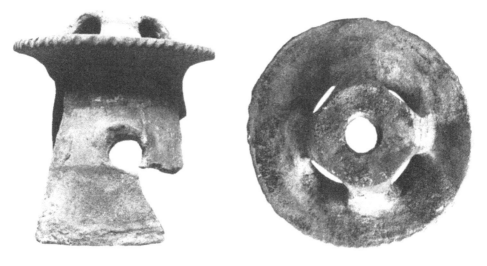

Figure 4.10 Ceramic cooking stand from the Roman forum, seventh century BC (Courtesy of the American Academy in Rome).

Tripod cooking stands made of iron have been found at Pompeii and likely served the same purpose as the ceramic examples (Stefani, 2005, n. 86).

Utensils

Although Roman knives and spoons have been found on archaeological sites throughout the Mediterranean, much like metal vessels, they are most prevalent in deposits at Pompeii, in hoards, and less frequently in tombs. Little systematic study of these utensils has been undertaken beyond cataloguing. In Roman Britain, where there is a strong tradition of artefactual analysis, particularly of metal objects, the most detailed studies have been undertaken. Typologies of spoons in precious metals have been articulated as well as studies of use wear (Johns, 2010; Mould, 2011). A recent study of traces of wear on 339 spoons of bone, silver, and pewter from Roman Britain used 3D-scanning to record and assess wear on the surfaces of the spoons and determine what activities they may have performed. The analysis convincingly demonstrates that spoons of different shapes and size had been used for different activities: some likely not associated with eating, but perhaps with measuring spices or medicine, others for stirring and scooping contents from a bowl for consumption. For example, certain spoon forms consistently have graduated wear along one edge (see Figure 4.11). In one case, a spoon's edge is deformed to precisely match the shape of a bowl found in the same hoard (Swift, 2014, 218–223).

To the author's knowledge, no synthesis or typology of Roman knives has been published. In general, Roman knives for domestic use have narrow slightly curved blades of iron and wooden handles. In a series of knives examined from the Egyptian Fayum from about the first to the third centuries AD, the blades and handles' combined length ranges from 8 cm to 34 cm in length (Harcum, 1921, 51) (see Figure 4.12).

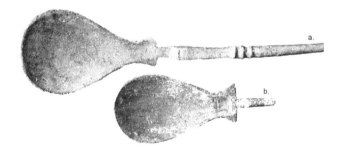

Figure 4.11 Fig-shaped copper-alloy spoons with graduated wear (Swift, 2014, fig. 11; Courtesy of E. Swift and the Journal of Roman Archaeology).

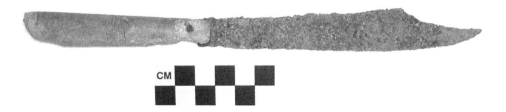

Figure 4.12 Knife from Karanis, Fayum, Egypt (photo by author; Courtesy of Kelsey Museum of Archaeology, University of Michigan).

Conclusions

The material record provides an essential component to the study of the Roman diet. Following the trajectory of daily life studies in the Roman world in general, the study of artefacts to consider questions of what and how people ate has developed into a systematic discipline only in recent decades. Combining techniques of morphological and material study with those of use wear and residue analysis can produce fruitful results suggesting which foodstuffs may have been used and combined and how they were cooked and served.

Notes

1   Ceramic kilns in ancient Italy would have reached "sufficient temperature" at about 850°C, and 900°C was common. Hotter than this was used for glossy vitrified or sintered vessels like Italian *terra sigillata*, but would have created too little flexibility in utilitarian cooking wares and preparation vessels (Olcese, 2003, 22–23; Cuomo di Caprio, 2007, 497).

2   This is often combined with isotopic analysis. Although GC-MS has been the most common method for residue analysis, liquid chromatography-mass spectrometry as well as inductively coupled plasma-mass spectrometry is also increasingly used, depending on factors such as the condition of the sample and the chemical compounds being tested.

3   For all the sites with sunken *dolia* in Italy, see Rossiter, 1981, 353.

4   Curtis, 1984, 561, also discusses *tituli picti* of fish sauce on a small amphora-like vessel called an *urceus* at Pompeii.

5   For example, KOR OPT for "optimal Corcyran wine" (*CIL* 4.2589) or RVBR VET . V (with a line over it) P . CII perhaps meaning "Red Vesuvian vintage, weighing 102" (*CIL* 4.2616). The complications surrounding the original labeling and relabeling of amphorae is treated by J.T. Peña, 2007, 99–114.

6   This is Cato, *Agr.* 81 and Apicius 4.2.1. Galen mentions the consumption of *oxygala* with honey, which we might understand to be yoghurt or cottage cheese (Galen, *Alim. Fac.* 3.15, see Dalby, 1996, 66, and Galen, 2002, trans. Powell 182).

7   Their study began in the early twentieth century with the examination of *terra sigillata* and black gloss vessels from Italy and continued to develop with the introduction of archaeometric analysis. For summaries see Banducci, 2014b, 1327–1331; Crawford, 2014, 1307–08.

8   These can be seen in the House of the Iulia Felix at Pompeii, and the villas at Oplontis, and Boscoreale (Stefani 2005, 1, 8, 17).

5

INVESTIGATING ROMAN DIET THROUGH ARCHAEOBOTANICAL EVIDENCE

Alexandra Livarda

Food plants and the Roman world

Food plants formed the bulk of Roman diet as they did and still do for the majority of populations across the world. A wide range of cereals, pulses, vegetables, fruits, herbs, nuts, but also oil-producing plants and various spices were available and some of them would be part of the everyday Roman diet. Staples, such as certain cereals and legumes, are the 'centrepiece' in several recipes of the most famous collection of the period, *Apicius' De Re coquinaria*, to be served with more or less elaborate seasonings and sauces. Concerns for their provision and supply were high on the Roman agenda, impacting not only on economic but also political strategies. One has to think, for instance, of the acquisition of cereals through taxation of provinces like Egypt for the supply of Rome's army and civilian population that became an instrument in its internal affairs (e.g., Erdkamp, 2000). Rome's various ceremonies associated with agriculture, celebrating the harvest, sowing, first baking and so on, further highlight the central role of staple food plants in Roman society. More exotic spices were entangled in other spheres of economic pursuits and sociopolitical agendas, very much related, for instance, to the exploration of new lands, the discovery of trade winds that allowed sailing to India, wealth and social aspirations. No matter how mundane or special, different food plants were thus important, often indirect, players in the fates of the empire. But food plants were also part of everyday decision-making for all classes and people to sustain both the physical and social individual. Therefore, plants can inform on diet, cuisine and by extension to all aspects of Roman life. This chapter explores the plant evidence in archaeology, the methods employed in their study, and the limitations and the possibilities of this line of inquiry, with the aim of shedding light on the great potential of archaeobotanical research with a particular focus on the Mediterranean.

Nature of evidence

Archaeobotany or palaeoethnobotany, as it is better known in the Americas, is a discipline that was fully formed in the 1970s with the introduction of rigorous methods for the collection of plant remains from archaeological contexts, although plants had been noted and occasionally recovered and studied since the mid-nineteenth century. In a broad sense archaeobotany refers to all types of plant remains, both micro- and macro-fossils, but strictly speaking its focus is on those that are visible to the naked eye, such as charcoal, seeds, fruits, leaves and so on. With the development, however, of better analytical methods, the study of charcoal has developed into a discipline in its own right. Here the nature of macro-remains other than charcoal will be explored and the term archaeobotany will be used thereafter to refer only to studies of this material.

Plant remains once deposited in the ground will decay due to the actions of micro-organisms, which only if they are arrested will allow plant preservation. There are six main ways that this can be achieved: under anoxic conditions (principally waterlogged environments), in very dry (anhydritic) or freezing environments, when the material turns to an inert form after charring, when plants are in environments saturated with salts or metals that poison micro-organisms, and finally when they come into contact with diluted minerals and their organic tissues are replaced by inorganic substances.

In the Mediterranean, carbonisation is the most common preservation mode of plant macrofossils, followed by mineralisation. The latter usually takes place when the organic remains are significantly decayed, the conditions are periodically waterlogged and a source of soluble minerals is available (e.g., Carruthers, 2000, 75–84; McCobb and Briggs, 2001, 939). In the Mediterranean, mineralisation often occurs when the substrate is rich in carbonates/calcite, but mineralised seeds are generally found in low numbers. The chemical composition of the seed coat and its structural features, such as its permeability, are key factors that determine the extent of mineralisation of a taxon (McCobb et al., 2003). Some species, like the gromwells (*Lithospermum* spp.), tend to be preserved almost exclusively in a mineralised form. These can produce carbonates in their fruit pericarps, a process known as biomineralisation, rendering them resilient to decomposition (Shillito and Almond, 2010). The antiquity of such species has been often questioned but several techniques (e.g., FT-IR and SEM-EDX) are now available that when carefully applied in conjunction with tight contextual information can help resolve such concerns (Shillito and Almond, 2010).

Waterlogged deposits are found in areas and contexts with deep stratigraphy or when the water table is high, and allow the preservation of a wide range of plants and plant parts. In the Mediterranean such deposits are rare and have been encountered in exceptional circumstances. Examples for the Roman period include various deposits at the harbours of Portus, Pisa and Naples in Italy (Pepe et al., 2013; Sadori et al., 2015), two wells from the site of Gasquinoy at Béziers (Figueiral et al., 2010) and another one at Nîmes (Bouby et al., 2011) in southern France.

In the southern part of the Mediterranean, in areas with dry climates, plant material is also commonly found in desiccated form. Examples of such Roman assemblages include those recovered at the quarry settlements of *Mons Claudianus* and *Mons Porphyrites*, and the port of *Myos Hormos* in Egypt (Van der Veen, 1998a; 2001; 2011; Van der Veen and Tabinor, 2007). Desiccated remains are very robust and even the most delicate plants or plant parts, such as hairs and tissues, are often preserved and usually in large amounts; the range of material being similar to that of waterlogged assemblages (Van der Veen, 2007).

Different preservation modes dictate the recovery methods of plants in archaeological sites and impact on the type of information the material carries. In the following section the formation processes of archaeobotanical assemblages are critically discussed, outlining the methodologies involved in their study and highlighting their limitations.

'Dissecting' plant assemblages

Every concentration of archaeobotanical material is the end result of a long chain of events in which various agents are actively involved. These include (1) the people who managed and were involved in the deposition of the plant resources, (2) the natural environment, and finally (3) the archaeologists and their decisions regarding processing and treatment of the plant material. A series of cultural and natural factors thus act as filters that dictate the final composition and preservation of plant assemblages, which are normally a partial reflection of what was originally present.

Cultural factors: past decisions

Cultural elements, such as procurement, consumption, processing and deposition practices of past people are the first filter of the available plants and underlie the sociocultural, economic and even political approaches of a given group. Food plant remains, therefore, hold the potential to shed light on all aspects of past lifeways, addressing mainstream archaeological questions. To do so, all factors contributing to the *composition* of an assemblage must be first disentangled.

Past everyday choices impact on the likelihood of food plants to be preserved. For instance, plants that needed to be processed using fire, such as in the case of parching to remove inedible parts, have higher chances of being preserved in archaeological contexts in the Mediterranean where carbonisation is the dominant preservation mode. Cereals and legumes that need to be cooked before consumption are mostly preserved by charring, whereas fruits, vegetables, condiments and oil-rich crops are usually found in waterlogged environments (e.g., Jacomet, 2012; Jacomet and Kreuz, 1999; Willerding, 1971; 1991). Research on the formation processes has further shown that carbonised plants represent a rather low proportion of what was originally present in the archaeological deposits in contrast to waterlogged or desiccated material (Van der Veen, 2007). The type of food plants that can be potentially present or missing can be roughly assessed using data from central and northern Europe that allow insights into the whole spectrum of archaeobotanical finds, due to the prevalence of both carbonised and waterlogged conditions. A detailed study investigating the distribution of food plants other than staples in northwestern and western Europe has highlighted the typical preservation mode of various taxa (Livarda, 2008a; 2008b; Livarda and Van der Veen, 2008). Figure 5.1 shows the most common such archaeobotanical finds in the Roman period and demonstrates, in accordance with previous observations, that the vast majority of fruits, vegetables, herbs and spices are found predominantly in waterlogged conditions, whereas legumes are encountered mostly carbonised. Nuts have high chances of preservation in both carbonised and waterlogged conditions. Interestingly, however, there are also exceptions that reveal a more complicated picture. Dates are such an example as, unlike other fruits, they are found mostly charred. The investigation of the reasons behind these outliers can shed light on specific cultural practices of the period.

Taphonomic processes

Taphonomy is literally translated as 'the laws of burial' and refers to all those processes that act on the material during deposition and burial until their recovery by the archaeologists, and these are examined here.

Differential preservation is also due to physiological factors. Within the same category of plants some preserve more readily than others and certain parts of the same plant preserve better. Focusing on charring, each species reacts differently to fire according to its size, shape, molecular properties, chemical content, and the amount of moisture present, resulting in

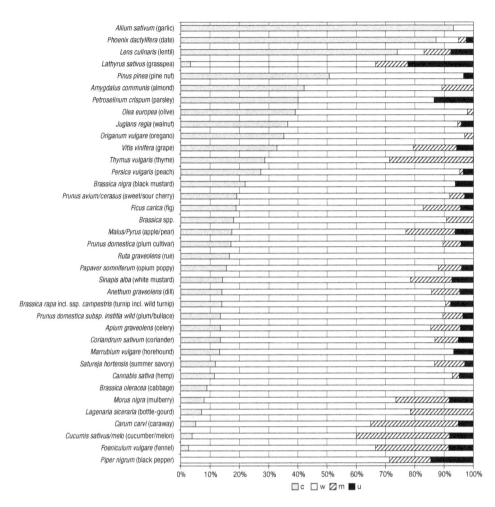

Figure 5.1 Relative proportion of the preservation mode of species with >5 occurrences across northwestern Europe in the Roman period (c=carbonised, w=waterlogged, m=mineralised, u=unknown) (Livarda, 2008a, unpublished results).

various survival rates, and therefore, absence does not necessarily reflect low or no usage (e.g., Wright, 2003). Seeds and fruit stones are much more robust compared to leaves, stems, roots and other soft tissues. For cereals, charring experiments indicated that straw is the first component to be destroyed, followed by rachis, glume bases of glume wheats, and finally seeds (Boardman and Jones, 1990; see Figure 5.2).

Furthermore, the survival rate of a plant or plant part varies according to the charring conditions (e.g. Boardman and Jones, 1990; Braadbaart and van Bergen, 2005). For instance, the combination of the duration of exposure to fire, the temperature and the reducing or oxidising atmosphere determine the degree of carbonisation and destruction of different components, with higher temperatures and oxidising conditions having generally the greater impact (Boardman and Jones, 1990). Evaluation of the charring conditions is possible by assessing the degree of preservation and distortion of the material. Hubbard and Azm (1990) first attempted a categorisation that would allow quantification of these two attributes by

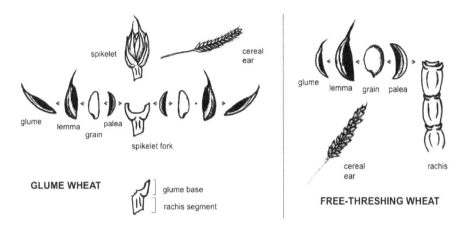

Figure 5.2 The basic components of glume and free-threshing wheat (drawing by Leslie Bode).

considering the amount of the plant epidermis preserved and the degree of puffing, fusion and other morphological changes of each specimen. Such evaluations can provide information on whether the absence of more fragile plant parts is likely to be due to thermal exposure or not, allowing more realistic interpretations of an assemblage. In the case of waterlogged environments the consistency with which they remain wet dictates the degree of preservation of plants. Desiccated material, on the other hand, is quite robust and can withstand repeated re-deposition, resulting in an impressive preservation that resembles modern material even in colour, albeit in darker and brownish hues.

More biases may be added, for instance, by the pH of the buried environment, as plants in general survive less well in alkaline conditions. Braadbaart et al. (2009) conducted a series of experiments to test the effect of alkalinity on charcoalified material that indicated increased fragmentation into small, potentially unrecognisable pieces, the size of which varied according to the degree of the initial temperature, and suggesting potential loss of plant material. Other physical factors, such as the permeability of the soil, also seem to affect preservation (Braadbaart et al., 2009), and negative evidence must therefore be considered within the framework of the physical environment during deposition, rather than taken at face value. Other factors that may introduce biases include the time of exposure of an assemblage after deposition, with longer periods increasing the potential of weathering, greater activity of rodents and other organisms, and mechanical damage due to trampling. Careful assessment of the state of preservation holds the key to a better understanding of an assemblage.

A final important consideration is the degree of perturbation. This is particularly significant in the case of low quantities of material and early or first occurrences for the study period. Due to their small size, plant macro-remains can easily move through the sediment resulting in the potential inclusion of residual or intrusive material influencing interpretations. The identification of a few asparagus (*Asparagus officinalis* L.) seeds from the Roman town of Alcester, Warwickshire, the earliest such find in Roman Britain (Moffett, 1996), may be such an example. Pelling et al. (2015) challenged the validity of their dating on the grounds of the history and land use of the area, and suggested that they were probably post-medieval intrusions. Targeted radiocarbon dating of exceptional finds can help identify potential biases or indeed early trade of food plants under the Roman Empire. For more regular finds, an evaluation of the degree of perturbation can be achieved by recording other types of intrusive material, such as modern uncharred vegetation, rodent faeces, certain molluscs and insect remains.

Cultural factors: archaeological methods

Archaeological procedures for the collection and study of archaeobotanical material pose their own biases but careful planning allows a level of control that can minimise them.

Sampling

Unless exceptional deposits, such as burnt storage rooms, are encountered plant remains are hardly visible to the naked eye. Specialised methodologies are thus required for their recovery, involving the collection of soil samples, which are subsequently treated for the separation of plant macro-remains. Several soil sampling strategies have been developed, including random, interval, judgement and systematic sampling (e.g., Pearsall, 2000). In practice it is usually judgement and, less commonly, systematic sampling that are employed nowadays. The former refers to the collection of soil samples from selected contexts of particular interest or with good potential to yield plant remains, following the judgement of the archaeologists, and the latter involves collection of soil from every excavated unit. Each method has its own advantages and disadvantages and its planning should be integrated into the initial design of a project to maximise the potential information that can be gained by archaeobotany.

Systematic sampling ensures good representation of the material across a site, both vertically and horizontally, and allows insights into both positive and negative evidence that can better inform on the use of space through time. On the downside, such large-scale sampling implies investment of a considerable amount of time, increased personnel and more resources and money. It is for this reason that judgement sampling is preferred, especially in developer-funded archaeological excavations or in those directed by archaeological services with limited resources (but see, for example, Livarda and Kotzamani, 2014, 21). In this case the number of samples taken is crucial in guaranteeing the recovery of enough material to allow intra- and inter-site comparisons. A detailed review of the state of archaeobotany of Roman Britain illustrates the significance of this parameter. Assessment of all available archaeobotanical records suggested that datasets classified as 'good' in regards to their potential to provide a good level of information on agriculture and/or diet were generally related to larger sample numbers (Van der Veen et al., 2007). It was thus suggested that a minimum of 30 samples per phase and site type (if multiple in an excavation) is necessary, provided the information they contain is usable. As best practice Van der Veen et al. (2007) recommend that all closely dated and well-sealed deposits and all feature types should be sampled, the latter in multiple occasions if large enough.

Other factors that need considering are how to sample a context (e.g. from its centre, amalgamation of soil from various points, etc.; for a good summary see Pearsall, 2000) and how much soil to collect. The amount of soil varies according to the nature of the deposits. Waterlogged and desiccated material is usually very rich, and therefore, smaller volumes are required compared to carbonised assemblages. Generally, roughly 5–10 litres of soil is needed for waterlogged material and 40–60 litres for the recovery of carbonised remains to maximise the potential for yielding a statistically significant number of remains.

Several methods have been proposed for the measurement of the sediment, which can be more, or less accurate (e.g., Jacomet and Kreuz, 1999; Pearsall, 2000). The most common ones involve the use of calibrated containers, measurement of the sediment weight or of the context's volume *in situ*. An evaluation of the different methods in dry environments was conducted by Wright (2005) and indicated that calibrated buckets give more reliable results for loose, sandy sediments while *in situ* measurements are more suitable for very compact sediments, although it is always preferable to combine both techniques as control measures. For waterlogged deposits, experimental work by Antolín et al. (2015) recommended measuring the displacement volume for samples with roughly the same degree of wetness as the best method, but also suggested that the use of calibrated buckets does not introduce any significant error. Such studies have provided fundamental insights into archaeobotanical procedures, as accurate measurement of the volume is crucial for the calculation of the density of plant remains (number of specimens/sediment volume). Density can be then used as a means of data standardisation that can allow rigorous intra- and inter-site comparisons.

Recovery

Recovery methods vary according to the nature of the remains. The most common method in the Mediterranean is flotation, which is based on the separation of the heavy organic and inorganic material from light remains with the aid of water. In practice this involves a set of tanks with notches to control the inflow and outflow of water (see Figure 5.3). A soil sample is poured into the main tank and into a mesh and an operator facilitates the disintegration of the sediment during which process any light organic part floats on the water's surface. With an increase of the water inflow, this material is then gently pushed into sieves or meshes for its recovery. Both the light and the heavy fractions are collected and left to dry. In waterlogged contexts, wet-sieving is usually employed as the water-saturated organic material does not float as readily. In this case the soil is placed on the top of a stack of sieves with different apertures and water is continuously poured over the sample to break down the sediment and free the various remains. Experiments, however, have suggested that there is a high degree of variation in the recovery rate of material according to the operator. Round and robust material are generally unaffected but more fragile plants and plant parts are either lost or reduced when the intensity of agitation of the sediment in the sieve is increased (Hosch and Zibulski, 2003). The wash-over technique has been put forward as a less destructive alternative (Badham and Jones, 1985; Hosch and Zibulski, 2003; Tolar et al., 2009) whereby the soil sample is placed in a small container in which water is added. The operator disaggregates the soil by gentle agitation, then pours the material onto a sieve(s) and repeats the procedure until all the floating material is emptied. The residue is then poured into a separate set of sieves and is processed as in the wet-sieving method (e.g. Kenward et al., 1980). Further experiments on the effect on sample composition of different operators using the wash-over technique showed that variability is mainly observed in the case of small-seeded macro-remains in the larger fractions (sieves with apertures of ≥ 2 mm) but with initial small-scale tests this can be minimised (Steiner et al., 2015). Waterlogged material must be stored in a constantly wet environment as otherwise there may be damage, particularly of the most fragile parts (Jacomet, 2012). Processing of desiccated material is limited to dry-sieving as contact with water can destroy the plant remains. Finally, it should be noted that the aperture size of the last sieve for the collection of macro-remains needs to be 0.3 mm or 0.25 mm to capture small-sized material and avoid biases. Reporting on the exact method and the equipment employed for the recovery of plant remains is imperative to allow an evaluation of the reliability of the results and to provide necessary information for their informed comparison with those from other sites.

Processing and identification

Collection of soil samples should ideally aim at the creation of a large data bank since the excavation process is irreversible. Once at the laboratory, however, time, money and research priorities need to be balanced, often resulting in the selection of a smaller dataset for full

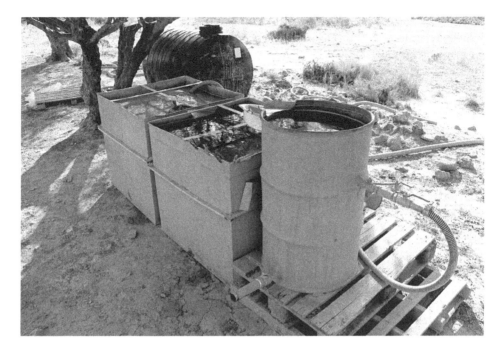

Figure 5.3 Flotation machine with tanks for water recycling (photo by Sevastos Giannakidis).

analysis. The selected samples are studied under a stereomicroscope to sort out all plant items that are identifiable and quantifiable.

Identification of plant remains is carried out on the basis of their morphology with the aid of modern plant reference collections and atlases. The level and accuracy of identifications are highly dependent on the availability of such resources and the expertise of the archaeobotanists. Cereal grains and chaff are the best-studied plant remains and robust criteria exist for their identification (e.g., Jacomet, 2006). In contrast, only few resources are available for the identification of leaves, stems, roots, tubers, fungi and other softer elements (but see, for example, Tomlinson, 1991; Hather, 1993; 2000). Identification can be also hampered if plant remains are broken into smaller, unrecognisable parts as a result of past preparation techniques, such as grinding of spices (Livarda, 2011). New approaches and tools are increasingly tried out, such as DNA analysis, SEM and geometric morphometric analysis, along with more experimentation to refine identifications of plant remains and their processed products with promising results (e.g., Marinova et al., 2011; Ros et al., 2014). Overall, however, there is still a potential imbalance regarding the type of food plant resources that are reported in archaeobotanical literature, and therefore, negative evidence should be treated with caution in the light of the current limitations.

Quantification

Plant material needs to be present in large enough numbers to allow statistically significant analysis. The seminal study by Van der Veen and Fieller (1982) established thresholds for sample size according to which generally a 95 or 98% chance of estimating a percentage content of a species to within 5% accuracy (in absolute terms), assuming an infinite 'target population', is adequate. In other words, using statistics they estimated the minimum number of plant items that needs to be present in a sample to allow meaningful interpretations, which according to their calculations is 138–384 and 195–541 plant items respectively. Samples here are defined as discrete contexts, and thus stratigraphic information is essential to understand their provenance (see Jones, 1991, for detailed definitions).

Various quantification methods can be employed to examine datasets and these have been fully described in the literature (e.g., Jones, 1991; Miller, 1988; Popper, 1988). Absolute counts should be the first level of quantification to provide the basis for comparisons between datasets. Waterlogged material, due to its richness, is often reported using abundance scales that provide ranges of quantities (e.g., x=1–10 items, xx=11–50 items, and so on), which can limit interpretations as they do not allow direct numerical comparisons. Regardless of the method employed it is imperative to first define the quantification unit. In archaeobotany the basic unit employed is the minimum number of individuals (MNI), whereby only a diagnostic part of a plant item is counted, usually the most robust one, such as the embryo end of cereal seeds, to avoid potential number inflation. Antolín and Buxó (2011) proposed an alternative method for the calculation of the MNI for cereals that takes into account fragmentation and various taphonomic processes, but also economic aspects, such as processing before deposition. This method is more time-consuming but has the advantage that it provides a much more nuanced picture of assemblages, shedding light on both natural and cultural formation processes. Once plants are quantified, critical 'reading' of their numbers is necessary by considering the nature of each plant remain. For instance, some fruits, such as fig, produce several hundred seeds whereas others, like cherry or plum, include only one stone, and therefore, numerical superiority of the former in an assemblage does not necessarily mean their increased importance/use compared to the latter.

Archaeobotanical analysis and the study of diet and plant resource management

To disentangle the meaning of plant assemblages, the various routes of entry of plant remains need to be considered, and these have been fully outlined for carbonised and desiccated material by Van der Veen (2007) and for waterlogged material by Jacomet (2012). Carbonised plants, particularly relevant to the Roman Mediterranean, are incorporated into archaeological contexts in several ways: as fuel (including dung); accidentally charred during food preparation; if there was a fire destruction of stored crops either deliberately or accidentally (Van der Veen, 2007). To these, deliberate burning of plants as offerings in rituals can be added as another route of entry. Jacomet (2012) suggests that decaying wall plaster, insulation, and roofing material can also contribute to plant assemblages and this is also true in some instances for charred material. Careful consideration of contextual information is essential to better understand these processes.

Questions that need to be addressed at the beginning of a study are whether an assemblage is a primary (*in situ*) or secondary (material that has been re-deposited away from its original use context) deposit, and whether it is a pure concentration of largely one taxon or a mixture of material. Primary deposits can inform on the use and organisation of a particular context or space in general, such as, for instance, food preparation and storage areas. They are snapshots of certain activities and they are usually rare. Secondary deposits normally include mixed material and they represent the most common archaeobotanical finds. The degree of purity of assemblages can be used as a starting point in the investigation of food systems, among other research avenues. Pure concentrations of food plants hold information on agricultural practices and consequently on dietary regimes. In case of pure crop plant assemblages with no chaff or weed admixtures, stable isotope work can add important information on their management and add a missing dimension on trophic chain studies. Research has shown that the application of animal manure to increase soil fertility impacts on the $\delta^{15}N$ values of cereal grains and chaff, and to some extent, of pulses, and therefore, consumption of manured crops results in similar values to those observed when diet consists primarily of herbivore meat (e.g., Bogaard et al., 2007; Fraser et al., 2011). Combining, thus, the $\delta^{15}N$ values of crops, with those of animal and human bones at a site level holds the potential to unlock past dietary regimes (e.g. Bogaard et al., 2013; Fraser et al., 2013). Work on other stable isotopes can reveal information on various aspects of agronomy, which in combination with contextual and sample composition evidence can be used to put forward hypotheses concerning resource management, including past practices of long or short-term grain storage, cultivation of crops in the same fields, and crop mobilisation (e.g., Heaton et al., 2009). Discrete crop concentrations also provide indications of which species were consumed, although the possibility that some of them were used for fodder must be also considered. In fact, ethnographic work has indicated that oftentimes the definition of food and fodder is blurry and depends on multiple factors that can vary from year to year. For instance, in a good harvest year there may be a complete separation of crops for food or feed but in a bad year, a mixture of the two may be used for human consumption (Jones and Halstead, 1995). An infested crop aimed initially for human consumption may be given to animals and so on. Although not always possible, contextual information can help illuminate this issue.

Mixed assemblages of grain, chaff and wild species can also shed light on agricultural and dietary regimes, but in this case the key lies in the proportion of the different components and the ecological characters and attributes of the wild plants. Ethnographic work has shown that, in the absence of modern machinery, there is a standard set of steps for crop processing from harvesting to its final preparation for consumption (Hillman, 1981; Jones, 1984). Each step results in certain products and by-products of the different plant components (grains, chaff, weeds). Calculation of the proportion of these components in an archaeobotanical assemblage can indicate the crop processing stage. Classification of wild species according to their properties (size, weight and aerodynamic qualities) is another way to investigate this (e.g. Jones, 1987). This information can be used to allow comparisons of samples from the same processing stage to minimise biases introduced by such differences, and to provide insights into the range of cultivated crops and other agronomic information. Wild species that entered into an assemblage as weeds of cultivation are useful as indirect indicators of the conditions in the field, and can thus be employed to infer past plant husbandry regimes (e.g. Jones, 2002; Jones et al., 2010). Mixed assemblages may also represent fodder as both seeds and chaff can pass through the animals' digestive track in an identifiable form. Experimental work is advancing, helping distinguish plants eaten by animals (e.g., Valamoti, 2013; Wallace and Charles, 2013) and producing a range of criteria to identify dung material (e.g. Charles, 1998; Jones, 1998).

Waterlogged and desiccated remains due to their nature allow the investigation of a greater suite of plants and provide more holistic observations of diet, but also horticulture and arboriculture. The downside is that such assemblages can contain intrusive plants from the natural environment and it is often difficult to distinguish these from those deliberately collected, so scrutiny of the formation processes becomes essential. Overall, the various analytical tools employed to unravel plant assemblages add depth to archaeobotanical interpretations and contribute to a more nuanced understanding of past choices regarding food and its management, which are ultimately culturally defined, opening windows into the past. In the following section selected studies are showcased to highlight the potential of archaeobotany in the investigation of Roman diet.

Case studies: Archaeobotany and food in the Roman world

Far fewer archaeobotanical studies exist on the Roman period for the Mediterranean compared to central and northern Europe (see also Kaszab-Olschewski in this volume). This is due to a variety of reasons including the general reluctance of classical archaeologists in the Mediterranean to incorporate the study of organic remains in their projects, although this is gradually changing. In central and northern Europe the long tradition of bioarchaeology has led to large enough datasets that can be synthesised, providing better insights into food patterns under the empire.

Archaeobotanical work on the northern provinces, for instance, has identified the introduction of several new food plants at the onset of the Roman period, the study of the distribution of which allowed a better understanding of the Roman economy and sociocultural attitudes to food. For central Europe, Jacomet et al. (2002) and Bakels and Jacomet (2003) reviewed a number of these new additions by phase and site type. Their results suggested that species that could only be cultivated with considerable investment or had to be imported, such as rice, almond and pomegranate, remained luxuries and disappeared with the collapse of the empire. Most of them were initially associated with the military and only in the last phase of the empire did some appear in civilian sites in the southern part of the study area. Other food plants that could be locally cultivated lost their initial exclusive status and were taken up into the local diet and agricultural and horticultural regimes (Bakels and Jacomet, 2003). A similar contextual approach was employed for the study of all possible introductions into northwestern provinces and provided a more nuanced picture of their access and distribution (Livarda, 2008a; 2011; Livarda and Van der Veen, 2008). True imports were restricted, being recorded mostly in military and urban sites, highlighting the key role of the army and the markets for their dissemination. Their consumption seemed to be tightly linked to certain manners and eating habits, aiming to convey distinct social identities, such as elite tastes of cosmopolitanism brought together by an expanding central power (Livarda, 2011; 2017).

Contextualised archaeobotanical work has also demonstrated that although several imports were introduced with the army, pine nuts and dates for instance, entered into the Roman world through their strong relation to rituals (e.g., Bouby and Marinval, 2004; Zach, 2002; Kreuz, 2000; Livarda, 2013). The distribution of archaeobotanical remains of dates across the empire indicates that these were employed in certain occasions and ceremonies; for example, as offerings in temples and graves. Dates have also been found as part of a foundation offering at a storehouse at the port of Lattara in south France, but this is a rare discovery (Rovira and Chabal, 2008). The fruit also seems to have been employed in mystic cults, including that of Isis, and possibly as a symbol of resurrection, afterlife, fecundity and longevity (Rovira and Chabal, 2008; Livarda, 2013). Its inclusion in aspects of diet was thus largely entwined with its role and meaning in certain contexts. A good example in the Mediterranean are the date remains recovered from first century AD deposits at the House of Amaranthus and the tavern kitchen at the House of the Postumii in Pompeii, alongside other foods, such as pine nuts and olives, which were interpreted as part of the meal aimed at domestic worship and offerings to gods (Robinson, 2002). Charring of fruits and nuts as part of the ritual has, therefore, provided a window into aspects of diet that would otherwise be elusive, as such foods do not normally come into contact with fire during their processing for consumption.

At a smaller scale, archaeobotanical datasets can be useful in providing comprehensive readings of the diet and its organisation at specific sites. Several urban centres of the Roman world are particularly well studied, partly due to the continuous building and infrastructural projects requiring archaeological assessments prior to construction. This is particularly relevant to central and northern Europe, as in the Mediterranean archaeobotanical work is rarely included in rescue excavations due to lack of relevant legislation. A good example of the potential of archaeobotanical studies of urban centres is Roman London. Systematic recovery of plant macro-remains for several decades has resulted in a robust dataset that allows tracing of the dietary preferences and trends of its inhabitants during Roman rule. Using network and spatial analyses Livarda and Orengo (2015), for example, have demonstrated that London was predominantly a consumption centre of exotic food plants since its very beginning, but from the second century AD and until its final decline at the end of the Roman period became largely a redistribution centre of such goods to other areas in Roman Britain. Their analysis suggested that although in the beginning of the Roman period exotics, such as figs, olives and a wide range of other fruits, nuts, condiments and other food plants, were widely accessed within the city, during the middle Roman phase (second/third centuries AD) they were found increasingly near the port area, which was their first point of entry. From there they seem to have been transported to certain other areas for their distribution, such as areas at the west part of the city, the upper Walbrook valley and Southwark. Increased commercial activities in these areas and/or potential changes in their social make up seem to have contributed to this pattern, with upper Walbrook valley, for instance, seeing the settling of new skilled craftsmen and other people. During the last phase of the Roman period (fourth century AD) exotics were found in previously marginal, in terms of their consumption, areas of the city, such as the eastern and western suburbs (Livarda and Orengo, 2015). This research has thus provided a detailed culinary map of exotics within the city through time and added new interpretations in relation to their trade, highlighting the maintenance of their social value for certain groups in Roman Britain.

In the Mediterranean, archaeobotanical work at Roman urban centres has also lead to some very interesting insights into dietary systems. A prominent case study is Pompeii, which due to its exceptional status has provided some excellent opportunities for plant analyses (e.g., Meyer, 1980; Robinson, 2002; Ciaraldi, 2007; Matterne and Derreumaux, 2008). Archaeobotanical finds include whole charred bread loaves and fruits from AD 79 but also others systematically collected that allowed more in-depth insights into culinary regimes and agriculture. The Anglo-American project in Pompeii, for instance, excavated a whole *insula* block with blanket sampling, revealing a general lack of crop processing by-products and thus related activities within this part of the city, and supporting the view that Pompeii was fully urbanised by the first century BC (Murphy et al., 2013). Most plant remains were interpreted as kitchen debris and table waste, allowing glimpses into everyday cooking and consumption. Several types of wheat, barley, millet, various pulses and fruits were frequently eaten in the city while olive cultivation and consumption seemed to increase in the first century AD and this was attributed to Roman influence (Murphy et al., 2013).

Life in other parts of the Roman world, in rural areas, industrial sites and harbours, has also been studied using plant data, adding to the picture of consumption patterns and trade of food plants, production and management systems. Primary plant data are in fact indispensable for more complete readings of past foodways despite the availability of historical sources for the period, as the latter can often be selective. Comparison of archaeobotanical material from the Roman port of Berenike on the Red Sea coast (see also Clarysse in this volume, reporting on selected food plants found archaeologically) with written sources, for instance, highlighted a number of discrepancies between the two sources of information that together provided a more nuanced picture of life and trade at this settlement (Cappers, 2006, 166–167). Several of the recovered plant macro-remains are not mentioned in the available sources (such as the Alexandrian Tariff and *Periplus*), and these represented both products intended only for the inhabitants of Berenike and others that were traded items, including coconuts, mung beans and Job's-tears. In addition, the absence of plants mentioned in the texts was also useful in providing other information for the reconstruction of Roman trade. Some of these, such as amomum, were possibly highly valued luxury foods and were transported beyond Berenike while others, like long pepper, were interpreted as minor trade foods, as Roman commerce focused more on the southwestern coast of India compared to the northwest, where long pepper was the main product of interest (Cappers, 2006). As these case studies illustrate, archaeobotany can thus add new dimensions to the study of past food practices and related activities.

Conclusions

Archaeobotanical work, although still not fully integrated into archaeological research in the Mediterranean, can significantly contribute to the revelation of new, different aspects of diet and consumption patterns of the Roman world and their cultural implications and meanings, as is already the case in research focusing on the northern provinces of the empire. The selection of case studies presented in this paper highlights the great potential of this line of evidence to amplify historical and archaeological interpretations by incorporating plant remains in research questions that move beyond mere plant lists and help explain past decisions and ways of life. Similar to all other lines of enquiry, archaeobotanical analyses have their own limitations that are conditioned by a number of natural and cultural parameters. In-depth understanding of the nature of the evidence and of the formation processes that dictate the presence and absence of plant remains in archaeological contexts, and the employment of robust methodologies for their study can help minimise or take into account several of the weaknesses of the discipline. Ultimately, it is the integration of archaeobotanical research alongside all other available sources of data into research designs that holds the key to more holistic insights into the past.

6

THE CONTRIBUTION OF ZOOARCHAEOLOGY

Paul Halstead

The role of animals in Roman diet and nutrition was multifaceted and variable, posing a wide range of questions: what products were eaten of which types of animal, by whom and on what occasions? How were they prepared and distributed for consumption? In what relative and absolute quantities were they consumed and to what extent did they meet the cultural aspirations and nutritional needs of different demographic and social groups? Zooarchaeology, in the conventional sense of the study of animal remains – and especially the macroscopic study of durable skeletal remains – is a rich and essential tool for addressing such questions. Skeletal remains are available far more widely, not only temporally and geographically but also across different social groups, and are less subject to the promotion of idealised visions of consumption than the iconographic and written records on which work in this field was primarily dependent until recently. Moreover, with ongoing excavations and advances in macroscopic, microscopic and biomolecular analytical methods, the volume and resolution of skeletal data are increasing – and will continue to increase – much faster than the discovery of new images or texts. In common with images and texts, however, osteological evidence requires careful source criticism to realise its potential without falling foul of its limitations and ambiguities. Accordingly, the first section of this chapter outlines how the zooarchaeological record is formed and how zooarchaeologists extract meaning from it by 'identification' and recording of physical remains and then analysis and interpretation of recorded data. The second section then evaluates the potential of zooarchaeology to answer the questions listed above.

Zooarchaeological formation processes, analysis and interpretation

Two hypothetical examples, representing contrasting forms of animal consumption, may illustrate the nature of zooarchaeological formation processes and the potential and limitations of macroscopic study of skeletal remains. The first example concerns a sacrifice to a celestial deity in a newly constructed temple at a small, short-lived settlement of the late first century AD. Amid prayers and libations, a priest removes and burns a few hairs from a young all-white bull that is led uncomplaining to slaughter. The lifeless victim is opened up and inspection of its innards confirms that the ritual can safely proceed. The head and feet are removed for burial adjacent to the temple, the innards are burnt in offering to the deity, and the dressed carcass is butchered and cooked for a feast within the temple precinct attended by local dignitaries, each of whom receives a share befitting his status. After the diners discard bones stripped of meat, a few are scavenged by a pet dog, but most are collected for on-site burial in a second pit. Soon after, a catastrophic flood buries the temple under alluvium until modern ploughing turns up an inscription recording a dedicatory sacrifice. The resulting well-resourced research excavation practises intensive recovery, including systematic sieving of all clearly defined contexts.

The second hypothetical example focusses on a long-lived and densely inhabited town of the same date. With minimal ceremony, a butcher slaughters two elderly ewes from a local flock, delivering the skins with a few attached foot bones to a tanner. He sells the rest of the carcass as small joints to nearby households, where the larger limb bones are broken open before or after cooking to access marrow. Some bone fragments from meals are thrown with other domestic refuse into any open pits, but many are discarded in yards and streets, to undergo more or less severe attrition from gnawing, trampling, and weathering. Soon after, fire destroys the town, but it is rebuilt. During continued occupation over subsequent centuries, a medieval ditch obliterates the first-century butcher's shop and tannery, while repeated cutting of pits and foundation trenches further scatters the sparse remains of our two sheep before eventual retrieval without sieving in rescue excavations preceding modern redevelopment.

The temple site's zooarchaeologist examines bones from two pits close to the temple foundations. All are from large animals and those identifiable to species from cattle. A few specimens exhibit fresh breaks, inflicted during excavation, and an incomplete limb bone has traces of ancient gnawing. Otherwise, the more robust bones are intact and form matching left-right pairs and/or articulate smoothly with anatomically adjacent elements, showing that one pit contained the head and feet and the other the remainder of the same individual skeleton. In the mandible (lower jaw), permanent (adult) premolars are in the course of replacing their deciduous ('milk') precursors and the third molar at the back of the tooth row is just coming into wear, so the animal died at around three years old. Likewise the limb bone epiphyses (articular ends) expected to fuse to the diaphysis (shaft) at around three years of age are partly fused, while those expected to close at a younger or older age are fully fused or fully unfused, respectively. Preserved bone dimensions, especially sexually dimorphic forelimb breadth measurements, are larger than many fully adult specimens from contemporary sites nearby, suggesting a male animal. A deep axe or cleaver chop mark into a neck vertebra may have caused death, while similar blows had parted the vertebral column into sections. The limbs were dismembered by a smaller knife that left finer cut marks transversely around articulations, while the absence of longitudinal or diagonal cuts to shafts suggests that raw meat was not filleted from the bone (the carving of *cooked* meat, requiring less force, is less likely to leave traces). Meat was apparently roasted 'on the bone' as several dismembered specimens exhibit light burning on the exposed articular surfaces but not the protected shafts. Unusually, since most bones are unbroken, no attempt was made to retrieve bone marrow or grease, while the lack of cuts on the intact skull or mandible suggests that meat from the head, including tongue and brain, was discarded. Lack of gnawing implies rapid burial of the head and feet, while the rest of the carcass, although discarded within reach of dogs that damaged a few bones and perhaps destroyed or removed a few missing specimens, was subsequently gathered up and buried. The wasteful consumption and careful disposal of a large and prime-aged animal implies a significant commensal episode, which context suggests was probably preceded by sacrifice – although the associated rituals are osteologically invisible (cf. A. King, 2005).

The urban site has yielded more challenging material of variable date from several modern construction sites, although a widespread conflagration sealed, and therefore identifies as broadly contemporary, a series of late first-century AD surfaces and fills. The overwhelmingly fragmentary bones in these deposits are mainly of sheep/goat (of which all those identifiable to species are sheep), pigs and cattle. The representation of body parts is very uneven and differs between these three taxa, but ease of identification and likelihood of recovery and survival also vary significantly and must be considered before claiming selective treatment of carcass parts or species by Roman butchers and consumers.

Working backwards through potential biases, in a heavily fragmented assemblage some body parts especially (e.g., the more robust 'long' limb bones of cattle) yield multiple, durable and identifiable pieces and so are overrepresented by total numbers of identified specimens (NISP). Accordingly, the zooarchaeologist has recorded presence or absence of 'diagnostic zones' within body parts, to estimate the minimum numbers of bones represented. Next, excavation without sieving tends to miss small body parts, such as phalanges (toes) and tarsals (ankle bones) especially of smaller species. Here pig and sheep phalanges and tarsals are very underrepresented, but not so the larger and anatomically intervening metatarsals (upper foot bones), suggesting that the tarsals at least were not discarded during slaughter and skinning, but missed during excavation. The phalanges and tarsals of cattle are much larger and only the former are underrepresented, probably removed elsewhere during primary butchery rather than lost during excavation; a later pit, outside a non-residential building, contained numerous unbroken cattle and sheep phalanges, perhaps removed with the hide and then discarded during hide working. Lastly, among the larger limb bones, the robust distal (lower) humerus is far more frequent than the fragile proximal (upper) part, suggesting that attrition by dogs (below) and perhaps trampling has significantly shaped the surviving assemblage.

Any remaining irregularities in assemblage composition may reflect ancient human choices. Whereas pig and sheep jaws are well represented and were probably distributed 'on the bone' with the rest of the dressed carcass, those of cattle are surprisingly scarce, suggesting discard of the heads elsewhere (perhaps stripped of edible matter by the butcher). Otherwise, with allowance for expected biases, body part representation is fairly even, with no evidence of differential access to meat-rich cuts between excavated neighbourhoods, although the larger houses yielded higher proportions of pig bones.

Traces of gnawing were frequent in pig, intermediate in sheep, and infrequent in cattle, whereas breakage with cleavers exhibited the opposite pattern. Moreover, among fragments preserving all or part of the articulation, younger (unfused) specimens were more often gnawed than chopped and older (fused) ones the reverse, even though the vulnerability of young specimens to attrition favours the opposite outcome. After primary butchery, therefore, the larger bones of cattle and adults were chopped up, for pot-sizing and/or to extract marrow and grease, whereas those of smaller species and younger individuals were often cooked intact and so were more attractive to dogs after discard. The extensive use of heavy cleavers and fairly standardised placement of cleaver marks, especially on cattle, suggest carcass processing by specialist butchers, rather than on a domestic scale. The lack of likely paired or articulating bones is also consistent with this interpretation, although heavy fragmentation and attrition greatly reduce the likelihood of recognising such matches.

As already hinted, the degree of epiphyseal fusion between limb bone articulations and shafts suggests that pigs were slaughtered young, sheep as a mixture of juveniles and adults, and cattle mainly as adults. The more precise evidence of dental eruption and wear confirms this picture for pigs and sheep, but suggests younger slaughter for cattle – perhaps because the 'missing' jaws (above) were mainly from adults. Biometric data (bone measurements) suggest slaughter of immature male and adult female sheep, but are uninformatively sparse for pigs (because of young deaths and frequent gnawing) and cattle (because of intensive chopping). The combined sex and mortality data imply that the pigs and many of the sheep consumed in the town were reared for meat, but that cattle were culled after working, breeding or being milked for several years. A few fragments from the proximal femur (hip) and distal metacarpal (fore-foot) of cattle exhibit degraded articular surfaces potentially attributable to 'traction stress' and thus compatible with use as draught animals.

These two 'case studies' share important common ground. First, zooarchaeological 'identification' includes a long list of variables related to depositional history (gnawing, weathering), preparation for consumption (cut marks, fragmentation) and husbandry (sex, age at death, biometry, pathology) as well as body part and taxon. Second, these variables are diagnosed by comparison with present-day specimens of known identity or history. Third, the proportion of 'identifiable' specimens differs between variables: depositional history, body part, and taxon are determinable more frequently than variables relevant only to certain body parts (e.g., dental evidence for age, morphological evidence for sex) or relatively complete specimens (e.g., biometry). Fourth, careful consideration of assemblage formation processes is a precondition of reliable insight into ancient consumption practices.

The case studies also exhibit strong contrasts. The temple assemblage comprises most parts of a single animal, for which butchery, consumption and discard history can be reconstructed in considerable detail. Conversely, in the urban assemblage, anything that has survived of our original two elderly ewes is irretrievably mixed with the scattered, fragmented and often poorly preserved remains of many animals. Based on the most abundant parts (durable distal humeri of cattle and mandibles of smaller taxa), the minimum number of individuals (MNI) represented in excavated deposits underlying the burnt destruction is about 100, but no plausible left-right pairs or articulating elements were observed, so each of the approximately 5,000 identified and recorded specimens *could* be from a different individual. Even this figure, equivalent to only 100 animals slaughtered per year over the five decades during which the relevant deposits accumulated, may be a significant underestimate. The large size of this urban assemblage enables useful insights into how different species were butchered and their carcasses dispersed across the city, but these are aggregate patterns of multiple slaughter and consumption episodes over many years and in a variety of commensal contexts.

Unfortunately, while zooarchaeological material of benign formation processes and high contextual resolution is encountered, the hypothetical urban case (or worse) is much closer to the norm.

Questions about diet and nutrition: the potential of zooarchaeology

What can we reliably infer about diet and nutrition from zooarchaeological assemblages of variable formation history and contextual resolution? The questions posed at the beginning of this chapter are here addressed in ascending order of difficulty.

First, which types of animals were eaten? A few animals found on Roman habitation sites, often as more or less intact skeletons, may represent later intrusions (e.g., burrowing species and their prey) or commensals attracted by human stores or refuse (e.g., small rodents at York – O'Connor, 1988, 117), while others may have been exploited only for their pelts or discarded/buried intact as unfit to eat (e.g., dogs and horses at Ribchester fort, northwest England – Stallibrass, 2000). For the most part, however, Roman faunal assemblages overwhelmingly comprise disarticulated bones variously bearing knife or cleaver marks or localised burning traces and exhibiting fragmentation patterns or anatomical frequencies that in combination suggest the remains of carcasses processed for human consumption. On this basis, it seems clear that cattle, goats, pigs and sheep were routinely eaten, as also, albeit less clearly for reasons of smaller sample sizes, were chickens and a more or less broad range of wild species. The same was sometimes true for horse, donkey, mule and dog, although sparse butchery and fragmentation indicate much lower 'edibility' (e.g., Dobney et al., 1996, 46–47; Peters, 1998, 287; Lauwerier and Robeerst, 2001).

Second, which animal products were consumed? Butchery marks, bone breakage and localised burning may provide fairly direct evidence for removal or cooking of meat *sensu stricto* (flesh or muscle), tongue, brain, marrow and grease, but exploitation of offal (other than brain and tongue), blood and milk leaves no direct macroscopic osteological trace. The intestines, internal organs and blood from slaughtered animals, consumption of which is recorded in Roman literary sources, were traditionally used for culturally significant dishes in many regions of Europe, while bleeding of *live*stock in the recent past (e.g., in highland Scotland) could mitigate food scarcity. Milk products too were culturally significant in antiquity: written sources cite regional cheeses, used in elite cuisine, while drinking milk could be a sign of rustic backwardness. Milk is especially significant nutritionally, however, because milking of female domestic ruminants can potentially yield far more protein and energy than eating both them and their offspring (Legge, 1981, 89). Lipid traces in pots may identify the heating of milk (e.g., for Iron Age Britain – Copley et al., 2005), but not processing in organic containers nor probably consumption of fresh milk, while whey proteins preserved in human dental calculus may identify both individual consumers and the source species (Warinner et al., 2014). More indirectly, macroscopic zooarchaeology may reveal whether male domestic ruminants died in infancy and so consumed very little maternal milk or survived long enough potentially to compete for milk with humans (Payne, 1973; Legge, 1981). In the latter case, analysis of changing nitrogen isotope ratios during first molar development may reveal whether early weaning made milk more available to humans (Balasse and Tresset, 2002). Both mortality and weaning patterns measure dairying *potential*, but do not demonstrate milking (Halstead, 1998), so they complement ceramic and dental calculus evidence, which document the practice but not its scale or intensity.

Third, how were animal products prepared and distributed for consumption? Although blind to the use of milk, blood and most forms of offal, osteological traces of cutting, breakage and burning, coupled with more or less selective anatomical representation, may reveal interesting qualitative details of the processing and preparation for consumption of the rest of the carcass, including some striking differences between both species and depositional contexts. Carcass processing sequences (O'Connor, 1993) are clearest on urban settlements, where anatomically selective dumps, especially of cattle bones, are reasonably commonplace and widespread (Maltby, 1985, 52; Lignereux and Peters, 1996; Peters, 1998, 258–268; Lachiche and Deschler-Erb, 2007; Lepetz, 2007; De Cupere et al., 2015). Such dumps attest to the temporal and sometimes spatial segregation of primary butchery (heads and feet discarded) and hide- and horn-working (toes and horncores discarded), while consumption of dressed carcasses involved extensive filleting of meat for distribution off the bone, preserving (probably by smoking or brining) of shoulders perforated for hanging (sometimes distributed off the bone), and systematic chopping of long bones for production of marrow and broth and perhaps glue (see Figure 6.1).

Compared with rural sites and earlier periods, urban carcass processing used cleavers rather than knives and consistent time-efficient methods that, together with anatomically selective discard, imply specialist butchers working on a large scale (Seetah, 2006; Lachiche and Deschler-Erb, 2007; Lepetz, 2007; Maltby, 2007). Less consistent methods and anatomically less selective discard on rural sites may reflect household rather than specialist carcass processing, but are also reported for sheep(/goats) and pigs on urban sites, perhaps partly because smaller carcasses were more often (as today) distributed on rather than off the bone. Nonetheless, some anatomically selective deposits also reveal large-scale processing of pig carcasses, with preserved hams perhaps

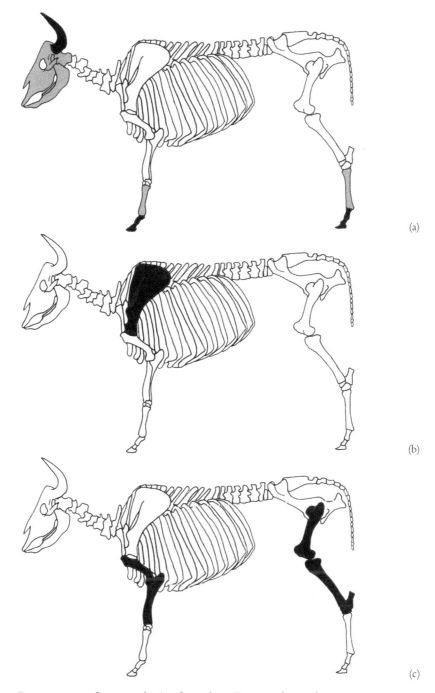

Figure 6.1a–c Frequent stages of carcass reduction for cattle on Roman urban settlements

    (a) heads and feet (shaded) discarded in primary butchery; horns and toes (shaded black) discarded during horn and hide working, respectively

    (b) shoulder (shaded) cured in brine or smoke

    (c) long bones (shaded) chopped to extract marrow, grease or glue exported from Iron Age and Roman rural sites in France (Frémondeau et al., 2015) and England (Maltby, 2006). Table waste tends to be particularly elusive, because of piecemeal discard, but plausible examples include concentrations of fish or bird bones with ribs and vertebrae of pigs or sheep (all difficult for butcher or cook to strip of meat) at Roman Caerleon and York in southern Britain (O'Connor, 1993). Likewise, in an early Roman tavern at Lattes, southern France, the floor of the dining room yielded vertebrae, but the adjacent food-preparation area heads and scales, of fish (Luley and Piqués, 2016). The tavern also served meat of cattle and sheep, as well as bread and abundant drink, and a votive deposit in this otherwise secular setting included a millstone, plate, drinking bowl and cuts of meat. A stark contrast in scale and context of consumption is afforded by the sanctuary of Mercury atop the Puy de Dôme, central France, where simultaneous dumping of parts of at least 112 pigs apparently followed *in situ* butchery and cooking of the hams, but discard of intact lower limbs (Méniel, 2014) – 'gourmet' behaviour very different from parsimonious urban broth making.

Fourth, by whom and on what occasions were animal products consumed? Particular occasions of consumption can sometimes be identified, for example at Great Chesterford temple, southern England, where rapidly buried mandibles and feet from accurately ageable first-year lambs suggested mass slaughter in spring and autumn (see Figure 6.2); while most toes (presumably attached to skins) and meatier parts were removed, a few exclusively right-sided forelimbs, also deposited within the precinct, have plausibly been identified as the priest's portion (Legge et al., 2000). Distinctions are apparent *within* sites between groups of consumers. At South Shields fort, northeast England, the fourth-century AD commandant's house received proportionally more beef (especially meat-rich upper-limb cuts), chicken, goose, duck and hare than the third-century soldiers' barracks, where more pork and especially mutton and all parts of cattle carcasses were consumed (Stokes, 2000). In the Rhineland villa at Bad Kreuznach, guests consumed a range of wild species rarely encountered in the domestic quarters (Peters, 1998, 249), while on a larger scale the higher-status central *insulae* of urban Augst, Switzerland, enjoyed better access to pork and poultry than did poorer outlying neighbourhoods (Schibler and Furger, 1988; cf. Furger, 1994). On a larger scale, differences are widely reported between regions, periods and site types in the relative abundance of the common domesticates. The consistency of some such trends is perhaps surprising, given the sometimes considerable differences between sites in the quality of bone preservation and types of depositional contexts (and hence perhaps pre-depositional activities) sampled, between excavations in recovery standards, and between zooarchaeological specialists in quantification protocols. These complicating factors, however, are far more likely to have obscured than created the observed regional, temporal and contextual trends in taxonomic composition. Thus, for Late Iron Age to Late Roman Britain, there is no reason to doubt a trend from sheep towards cattle and pigs that was more marked on military and urban than less 'Romanised' rural sites, although there is no consensus whether this represents adoption of Roman or at least continental culinary preferences (King, 1978; 1999) rather than practical corollaries of increasing urbanism and trade (e.g., Albarella, 2007; Albarella et al., 2008).

Fifth, in what relative quantities were animal products consumed? Despite some broadly consistent trends in species frequencies among recorded bones, converting these to frequencies among bones originally discarded is more problematic. Without intensive sieving, small anatomical parts of sheep, goats and pigs (and even more so of many bird and fish species) are almost inevitably underrepresented relative to those of cattle. In assemblages subject to significant canid attrition or trampling, bone survival is likely to be much poorer in species slaughtered young, as is common with pigs, than in those culled at a greater age, as cattle especially tend to be. The larger limb bones of cattle were often chopped into more numerous pieces than

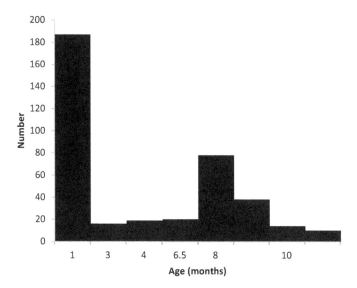

Figure 6.2 Numbers of mandibular first molars (vertical axis) at successive stages of eruption and wear (horizontal axis), with approximate ages in months (after Jones, 2006). Assuming spring lambing, peaks around 0–2 and 8 months of age imply slaughter in spring and autumn.

those of the smaller domesticates, potentially resulting in either over- or underrepresentation of the former, depending on how assiduously fragments are identified and how conservatively they are quantified. While the *direction* of such biases is quite predictable, however, appropriate correction factors are not easily defined (e.g., Maltby, 1985, 40–49; O'Connor, 1988, 75). Estimates of minimum numbers of individuals (MNI) generally dampen the effects of interspecific differences in survival, recovery and butchery, as well as controlling for differences in anatomical structure (e.g., variable numbers of foot bones in complete skeletons of different species), but exaggerate the abundance of rare species and may be very inaccurate if calculated from numbers of identified specimens (NISP) rather than estimated minimum numbers of body parts. Taking account of variables such as side of body, age and size, MNI is usually assessed from the best represented body part, which is often the mandible, and so may underestimate species with older age profiles (and thus less precisely ageable mandibles) and even more so any whose heads are discarded during primary butchery off-site.

To convert any quantified estimates of species composition into relative contribution to overall meat intake requires allowance for differences between species in carcass size. Ideally, this exercise should take account of age at death and sex ratio of each species and of biometric evidence for the size of local breeds (e.g., Vigne, 1991), but coarser approximations are more usual and perhaps more appropriate given the resolution of the underpinning zooarchaeological data. That meat weights are usually estimated for whole animals may also be problematic, given that part-carcasses (e.g., smoked shoulders – Deschler-Erb, 2013; Lachiche and Deschler-Erb, 2007) were sometimes introduced to particular sites or contexts. Potentially most problematic in using consumption debris to estimate different species' dietary importance is again the low zooarchaeological visibility of milking. While ceramic residues may confirm the use of milk and perhaps also its conversion to more storable cheese (e.g., Copley et al., 2005), our best guide to the intensity of milking is arguably the extent to which mortality patterns or isotopic weaning records suggest management maximising the *potential* for specialised dairying (Halstead,

2014a). If (some) domestic ruminants were milked, therefore, butchered animal bones may offer an extremely incomplete picture of the contribution of different species to human diet, especially if consumption of milk tends to be more egalitarian than that of meat (Stegl and Baten, 2009). Yet more challenging, even disregarding the lower visibility of dairy than carcass products, is zooarchaeological assessment of the combined dietary contribution of animal foods, because the formation processes of bones and plant remains are so different that their quantified records cannot meaningfully be compared. Fortunately, much of the human population of the Roman world lived in urban aggregations sufficiently large that dietary dependence on staple grain crops seems inevitable, but for smaller rural communities, especially in upland regions, such dependence should be demonstrated rather than assumed.

Sixth, in what absolute quantities were animal products consumed and to what extent did they meet the cultural expectations and nutritional needs of different demographic and social groups? Under favourable recovery, preservation and especially discard conditions, absolute quantities of carcass products prepared or consumed in particular events may be inferred from short-lived depositional episodes. Striking examples, albeit of meat ultimately 'wasted' are a pot filled with 28 thrush breasts at Nijmegen (Lauwerier, 1993a), the Lattes tavern votive deposit (above) and numerous grave offerings (e.g., Lauwerier, 1993b). Sanctuary deposits, such as at Puy de Dôme and Great Chesterford (above), are much larger-scale and probably reflect actual rather than symbolic consumption, although single depositions might include curated remains of multiple feasts. Given the multiple obstacles outlined above to even *relative* quantification, the difficulties of more generalised absolute quantification from zooarchaeological data are plain. Moreover, to assess the extent to which consumption meets cultural expectations or nutritional needs, it needs to be quantified per person and ideally for individuals of known age, gender, social standing, cultural identity and life history. This demands human skeletal analysis of isotopic and biometric proxies for dietary quality, the compatibility of which with zoo-archaeological evidence requires comment. Nitrogen isotope ratios in human bone measure fairly directly, on the same basis as they detect weaning, animal protein (meat or dairy) intake, although values can be raised by consumption of manured cereal grain (or animals that have eaten manured cereals) and depressed by consumption of pulses. Osteological estimates of human stature have underpinned several recent studies of diachronic trends in nutritional quality in various regions of the Roman world (e.g., Koepke and Baten, 2008), but stature is a more indirect proxy measure of diet than is bone chemistry and may be heavily influenced by disease and thus hygiene (e.g., Hatton and Bray, 2010), in addition to possible regional differences in genetic potential. Perhaps most seriously, both isotopic and biometric evidence for changing dietary quality may be misleading if the funerary record over- or underrepresents social groups living under atypical conditions of diet, physical exertion, hygiene and so on. For example, at Gloucester, southern England, single and mass burials, plausibly attributable to individuals of higher and lower status respectively, exhibited contrasting nitrogen isotope ratios implying differences in protein intake (Cheung et al., 2012). It is highly improbable that the extant skeletal record includes a similar proportion of both burial/dietary groups and inevitable that remains of some groups – here or elsewhere – have not survived or been recovered at all. Moreover, human isotopic proxies are interpreted relative to local crop and livestock 'baselines', also subject to risks of unrepresentative sampling. Thus, any apparent contradictions between zooarchaeological and human skeletal evidence for consumption of animal products may offer valuable hints that the two data sets are sampling different social groups or different dimensions of consumption. For example, the human body absorbs (and isotope ratios thus reflect) frequent small intakes of animal protein far better than rare episodes of excess, whereas the zooarchaeo-logical record is probably biased towards the latter – if only because remains from large-scale carcass processing are more likely to be buried rather than exposed to attrition on surfaces (e.g., Maltby, 1985, 60) while dogs favour fresh bone and hence piecemeal discard. Abundant evidence for butchered animals coupled with low nitrogen isotope ratios in human skeletons might, therefore, reflect meat consumption in rare events of ostentatious carnivory, while the converse might reflect consumption of animal protein primarily as dairy produce. In this case, while the isotopic evidence sheds most light on human health or dietary quality, the zooarchaeological record may be more revealing of the commensal politics of meat eating.

In closing, the difficulty of quantifying consumption of animal products is illustrated by consideration of Jongman's (2007a; 2007b) recent use of the macroscopic zooarchaeological record to measure living standards or economic performance in the Roman world. Jongman persuasively justifies meat consumption, as his preferred metric, in terms of the income elasticity of demand: 'we need to look at goods that are too expensive for the very poor, attractive and potentially affordable for those who lived somewhat above subsistence, but not something the very rich could consume in huge quantities. Meat is a suitable indicator of intermediate prosperity' (Jongman, 2007a, 613). From published syntheses, Jongman charts numbers of mammal bones deposited per century, as avowedly rough proxies for the scale of meat consumption, between the sixth century BC and the eighth century AD (see Figure 6.3). In Italy, deposition rises and then falls over this period, with peaks in the first and fifth centuries AD separated by a trough in the third century AD, while in the provinces of the Roman Empire (overwhelmingly represented by assemblages from north of the Alps) heavy deposition is more narrowly restricted to the first century BC–fourth century AD period of Roman rule with a peak in the second century AD. Perhaps encouragingly for Jongman (but cf. Scheidel, 2009; Wilson, 2009), heavy deposition roughly matches other proxies (e.g., shipwrecks, lead pollution) that suggest a rise and fall in aggregate economic activity over the Late Republican-imperial period (Jongman, 2014). Moreover, although bone deposition curves are a proxy for *aggregate* meat consumption, their match with a proposed late first–early second century AD peak in living standards, inferred from human femoral lengths (Jongman, 2007b, 194 fig. 7), is compatible with increased consumption *per caput*. Other scholars, using slightly different biometric protocols and perhaps skeletal samples, have in fact proposed a decrease in human stature at this time (Giannecchini and Moggi-Cecchi, 2008), but the focus here is on the analytical and formation processes underpinning Jongman's *faunal* data.

First, total bone counts exaggerate changes in meat consumption in Italy, given a 'Roman' predilection for small suckling piglets (King, 1999), and understate them elsewhere (especially Britain), where 'Romanisation' apparently involved increased frequencies of cattle. Conversely, as Jongman notes, allowance for the large size of some Roman livestock breeds would accentuate his suggested trends. In estimating meat consumption, therefore, bone counts should ideally be 'corrected' for species, breed and age, which is neither easy nor accurate, but also unlikely to neutralise or reverse his suggested trends. Second, identification and quantification protocols, retrieval standards, and excavation priorities have certainly varied, but are unlikely to correlate strongly with date of deposition. By default, the bone deposition data may be broadly representative of fluctuating numbers of surviving bones encountered in layers of different date. Third, other things being equal, the likelihood of archaeologists finding deposits of a particular century should be roughly proportional to the number and extent of sites occupied and thus to human population size. In Italy, census records have been interpreted as indicating rising late Republican–early imperial population, but only the steepest of the alternative suggested trends (Scheidel, 2007, 31, fig. 2) matches, and so potentially accounts for, the increased bone deposition. Fourth, even given a constant rate of bone discard over time within an inhabited area, the rate of *in situ* bone survival is likely to be very uneven. For example, while bone on

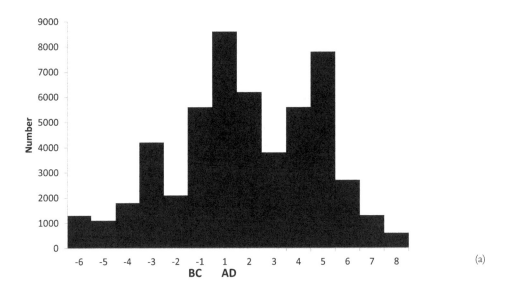

(a)

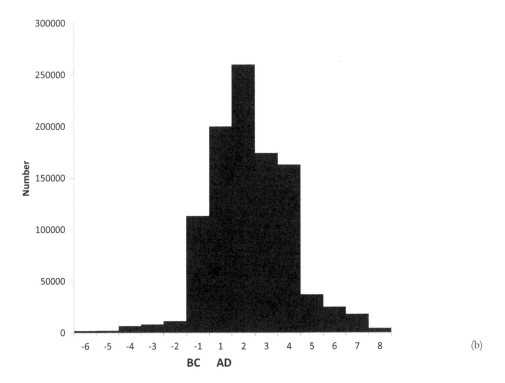

(b)

Figure 6.3 Numbers of identified and recorded animal bones by century for sixth century BC–eighth century AD in (a) Italy, (b) provinces (mainly transalpine) of the Roman Empire.

stable occupation surfaces is susceptible to attrition or removal for off-site discard, large-scale rebuilding may create extensive fill deposits that trap and preserve bone in large quantities. Jongman notes that public building projects in Italy peaked in late Republican–early imperial times, declining in the late second century AD before a temporary recovery (2007a, 616), while dated wood remains from Germany indicate a marked pulse in construction activity in the first century BC to second century AD. Increasing population and the surge in building could alone account parsimoniously for the observed temporal trend in aggregate bone deposition without any change in *per caput* consumption. Any increase in human stature, if not an artefact of the geographical or social structure of the human skeletal sample, could be due to improved hygiene or consumption of protein on a more regular or egalitarian basis rather than in larger aggregate quantities. Choosing between these and other alternatives requires analysis of *multiple* proxy datasets.

Conclusion

Animal bones are far more ubiquitous, and also more amenable to quantitative analysis, than all other sources for Roman consumption of animal food resources. They are also much less likely to represent cultural ideals rather than routine practice, although structured deposits with a normative message are widely encountered. On the other hand, routine 'non-structured' refuse is perhaps less likely to be buried rapidly and so more likely to undergo severe attrition and mixing of by-products from diverse activities. Accordingly, all faunal deposits require careful 'source criticism' of the discard practices and survival conditions, as well as retrieval and analytical methods, that have shaped published data. The biases introduced by formation processes are often predictable in direction, but not in degree. Accordingly, zooarchaeology can rarely provide *absolute* quantification of, for example, meat consumption in a particular historical context, while even *relative* quantification of, say, the dietary contribution of different species must often be treated with caution. On the other hand, zooarchaeology can offer relative quantitative comparisons between periods, regions, site types, intra-site contexts and species and also a wealth of qualitative insights into animal carcass processing and consumption.

Integration with other classes of evidence greatly enhances the value of the macroscopic faunal data on which this chapter has focussed. For example, textual and iconographic sources reveal culturally important detail regarding the ritual and symbolism of sacrificial slaughter (e.g., Aldrete, 2014), but zooarchaeology clarifies the extent to which the Romans consumed 'profane' as well as 'sacred' meat (Scheid, 2012, 90; Lachiche and Deschler-Erb, 2007; Lepetz, 2007). Iconographic representations of butchery and slaughter, coupled with finds of the tools depicted and with experimental replication have shed rewarding light on the methods, traditions, aims and constraints of urban, rural, military and civilian carcass processing (Lignereux and Peters, 1996; Deschler-Erb, 2006; Seetah, 2006; Maltby, 2007; Monteix, 2007). Archaeological context is invaluable in disentangling the practical, social and symbolic dimensions of carcass processing and consumption, without making potentially circular assumptions about the cultural value of different species, ages and cuts of animals (Ervynck et al., 2003). For example, the second century AD communal dining structure at Sagalassos, Turkey, was identified as such primarily from the functionally restricted ceramic vessels in an adjacent dump, while poor-quality tableware attributes the associated faunal material to low-status dining (De Cupere et al., 2015, 191–195). Such high-resolution and closely contextualised zooarchaeological 'windows into the past' are now quite numerous, but – in terms of potential for quantification – are perhaps comparable with 'anecdotal' literary and iconographic evidence.

Finally, this chapter has focused on macroscopic rather than microscopic and biomolecular analyses of faunal remains, partly because the former dominate study of the *consumption* of *dead*stock, while the latter primarily shed light on the *husbandry* of *live*stock. Husbandry histories are also relevant, however, to the distribution and consumption of animal products. For example, at Owlesbury in southern England, strontium isotope analyses of cattle teeth are compatible with local rearing of cattle consumed in the Iron Age, but indicate more distant sources in the Roman period (Minniti et al., 2014). At Roman Sagalassos, linear enamel hypoplasia defects in pig teeth suggest seasonal growth checks in free-ranging animals, but dental microwear indicative of a soft diet suggests a final period of stall-feeding and fattening (Vanpoucke et al., 2009). Dental microwear, reflecting diet in the days or weeks before death, may thus shed light on the culturally and nutritionally critical, but otherwise obscure, issue of whether animals were killed in prime (fat) or poor (lean) condition. Finally, at Late Iron Age Levroux les Arènes in central France, sequential analysis of temperature-sensitive Oxygen isotope ratios in pig teeth indicates births at various times of year, with the implication that the concentration of deaths during a short period in the animals' second year represents slaughter not in a particular season but at a consistent age. This in turn may reflect a desire for hams of a standardized size, export of which has been inferred from the underrepresentation of pig femurs (thigh bones) (Frémondeau et al., 2015). Increasing application of such approaches to animals consumed in different contexts has the potential to determine, for example, where and how sacrificial victims were reared (A. King, 2005) and whether their husbandry histories differed from those of animals distributed through urban butchers.

Zooarchaeological data and methods are revolutionising our understanding of Roman animal management, distribution and consumption, and of the contribution of animal produce to Roman nutrition, cuisine and social dynamics. Together these insights are shedding a wealth of piecemeal, qualitative light on ancient historians' questions concerning the structure and performance of the Roman economy, even if quantified zooarchaeological assessment of economic performance is unattainable.

Acknowledgements

Many thanks to the editors for their considerable patience, to Valasia Isaakidou for comments on various drafts and help with figures, and to many zooarchaeologist and ancient historian colleagues for making their invaluable work accessible; among the historians, Wim Jongman's contribution was productively thought-provoking, even if I remain sceptical!

7

THE BIOARCHAEOLOGY OF ROMAN DIET

Chryssi Bourbou

Eheu nos miseros, quam totus homuncio nil est!
Sic erimus cuncti, postquam nos auferet Orcus.
Ergo vivamus, dum licet esse bene.

(*Petronius*, Satyricon, 34.10)

Food and the pleasures of life

Trimalchio, a *nouveau riche* host of a dinner party exclaims this poetic commentary, joyfully tingling on the table the small silver skeleton brought out by one of the slaves between courses. This skeleton miniature, called *larva convivalis* by the Romans, frequently used in dining settings as a blending imagery to emphasize the need to grasp the pleasures of life while still able, can be considered as the ideal introduction for a chapter discussing the bioarchaeological data on Roman dietary habits (see Figure 7.1). Roman diet is largely known through existing documentary and archaeological evidence, which is, however, not representative of the diet that the average inhabitant of this vast and heterogeneous empire ate. Textual evidence produced by and directed to the elite rarely gives us a thorough idea about the diet of the common people (Faas, 1994; Garnsey, 1999; Dalby, 2003; Alcock, 2006; Cool, 2006; Beerden in this volume). Documentary evidence, in general, allows us only a shallow glimpse of the diet of the lower strata (for example, Cato the Elder in the *Agricultura*). Similarly, the kind and amount of products like meat, fish or legumes consumed by average people remains unclear and debatable (Beer, 2010; Garnsey, 1991; 1999; Purcell, 2003; Wilkins and Hill, 2006; for discussions on specific foodstuff see in this volume Marzano, Heinrich and MacKinnon). Hence, reconstructing the Roman diet is a difficult task and cannot be undertaken solely based on documentary and artistic evidence, especially since numerous variables, i.e., social class, have played an important role.

This chapter aims to explore the contribution of bioarchaeology to the reconstruction of adult Roman dietary patterns, through the study of specific pathological conditions (i.e., oral pathologies and hematopoietic conditions), and stable isotope analysis. Due to the scarcity of available studies and constraints of the chapter's length, the main focus will be the Mediterranean area, but reference to work in other parts of the Roman world, relevant to the discussion, will be also made.

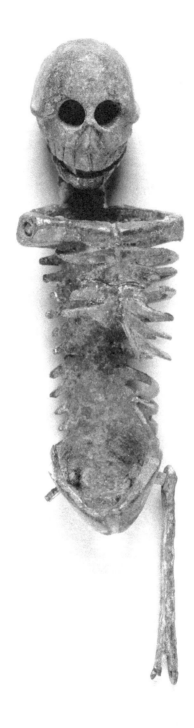

Figure 7.1 Miniature bronze skeleton (*larva convivalis*), first century (J. Paul Getty Museum, Villa Collection, Malibu, California).

The bioarchaeology of Roman populations

Bioarchaeology is the study of human skeletal remains contextualized within the available archaeological and/or relevant documentary evidence when dealing with historic populations (see, for example, Larsen, 2002; Buikstra and Beck, 2006; Baadsgaard et al., 2011).[1] Bioarchaeologists begin with the macroscopic study of the human skeletal remains that includes estimation of age and determination of sex, as well as recording of the observed pathological conditions (paleopathology). This first step is usually accompanied by imaging methods, such as plain radiology or computed tomography that has lately demonstrated a significant increase in its application (Wanek et al., 2012). In the last decades, bioarchaeological studies have benefited from the development of new methodological tools of investigation, which although of destructive nature and costly, have enabled the researchers to answer complicated questions about life in the past (i.e., ancient pathogen DNA analysis, Spigelman et al., 2012; histological analysis, Schultz, 2001). In particular, the application of stable isotope analysis and more widely carbon and nitrogen analysis (see below) has been a significant contribution to the investigation of dietary patterns in past populations.

However, trying to infer characteristics of the living from the dead is a tricky attempt. The seminal paper by Wood et al. (1992) provoked much skepticism on the limitations of bioarchaeological studies (what is known as the *osteological paradox*), and after more than 20 years it still remains a topic of discussion among researchers (Wright and Yoder, 2003; De Witte and Stojanowski, 2015). Representativeness and sample sizes, poor preservation of the human remains and selection biases influenced by mortuary practices are widely accepted as significantly limiting challenges in any bioarchaeological research (Waldron, 1994; Pinhasi and Bourbou, 2008; Jackes, 2011; Brickley and Buckberry, 2015). Furthermore, not all diseases affect the human skeleton, and in many cases it is only possible to attribute the observed lesions to a broad "category" of pathological conditions or offer a number of possible differential diagnoses, which considerably narrow our inferences about health patterns in the past (Ortner, 2012; Roberts, 2013). Added to this, problems related to inconsistencies in diagnostic criteria and terminology applied among researchers further complicates the interpretation of the biological data. Despite these limitations, bioarchaeology is constantly making significant steps towards the development of more standardized methodological protocols and research strategies that permit a thorough interpretation of environmental and cultural influences on living conditions and health status in the past.

The bioarchaeological study of Roman populations is a relatively new field of investigation and still does not consist of a solid bulk of comparative material (see an overview in Killgrove, 2014). The majority of these publications focus on Italy and Britain. Britain especially is at the front stage of Roman bioarchaeology and a valuable overview has been conducted by Roberts and Cox (2003, 107–163), who have reported on 52 sites and a total of 5,716 individuals. Such a synthetic study, contextualizing the human remains in the specific context of the era, providing crude prevalence rates (the number of individuals affected by a pathological condition) and true prevalence rates (the number of skeletal/tooth element affected), and thus making a useful dataset of comparative material, is not available – to that extent – for other regions of the Roman world. In most cases data presented are limited to small samples where only general overviews of the pathological conditions are presented, or with only scattered references to their prevalence. The analysis of Roman populations from Greece, for example, has only a handful of studies to present, usually referring to small samples and briefly commenting on the health status of the populations (i.e., Lagia, 1999; 2000). Larger population studies are rare (i.e., Malama and Triantaphyllou, 2002; Bourbou, 2005; Fox, 2005; Ubelaker and Rife, 2011).

In addition, most researchers acknowledge the absence of relevant comparative data or their inability to utilize them due to the use of different criteria for scoring the observed pathological conditions.

The human skeleton serves as a repository that potentially displays various aspects of the life of an individual, including their dietary habits; as such, the contribution of bioarchaeology is essential. Eating is a fundamental biological need and in order to maintain a healthy organism a number of requirements need to be met, such as the minimum intake of substantial nutrients for numerous bodily functions. Thus the quality and quantity of foodstuff consumed can influence the development of specific pathological conditions. For example, dental disease (i.e., dental calculus and carious lesions) has been widely studied as a reflection of dietary changes, and hematopoietic conditions (i.e., cribra orbitalia and porotic hyperostosis) have been also extensively used to identify nutritional stress in past populations. These two categories are also used in the current discussion on Roman diet, as they are sufficiently recorded in the available publications and offer a first-hand insight into the variables affecting the reconstruction of dietary patterns.

Dental calculus is mineralized bacterial plaque, and more protein intake has been associated with its development. Microscopic examination of dental microware, i.e., the presence of starch granules in archaeological dental calculus (Hardy et al., 2009), is another methodological tool that has potentials for dietary reconstruction, but it has not been extensively applied.[2] Carious lesions (see Figure 7.2) are characterized by the local demineralization of dental hard tissues by organic acids produced by bacterial fermentation of dietary carbohydrates, especially refined sugars (Lukacs, 1989; 2012; Hillson 2001). Foodstuffs high in sugar promote bacterial

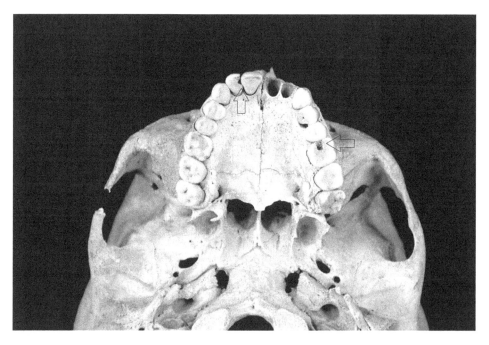

Figure 7.2 Carious lesions (arrows) on the right lateral incisor and left first molar of the maxilla. Middle adult (35–50) female, Oplontis (Italy, AD 79). Photo courtesy by Dr. Kristina Killgrove.

Table 7.1 Frequencies of carious lesions in archaeological populations from Italy

Site	Date	% of carious lesions per tooth
Vallerano	second–third centuries AD	2.5
Isola Sacra	first–third centuries AD	4.0
Lucus Feroniae	first–third centuries AD	6.1
Casal Bertone	second–third centuries AD	4.9
Castellaccio Europarco	first–third centuries AD	8.3
Quadrella	first–fourth centuries AD	15.0

activity and thus the development of carious lesions. Roman texts attest a wide range of foods rich in sucrose that have been consumed or used as sweeteners, for example, honey and *sapa* (reduction of must). Roman texts also refer to dental hygiene, for example the use of toothpicks made from organic material such as splinters of wood, or the preparation of toothpastes made of a variety of substances, such as eggshell, but it is uncertain to what extent people cared for their dental health – perhaps individuals of higher status did so (Bennion, 1986; Jackson, 1988; Cruse, 2004; Fejerskov et al., 2012). It should be noted, however, that although diet plays an important role in the formation of oral pathologies, the mechanisms controlling their prevalence are more complex, and diet should be considered as one of a number of possible causative factors, along with tooth morphology, food process techniques, and conditions in the oral environment (i.e., Lukacs 2012; Lieverse, 1999).

A number of publications on Roman populations from Italy, mainly from the first to the fourth centuries AD, are gradually shedding light on the prevalence of dental diseases and their association with the consumption of specific foodstuffs (see Table 7.1). Taking as an example the prevalence per tooth of carious lesions, which is provided in all these publications, we can have an insight into the dietary choices that led to their formation. The Quadrella population (first to fourth centuries AD), from an extra-urban area of Aesernia, demonstrated the higher frequency of carious lesions (15%), suggesting that carbohydrates formed a large part of the diet, as well as a lack of oral hygiene (Bonfiglioli et al., 2003; Belcastro et al., 2007). The population of Castellaccio Europarco (first to third centuries AD), a largely agricultural area in the suburbs of Rome, is the second sample exhibiting a significant amount of carious lesions (8.3%), attributed to the consumption of more carbohydrate-based foods, as well as poor dental hygiene (Killgrove, 2010a).[3] Lucus Feroniae (first to third centuries) was a relatively poor rural center close to Rome, inhabited mainly by war veterans, slaves and free slaves (Manzi et al., 1999). A similar dependence on foodstuffs rich in carbohydrates can be suspected for this population, resulting in a frequency of 6.1%. Isola Sacra (first to third centuries AD), a key maritime trading port (Portus Romae) for Rome during the imperial age (Manzi et al., 1999),[4] and Casal Bertone (second to third centuries AD), an agricultural and industrial area just outside the walls of Rome (Killgrove, 2010a), have lower frequencies (4.5% and 4.9%, respectively). Both populations might have been eating less cariogenic foods and/or more meat, as suggested for Casal Bertone. At the latter, the presence of a *villa* and a fullery or tannery points to a skilled workforce; individuals, either free or slave, practicing a skill during the Roman period were considered of higher status and enjoying a better income than, for example, farmers, (i.e., Garnsey, 1988), and perhaps enjoying a better diet. The lowest frequency of carious lesions (2.5%) was attested for the population of Vallerano (second to third centuries AD), at the *suburbium* of Rome. This population represented the working force of the nearby *villa*, although members of wealthy families were also interred in the same necropolis (Cucina et al., 2006). The authors argued that the overall low frequency of oral pathologies was suggestive of a high meat consumption completing a diet rich in agricultural products, but presumably low in refined carbohydrates.

Using as an example the frequencies of carious lesions recorded in these Italian series, the observed dental patterns clearly indicate that the consumption of a diet rich in carbohydrates and the lack of regular dental hygiene played a significant role. It is also evident that socioeconomic factors and geographical location might have also influenced access to specific foodstuffs, thus shaping the observed dietary patterns.

Cribra orbitalia (porous lesions on the orbital roof), and porotic hyperostosis (porous lesions on the cranial vault) are the result of marrow hyperplasia, and although better viewed as descriptive rather than diagnostic terms, they have become almost synonymous with iron-deficiency anemia in the bioarchaeological literature. Walker and colleagues (2009), however, have argued that for the presence of cribra orbitalia and porotic hyperostosis as a result of marrow hypertrophy, a vitamin B_{12}-deficient diet[5] is much more likely to be the key nutritional component in a set of various interacting variables that should be taken into consideration (e.g., parasitic load, and environmental conditions).

Angel's hypothesis (i.e., Angel, 1966; 1977), that these lesions reflect thalassemia genotypes as a response to endemic malaria in Mediterranean populations has strongly influenced the accelerated interest in their frequencies in Roman populations from the Italian peninsula. Differentiating between genetic and acquired anemias is, therefore, particularly important, considering the presence of malaria and the diffusion of thalassemic genes in the area. The study by Gowland and Garnsey (2010) discussing the available data on porotic lesions (and dental enamel hypoplasias), argued for the significance of malaria in the presence of cribra orbitalia, also highlighting the fact that multiple factors might have contributed to their presence.

All available studies (i.e., Salvadei et al., 2001; Facchini et al., 2004; Cucina et al., 2006; Belcastro et al., 2007; Killgrove, 2010a), suggest that in the absence of lesions pathognomonic to genetic anemias, the most plausible explanation of the observed cases of cribra orbitalia and porotic hyperostosis in the Italian populations under study is a chronic acquired anemia, while also recognizing the interaction of deficient diets, parasitic load and environmental conditions (see Table 7.2).

Roman diet was primarily cereal-based and cereals are low in iron; they also include phytates that inhibit the intestinal absorption of iron. A diet rich in agricultural products (although low in refined carbohydrates, thus explaining the low frequency of carious lesions) in conjunction with harsh living conditions can explain why the Vallerano sample presented the higher frequency (69.2%).[6] As noted above, the people of Vallerano represented the work force of the

Table 7.2 Frequencies of cribra orbitalia in archaeological populations from Italy

Site	Date	% of cribra orbitalia per adult individual
Vallerano	second–third centuries AD	69.2★
Lucus Feroniae	first–third centuries AD	19.4
Casal Bertone	second–third centuries AD	9.1
Castellaccio Europarco	first–third centuries AD	6.6
Quadrella	first–fourth centuries AD	22.8
Ravenna series	first–fourth centuries AD	59.3
Rimini (via Flaminia)	second–third centuries AD	30.8

★ Including non-adult and undetermined individuals

nearby *villa*. Living conditions for the working class in Rome were harsh but socioeconomic mechanisms might have been buffering the people of Rome from famine crises (see Erdkamp and Holleran in this volume). For their counterparts in the *suburbium*, however, the situation was more difficult as they had to develop their mechanisms to cope with difficult situations. Environmental conditions also play an important role in the formation of the observed lesions. Swamps, for example, such as those that existed in the Ravenna area might have put the population at high risk of contracting malaria or any other parasitic infection. Both Adriatic samples, and in particular the Ravenna sample (59.3%), had higher frequencies than Quadrella (22.8%), located at the mountainous area of Molise (Belcastro et al., 2007).

It is thus likely that numerous variables, including geographic location, climate, disease ecology, differential access to foodstuff, and sanitation levels, contribute to the development of porotic lesions. Moreover, every setting is marked by its specific characteristics and population attributes, and it should be taken under consideration that most probably all these variables share an interdependent relationship and none of them acts alone.

Isotopic analysis of Roman populations

Traditionally, textual (such as medical writings) and archaeological evidence (that is plant and animal remains, food preparation utensils, artistic representations), have been used to reconstruct the diet of the Romans. However, the eclectic nature of the written testimonies and the fact that the preservation of actual food remains in archaeological contexts (animal bones, carbonized seeds, phytoliths, etc.) heavily depends on numerous factors (e.g., taphonomic, food processing and discarding methods), limit our knowledge of Roman dietary habits.

Over the past decades, stable isotope ratio analysis has been an invaluable addition to these data sets, providing information on a wide range of dietary topics for different cultures, such as differential access to foods dependent on occupation, social status or lifestyle, intra and inter populations dietary variation, the proportion of marine versus terrestrial food in diet, age and/or sex based differences in diet, or temporal changes in diet (for thorough reviews see Sealy, 2001; Lee-Thorp, 2008; Katzenberg, 2008; 2012; Eriksson, 2013; Reitsema, 2013). Foodstuffs vary in their isotopic composition, so chemical analysis of human bone collagen, the major component of bone, provides long-term dietary information about the foods that an individual consumed during life; in short, the isotopic signatures of foods consumed are reflected in the tissues of the consumer. Carbon isotopic ratios, expressed as δ^{13}C values in per mil (‰, meaning per thousand) relative to Vienna Peedee Belemnite (VPDB), are used to distinguish between plants that follow different photosynthetic pathways and between marine and terrestrial food webs (marine resources are enriched in ^{13}C by ~ −7‰ compared to terrestrial foods). C_3 plants, like wheat and barley, have δ^{13}C values ranging from −20‰ to −35‰, while C_4 plants, like millet and sorghum, have δ^{13}C values ranging from −9‰ to −14‰ (Smith and Epstein, 1971; Deines, 1980). Nitrogen isotopic ratios, expressed as δ^{15}N values in per mil (‰) relative to atmospheric N_2 or the ambient inhalable reservoir (AIR), primarily reflect the position of an organism in the food chain, with an increase of approximately 3–5‰ in each step of the trophic level; for example, carnivores have δ^{15}N values that are 3–5‰ higher than those of the herbivores they consume, and respectively herbivores have values that are 3–5‰ higher than the plants they consume (DeNiro and Epstein, 1981; Schoeninger and DeNiro, 1984; Schwarcz and Schoeninger, 1991; Bocherens and Drucker, 2003; Reitsema, 2013). δ^{15}N values from about 5‰ to 12‰ are typical of terrestrial diets, while δ^{15}N values ranging from 12‰ to 22‰ indicate protein from marine foods (Schoeninger and DeNiro, 1984; Walker and DeNiro, 1986). In coastal areas where populations may have been consuming both marine resources and

C_4 plants, the combination of nitrogen and carbon isotopes values are particularly useful in distinguishing between dietary protein derived from marine resources versus terrestrial foods. It should be noted, however, that nitrogen comes from dietary protein (both from animal and plant), and nitrogen ratios provide information on the source of protein but not its amount.

Although a powerful methodological tool in many different contexts, some limitations should be taken under consideration when applying stable isotope analysis in past populations, basically oriented to issues of interpreting quantity, representation and reliability (Lee-Thorp, 2008). An issue that has constantly puzzled researchers was to what extent isotopic ratios measured in ancient bones and teeth are reliable or subjected to post-depositional contamination (diagenesis). Ongoing studies on sample pre-treatment protocols, specific methods to identify diagenesis and technical advances in mass spectrometry (which enabled process of a larger volume of samples, also at a lower cost) provide the necessary confidence that isotopic results can be reliable (Makarewicz and Sealy, 2015). On the other hand, specific cultural treatments of the human bones, like cremation, makes it impossible to apply stable isotope analysis in burned bone or teeth as heating alters the structure and isotopic values of collagen and bioapatite (Eriksson, 2013).[7]

When comes to nitrogen isotopes, in particular, it should be noted that the trophic level shift of 3–5‰ discussed above is not constant,[8] and although why this variation occurs is not yet fully understood, this is a subject of continuous research (Poupin et al., 2011; 2014; Katzenberg, 2012). Nitrogen isotopes offer an insight into protein intake in a diet, but their distribution in the ecosystem and the way dietary nitrogen values are incorporated in the human tissue and consequently expressed in collagen values are more complex than originally thought. For example, diversity of nitrogen values in different wild and domestic herbivores depend on animal physiology (e.g., digestive physiology), environmental factors (e.g., seasonality of available food resources) and anthropogenic activity (e.g., manuring of the fields). These factors have been currently recognized as playing an important role and the need to establish the extent of nitrogen isotope variation within and in between species so to provide better means of nitrogen values in consumers is well understood (Makarewicz and Sealy, 2015). In general, it is essential to improve our understanding of the stable isotopes natural distributions in different kinds of ecosystems and conditions. The idea to perform more regional contextual studies is a difficult goal to accomplish because many regions have been completely altered by millennia of human activity (e.g., agricultural activity). In addition, faunal material derived from archaeological contexts is often limited to a few species (primarily domesticated animals), thus reducing our ability to have a broader idea of any given ecosystem (Lee-Thorp, 2008).

Every analytical process in archaeological research starts with a question that will ideally end with some type of answer based on new information; however, the answer that throws light on that question quite often generates innumerable new questions. As Eriksson underlines (2013, 141) "stable isotope data should be considered and treated like any archaeological data. They are not intrinsically more 'true', more exact, better of greater scientific value than traditional archaeological data." Therefore, if isotopic analysis is carefully employed, it can serve as an additional data set to traditional archaeological evidence, providing new and original information on past practices, including dietary choices. Isotopic analysis cannot be used to rule out the consumption of any foodstuff but it may outline at a specific time period and site the dominant components of the diet, and suggest the proportions of each component in the diet of the individuals.

In this chapter, our discussion will focus on the valuable contribution of isotopic studies to the adult diet, tackling issues like fish protein and millet consumption, and sex-based or occupation-related variations in the diet during the Roman era. Current isotopic data on

Roman diet is still limited but presents considerable variation, suggesting that there was no singular "Roman diet" and to the so-called "Mediterranean trinity" of cereals (especially wheat), olives and wine, meat, legumes, marine protein (freshwater and seawater species) were added, as well as C_4 foods, such as millet.[9] Why did the diet of populations living in coastal sites present variations in marine consumption? Did males have better access to higher trophic level foods such as meat and fish? To what extent did people consume millet, which was largely considered a lower quality crop? Some of the isotopic work conducted addresses these issues and it seems that we are only now beginning to understand that the observed intra- and inter-population dietary variation is strongly influenced by the complex interaction of, for example, socioeconomic status, occupation, age, sex, and geographical location.

Actual fish consumption in Roman times is rather unclear and evidence in the sources is controversial: was it an easily accessible product, especially to the coastal populations, or a luxury item restricted to the elite? Fishing and the trade of fish and its by-products, such as *garum*, were important economic activities, especially at the ports of Rome, as evidenced by the existence of corporations of fishermen and fishmongers along the Mediterranean coasts (for example, at Ostia). Salted fish and fish sauces were also available, with *garum* being widely cited in both cooking and medical recipes (Curtis, 1991). Freshwater fish, on the other hand, was raised in fishponds already in early imperial times (Higginbotham, 1997), and must have been a popular foodstuff since it was easily accessible and affordable. Its popularity must have led Galen in the second century AD to oppose fish consumption from the contaminated river Tiber (Nutton, 1995). Although during the Roman period C_3 terrestrial resources predominated in the diet at sites where isotopic analysis is available, in Italy (see below for a thorough overview), Britain (i.e., Richards et al. 1998; Müldner and Richards 2007; Chenery et al. 2010; Redfern et al. 2010) and Croatia (Lightfoot et al., 2012), there is evidence for the consumption of some marine or freshwater protein. To what extent, however, the site location, environmental and socioeconomic conditions might have influenced dietary choices still remains unclear, as it is not fully understood whether marine consumption represents a necessity or choice. However, it is interesting to note the changes seen in the diachronic survey for dietary patterns in Croatia (Lightfoot et al., 2012): the marine component to the diet increases from the Iron Age to the Roman period and then declines (or becomes too low to be isotopically detected) from the Roman to the early medieval period.

The isotopic study of the population from the necropolis of Isola Sacra, showed that marine resources must have constituted an important part of their diet (Prowse et al., 2004). Although terrestrial resources (C_3 plants and animals) formed the bulk of diet, the strong marine signal cannot be explained by the widespread consumption of *garum*, but rather of higher trophic level marine resources. This is further explained based on the isotopic analysis of some *garum* samples retrieved from amphorae, which was also performed by the researchers (Prowse et al., 2004).[10] The low nitrogen values of these samples (with a mean $\delta^{15}N$ value of 6.5±1.7‰), suggest that *garum* must have been prepared from low trophic level organisms (small fish like sprat or smelt, possibly some shellfish too), a composition also attested in the documentary evidence (see, for example, Curtis, 1991). Thus, *garum* could not have contributed significantly to the high nitrogen values seen for the Isola Sacra samples, suggesting the consumption of marine organisms at a much higher trophic level, such as tuna and salmon.

The results of this study were further compared with a smaller sample from the nearby inland site of ANAS that exhibited dietary variability in the form of two distinct clusters: a cluster with isotopic values similar to that of Isola Sacra sample, that is with notable marine protein intake, and a cluster where isotopic values fall within the range expected for a terrestrial diet. The authors suggested that the variability of the isotopic values possibly indicate status difference within the population, as well as that the individuals with isotopic values similar to Isola Sacra may have been migrants working on the coast and thus consuming a diet higher in marine protein in contrast to individuals living further inland and engaged to agricultural activities and thus consuming a more C_3 based diet (Prowse et al., 2004, 270–271).

The isotopic analysis of another coastal imperial Roman population (first to second centuries AD) interred near the port of Velia in south Italy, revealed a diet high in cereals, relative consumption of animal and only minor consumption of marine protein. However, a number of individuals at the site, predominantly but not exclusively males, appeared to have had greater access to marine resources and especially high trophic level fish (Craig et al., 2009). When comparing the two coastal sites, the population at Velia seemed to eat less fish than the population from the necropolis of Isola Sacra. Since in both sites no evidence of differential social status is present, Crowe et al. (2010) turned to the investigation of a possible connection between dietary patterns and occupational activities. Their study revealed high rates among male individuals (21.1% in Isola Sacra and 35.3% in Velia) of external auricular exostosis – a condition consistent with long-term and habitual exposure to cold water or water-deriving wind chill. Most probably, the development of the condition in both these coastal populations is indicative of some sea-related occupation such as fishing; this seems to be particularly the case for those individuals at Velia presenting a higher prevalence of the condition and very high nitrogen values indicative of more marked marine consumption. However, this direct link between diet, occupation and pathology is less easy to establish for the population of Isola Sacra: although the pathology was present, albeit in a lesser prevalence so to justify the engagement with sea-related activities, it should be taken into consideration that Portus Romae was a far more significant port than Velia and fish consumption was more widespread as imported fish was also present.

A mixture of marine and terrestrial diet, where legumes and C_4 plants appear not to have been important sources of protein, is evidenced through the isotopic analysis of the Late Roman (second to fifth centuries AD) population from Leptiminus on the Mediterranean coast of Tunisia (Keenleyside et al., 2009). However, a significant amount of dietary protein was obtained from marine resources, and indeed in a larger fraction in comparison with the individuals buried at Isola Sacra. Although in the recent past the population living at the coastal region of Leptimimus and modern-day town Lamta considered meat, for example lamb and mutton, to be a more desirable and prestigious food than fish (Keenleyside et al., 2009, 53), the enriched collagen in both ^{13}C and ^{14}N values clearly indicates significant marine consumption. As with the population of Isola Sacra, the authors suggest that marine signature cannot be explained by the consumption of *garum*; rather it is indicative of consumption of higher trophic level marine species.[11]

Rutgers et al. (2009) have for the first time attempted to isotopically investigate the diet of Rome's early Christians. Their sample was derived from the Liberian Region in the Christian catacomb of St. Callixtus (mid-third through early fifth centuries AD), and it has been an important contribution to the investigation of fish consumption in the Roman diet, and especially freshwater riverine fish. The isotopic evidence for the consumption of freshwater fish in this population now questions the general view that did not consider freshwater fish as an essential ingredient in the typical Roman diet. It further addresses cultural attitudes, namely the intertwining of religious and secular aspects: fish was not only a widespread symbol of Christianity, but also a possible regular foodstuff included in the menu of Rome's early Christians. However, the authors argue that since a uniform ecclesiastical ideology on fasting has not developed yet, it seems most possible that practical reasons (easy access and low cost) must have outweighed religious ones (Rutgers et al., 2009, 1133).

The consumption of C_4 plants, and especially millet, has been only sporadically identified in Roman diet, and there is still a lot of work to be done on the importance of millet in the economy and diet of the era. Documentary evidence presents ambivalent information on the actual consumption of millet; millet was largely considered to be the food of the poor and was usually associated with periods of famines and shortages (Spurr, 1983; Garnsey, 1988). The perception of millet as a substandard grain may have contributed to the assumption that it was primarily used as animal fodder rather than for human consumption. The study by Tafuri et al. (2009) on millet consumption in Bronze Age Italy (sixteenth to twelfth centuries BC) demonstrated that northern populations consumed significantly more C_4 resources than southern populations, although both geographic groups also consumed C_3 plants. Killgrove and Tykot (2013) analyzed samples from two inland sites in close proximity to Rome: Casal Bertone and Castellaccio Europarco. Both sites suggested a diet composed of mostly terrestrial protein: primarily from C_3 foods for Casal Bertone with some marine protein intake, while consumption of more C_4 foods, most probably of millet, was attested for Castellaccio Europarco. This difference is not surprising as the population at the latter site was likely associated with a large agricultural area, in contrast to Casal Bertone where the population comes from a periurban cemetery, just outside the city walls of Rome. Individuals having a significant input of dietary C_4 protein have also been reported for Roman Britain (Müldner et al., 2011; Pollard et al., 2011), adding to the discussion for the presence of people consuming such diets and the importance of millet during the Roman era. These outliers in the isotopic graphs point to the existing diversity of diet in the Roman world and the movement of people from areas that had a tradition of growing millet.

Access to food is not only a matter of biological need; it is influenced by social attitudes towards the status of males and females in both the household and the society. As such, males in Roman society had a higher status and power than females, and most likely better access to a greater variety of food items, including luxurious and prestigious ones. Few isotopic studies have addressed the possible existence of sex-related variation in diet. The study by Prowse et al. (2005) for Isola Sacra has traced such sex variation, albeit the differences were comparatively small. Females had a more C_3 plant-based diet, while males whose values were more variable, possibly suggestive of access to a larger variety of food items, had a comparatively larger proportion of marine protein in their diet. Sex differences (albeit subtle, <1‰) were also attested for Velia, as males seemed to have better access to high trophic level foods like meat and fish (Craig et al., 2009). Such sex-based variation, however, was not present in the Leptiminus sample and the authors argue that either such a difference cannot be detected isotopically or simply both males and females were eating the same food, despite textual evidence to the contrary (Keenleyside et al., 2009, 60). Similarly, no such evidence was found in the study by Killgrove and Tykot (2013) for Casal Bertone and Castellaccio Europarco. Since some women consumed significant quantities of meat and fish (for example at Velia), likely differential access to foods was not strictly adhered to. A better explanation of the observed isotopic differences between the sexes may be accounted for by occupational activities, particularly related to the involvement of males in the procuring and processing of meat and fish, and cultural restrictions of certain foods opposed to females in respect to health issues.

Chemical analysis on distinct groups of Roman populations has recently offered insights into the diet of gladiators, whose remains were retrieved from a cemetery in Ephesus (Turkey), dating to the second and third centuries AD (Lösch et al., 2014). Gladiator and non-gladiator individuals from other burial complexes were chemically tested in order to detect possibly dietary differences and restrictions between this group and contemporary inhabitants of Ephesus. The occupational group of gladiators, primarily derived from the lower strata of the Roman society, are referred to in the texts as consuming a specific diet (*gladiatoriam saginam*), including barley and beans, which gave them the nickname of *hordearri*, "barley eaters" (Lösch et al., 2014, 1, 3, 9). Although this dependence on specific foodstuffs attested in the sources, such as C_3 staples and legumes, was chemically evidenced, the data obtained indicated that gladiators' diets did not significantly differ from other groups. Furthermore, gladiators were a very heterogeneous group who consumed different kind of foods: for example, one gladiator had a strong signal for C_4 plant consumption, another a mixed signal of C_3 and C_4 consumption, and two others exhibited the highest nitrogen values indicative of regular consumption of animal proteins and a lower intake of legumes.

Clearly Roman diet was cereal-based and enriched according to a number of variables: social stratification, gender, occupation and origin, giving this image of Roman populations as a splendid human mosaic with distinguished dietary patterns. It is still difficult to assess whether the observed patterns are shaped by necessity or choice; however, the more pieces we gather, the clearer appears this puzzle of the Roman diet.

Ab ovo usque ad mala: Roman diet in a multidisciplinary context

Understanding Roman dietary patterns is a complex task and, as evidenced, their reconstruction greatly benefits from multidisciplinary approaches drawing from a variety of data sets: documentary and archaeological evidence, paleopathology and chemical analysis. The researcher working with historic populations has the advantage of drawing evidence from the textual record. Despite the problems inherent to the type of information provided, as Roman texts are produced by and for the elite, they still form a solid background against which other data sets can be projected and evaluated. Roman historians and specialists working on human bones, fauna and flora from archaeological contexts should closely collaborate and promote shared and combined research, in order to have a holistic image of the variety of natural resources available and consequently consumed during the era in question.

Stable isotope analysis, and in particular carbon and nitrogen as tracers of foodstuffs, has revolutionized our understanding of past diets – at the very least, it identifies the role played in the diet by isotopically different foodstuffs and broad similarities and differences in diets in a temporal and regional level. As such, it is a powerful methodological tool that needs to be further applied to Roman populations, also focusing on the link between diet and disease (see Katzenberg, 2012; Olsen et al., 2014; D'Ortenzio et al., 2015). The study by Killgrove (2017) is an excellent example of the potentials of biochemical analysis for the understanding of the presence of porotic lesions in Rome and its *suburbium* during the first to third centuries AD. Carbon and nitrogen analysis for the reconstruction of dietary patterns included the analysis of individuals exhibiting these lesions (Killgrove and Tykot, 2013); since only one individual out of the seven with porotic lesions demonstrated lower $\delta^{15}N$ value than the mean for the site, a hypothesis based on a low animal protein diet cannot sufficiently explain their presence in the samples of Casal Bertone and Castellaccio Europarco. Similarly interesting is the combination of the results obtained from the analysis of lead concentrations in samples with and without porotic lesions from the same sites (Montgomery et al., 2010).[12] Lead is known to have been extensively used by the Romans (e.g., pipes of the water system, food and beverage containers). Concentrations higher than 0.5 mg/kg can result in lead poisoning, which consequently can cause hemolytic anemia evidenced by the presence of porotic lesions. Individuals with porotic lesions have high lead concentrations and thus a hemolytic anemia can be suspected, although high lead concentration might have been one of the many variables that can be accounted for the presence of these lesions.

Currently, studies on diachronic changes in Roman diet are scarce; however, a topic gaining significant attention among researchers is the possible identification of changes in alimentary patterns and living conditions during the transition from the Roman to the early medieval period. During this passage, the attested social and economic transformations were usually interpreted as an actual cultural discontinuity. Manzi et al. (1999) and Šlaus et al. (2011) argued that in Italy and Dalmatia, respectively, the transition from the Roman times to the early medieval period was marked by an evident deterioration of oral health. The frequency of carious lesions, for example, is significantly higher in the early medieval series, suggesting markedly different dietary habits and an early medieval diet richer in carbohydrates. However, the study by Belcastro et al. (2007) suggested that in the Sannio area of Molise there was substantial continuity of the dietary habits from the first to the seventh centuries AD, marked by high consumption of carbohydrates during both the Roman and early medieval period. A comparison of their samples with other Roman and early medieval populations who lived close to Rome and probably enjoyed better living conditions, demonstrated that the transition occurred at different times and in different ways in Italy.

Standardization of the criteria and the methodology applied in the study of Roman archaeological populations will minimize the disparities in the observed frequencies, thus providing sufficient comparative data and contributing to a synthetic reconstruction of lifestyles and dietary patterns. As an increased interest is expressed in the study of Roman populations it is hoped that more multidisciplinary approaches will appear in the near future.

Acknowledgments

I deeply thank the editors of the volume for their invitation to participate in this volume. I am also grateful to Dr. K. Killgrove (University of West Florida) for our fruitful discussions on the topic and for sharing her data and photographs with me, and to my dear colleague Dr. B.J. Fuller for years of research in stable isotope analysis.

Notes

1 For the term "bioarchaeolgy", see Buikstra, 2006, pp. xvii–xx.
2 For the Roman population the study on phytoliths (microscopic remains originating in plant tissues) observed in the dental calculus of a sample from Tarragona, Spain (c. AD 300–550) revealed that most of the phytoliths identified on the enamel and the dental calculus belonged to the family of Poaceae (Lalueza Fox et al., 1996).
3 Similar high frequency (9.7%) of carious lesions is also observed for a series of Roman populations from Croatia dating from the third to the sixth centuries AD (Šlaus et al., 2011); from continental Croatia there is also a study of a skeletal series from a settlement at the Danubian limes, and "non-limes" skeletal series from settlements to the west of the limes (Šlaus et al., 2004).
4 Manzi et al., 1999 reported on a sub-sample from Isola Sacra. A larger sample was studied by Prowse (2011), however the latter did not provide prevalence of dental pathologies per tooth but per age/sex category and thus is not included in the discussion.
5 Vitamin B_{12} is found in foods that come from animals, including fish and shellfish, meat (especially liver), poultry, eggs, milk, and milk products (WHO, 2004, 279–280).
6 It should be noted that this percentage does not represent only adult individuals; however frequencies in adult sexed individuals were high: 85.7% for females and 50% for males.
7 This is a considerable setback to the study of Roman populations, since although inhumation never stopped to be practiced throughout the Roman era, cremation was the dominant practice, for example, during the Republican period.
8 Variability is due to the amount and quality of protein consumed; for example, high protein diets have lower trophic spacing, while poor quality protein (like in plants) has higher trophic spacing.

9　The study of dietary patterns at Sagalassos (Turkey) by Fuller et al. (2012), combining isotopic and zooarchaeological/archaeobotanical evidence when available, presented interesting data on animal husbandry practices during the early to middle imperial (25 BC–AD 300) and late imperial (AD 300–450) period. The bulk of the analyzed samples consisted primarily of animal bones, while the three human bone samples analyzed from the late imperial period, revealed a terrestrial C_3 diet.

10　The samples consisted of small fish bones, brown flakes (probably dried fish), and shells. However, the authors advise caution as the values of the *garum* samples cannot be representative of the range of isotopic composition for this product.

11　Keenleyside et al. (2009) have not tested any *garum* samples; their assumption that *garum* must not have made a significant contribution to the higher $\delta^{15}N$ values seen at the Leptiminus sample, which can be better explained by consumption of higher trophic level species, is following the results of the study at Isola Sacra (see above, and also note 10).

12　A similar chemical analysis for lead concentration was performed in the Ravenna and Rimini series (Facchini et al., 2004).

PART II

Food and drink

8

ROMAN MEALS IN THEIR DOMESTIC AND WIDER SETTINGS

John Donahue

Introduction

A popular method of ancient education called for children to memorize various commands in order to improve their Latin and Greek. In the following excerpt we find a child practicing for the role of the head of a household, a position that he would one day be expected to fill:

> Bring the cups and a dish, a candelabrum, decorate the table, sprinkle flowers in the dining room, set out charcoal and the incense burners, have everything prepared. Tell your fellow slave to make the food tasty, as I have important men as guests.
>
> *(Dionisotti, 1982, in Osgood, 2011, 75–76)*

For the student of ancient dining practices this passage is especially significant, for in the space of a few lines it contains many of the elements that defined a meal among friends: careful attention to dinner service and setting; the presence of slaves; the necessity of fine fare; and important men as guests. We note another feature as well. The dinner ritual was routine enough to be included in schoolboy exercises but important enough to demand careful attention to detail, as these lines confirm. Furthermore, if we look more closely, we find evidence of larger issues – the reality of slavery versus freedom, and the inevitable risk to one's reputation in putting on a dinner of this sort. Thus do we have an entry point for considering in the pages ahead not only meals of this sort but also eating and drinking across a broad spectrum of the Roman world and the issues associated with this activity during the imperial period, both in domestic and wider settings.

History and terminology

The history of social customs in antiquity is often difficult to trace, and Roman dining is no exception. In contrast to ancient nutrition, where we tend to be better informed about medical thinking on the topic than we are on how closely individuals may have conformed to such theory (Donahue, 2016), Roman dining is better known in its everyday aspects than in its historical development. On the historical side, we see this reality most clearly in the practice whereby participants reclined on couches when eating and drinking. Most likely, this convention found its way to archaic Italy through the Etruscans, who have preserved much evidence through tomb paintings and cooking and dining utensils (Pieraccini, 2000; Spivey, 1997) and who, according to a recent interpretation, were ultimately influenced not by the Near East, as conventionally thought, but by the drinking celebrations (*symposia*) of Greece, which date as early as 800 BC (Wecowski, 2014). Even so, reconstruction of the Roman practice has remained elusive, especially for the period of the early Republic.

We are on firmer ground by the early second century BC when Roman control of the Hellenistic East brought Greek values to bear on Roman social life, including customs related to dining. Here we begin to witness the paradoxical nature of Roman festal ideology, as Greek ideals of equality and participation by the community inevitably came into conflict with Roman concerns with rank and status among the political elite. In terms of dining, it is within this context that we start to see the appearance of various sumptuary laws (*leges sumptuariae)* and their limits on festal foods and display. For example, the *lex Aemilia* of 115 BC, one of at least a dozen laws proposed or enacted from the mid to late Republic to place limits on exotic dishes and expensive tastes, banned dormice, shellfish and imported birds from Roman banquets (Plin. *HN* 8.82.223). Nevertheless, excessive festal display and consumption by elites continued unabated, with the rationale for these laws having as much to do with protection from political competition as with the pursuit of luxury (Zanda, 2011). Even more compelling were feasts provided by Roman dynasts of the late Republic, such as the banquet provided by Julius Caesar to celebrate his four-fold triumph of 46 BC, which featured an enormous public feast throughout the city of Rome but a more private (and luxurious) meal for his elite comrades (Dio Cass. 53.19–23; Plut. *Caes.* 55; Meier, 1997). By the time of the Principate these social divisions at the table had become standard. Thus do we find Pliny speaking about a dinner he attended in which the host reserved the best dishes for himself and a select few while the rest of the company had to be content with nibbling on cheap scraps of food (Plin. *Ep.* 2.6); similarly, the poets Juvenal and Martial complain bitterly about the stingy meals furnished to clients by their arrogant patrons. (Mart. 3.60; Juv. 5) Although evidence of this sort has the feel of a literary *topos*, it also indicates the power of food and drink to exploit some of the tensions that inevitably existed between persons of unequal status in the Roman world.

Closely tied to Roman festal behavior was a distinctive vocabulary of meals, which, although equally difficult to trace historically, nevertheless helps us to understand more fully the ancient dining experience. These terms were not rigidly fixed, a situation akin to modern Britain, where "lunch" might mean "dinner" and "dinner" might mean "tea," depending on the region. Furthermore, the fluidity of such terminology perhaps suggests a Roman mindset more focused on the impact that such meals had on the reputation of the donor or on "atmospherics" such as setting and service than on concerns over strict usage of the terms themselves. This kind of imprecision marks the term *sportula*, where it is not always clear if the Romans meant a handout of cash, its equivalent as a meal, or a combination of both (Vössing, 2004). The remaining terms are utilized to describe meals in a variety of circumstances and settings. The *cena*, as the main meal of the day, was the most widespread term and one with a wide variety of meanings. It could take place at home, on the streets or among invited guests, whether at the imperial palace as a formal dinner (*cena recta*) or in the dining rooms (*triclinia*) of the elite. In the hands of a clever host, the *cena* helped to reinforce a code of elite values while providing the modern reader with useful insight into social relationships in ancient society. *Cenae* also celebrated rites of passage, including the coming of age ceremony, marriage and funerary rites, and accession to political office (Donahue, 2004a). The *epulum* was the most widely attested eating event in the ancient sources and the meal of choice at large public gatherings, such as those sponsored by the emperor in the Colosseum and by municipal elites, who eagerly recorded such acts of generosity in numerous honorary inscriptions, especially in the Roman West. The *epulum* might also be a cash handout that could be used to purchase food on occasions such as these (Slater, 2000). The *convivium* too was a dinner, often for large numbers of guests. Candidates running for office often provided *convivia* to potential voters, a form of bribery that was difficult to control (Plin. *Ep.* 6.19) On the other hand, we find *convivia* on community calendars (*CIL* 11.1421=*ILS* 140), and commemorative inscriptions, indicating the difficulty of separating public from private or legal from illegal in Roman everyday practice. *Convivia* might be staged by emperors for their guests, often times elaborately and at great expense (*SHA, Verus* 5.1; *SHA Elagab.* 19). The latter evidence, closely connected to issues of imperial reputation, rank, and anxiety about the proper role of food and drink in ancient society, will receive additional treatment below.

The Roman family at table

For nearly 30 years the ancient family in Italy has been the focus of intensive study (Rawson, 1986; 2010; Rawson and Weaver, 1999; Kertzer and Saller, 1991; Dixon, 1990; 1992; Gardner, 1998; George, 2001; Osgood, 2011). What has emerged, among other findings, is a closer scrutiny of what the term "family" actually means and, more specifically for our purposes, a deeper appreciation of imperial and elite intrusion into family life through mechanisms such as handouts of food or money (*congiaria*) and food support programs (*alimenta*) for children (Rawson, 2010; see also Holleran in this volume). Largely missing from this research, however, has been any treatment of "ordinary" everyday domestic meals due to the fact that such meals are simply not very well understood. We can gain some glimmer of insight through funerary reliefs such as imperial-era sarcophagi, which typically depict a family member (most often the male head of an elite household) reclining amid a banquet scene (Dunbabin, 2003, especially chapter 4). Yet even here the need to express individuality had to be balanced with the need to connect with external viewers, who had to rely on visual terms that could be easily understood. As a result, these scenes tend to be highly contrived rather than casual and genuine, even if they appear so (Huskinson, 2011, 522).

Perhaps the closest we can get to the domestic meal is through the terms associated with various mealtimes. The *cena*, mentioned earlier, was the main meal of the day taken in the evening. Additionally, the Roman *ientaculum*, or breakfast, was typically comprised of bread and cheese (Mart. 13.31; Apul. *Met.* 1.18; on the fiction of Apuleius as a source for the historical Roman family, see Bradley, 2000), while the *prandium*, a light lunch, might include bread, vegetables, cold meat and fruit, along with wine (Plin. *Ep.* 3.5.10; Hor. *Sat.* 2.4.22; Mart. 13.13.1–2). We even have evidence of the *merenda*, an afternoon snack, which, for the abstemious Stoic emperor Marcus Aurelius, consisted of simple bread, and for the more voracious eaters, beans, onions and herrings full of roe (Fronto *Ep.*, vol. 1, p. 182 Haines [Loeb]). What is clear from this evidence, however, is that these were meals that could be eaten without a table or hand-washing (Dalby, 2003) and thus were perhaps closer to meals eaten on the street (see below) than to family-centered meals. Consequently, it is difficult to know if it was even the norm for families, whether elite or sub-elite, to eat together on a daily basis, a reality that should give fair warning to any attempt to impose modern notions of "the family dinner" upon the ancient evidence. Instead, we tend to see the Roman family at dinner through the interpretative lens of elites, whose main concern was how family members prepared for their place in society through formal education as well as through instruction in etiquette, attire and the proper control of emotions (Osgood, 2011; Bradley, 1998). In this aspect we are reminded of the image in the literary sources of the Republican values of self-restraint and modesty in meals and general comportment as established by Augustus for the imperial family (Suet. *Aug.* 72–78). Finally, it is not easy to determine on what basis such elites chose to dine with family members or if the latter were even guaranteed as the first choice on any given day, especially since ties of kinship and patronage among Roman elites during the imperial period would have provided the status-conscious dinner host with a ready source of desirable dining companions beyond his immediate family (Bradley, 1998).

Eating and drinking in the streets

In contrast to family meals, we are better informed about those meals consumed along the streets of the city, most notably in Ostia, Pompeii and Herculaneum. Here inscriptions, wall paintings, reliefs, archaeological remains and literary evidence combine to reveal a vibrant and colorful café culture. Critical to this portrait was the *taberna*, or bar, an establishment easily identified in the archaeological remains by its L-shaped counters, one arm of which faced the street to catch pedestrians, with the other extending inward for customers inside the shop. The counters themselves often contained braziers for hot food as well as inset storage jars. The latter, traditionally thought to have contained wine, more likely held a variety of dried goods, such as fruits, nuts and vegetables; wine was perhaps stored in jars on the floor or in racks on the walls, although the evidence for this is very limited (Holleran, 2012, 135–143). An inscription of food items bought and sold as preserved in an atrium close to a Pompeian bar featuring the type of serving counter described above sheds additional light on what the typical customer might have consumed: bread, oil, wine, onions, cheese, leeks, porridge, small fish, dates and sausage (*CIL* 4.5380, in Cooley and Cooley, 2014, 238–239). Evidence of such variety suggest that the neighborhood bar provided a respite from the typically bland regimen of grain, olive oil and vegetables, and even raises the possibility that some of these establishments may have functioned not so much as fast-food taverns but more in the manner of corner grocery stores (Beard, 2010, 225–233).

Additionally, it is clear from the sources that the rather generic term *taberna* was supplemented by other terms with more specific meanings. The *caupona* seems to have primarily denoted an inn featuring accommodations but also food and drink for guests and other customers. The *popina* was not associated with lodging but did sell a variety of foods, including sausages, smoked ham, tripe and other meat. Indeed, the remains of hearths in many of these establishments confirm that cooked food items were popular. Furthermore, supplementing the sale of these items from fixed locations were hawkers or traders, who sold all kinds of foods as ambulatory vendors (Holleran, 2011, 254–255). The sale of wine too is well attested, highlighting the importance of the *taberna* in the diffusion of a thriving urban wine culture in imperial Italy (Holleran, 2012, 140–147).

Beyond their capacity to provide food and drink to a bustling urban population, *tabernae* were closely associated with leisure and relaxation. Scenes of drinking and gambling on wall paintings, advertisements for bars, pricing information for different varieties of wines (Cooley and Cooley, 2014, 230–233, 235–246) and coins and dice boxes for gambling (Laurence, 2007, 99–101) confirm this impulse for sociability. At the same time, such pursuits were met with scorn in the literary sources, which took a dim view of street life in general, and taverns and inns in particular, typically associating them with sex, prostitution, crime, noise and corrupt proprietors (Holleran, 2012, 147–149). Juvenal associated the inn with gossip (Juv. *Sat.* 9.102); far worse, laws concerning rape and adultery could not be enforced there, underscoring the strong male presence at these places, the dangers for women, and the impulse for elites to exert control over those whom they perceived as their moral inferiors (Laurence, 2007, 92–101). Thus did elite control extend not only to the recipients of meals but also to the establishments themselves where food and drink was made available to the urban masses. In the context of public policy, this latter feature was also present in periodic attempts by several first-century emperors to close some taverns or prohibit the sale of certain foods, such as hot foods (and the threat of fire that they posed), in an attempt to preserve public order at Rome (Suet. *Tib.* 34; Dio Cass. 60.6.7; Suet. *Claud.* 38–40; Suet. *Nero* 16.2; Dio 62.14.2). Ammianus Marcellinus indicates that this ideology continued at Rome into late antiquity (Amm. Marc. 28.4.4) Thus, as with *collegia* (see below), the neighborhood tavern was seen as a potential source of civic disruption.

While it is difficult to imagine that the inn and the tavern were always trouble-free, the streets may have been less lurid than our sources care to admit. As Laurence has noted, the largest inn at Pompeii provided a small garden for relaxing, a larger one for supplying food, and a dining room (*triclinium*) for guests (Laurence, 2007, 94). Even so, these amenities contrast with the reality that this same establishment was situated opposite the city's largest brothel, suggesting that the world of vice was never more than a few steps removed from that of eating and drinking. Finally, in terms of social values, what seems most important for the modern observer is to recognize the gulf that existed between elites and their inferiors concerning activities of the street. Elites would have never frequented the inn or the tavern, or so they would have us believe, given the scorn they typically cast upon these venues. Indeed, when they dined, they were expected to do so in the privacy of their own homes (Holleran, 2012, 148). To be sure, the emperor Augustus once signaled as much when he reminded an *eques* who was spotted at a *popina* that when he himself wished to eat, he went home (Quint. 6.3.63). Nevertheless, the *taberna* provided an important venue for social interactions of all kinds, and it is equally clear that it was an essential outlet for providing food and drink to a significant portion of the urban population on a daily basis.

Meals among associations (*collegia*), slaves and soldiers

Patrons of the *taberna* are not the only ordinary Romans whose eating and drinking habits are known to us. Slaves, soldiers and members of *collegia* are able to provide additional perspective. For slaves and soldiers, food rations (*cibaria*), typically consisting of grain, were common. Turning first to slaves, agricultural slaves, about whom we are best informed, could expect their rations to be closely monitored by the attentive owner, who would adjust his distributions based on the time of year and the labors to be performed (Cato *Agr.* 56) as well as the health of the slave (*Agr.* 2.4) Soldiers, on the other hand, carried their own provisions (Cic. *Tusc.* 2.37), with amounts varying according to the nature and duration of the expedition (Caes. *Gal.* 1.5.3; 6.10.2). Rations might even factor into military punishments, as when Galba starved to death a soldier who had sold some of his leftover rations for cash amid a shortage (Suet. *Gal.* 7.2; more generally, Phang, 2008). Meals among *collegia*, known primarily through inscriptions and archaeology, are especially well known and require more detailed treatment.

Collegia were societies organized on the basis of voluntary membership and were especially popular among workmen and worshippers during the Principate (Perry, 2011). Although the nature and goals of these groups have not always been obvious, there is ample evidence that commensality in many forms and settings was a common feature (Ascough, 2008) – and so too the impulse for men of shared religious belief or a common occupation to socialize through food and drink (MacMullen, 1974; Alföldy, 1985). A handful of specific groups helps to sharpen our understanding of collegial feasting in useful ways. The association of the Arval Brothers, an exclusive aristocratic group with its own temple outside of Rome, enjoyed ritual feasts over the course of several hundred years as preserved in a long fragmentary series of inscriptions (Scheid, 1990). Among non-aristocratic groups, the college dedicated to Diana and Antinous at Lanuvium in the second century AD devotes nearly half of its regulations to its schedule of banquets and conduct on festal occasions. Here we learn that each supervising magistrate was to provide "good wine," bread for all the members, sardines and specific dining accoutrements (*CIL* 14.2112=*ILS* 7212; Donahue, 2004a). Indeed, in order to make for a more memorable occasion, it is not unrealistic to suppose that the patron of this *collegium*, whose relatives' birthdays were celebrated by the association, might have periodically contributed an animal (or more) to be sacrificed and subsequently eaten. We also learn that a member could not take another seat at a festive dinners other than the one assigned (*CIL* 14.2112, col 2, l. 25), an indication that helps us to appreciate the importance attached to seating placement as a way to reinforce hierarchy and monitor proximity to the host or special guests. Finally, at Rome, the college of Aeculapius and Hygia, also dated to the second century AD, featured seven fixed banquets per year, a number likely supplemented by many additional opportunities for feasting (*CIL* 6.10234=*ILS* 7213; Donahue, 2004a). Striking here is the emphasis on rank within the group as a determinant for the level of benefits conferred, confirming that even among ordinary *collegia*, concerns over rank and status were ever present at the meal table.

Two additional features are noteworthy. First, officials of these groups often went to great lengths to enforce codes of conduct and to publicize this fact in their regulations. At the college of Diana and Antinous, penalties were imposed for rowdiness at meetings on a sliding scale, with the most costly infraction imposed for insults or abuse directed toward the group's leader. Such regulations suggest that the group was willing to accept, and advertise, civic values but that decorum was often difficult to maintain, especially within a system where strict hierarchical distinctions prevailed. Given this situation, it is easy to see how periodic violence erupted, contributing to the image of the *collegium* as potentially disruptive to the political order of the city at times (Nippel, 1995; Lintott, 1999). Second, new approaches are allowing us to reassess the nature and significance of the meeting places (*scholae*) utilized by *collegia* within the wider urban landscape. At Ostia, a theoretical model for spatial analysis known as space syntax has determined that *scholae* were deliberately situated along the most easily accessible streets and public spaces in order to increase the potential for promoting contact and communication. In this way, *scholae* contributed to the "urban buzz," where a large number of different activities coincide within the same space (Stöger, 2011, 239–242). Such approaches are allowing us to assess *collegia* and activities such as feasting in new ways within a broader urban framework.

Social dining: elites and emperors, venues and victuals

The sights and sounds of eating and drinking in the streets existed alongside the social meals of private individuals and the emperor himself, about which we are generally well informed through literary and archaeological remains. Here the energy and excess of street-level food and drink gave way to the refinement of the dining room, where setting, status and even dining posture combined to form a ritual that, perhaps more than any other social practice, helped to advertise identity and reinforce elite values.

At the center of these meals was the dining room itself, most commonly known as the *triclinium*, after the three-couch arrangement that had become the standard feature of dining rooms by the end of the Republic. The term also applied to the room designated for this type of dining, whether indoors or outdoors. These couches were arranged around tables set in the center, upon which the waiters, typically handsome boys and slaves from the kitchen staff, placed the food and drink. Guests, typically three per couch, took portions of food with their right hand while reclining on their left elbow. As we saw earlier with *collegia*, seating arrangements remained critically important. Guests were arranged in positions of varying status in relation to the host and his guest of honor, who were recognized as the most significant attendees and who typically reclined in specific places within a scheme where each seating position had its own name. Even so, custom was not always followed, at least according to Horace and Petronius, who reveal that the host might take a different seating position based on circumstance or preference (Hor. *Sat.* 2.8; Petron. *Sat.* 31; Dunbabin, 1991).

While venue was important, so too were the diners who occupied such space. Especially noteworthy is the presence of women of all classes at Roman social banquets, a clear departure from formal Greek symposia, where women appear to have been absent. Here, women of every status did not sit when dining but frequently reclined like their husbands (Roller, 2006, chapter 2); at other times they were known to dine separately from men, such as at the dedication of a statue to Augustus in AD 14 when Tiberius feasted with senators and knights while Livia entertained the wives (Dio Cass. 57.12). Even so, there is little else recorded about events of this sort, although, as mentioned earlier, they display an emphasis on Republican virtue that was an important focus of the early Julio-Claudian emperors. Children, the object of much scholarly attention in recent years (Rawson, 1991; 2003; Dixon, 2001; Laes, 2011; see also Laes in this volume) are also attested at formal family meals (Bradley, 1998), where they might sit or recline, although boys would have reclined once they reached manhood (Roller, 2006, chapter 3).

Finally, the social dining experience would have been incomplete without the host's attention to menu, apparatus and entertainment. Concerning the menu, an extensive technical literature on viticulture attests to a Roman interest in wine that was much greater than that of the Greeks and that grew into true connoisseurship on the basis of a careful ranking of vintages from Italy and abroad (Tchernia, 1986; Unwin, 1996; see also Broekaert in this volume). In fact, wine was so valued at the dinner party that each guest could make his own decision about how he would receive it, a custom that was in sharp contrast to the Greeks, who decided as a group at the start of their symposia on the proportion of water to wine (Dunbabin, 1993). When it came time for the food itself, various recipes for rich sauces and rare birds (Solomon, 1995), such as those gathered in the cookbook under the name of Apicius, the famous gourmand of the first century AD, would have helped to distinguish the ambitious dinner host from his lesser rivals. Essential too was service apparatus that was consistent with the overall quality of the dining experience, as seen in the first-century wall painting of elaborate silverware for a banquet from the tomb of Vestorius Priscus at Pompeii (Dunbabin, 2003, fig. 44). This did not mean that the accoutrements were always tasteful, however. The garish serving pieces at Trimalchio's feast in Petronius' *Satyricon* come to mind (Petron. *Sat.* 31, 35), although Trimalchio's misreading of the art of display is surely part of the point here.

Public feasts

As a final dining experience to consider, public banquets offered by the emperor or private benefactors formed a colorful and important strand in the festal tapestry of the Roman world. Turning first to the emperor, his public feasts likely had their origins in the banquets furnished by Hellenistic monarchs. As mentioned earlier, these feasts were later incorporated into the political programs of Republican dynasts like Julius Caesar. With his defeat of Antony in

31 BC and subsequent rule as Rome's first emperor, Augustus ensured that the public feasts of the Hellenistic monarch and the Roman dynast would find a permanent place in the Roman world as a means to display imperial munificence to large numbers of people.

The nature of imperially sponsored public feasts depended largely on the interests and personality of the sponsoring emperor and how the sources chose to portray such munificence. For a thoroughly flattering portrayal, we cannot overlook Statius' account in *Silvae* 1.6 of Domitian's banquet for the *populus* of Rome at the Colosseum to celebrate the Saturnalia, one of many occasions on the Roman calendar where feasts or sacrificial meat would have been available to the people (Beard et al., 1998, vol. 2, chapter 5). Here we find a large and enthusiastic crowd and the distribution of fine foods by means of ropes dramatically suspended above the gathered masses (Stat. *Silv.* 1.6.9–20). Furthermore, handsome stewards deliver finer food and wine, presumably to the elites (Stat. *Silv.* 1.6.28–32), suggesting that the attendees did not share the same food, despite Statius' claim to the contrary (Stat. *Silv.* 1.6.43-5) To be sure, the seating scheme of the Colosseum, segregated by class (Claridge, 2010), would have reinforced this practice of differential food based on social status.

Beyond the public feasts of the emperor at Rome, community-wide banquets, preserved in numerous dedicatory and honorary inscriptions from Italy and the Roman West during the Principate, allowed benefactors to advertise their generosity and to enhance their social standing within the Graeco-Roman world of privately sponsored philanthropy known as *evergetism* (Donahue, 2004a). Most common was the scenario whereby a municipal notable provided a meal, cash for a meal, or a bit of honey cake and sweet wine for the townsfolk, perhaps to mark a statue dedicated in his honor or at the completion of a public works project for which he or she had paid. A key feature of this system was the practice of linking the quality of a meal or the amount of cash for a meal to the social status of the recipient. In this way, local senators typically received the best meal or most funds for a feast, followed by the local priests or members of various *collegia* (van Nijf, 1997), and then the townspeople. As with the emperors' feasts at Rome, local benefactors displayed a similar concern with rank and status.

A significant aspect of this phenomenon was the opportunity it presented for donors of lower standing but of sufficient means to distribute largess. Thus do we find a freedman and priest of Augustus from municipal Italy providing banquets and distributions of meat to his fellow residents at a statue dedication marking his service to the town (*CIL* 11.5965). This system allowed for female participation as well, evident in the striking generosity of a certain Junia Rustica from first-century Roman Spain, who financed public repair projects, the town's tax burden and family statues, while providing a feast to the residents at the statue dedication recognizing her munificence (*CIL* 2.1956 = *ILS* 5512; Donahue, 2004b). Finally, testamentary options helped to guarantee public feasts on an annual basis, as at Rudiae in southern Italy during the second century where a father set up an endowment of 80,000 sesterces, the interest from which was to provide a distribution of meat each year on his son's birthday (*CIL* 9.23 = *ILS* 6472). The endowment was modest in comparison to similar foundations, which were capitalized with as much as 250,000 sesterces, nor can we really know how many recipients it supported owing to our lack of demographic data. Even so, we can suppose that the distributions of this sort played an important role in the local economy and would have been most especially welcome to the lower classes (Liu, 2008).

9

CEREALS AND BREAD

Frits Heinrich

Introduction

Within the study of Roman diet, hardly any category of foodstuffs has received as much attention as the cereals.[1] This is quite unsurprising as cereals were the most important staples of the Roman world, as they are today. All cereals (including rice and maize) are grasses, and hence members of the Poaceae (formerly Gramineae) family. If cultivated for human consumption, their seeds (also grains or kernels) are the primary product, which makes them the eponymous grain crops.[2] Other grain crops include pulses (see Heinrich and Hansen, this volume) and various other non–Poaceae species, sometimes referred to as the pseudo-cereals (e.g., quinoa and buckwheat). Grain crops are very suitable as staples because they produce high yields per area unit, contain a high energetic value per weight unit, can be efficiently and cheaply produced, processed and transported, and can be stored efficiently and have a long shelf-life. Of all cereal preparations, bread is perhaps the most iconic and culturally most significant as well as the most highly preferred consumption mode, certainly in the wider Mediterranean.

Cereal nutrition and cereal and bread consumption are multifaceted topics and no single chapter can hope to be complete. I will therefore focus on aspects that have featured less prominently in the discourse, especially cereal taxonomy and nutritional biochemistry, and less so on the classical sources, which have often been expertly discussed (e.g., Moritz 1958; White, 1970; Frayn, 1979, Spurr, 1986; Sallares, 1991; Wilkins et al., 1995; Garnsey, 1999; Erdkamp, 2005; Wilkins and Hill, 2006). Historians and archaeologists have increasingly been using nutritional, biochemical and genetic data over the past two decades (e.g., Sallares, 1995; Garnsey, 1999; Thurmond, 2006). Due to the dependence of the majority of the world's human and livestock populations on cereals, and the great commercial importance of wheat and bread in particular, the wealth of modern scientific research into these topics is virtually boundless and developments continue at a fast pace.[3] Therefore some new insights have not yet been applied to the study of ancient diet. On the other hand, some insights that were used have since been updated or have become obsolete. In this text I will highlight several examples that are of importance when modelling the ancient diet.[4]

One aspect that I will try to nuance in this chapter is the often assumed superiority of bread wheat over other types of wheat in bread-making due to its high gluten content. I will show that gluten content can be highly variable at any taxonomic level and that other variables besides genetics affect gluten content. Another aspect I will redress is the somewhat negative nutritional appraisal of cereals. Historians of any era are often concerned about the centrality of cereals in the diet on account of their alleged nutritional deficiencies and the presence of anti-nutrients. Peter Garnsey, for instance, in his *Food and Society in Classical Antiquity*, implicitly paints the picture that the centrality of cereals in the ancient diet helped cause endemic, chronic malnutrition and a subsequent array of diseases (Garnsey, 1999). While appreciating their role as energy-suppliers, providing carbohydrates (primarily as starch), fat and protein, Garnsey added that they were limited in certain essential amino acids and vitamin B2, while vitamins A, D and C were absent. Garnsey argued that minerals such as zinc, iron and calcium were present, but largely useless due to the presence of anti-nutrients. Those who have instead argued that the Roman diet was healthy and wholesome (or perhaps even better than most other premodern diets) generally did so not by exonerating cereals, but by arguing in favour of the more generous addition of other (protein-rich) foodstuffs to the diet (e.g., Jongman, 2007a; Kron, 2008a). Dietary variation is indeed quintessentially important for good health, as no category of foodstuffs alone meets all our dietary requirements. However, this in itself does not justify a negative assessment of cereals. I will therefore review the validity of some of the nutritional concerns that have been raised against cereals, using recent biochemical insights. I will also show that biochemical and nutritional data obtained from modern, modified cultivars may lead us to underestimate the nutritional value of cereals in the past. In addition, I will assess the effect of several traditional preparation techniques that have been shown to increase the nutritional value of cereals and negate anti-nutrients. First, however, I will briefly touch upon cereal taxonomy and discuss the range of cereals and consumption modes available to the Roman consumer.

Roman cereals

What's in a name?

Much of the discourse on cereals in Roman diet and agriculture has been delivered using imprecise categories. While it is sometimes useful to use categories such as 'cereals' or 'grain', 'wheat' and 'barley', they are often too general; the term 'millet' or 'millets' is even more problematic.[5] Important morphological and other differences with crucial economic consequences, for instance, tend to occur on the (sub)species level.[6] Generalization may also lead to confusion. In the literature on the Roman diet, it is for instance not uncommon for 'wheat' and 'emmer' to be implicitly contrasted (wheat being suitable for bread-making while emmer is not). Emmer, or more precisely emmer wheat (*Triticum turgidum* ssp. *dicoccon*), however, is a wheat too. A possible explanation for such generalizations and misunderstandings is that in most nutritional or biochemical literature the studied (sub)species of wheat is not specified. More often than not, it is assumed that the intended audience will understand that by 'wheat' (any (sub)species in the genus *Triticum*) *specifically* bread wheat (*Triticum aestivum* ssp. *aestivum*, a subspecies of *Triticum aestivum*) is implied, unless otherwise specified.[7] This is because at present bread wheat is economically by far the most important type of wheat: it accounts for about 95% of all wheat cultivated. The remaining 5% consists largely of hard wheat (*Triticum turgidum* ssp. *durum*), primarily to cater to the pasta industry (Shewry, 2009). The other wheats listed in Table 9.1 have been economically marginalized in the nineteenth and twentieth centuries, although recently the demand for them by the health food industry has caused an increase in their cultivation. For a further discussion of the cereals listed in table 9.1 and geographic distribution, see Heinrich, 2017.

Table 9.1 List of cereals available for consumption to the Romans

Scientific name	Common name	Hulled (H) or naked (N)
Barleys		
Hordeum vulgare ssp. *distichum*	2-Row barley (hulled)	H
Hordeum vulgare ssp. *distichum*	2-Row barley (naked)	N
Hordeum vulgare ssp. *vulgare*	6-Row barley (hulled)	H
Hordeum vulgare ssp. *vulgare*	6-Row barley (naked)	N
Wheats		
Triticum monococcum ssp. *monococcum*	Einkorn wheat	H
Triticum aestivum ssp. *aestivum*	Bead wheat	N
Triticum aestivum ssp. *spelta*	Spelt wheat	H
Triticum turgidum ssp. *dicoccon*	Emmer wheat	H
Triticum turgidum ssp. *durum*	Hard wheat	N
Other cereals		
Avena sativa	Oats	N/H
Oryza sativa	Rice	H
Panicum milliaceum	Common millet	H
Pennisetum glaucum	Pearl millet	H
Secale cereale	Rye	N
Setaria italica	Foxtail millet	H
Sorghum bicolor	Sorghum	H

Recognizing diversity in Roman cereal consumption

There are several methods besides studying the written sources to detect the consumption, and sometimes the relative importance, of specific cereal (sub)species within the Roman diet. Archaeobotany (see Livarda, this volume, cf. Van der Veen 2018) offers the most potential by identifying plant remains to species or subspecies level. Stable isotope analysis can also be useful as it can recognize (or note the absence of) the consumption of the group of so-called C_4 cereals (for the Old World the 'millets' and sorghum). These C_4 cereals use a different photosynthesis pathway than the C_3 cereals (all other Old World cereals), which affects the ratio of the $^{12}C/^{13}C$ isotopes in the plant tissue. Simply put, this ratio is routed into the tissues of the animal that consumes the plant or the human who either consumes the animal and/or the plant and can subsequently be discerned in archaeological bone material (Pollard et al., 2011; see Killgrove and Tykot, 2013; 2018 for Roman examples).[8]

Roman cereal selection

Spurr (1986) aptly defined Roman cereal cultivation as a 'highly diverse polyculture' and, as a consequence, Roman cereal consumption was no less diverse. Table 9.1 provides an overview of cereal (sub)species used as food crops by the Romans. Within environmental constraints, at least several of these could be cultivated in any region of the Roman Empire. This is evident from the fact that in almost any archaeobotanical context multiple wheat (sub)species are encountered alongside barley and sometimes other minor cereals. Cultivating multiple crops can be motivated by a desire for risk-reduction or by the different functions fulfilled by different cereals. Which crops were actually chosen could depend on (the farmer's perception of) a myriad of environmental, cultural and socioeconomic circumstances. Creating crop chronologies and analytical crop selection models may assist in noting and explaining patterns and changes in crop selection.[9] Regional and local variation in which (sub)species were chosen or were dominant widely occurs. Urban centres tend to show even greater diversity in available cereals than rural sites as cities would obtain cereals from multiple producers within their hinterland, or in the case of Rome, from far beyond (Heinrich, 2017). A general trend that various authors have observed in archaeobotanical data from the wider Mediterranean is a gradual shift from hulled wheats (especially emmer wheat) towards naked wheats (especially hard wheat) before and during the Roman period. This change has been explained in terms of the advantages naked wheats offer with regard to yield, ease of processing and transportability.[10]

Cereals and the Roman diet

Roman staples

Cereals were the main staple in the Roman diet, but other grain crop staples were also available. Of these, the pulses, which would be processed and consumed in similar modes as the cereals, were most important (Heinrich and Hansen, this volume). Locally, tree seeds such as acorn (*Quercus sp.*) and sweet chestnut (*Castanea sativa*) were important staples. Mason (1996), using ethnographic data, has argued in favour of acorns as rural staples rather than famine foods. Similarly the chestnut was the dominant rural staple in several European regions until the late nineteenth century, especially in parts of France (Fauve-Chamoux, 2001). Recent ethnographic studies in Tuscany have shown that the populations of some villages still depended on chestnuts for about half the year and for the remainder on emmer wheat (Pieroni, 1996). Interestingly, these tree seeds are used in a fashion similar to that of cereals and pulses: after 'deshelling' they are crushed, ground or milled and prepared as breads, porridges and soups. These similarities in processing and preparation are conducive to the practice of mixing. Using flours that possess different chemical qualities may be functional or enhance taste and texture. Traditional Italian pizza dough, for instance, is still made of equal parts of emmer and hard wheat and similarly the modern food industry often mixes lupine and soybean flours with wheat flours. Mixing could also help to (surreptitiously) bulk up an expensive product with a cheaper one. Mixing is attested not only ethnographically, but also archaeologically (Mason, 1996; Renfrew, 1973) and in the classical sources (see Wilkins and Hill, 2006). Ethnographic evidence suggests that significant unintentional or tolerated contamination of up to 10% of total weight in the form of weed seeds may also have been common (Jasny 1942; 1944a; 1950).

While the different staples discussed above can be similarly prepared, their nutritional profiles are not as similar (see below). If mixing was common, the nutritional contribution to the diet that staples represent would be more balanced. Modern biochemical data on the nutritional value of cereals, however, does not account for mixing. Modern results arise from the analysis of clean, uncontaminated samples of specimens of the same (sub)species; 'real-world' Roman conditions would have deviated from this.

Consumption modes: semi-finished products and semiliquids

Cereals can be prepared as numerous final products or consumption modes. While some preparations are fairly simple (e.g. *frikeh*, roasted unripe barley or wheat, see Musselman and al-Mouslem, 2001), most require more substantial processing steps. Without processing, cereal kernels are not well-suited for human consumption. Processing may be mechanical (polishing, braying, grinding, milling, sifting), biochemical (fermentation, germination), thermal (roasting, puffing, steaming, boiling, parboiling, stewing, baking, frying) or a combination of the three. Mechanical processing may result in semi-finished products of different size-fractions such as groats and different grades of meal and flour. Parboiled kernels like bulgur (that are dried, broken and stored prior to final preparation) are also a semi-finished product. The Romans had separate names for different fractions of processed cereals and even for similar fractions from different (sub)species (see Spurr, 1986; Wilkins and Hill, 2006). Today flours are ranked on extraction rate: the weight percentage of the whole kernel that remains in the flour.[11]

In principle, material of any processing grade of meal and flour can be used to prepare any consumption mode (e.g., both coarse meal and fine white flour can be used to make 'bread', cf. Akroyd and Doughty, 1970). Using different processing grades in one dish (sometimes even from different (sub)species) is also common (cf. Cato *de Agri Cultura* 76 where groats and flour are used together to make *placenta*). I will divide Roman consumption modes into two groups: semiliquids that are fermented and/or boiled and solids that are fermented and/or baked or fried. Roman semiliquid foods ranged in thickness from beer (see below), and watery barley-waters and gruels (*tisana*) to porridges or mushes (most notably emmer porridge, *puls*) and soups, stews, purees and pottages of varying thickness. For a detailed discussion of semiliquid foods, see Heinrich and Hansen in this volume.

Leavened and unleavened bread

What is bread? The answer to this question is so obvious to most of us, that we tend to forget to ask it. Here I define bread as follows: all solid foodstuffs made out of any grade of fragmented cereal and/or other starchy staple that was mixed with a liquid to create a batter or dough and that has been solidified through baking or frying. Within this definition, breads come in two types: leavened and unleavened bread. In the debate these terms often cause some confusion in which (gluten-rich) fluffy loaves of bread wheat and hard flatbreads of any other cereal are contrasted. Leavening (a process) and flatbread (a shape) are however not dialectic terms, nor are they mutually exclusive. Leavening refers to the fermentation of the dough, which may occur regardless of the absence, presence or content of gluten. Creating a more aerated, softer structure is often the desired outcome of fermentation and gluten *do* play a key role in that. In traditional preparation methods this effect, however, is much smaller than in modern factory loaves, in the production of which variables are optimized and additional gluten are added. Many traditional leavened breads such as the *tannour* and *balady* breads of the Arab world, or the Ethiopian *injera* pancake breads, are for all intents and purposes *flat*-breads rather than loaves. Tannour is, moreover, traditionally made of a hard wheat and pulse mixture (Akroyd and Doughty, 1970). Most leavened breads in the Roman period will have been more similar to such traditional breads than to our modern loaves. In unleavened bread the dough is not fermented, but immediately baked or fried, as in the Indian flatbread *chapatti*. Regardless of gluten content, unleavened bread will not become aerated or fluffy.

Bread, fermentation and gluten

Gluten are storage proteins meant to nourish the seed's embryo after germination by providing nitrogen. They occur in all (sub)species of wheat as well as in rye and barley (although in smaller amounts). For humans, gluten are important in obtaining preferred qualities such as aeration and softness in leavened bread. The fermentation of dough is facilitated by microorganisms that are both naturally present in the environment or can be added purposely. These microorganisms can be either lactic acid bacteria that give bread a sour taste (e.g., sourdough bread) or yeasts (one-celled fungi). In non-sterile environments, the addition of naturally occurring yeasts and lactic acid bacteria is almost unavoidable and most Roman breads would have been somewhat sour (cf. Thurmond, 2006). Often fermentation starters or enhancers (leavening agents) are mixed into the dough. The Romans would use special grape must cakes (yeast occurs naturally on grape skins) or (fermented) cereal bran, crushed millets or pulse pastilles (*pastilli*). A bit of the previous day's dough could also be added as a starter. Pliny knew that the Iberians and Gauls used beer yeast to create exceptionally airy breads (*NH* 18.68), yet there is no evidence that the Romans used this technique.[12] During fermentation, dough 'rises' as the microorganisms consume part of the carbohydrates. The enzyme amylase, which converts starches into sugars that the microorganisms can consume, plays an important facilitating role in this process. It occurs naturally in cereals, but today it is added for better performance; traditional practices such as adding salt, however, also improve enzymatic action. As the microorganisms consume the sugars, they excrete alcohol (which is lost during baking) and carbon dioxide (CO_2). Because of their unique rheological properties (water absorption capacity, cohesivity, viscosity and elasticity, Wieser, 2006) gluten are able to catch this CO_2 in bubbles by stretching out, creating the desired airy, more voluminous bread.

Traditionally historians have assessed bread-making quality at the species or subspecies level on account of the genetically predisposed gluten content. Sallares (1995), for example, showed that bread wheat performs better than hard wheat, which again performs better than emmer wheat. All subspecies of wheat are typically said to perform better in this respect than barley or rye. While this ranking is not necessarily wrong, things have now been shown to be more complex. The gluten content of any subspecies of wheat is, for instance, affected by climate and season (e.g., summer vs winter wheat). Moreover, it can be significantly increased through manuring. Manuring makes more bioactive nitrogen available in the soil, which allows the plant to create more of the nitrogen rich gluten storage proteins in the grain kernel, so as to optimally support the embryo. Growing experiments have shown that even the protein content of an undomesticated taxon as wild emmer wheat (*Triticum turgidum* ssp. *dicoccoides*, the progenitor of domesticated emmer wheat) can be raised to over 40% (Vogel et al., 1978; cf. Shewry, 2009). Besides gluten content, gluten composition is important in bread-making. There are two main fractions of gluten, glutenins and gliadins, which in leavened bread function as a 'two-component glue' (Wieser, 2006). Gliadins can consist of more than 100 different components whereas the glutenin group is built up of aggregated proteins connected by inter-chain disulphide bonds of varying lengths. Both the individual compositions and the ratio of the two fractions, as well as the molecular weight of the so-called 'high molecular weight gliadin subgroup' (HMW-GS), have been shown to greatly influence baking quality and loaf volume. The underlying processes are, however, not yet completely understood (see Janssen, 1992; Shewry et al., 2002, Wieser, 2006). At this level great genetic and environmental variation may occur too.

Due to the combined effect of the variations described above, bread-baking performance can vary significantly between bread wheat cultivars. While bread wheat, if conditions were right, would on average have made the best leavened bread, a well-performing hard or even emmer wheat may have outperformed 'inferior' bread wheats or be deemed equally acceptable. Too generalized and stark statements on the functional application of certain cereals should therefore be avoided for the past.

Natural or induced fermentation can also be applied to a multitude of cereal products besides bread.[13] Examples include Near Eastern and Turkish porridges and semi-finished products, such as *khisk* and *tarhana*, in which lactic acid bacteria from milk or yoghurt facilitate fermentation.

In various Indian preparations (e.g., *idli*), cereal and pulse mixtures are soaked in water to facilitate fermentation by lactic acid bacteria from the atmosphere. In the traditional beer *bouza*, which is similar to ancient Egyptian beer, lactic acid fermentation also occurs, but then in a watery mixture of lightly baked breads and flour from sprouted kernels (Blandino et al., 2003). Most modern beers are produced differently, using yeast (cf. Pliny's mention of Gallic beer yeast above) and malted cereals.

Consumption mode selection and additives

Socioeconomic status, regional tradition, and economic factors such as the availability of labour and fuel as well as price may affect the choice of consumption mode, as the economics of producing each foodstuff interacts differently with these factors. Elsewhere (Heinrich, 2017) I have argued that in Roman Italy the choice between leavened bread, unleavened bread and porridge is primarily a function of the economics of production that vary under different levels of social organisation and urbanisation. Depending on context, the choice for any consumption mode can be the most economic choice.

The variation in recipes, local traditions, types, shapes, textures and consistency of any of the above foodstuffs would have been boundless (cf. Wilkins and Hill, 2006). The same goes for the range of additional ingredients that could be added to most consumption modes. This could include milk, oils, eggs, honey, herbs, fruits or even spices, meat and vegetables (especially in cereal soups and stews). Additives greatly influence the nutritional profile and culinary experience of a consumption mode.

Proportion of the diet

The proportion of cereals in the Roman diet (i.e., their energetic contribution) tends to be estimated at around 60% or even much higher (e.g., Garnsey, 1999). This may be rather high if the extensive mixing of cereals, pulses and other seeds (above) is considered.[14] Moreover, modern figures on the proportion of cereals in the diet of the poor may anachronistically exaggerate estimates for the past. In India, for instance, in the decades following the 'Green Revolution' – the rapid implementation of modified high yield cereal cultivars in the late 1960s – the production of pulses dropped over 20% in favour of cereal production, while the population doubled (Welch and Graham, 2000, for a discussion see Heinrich and Hansen, this volume). Even if very high cereal proportions could be substantiated for the past, this makes for a bit of a moot point. By definition staples are primary components of the diet and it is their function to supply the bulk of the required energy. Of course dietary variation is the key to good health, but that is no argument against a high cereal diet. Even if 80% of a person's energy requirements were provided by unmixed bread wheat, however, the diet is not *necessarily* unbalanced. For example, if bread wheat provides 80% of a 2,500 Kcal energy intake, there would be room to add 200 g of spinach (46 Kcal) and 756 g (about 11/4 pint) of whole fat goat's milk (454 Kcal) and still meet most daily requirements.[15]

Speaking of a single 'Roman diet' is problematic as great variation would have occurred. First, the nature and share of the cereal component in the diet would have varied geographically. In Egypt, Gaul and the North, for instance, beer consumption was common and would have added to cereal intake. Second, as a rule the poor rely more on staples of basic foods than the rich. However, poor rural populations are more likely to enjoy varied diets than the metropolitan poor. The former group would have had easier access to wild animal and plant resources and could pursue small-scale fruit and vegetable cultivation or livestock rearing. Metropolitan urbanites could not and would be dependent on purchasing or receiving food. For them this meant that they largely had to be content with foodstuffs that could be mass-produced and transported cheaply, including cheap olive oil and wine but primarily cereals. The urban poor would, therefore, likely have had the least varied diets and be most dependent on cereals and mixed grain-staples for both their energy and other nutritional requirements.

Cereals and nutrition: content and composition

Nutrients

The nutrients required by the body can be divided into two groups: the micronutrients (vitamins and minerals) that support bodily functions and the macronutrients that supply our energy. Macronutrients have different energetic values: carbohydrates and proteins both provide 16.8 kJ/g (4 Kcal) while lipids provide 37.8 kJ/g (9 Kcal). Carbohydrates are burned efficiently by our bodies, but cannot be stored except briefly and in small amounts as glycogen without being inefficiently converted into lipids. Lipids are both a source and store of energy for the body. Lipids are also important for obtaining and storing fat soluble vitamins (e.g., vitamin E) and the essential fatty acids. Lastly, protein is used to construct and repair cells and to support numerous vital brain and bodily functions. If necessary, proteins can be converted into glucose (a carbohydrate) and used as fuel.

In addition, there are also anti-nutrients (e.g., phytate) that reduce the bioavailability of nutrients. So-called promotor substances (certain amino acids and vitamins) can enhance the bioavailability of other nutrients (Welch and Graham, 2000). In the case of cereals, the different nutrients and anti-nutrients are not equally distributed over the kernel. Micronutrients and anti-nutrients, for instance, are concentrated in the outer layers of the kernel (colloquially called the bran), especially the aleurone layer (Haard et al., 1999). Therefore, choosing to only use part of the grain (like low-extraction white bread) negatively affects the nutritional value of bread. The nutritional content (both in energy and micronutrients) of an unprepared product (e.g., the wheat kernel) is only a potential. Processing, preparation and digestion ultimately determine which proportion of nutrients is or can actually be used. Identifying and understanding Roman processing and preparation methods is therefore quintessential for reconstructing the nutritional value of Roman foods.

Malnutrition

Malnutrition is the state of chronically not meeting nutrient requirements and is different from famine, which is a general scarcity of food. Different types of malnutrition can be distinguished. Energy-malnutrition is caused when individuals obtain too few calories, while protein-malnutrition is caused by obtaining either too little protein, or protein that is deficient in certain amino acids. Micronutrient malnutrition can result from obtaining too few micronutrients through the diet or from these micronutrients occurring in non-bioavailable forms (often caused by anti-nutrients). Malnutrition is still very common in the twenty-first century and is not limited to the developing world. Estimates suggest that at least two-thirds of the world population is deficient in at least one micronutrient. The most commonly deficient micro-nutrients are iron (Fe) and zinc (Zn), of which 30% and 35% of the world population are respectively estimated to suffer. Other common deficiencies occur in iodine (I), calcium (Ca), copper (Cu), magnesium (Mg) and selenium (Se) (Stein, 2010). High cereal diets with little variation have traditionally been held responsible for this (Stein, 2010; Ahmad et al., 2012). It is, therefore, understandable that historians and archaeologists have often projected these figures and causes onto the past or have assumed that matters were even worse in the past. While deficiencies of varying severity will certainly have occurred in antiquity, I will argue that malnutrition from the nineteenth through to the twenty-first century is categorically different from malnutrition in antiquity.

Malnutrition may cause a wide array of diseases and affect life expectancy, but also causes low immunity and lethargy. Malnutrition is also detrimental to labour productivity and subsequently earnings, and is thus a cause of poverty. The reverse, however, also applies (cf. Stein, 2010). Fogel (2004) for instance has argued that about 30% of the growth in per capita income in Britain over the past two centuries can be attributed to improved nutrition. Economic models for present-day India suggest that reducing iron deficiency in labourers could raise their productivity and subsequently their income by as much as 7–15% (Weinberger, 2003; Stein, 2010). Therefore, the nutritional qualities of the Roman diet are also relevant for the assessment of the performance of the wider Roman economy.

Variability in cereal nutrition

An impediment to concretely applying modern biochemical data on nutrition to past cereal consumption is the great 'natural' variation that may occur in most nutritional parameters. These occur at all taxonomic levels (species, subspecies and cultivars), but also between specimens of the same cultivar grown under different circumstances. This variation may occupy a wide range, and may occasionally mean the difference between a crop meeting human nutritional requirements or being deficient. Some of this variation, about one-third, is determined by genetics, while the remaining two-thirds are dependent on external factors such as soil conditions, season, year-to-year weather variations (rainfall, temperature) and anthropogenic actions such as manuring (cf. Shewry, 2009). With current methods we cannot hope to determine or reconstruct all these factors nor exactly differentiate between or assess the qualities of the different cultivars the Romans used. Like with gluten and bread-making performance, also with the nutritional profile we must assume a significant degree of regional and local variation.

The occurrence and intensity of at least one anthropogenic factor that significantly affects cereals and by extension human nutrition, namely manuring, can be attested archaeologically. From the textual sources we know that the Romans, like many societies before them, practised and valued manuring (cf. Kron, 2008a). Through stable isotope analysis of archaeobotanical specimens we can gain insights into manuring intensity. This is done through measuring and interpreting the ratio of $\delta^{14}N$ and $\delta^{15}N$ isotopes (higher ratios are associated with more intense manuring – see Bogaard et al., 2007). Unfortunately only few studies using this method are currently available. The only Roman example thus far is a comparison of barley and spelt wheat kernels from a British rural site with both Late Iron Age and Roman occupation. This study indicates that manuring intensity in the Roman period was high in absolute terms and significantly higher than in the preceding period (Heinrich, 2012). Taking into account what we established above on gluten content and manuring, this method could be used to tentatively suggest protein content and the baking quality of leavened bread (provided that was the local consumption mode) were higher at this site during the Roman period than in the periods before, when manuring intensity was lower.

Micronutrients: content

Micronutrients are a diverse group of essential dietary components consisting of trace elements ('minerals') and organic compounds ('vitamins') that the body requires in small amounts to grow and function properly. The number of essential micronutrients required for normal health and well-being is estimated at 25 (Stein, 2010). However, no single food category, including cereals, contains all of these: vitamins A, C and D are for instance not present in cereals. Wheats do however contain carotenoids, these act as pro-vitamin A, which the body can use to synthesize vitamin A on its own (Ortiz-Monasterio et al., 2007). Vitamins C and D, however, need to be obtained from other foodstuffs. Staples such as chestnut are rich in vitamin C, while pulses provide both vitamin A and C; vitamin D, in addition to being obtained through the consumption of certain foods (e.g. fatty fish, meat, cheese and eggs), can be synthesized by the body when exposed to sunlight.

Some mineral deficiencies in cereals are primarily geographic and are caused by a deficiency of the soil or the poor bioavailability of the compound in which the mineral occurs. Zinc, for instance, is a vital, yield-determining, plant micronutrient, but zinc deficiency is common in soils. Alkaline pH values and (semi-)arid climates may further reduce zinc bioavailability, as may high concentrations of magnesium and bicarbonate (HCO_3-) in irrigation water. It is likely that in the Roman Empire the (semi-)arid areas with irrigation-fed agriculture in Africa and the Near East were most prone to zinc deficiency; also at present ailments induced by zinc deficiency are most common in these regions. To counter soil mineral deficiency, soils can be enriched in bioavailable minerals through bio-fortification. An example of this with which the Romans were familiar is marling, which increases the soil's magnesium and calcium stores and increases nitrogen uptake in acid soils. It may however also reduce the bioavailability of zinc, adding to deficiency in humans (Ahmad et al., 2012). Manuring has, moreover, been shown to allow a greater uptake of iron and zinc by the plant, due to increased nitrogen availability (Monasterio and Graham, 2000). This effect has been strongly correlated with protein content (Camak et al., 2000).

Genetic predisposition also affects the uptake of minerals by plants considerably (Monasterio and Graham, 2000). Interestingly, over the past decades it has been firmly established that the semi-dwarf high yield variety (HYV) cultivars of bread wheat that are dominant today contain up to 30% less iron, zinc, copper and magnesium than nineteenth-century and other traditional, unmodified cultivars. Their development and rise to dominance in the 1960s was the great achievement of the so-called Green Revolution that has done much to alleviate and prevent famine since. Despite their advantages in, for instance, yield and disease resistance, these cultivars have been shown to be inefficient in routing minerals into the grain kernels (Shewry, 2009). In addition, high yield causes the dilution of minerals over more kernels, lowering mineral concentration per weight unit of consumer product. Moreover, these high-yield varieties may deplete soil minerals more quickly if mineral fertilization (which for farmers in developing countries is often too expensive) is not applied (Stein, 2010). The greater role of cereals in the post-Green Revolution staple diet (see above) further amplifies modern malnutrition. Therefore, if we focus on modern deficiency statistics or the nutritional profile of modern cereals, it is likely that we overestimate Roman micronutrient deficiencies for reasons that could not have existed in the Roman period. We may also be misattributing observed malnutrition (e.g. from osteological evidence) to the chemical composition of ancient crops rather than to other causes.

Micronutrients: bioavailability and anti-nutrients

Even if sufficient micronutrients are available in the soil and plants, anti-nutrients may prevent their uptake in the human body. Iron, zinc and calcium are traditionally held to be most susceptible to this in both cereals (cf. Garnsey, 1999) and pulses. This is because of the presence of phytate or phytic-acid, the quantity of which is variable and determined genetically (Raboy, 2000). Phytate chelates (i.e., binds) calcium, iron and zinc and hence reduces the bioavailability of these elements. Moreover, once consumed, the phytate may continue to do this with other foodstuffs in the digestive tract. As phytate is concentrated in the aleurone layer, wholemeal products contain more of it than 'white' flours. One way to reduce phytate content is to lower the extraction rate (Akroyd and Doughty, 1970). Low extraction rates can be easily obtained with modern steel roller-mills, originally a nineteenth-century Austrian-Hungarian contraption equipped with fine-meshed silk sieves, but in the premodern era such rates were harder to achieve. Moreover, most traditional techniques left at least some bran in even the 'whitest' flour (Akroyd and Doughty, 1970; Shewry, 2009). Nutritionally this was probably for the best, as most iron and zinc is bound to the phytate and therefore also located in the bran.[16] In this context obtaining a somewhat reduced share of a large amount of minerals is better than obtaining the total of a miniscule amount (Akryod and Doughty, 1970). Bio-fortification of wholemeal, especially with calcium is also a countermeasure used against the effects of phytate. It is legally required in England, though the need for this practice has been questioned for a long time (Akroyd and Doughty, 1970). The addition of gypsum ($CaSO_4 \cdot 2H_2O$), mainly as an adulteration or colorant of flour, has been attested for the Roman period (Braun, 1995) and may have unintentionally had a positive effect on calcium intake.

A far more effective solution than bio-fortification, however, is enzymatic hydrolysis of phytate by the enzyme phytase, which makes the minerals bioavailable again. This process naturally occurs in cereals during soaking, germination and fermentation (Hamad and Fields, 1979) and increases the availability of calcium, iron and zinc by several factors (Hamad and Fields, 1979; Blandino et al., 2003). Increases up to sevenfold also occur in the amount and availability of the B-vitamin complex due to biosynthesis (Campbell-Platt, 1994; Steinkraus, 1994). The proportion of fermented cereal and non-cereal foods in the Roman diet should not be underestimated. As discussed above, the Romans prepared various cereal (and non-cereal) dishes that were purposely or accidentally fermented or eaten with fermented products. Purposely fermented cereal foods include leavened bread, fermented porridge and beer; while some cereal dishes were mixed with lactic acid bacteria rich products (e.g., soft cheese in Cato's *placenta, De Agri Cultura* 76). Other foods may have been accidently fermented, for instance hulled cereals if soaked prior to dehusking (Thurmond, 2006) or any food through unsterile preparation conditions and unrefrigerated short-term storage of prepared products.

Even today 20–40% of the world food supply is fermented (Steinkraus, 1994); while it is impossible to assess the share of the Roman diet that was fermented, it is not unreasonable to assume that in an unrefrigerated world where fermentation was a cheap preservation method and where the importance of sterilization was not understood, this proportion would be similar if not higher.

Macronutrients and energy

Although some foods may only contain one macronutrient (e.g., olive oil), most foods (including cereals) contain all three. This makes considering cereals only as carbohydrate suppliers incorrect. The different wheats and rye contain 1.5–2% of crude fat; barley and the millets 3–4% crude fat; while oats may contain over 6% crude fat (Haard et al., 1999). More importantly, cereals contain fair amounts of crude protein, usually within a range of between 7–15%, but a higher range of 24–40% is also known to occur (Akroyd and Doughty, 1970; Shewry, 2009). Even the lower range of protein percentages does not compare unfavourably with the protein content of other dietary categories such as eggs (13%), meat (12–20%), fish (16–20%), pulses (18–43.5%;

see Heinrich and Hansen, this volume) and cheese (19–25%), let alone other staples such as potatoes (2%) (Akroyd and Doughty, 1970). Even today, the lion's share of the global protein demand is met by cereals (Shewry et al., 2002). The importance of cereal protein in Roman protein intake is therefore not to be underestimated.

Cereal protein composition: amino acids

Proteins are composed of amino acids. Nine of these, the essential amino acids, the body cannot synthesize and needs to obtain through the diet. Deficiencies in essential amino acids may result in reduced growth, and serious, even fatal, diseases. Although the main Roman cereal staples, wheats and barleys, are not deficient *per se* in any amino acid, lysine and threonine are the limiting amino acids. Lysine content varies between species (barley and rye on average contain slightly more than wheats), subspecies and cultivars (Chavan and Kadam, 1989; Haard et al., 1999). As has been widely noted, pulses are rich in lysine, while cereals are rich in sulphur-containing amino-acids that pulses are deficient in, which makes these two staples highly complementary (see Heinrich and Hansen, this volume). While manuring increases the total amount of protein in wheats (above), this increase consists solely of gluten and does not increase lysine content (Shewry, 2009).

In addition to the content of amino acids from a given protein source, the protein digestibility and protein absorption of this protein within the human organism also has to be taken into consideration (see Heinrich and Hansen, this volume). Processing and preparation methods can affect these factors. Various studies have shown that soaking, germination and fermentation may increase the amount and availability of lysine significantly (Hamad and Fields, 1979; Blandino et al., 2003 for an overview). Some baking or frying processes, depending on the duration and temperature of exposure, may lead to a (variable) reduction of the amount of lysine (Anjum et al., 2005), sometimes in favour of other amino acids (McKay and Baldwin, 1990). As discussed, the Romans consumed various fermented foodstuffs. Beer-drinkers and porridge-eaters, for instance, would have certainly benefitted from the improved lysine contents of their fermented foods; for bread-eaters this would have depended on baking conditions. Overall, the statement that a cereal-based diet is lysine deficient is far from a universal truth.

Conclusion

In this chapter I explored the nutritional value and functional properties of cereals, their role in the Roman diet, and their relationship with malnutrition. My aim was to assess whether the categorically sombre picture historians commonly paint of the nutritional value of cereals holds if tested against modern biochemical insights. Additionally, I aimed to reassess the statement that (only) bread wheat is well suited for bread production.

The negative appraisal of cereals springs from two causes. The first is the overestimation of the proportion of cereals in the diet and the role of cereals functioning as the main energy supplier while other foodstuffs functioned as micronutrient suppliers. The second is the underestimation and over-homogenization of the nutritional profile of cereals. While cereals were indeed the main Roman staple this fact tends to be misinterpreted, especially when it is expressed as a percentage. The correct premise that no single category of foodstuffs, including cereals, provides all nutrients humans require is often followed by the assumption that poor Roman consumers hardly ate anything else than cereals. The rationale is often that if cereals provided the lion's share of the energy requirement in the diet (>60%), then the non-cereal component would be too small to provide the nutrients that cereals lack in sufficient quantities.

The fact that cereals made up the bulk of the diet is a moot point: that is the function of staples. The rationale of the argument is not necessarily correct as many foodstuffs that nutritionally complement a high cereal diet (e.g., green leafy vegetables) hardly provide any energy at all. Moreover, as the other contributions to this volume indicate, many other groups of food-stuffs played important roles in the diets of most consumers. Cereals were of course also not equally important in all regions or for all socioeconomic groups within the Roman Empire. Rural populations and well-to-do urban dwellers would likely have had a more diverse diet in which cereals played a smaller role, while the urban poor would have been more dependent on cereals. Likewise in regions where beer-drinking was the norm, overall cereal consumption was higher. The category of staple foods was moreover more diverse than the group of cereals alone: dried pulses were consumed ubiquitously and tree-seeds such as acorn and sweet chestnut were important locally in the rural context. As similar semi-finished and finished products were prepared from the different staples, they were mixed liberally and sometimes surreptitiously. This mixing improved the nutritional profile of the consumed finished pro-duct as these staples have a different micronutrient makeup. We often do not consider such practices and their nutritional consequences when modelling premodern diets, but instead look at the biochemical analysis of cleaned samples consisting only of specimens of the same (sub)species, which does not capture the effects of processing and mixing. In addition, the more recently increased dependency on cereals in some diets in the developing world, following the Green Revolution, may have coloured our view of cereal dependency in the premodern world.

Cereals are a diverse category of crops that despite their relatively large morphological similarity may exhibit great variation in nutrient composition. The keyword in understanding cereal nutrition is variability: almost any nutritional parameter may vary at any taxonomic level or because of almost any environmental or anthropogenic factor. It is important to be aware of this when modelling the nutritional value of the cereal component of the diet. We should, for instance, aim to use the biochemical data for the specific subspecies of wheat that was used at a site or in a region (which we can establish through archaeobotanical analysis) rather than data on 'wheat', since much general data pertains only to modern cultivars of bread wheat. In fact, the use of such data has negatively and incorrectly influenced the reputation of cereals in historical research. Modern, commercial cultivars of bread wheat were genetically modified during the Green Revolution of the 1960s. While these modifications led to greater yields and better disease resistance, they inadvertently led to a reduction of around 30% in the uptake of important trace elements (Fe, Zn, Mg, Ca, Cu) into the grain kernels. Roman wheat cultivars may have had lower yields, but were also not subject to the nutritional effects of such modifications. Therefore, they probably contained greater quantities of micronutrients per unit of product.

When taking into account nutritional variability beyond the taxonomic level of the subspecies, more uncertainty comes into play. Though it is sometimes possible to *distinguish* between different cultivars and landraces of a (sub)species archaeobotanically, we still do not know the differences between their nutritional profiles. Much nutritional variation can be explained through environmental and anthropogenic factors. The most consequential of these factors is the agricultural practice of manuring of which the intensity may be reconstructed with the assistance of stable isotope analysis of archaeobotanical specimens. Modern research suggests that manuring may greatly increase the gluten content of any type of wheat. Therefore, archaeobotanical specimens with isotopic values indicating intensive manuring may be potential proxies for protein and gluten content. Although manuring raises the protein content, this in itself does not improve the biological value of the protein because the gluten do not comprise limiting essential amino acids. Manuring does increase the plant's ability to take up the trace elements Zn and Fe from the soil. More importantly, however, the greater amount of gluten in manured wheats makes them more suitable for baking better quality leavened breads. This effect can be significant and while bread wheat has the genetic predisposition for containing more gluten, other (sub)species of wheat, if manured well, would not necessarily have under-performed by comparison. This method requires further study, but potentially opens up an avenue to ascertain (and distinguish between) the potential bread-baking quality and protein content of Roman cereals from different locations. Lastly, it is important that not only the crude nutrient content of cereals is recognized, but also the effects of processing and preparation methods as well as the uptake of nutrients by the human organism. Recent biochemical research indicates that the effect of certain anti-nutrients, especially phytate, has long been overestimated as many common preparation methods would negate their effects. Preparation methods that were common in the Roman world, such as fermentation, play an important role in breaking down phytate. Moreover, fermentation has been found to significantly increase lysine (the limiting amino acid in wheat and barley) and vitamin B-complex content in cereals. The ratio between anti-nutrients and micronutrients would have been more favourable in the more nutritious Roman grains.

While cereals (like any category of foodstuffs) cannot provide all human requirements by themselves, they form a nutritionally adequate basis when supported by limited dietary variation, provided they are processed and prepared in a certain fashion. When studying the Roman period, we have to be careful when we use modern ethnographic, statistical or biochemical data. While some of the causes for rampant nutritional problems in the modern world could not have existed in antiquity, several countermeasures for the problems that existed would have been more widely applied in the past than today (even if unintentionally in some cases). Although it may be too bold to suggest that Roman micronutrient nutrition was much better than it was between the nineteenth and twenty-first centuries, the data presented above certainly do not support the contrary. Where there is evidence for malnutrition in the Roman world, different explanations need to be considered than an *a priori* assumed inferior nutritional quality of cereals. Many such alternatives may be associated with socioeconomic causes linked to lower overall standards of living, the unequal distribution of wealth or may follow from unhealthy dietary choices, diseases and parasites.

Notes

1 This chapter is intended as a diptych with Chapter 10 in this volume on pulses by Heinrich and Hansen.
2 Cereals also provide secondary products (also called by-products or rest-products) in the form of straw and chaff. The uses of these products include animal fodder and bedding, fuel (as binder in dung cakes) construction materials (temper in mud architecture, thatching for roofs), and temper in ceramics. See Van der Veen, 1999 and Hansen et al., 2017.
3 Shewry's (2009) review article estimates more than 20,000 publications on (bread)wheat biochemistry alone since 1945.
4 For a discussion of other aspects of importance when modelling ancient diet and nutrition, see Heinrich and Erdkamp, 2018.
5 The millets are a diverse group of small seeded cereals from a wide variety of genera. The name therefore has no taxonomic bearing, while the taxa considered a part of this group may differ (e.g., teff and sorghum are sometimes considered millets, although often not). Their domestication history and spread differs and is in some cases not yet well understood. The term might therefore best be used in the plural. For a discussion see Heinrich and Hansen, Forthcoming. For taxa relevant to the Roman period, see Table 9.1, cf. Spurr 1983; 1986; Thanheiser et al., 2002.
6 See Heinrich, 2017.

7 For example, Janssen, 1992; Shewry et al., 2002; Wieser, 2006; and Shewry, 2009 are all specialist publications on bread wheat, but only specify this implicitly or as an aside. Matters are made more complex by the fact that there is no common name for *Triticum aestivum*, the species of which both bread wheat (*Triticum aestivum* ssp. *aestivum*) and spelt wheat (*Triticum aestivum* ssp. *spelta*) are subspecies. If in archaeobotanical or historical literature *Triticum aestivum* is mentioned or found for the Roman Mediterranean, it is likely that specifically bread wheat was intended.

8 For an in-depth discussion of these and other examples of the use of stable isotope analysis with respect to Roman diet and the Roman economy, see Heinrich and Erdkamp, Forthcoming.

9 For a model of crop-selection and agricultural decision making in Roman Italy see Heinrich, 2017; cf. Jasny, 1942; 1944a and 1950. For examples pertaining to Egypt see Cappers and Neef, 2012; Cappers, 2013; Cappers et al., 2014. A general overview of crop selection trends is given in Van der Veen 2018.

10 See Heinrich, 2017, for an overview and historiography. For the application of some of these insights to quantitative case studies of hieratic papyri on grain transport in New Kingdom Egypt, see Heinrich and van Pelt, 2017a; 2017b and Van Pelt and Heinrich, Forthcoming. For alternative explanations of the shift, also see Van der Veen, 2018, who emphasizes the relationship between bread baking quality and cultural and religious preferences.

11 Jasny, 1944b and Moritz, 1958 did extensive work on Roman extraction rates.

12 For an overview of Roman fermentation starters, see Thurmond, 2006.

13 For an overview of traditional fermented cereal foods, see Blandino et al., 2003.

14 Many have argued general dietary variation was also greater, cf. Kron, 2008a; Jongman, 2007a; Wilkins and Hill, 2006.

15 Data on energetic value: De Jong, 2010. It should also be noted that not every daily recommended amount of (micro)nutrients needs to be consumed daily in order to remain healthy; it is more important that requirements are met over a longer period of a few weeks.

16 Bran itself is a good source of dietary fibre, which is important for digestive health and proper nutrient absorption. The industrialization of milling made white flour the cheap standard and bran a secondary product that could be sold to the fodder industry. The (urban) poor, who already enjoyed little dietary variation greatly suffered nutritionally from their switch to white bread (Akroyd and Doughty, 1970).

10

PULSES

Frits Heinrich and Annette M. Hansen

Introduction

Pulses are a group of crops in the Fabaceae family.[1] They have been an important element in the diet of all agricultural societies since the Neolithic Revolution. The Romans were no exception to this rule, as Roman names such as Fabius (from faba bean), Lentulus (from lentil) and Cicero (from chickpea) famously illustrate. More significantly, pulses feature prominently in the work of the classical agronomists and are attested archaeobotanically in every corner of the Roman Empire. Like their fellow grain crops, cereals, pulses would have been available to virtually any Roman producer and consumer and were a staple in the diet of most Romans.

The agricultural importance of leguminous crops as green manure, forage and fodder in past agricultural systems has often been stressed (Chatterton and Chatterton, 1984a; 1984b; 1985; Jones, 1990; Osman et al., 1990; Jones, 1998; Kron, 2000; 2004a; 2005c; Valamoti and Charles, 2005; Vaccaro et al., 2013). Compared to cereals, pulses have generated far less academic interest in terms of diet and nutrition. Although praised as the 'poor man's meat' because of their protein content, only the anti-nutritional and toxic qualities of some pulses (and associated maladies such as flatulence, favism and neurolathyrism) tend to be discussed in-depth. Due to this, and their alleged minor commercial importance and low or even famine food status, pulses have been underestimated in the debate on the ancient diet.

In this chapter we will look at the role of pulses in the Roman diet from a biochemical perspective. We will assess the nutritional profile of different pulses and will emphasize that they played a vital role in balancing the Roman diet. We will also discuss which pulses were available to the Romans and in what form they were consumed. We will pay particular attention to traditional food processing and preparation methods that affect nutritional values. We will first review the difference between Roman and modern definitions of what pulses are and how they should be categorized.

Roman pulses

Categorization of pulses and legumes

While by convention all pulses are in the botanical family of the Fabaceae, the word 'pulse' itself is not an official taxonomic designation, but a practical one. The FAO states that: 'the term 'pulses' is limited to plants that are solely harvested for dry grains [i.e., seeds]' (FAO,

2013). The word 'legume' is often used interchangeably with the word 'pulse'. While all pulses are legumes, any member of the Fabaceae family (formerly the Leguminosae family) qualifies as a legume. Besides pulses, this group includes plants that are practically categorized as wild, forage, fodder, vegetable, tree or oil crops (cf. Kron, 2004a). For example, fresh French beans are considered a vegetable, while dried navy beans are considered pulses; however, both are cultivars of the same botanical species, the legume *Phaseolus vulgaris*. Sometimes practical categorizations may seem contradictory. The peanut (*Arachis hypogaea*) is a leguminous crop of which the dry seeds are collected, but the FAO does not consider it a pulse since it is mainly used as an oil crop (FAO, 2013).[2]

The Roman categorization of groups of crops was as practical and confusing as our own. Unlike us, the Romans had no standardized botanical nomenclature nor knowledge of genetics and could only categorize using practical observations or visual characteristics. Legumes (*legūmen*[3]) were one of these categories, although its ancient meaning appears to have been more inclusive than ours. When summing up the most useful legumes, Columella (*Rust.* 2.7.1.) mentions many taxa that we would call legumes – and more precisely pulses – faba bean, lentil, pea, chickpea, lupine and *phasolus*, but also others that we would classify differently: barley 'of which tisane is made', common millet, Italian millet, sesame, linseed/flax and cannabis/hemp. Later, when discussing the category of cereals, Columella mentions the millets again. Realizing he had already categorized them as legumes, he argues they happen to fit in both categories (*Rust.* 2.9.17). Heinrich and Wilkins (2014) have noted that all of Columella's legumes share the characteristic of being primarily, or potentially, grain crops of which the seeds can be collected. We would like to add that the visual similarity between the pods (fruits) of legumes and the fruits of linseed, cannabis and sesame – colloquially also referred to as pods in modern languages – may further explain this classification. This does not explain the classification of millets and barley as pulses. Strong similarities, however, do exist between the processing and preparation methods of the grain crops listed by Columella (see below). The same can be said for their consumption modes: they can all be used to prepare semiliquid staple foods.[4] This interpretation of Columella's classification could be supported by Book V of Apicius' *De re coquinaria*: '*Ospreon*' (Legumes). In addition to recipes for fresh legumes in the pod and dried pulses, various cereal-based recipes with little or no actual leguminous ingredients (in the modern sense) are present. These include *tisana* (barley-gruel), *alica* (emmer-wheat gruel), other porridges and soups, lentil-chestnut mash, *tracta* (in this case functioning as a thickener – see Hill and Bryer, 1995, who relate it to *tarhana*), and *puls*,[5] the traditional Roman emmer wheat and pulse porridge.[6] Interestingly Apicius' categorization is as ambiguous as Columella's: some of the recipes in Book V (e.g., *tisana*) are also present in Book IV under a different title and dedicated to 'Miscellaneous Recipes'; this may, however, be an artefact of the work's compilation history. In summary, all our pulses and at least various other minor grain crops seem to have been considered legumes or pulses, either based on visual or practical similarities. In this paper we will use modern scientific convention and restrict ourselves to species within the Fabaceae family that are currently considered pulses.

Availability

Table 10.1 is a list of pulses that were available for consumption in the Roman Empire. The most important Roman pulses were all Neolithic founder crops that had been part of the Mediterranean farming curriculum since the arrival of agriculture: faba bean (*Vicia faba*), lentil (*Lens culinaris*), chickpea (*Cicer arietinum*), pea (*Pisum sativum*) and bitter vetch (*Vicia ervilia*). These species are frequently mentioned in classical literature and widely encountered archaeo-botanically.[7] A second, less important group, is comprised of vetchling (*Lathyrus cicera*), grass

Table 10.1 Range of pulses available for consumption to the Romans

Common Name	Scientific Name
Bitter vetch	*Vicia ervilia*
Faba bean	*Vicia faba*
Lentil	*Lens culinaris*
Chick pea	*Cicer arietinum*
Common pea	*Pisum sativum*
Grass pea	*Lathyrus sativus*
Vetchling	*Lathyrus cicera*
Spanish vetchling	*Lathyrus clymenum*
White lupine	*Lupinus albus*
Fenugreek	*Trigonella foenum-graecum*
Mung bean	*Vigna radiata*
Alfalfa	*Medicago sativa*

pea (or chickling) (*Lathyrus sativus*), and white lupine (*Lupinus albus*). These species are native to the wider Mediterranean and were domesticated locally long before the Roman period (Kislev, 1989; Peña-Chocarro and Peña, 1999; Kurlovich, 2002; cf. Heinrich and Wilkins, 2014). Spanish vetchling (*Lathyrus clymenum*) mainly had a local importance on Santorini (Sarpaki and Jones, 1990). The use of many other minor Eurasian vetches and vetchlings is sometimes suggested in translations of classical texts, though this is often difficult to prove since they are not always archaeobotanically attested.[8] Alfalfa (*Medicago sativa*) and fenugreek (*Trigonella foenum-graecum*) would have primarily been utilized as fodder crops rather than as pulses (cf. Chatterton and Chatterton, 1984a; 1984b; 1985; Kron, 2005c), although the latter was also used as a seasoning and pharmaceutical. Finds of the 'exotic' mung bean (*Vigna radiata*) from India are restricted to the Red Sea ports of Berenike and Myos Hormos and represent food stores of visiting trading ships rather than local cultivation or deliberate imports (Cappers, 2006; Van der Veen, 2011).

A controversy has long existed with regards to the Roman crop *phasolus* (often equated with the Greek crop *dolichos* (δολίχους)), a type of bean, whose identification was a subject of confusion even in antiquity (Galen, *De alimentorum facultatibus* 1.28). In modern times this crop has often been translated as kidney bean, a cultivar of *Phaseolus vulgaris*, which is incorrect since this is a Mesoamerican crop. Some classicists have interpreted *phasolus* as the subtropical *Vigna unguiculata*, either because it is currently present in Italy (Spurr, 1986), or because some archaeobotanists have claimed to have encountered it in (pre-)Roman contexts. Heinrich and Wilkins (2014) have shown that the cultivation conditions and sowing season for *phasolus* described by the classical authors are not suitable for *Vigna unguiculata*, and that the alleged principal archaeobotanical find of a *Vigna unguiculata* specimen could not be satisfyingly identified as such. They also suggest that the meaning of *phasolus* changed over time and could be both a generic name for 'beans' as well as a crop-specific name depending on context.

Pulses and the Roman diet

Post-harvest processing and consumption modes

Although in this chapter we focus chiefly on dry pulses as a product, it should be noted that most small producer-consumers would also have consumed part of the harvest of the same plants as a vegetable. When used as a vegetable, the fresh, sometimes unripe pods and/or the depodded seeds are roasted (famously chickpea as a snack – Akroyd et al., 1982), boiled or pickled (cf. Columella, *Rust.* 12.9.1). In addition to adding variation to the diet and creating an additional harvesting moment (hence spreading risk), consuming legume-vegetables is also nutritionally significant as their chemical composition is different from the ripe, dried seeds (see below). Legume-vegetables would have been something of a seasonal pleasure and likely to be consumed in greater quantities by rural populations with easy access or more affluent urbanites.

Even more so than cereals (Heinrich, this volume), pulses require processing prior to consumption. This is necessary to soften and detoxify the pulses, and make them digestible.[9] The main steps involved in this process are soaking or leaching, followed by rinsing and boiling. Soaking may take up to 12 hours, while boiling may take more than two hours. Ethnographic sources indicate that pulse dishes are often prepared for multiple days and reheated as needed to reduce fuel expenses (Akroyd et al., 1982). Dehulling pulses – removing the outer layers of the seed known as the seed coat – is optional and can be done either before or after soaking. Dehulling is often, but not always, combined with splitting the seed, as in Indian *dal* (any type of split pulse) or split-peas. The primary advantage of dehulling and splitting is that these processes greatly reduce cooking time and save fuel. Fermentation is another optional process that can reduce cooking time.[10] Both solid and liquid pulse preparations may also be fermented in order to change their chemical qualities (see below) and produce specific products (e.g., *tempeh*, *miso*, *sufu*, *natto*, soy-sauce, *ketjap* and *idli*). Allowing germination and engaging in malting after soaking increases pulse digestibility further and was a common preparation in India for post-weaning infant foods (Brandtzaeg, 1979). Boiling, draining and immediately consuming whole or split pulses is common. Parching, puffing or dry-roasting chickpeas and faba beans after soaking is widely attested in India and Africa (Kurien et al., 1972). An endless variety of semiliquid foods of varying consistency can be produced from pulses including: gruel, porridge, pap, puree, polenta, paste, potage, mush, mash, soup and stew. These dishes can serve as staples in the diet just like pea soup and pea porridge did in medieval Europe or *ful medames*, made from faba beans, still does in Egypt and Sudan.

Pulses can be made into a dry meal or flour through grinding or milling. These semi-finished products can be used to make all pulse dishes, such as Near Eastern and North African *falafel* or *taamia* (fried faba bean and/or chickpea) and pulse cakes (popular in sub-Saharan Africa). More commonly pulse flours are mixed with cereal flours. Traditional (unleavened) Indian *chapatti* bread for instance contains around 15% pulse flour, while the addition of considerable amounts of chickpea flour was standard in Near Eastern (leavened) *tannour* bread (Akroyd et al., 1982). In today's food industry, pulse flours are commonly added to baked goods, especially lupine and soybean. There is evidence that mixing different staples, especially pulses and cereals, was common in the Roman world (cf. Wilkins and Hill, 2006; Heinrich, this volume). While associated with adulteration by the classical authors (e.g., as the cheap faba bean flour, *lomentum* was by Pliny *NH* 18.30), conscious mixing was probably more common. Written sources report that even unprocessed mixtures of barley and lentils were sold (Bagnall, 1993). Cereals and small-seeded pulses that grow as arable weeds are often unintentionally mixed (contamination up to 10% being recorded) during the harvest. Ethnographic evidence shows that farmers do not always deem it cost-efficient or do not bother to remove such seeds (Jasny, 1942; 1944a; 1950).

Proportion of the diet

It is impossible to estimate reliably what proportion of the Roman diet consisted of pulses. However, given the amount of textual and archaeobotanical evidence, it is obvious that they were always eaten by everyone everywhere at least to some extent. This goes for both rich and poor, despite numerous references by the classical authors who considered pulses inferior goods (cf. Flint-Hamilton, 1999; Wilkins and Hill, 2006); even Apicius' elite cookbook still contains many recipes that include them. The cultural disdain seems to relate more to a reliance on pulses as a staple (in which capacity leavened wheat bread is preferred) or as the main protein supplier (in which case animal protein is preferred) than to pulses in general. This is a recurring theme in many societies throughout history, most notably the industrializing Western world where an inverse relationship between income and pulse consumption existed.[11] The fact that pulses were 'inferior goods' (i.e. less desired) and can be mildly toxic, however, may have contributed to the low valuation and low price of pulses (cf. Flint-Hamilton, 1999).

However, this in itself is an incomplete answer. Pulses are also cheap because their (*de facto*) production costs are lower. Pulses, unlike cereals, are not solely dependent on the amount of available bioactive nitrogen in the soil. Pulses live in a symbiotic relationship with nitrogen-fixing bacteria on their roots. These bacteria convert inactive nitrogen in the soil into a form that can be metabolized by plants. In return, the pulses provide the bacteria with glucose. This arrangement allows pulses to also thrive on poorer soils, without requiring manuring and without depleting the soil as much as cereals; this also explains why, if ploughed-in instead of harvested, pulses are a good green manure (cf. Kron, 2008a). Unfortunately pulses do not keep as well as cereals if stored long-term because they are vulnerable to predation by species-specific insects and other pests (cumulative seed loss of even up to 25–50% in warmer areas is not unheard of under traditional storage conditions; Akroyd et al., 1982). This relatively low bio-stability brings down the value and price of pulses. In addition, when pulses are stored their outer layers become harder, which may greatly increase cooking time and therefore fuel expense. The ethnographic observation that pulse consumption tends to be much higher in the months following the harvest (Akroyd et al., 1982) might be partly explained through this phenomenon, though a producer-consumer preference for legume-vegetables over pulses may also play a role. From a consumer perspective, pulses are more inconvenient and in some cases potentially more expensive commodities (both in terms of storage-loss and fuel) than cereals. This may have been of greater importance in cities, where fuel had to be purchased.[12]

Present-day (ethnographic) data on pulse consumption is not always the best tool to reconstruct the importance of pulses in the historical diet and may lead us to underestimate it. Following the Green Revolution of the 1960s, during which high yield cereal varieties had been developed (see Heinrich, this volume), there was a marked decrease in pulse production as the preferred bread wheat now significantly outcompeted pulses in terms of yield. Even in India where pulses were a preferred good, consumption dropped over 20% in a period during which population doubled (cf. Akroyd et al., 1982). However, over the following decades pulse yields were also improved through modification, though these higher yields inadvertently came at the expense of a lower nutritional value (see below). There is still a decline in pulse consumption today, both in the developed and developing world. This is a cause for great concern among nutritionists (Pastor-Cavada et al., 2014).[13] While such a concern is not warranted for the Roman world, an inverse relationship between income and consumption likely existed.

Pulses and nutrition: content and composition

Nutrients and variability

In this section the nutritional qualities of pulses will be considered. Macronutrients, micro-nutrients and anti-nutrients will be treated,[14] followed by a discussion of the toxic qualities (and associated diseases) of pulses. We will pay particular attention to traditional preparation methods and how these may negate the effects of anti-nutrients and toxins. As is the case for cereals, great variability occurs in almost any nutritional parameter between species, subspecies, cultivars or even specimens of the same cultivar grown under different conditions due to a variety of genetic, environmental and anthropogenic causes.

Macronutrients

The high protein content of pulses has been duly noted in most historical scholarship, even to the extent that the presence of other macronutrients is overlooked; Table 10.2 provides an overview of macronutrients in pulses, also in relation to processing and preparation methods. While most of the pulses available to the Romans were not particularly rich sources of lipids (typically containing 1%), lupine (5–13%) deserves an honourable mention. Similar to cereals, most pulses primarily contain carbohydrates (e.g. 50–75% for pea, chickpea and lentil), mainly occurring as starch. The protein content of pulses is variable with species available to the

Table 10.2 Modern macronutrient composition of major Roman pulses

Common Name	Scientific Name	Proteins (g/100 g)	Lipids (g/100 g)	Carbohydrates (g/100 g) or %
Bitter vetch[1]	*Vicia ervilia*	26.56	0.40	N.D.
Faba bean[2]	*Vicia faba*	19.3–27.8 (CP), 31 (HT); 31.9 (LT)	19 (HT); 20 (LT)	38 (HT); 44 (LT)
Lentil[3]	*Lens culinaris*	24.8–32.1 (CP), 26.6±0.50 (26.2±0.36 B); 28.6	N.D.	52%–75%
Chick pea[4]	*Cicer arietinum*	18.0–28.1 (CP), 23.64±0.50 (23.21±0.36 B)	6.48±0.08 (6.22±0.09 B)	41.10–47.42% or 43.97±0.93 (R), 40.62±0.65 (B)
Common pea[5]	*Pisum sativum*	21.0–32.3 (CP), 21.9±1.53	2.34±0.01	52.5±0.04
Grass pea[6]	*Lathyrus sativus*	25.6±0.20	1.67±0.18	72.91±2.95
Vetchling[7]	*Lathyrus cicera*	21.5±1.0, 21.7–33.0[7a]	0.7–1.4	N.D.
Spanish vetchling[8]	*Lathyrus clymenum*	21.6±1.8	N.D.	N.D.
White lupine[9]	*Lupinus albus*	38.48 (W), 43.57 (D)	7.91 (W), 10.23 (D)	8.35 (W), 10.43 (D)
Fenugreek[10]	*Trigonella foenum-graecum*	25.4 (W)	7.9	1.6
Mung bean[11]	*Vigna radiata*	20.0±0.50–22.8±0.10 (CP)	1.22±0.1–1.32±0.09 (CF)	68.2±0.4–71.3±0.5

B: Boiled; R: Raw; W: Whole; D: Dehulled; CP: Crude Protein. CF: Crude fat. HT: High Tannin. LT: Low Tannin. N.D.: Not determined. 1. Sadeghi et al., 2009. 2. Bahl, 1990 for CP. Crépon et al., 2010 for HT and LT. 3. Bahl, 1990 for CP. Hefnawy, 2011. Bhatty et al., 1976 and Bhatty, 1988. 4. Bahl, 1990 for CP; Alajaji and El-Adawy, 2006. 5. Bahl, 1990 for CP. 6. De Almeida Costa et al., 2006.; Tamburino et al., 2012. 7. Pastor-Cavada et al., 2011. 7a. Hanbury et al., 2000. 8. Pastor-Cavada et al., 2011. 9. Pisarikova et al., 2008. 10. Rao and Sharma, 1987. 11. Dahiya et al., 2013.

Romans typically ranging between 18% and 48%. The economically most important species (lentil, pea, faba bean, chickpea) have percentages of protein averaging around 20–25%. Minor pulses such as vetchling and chickling typically contain 20-30% of protein, while white lupine may contain 28–48% protein (Pisarikova et al., 2008). Under normal conditions, pulses contain more protein than cereals. Consumption mode may affect the per weight protein intake: if the seeds are eaten raw from the pod they obviously contain more water per weight unit than when they have been dried and have become pulses. In legumes of which the pod can also be eaten, the difference is even greater, as the pods contain less protein than the seeds. Processing methods may alter the actual protein content: soaking for instance causes a reduction in the solid mass of pulses; significant amounts of protein have been detected in the soaking wastewater. Unlike in some cereals, gluten are not present as storage proteins in pulses. Therefore, pulse flours that are used in bread production do not help create aerated bread (see Heinrich, this volume). The addition of pulse flours may still increase loaf-volume and the baking quality of commercial leavened white bread (Rizzello et al., 2014).

Perhaps more important than absolute protein content are the (essential) amino acid composition and protein digestibility, which together determine nutritional quality; Table 10.3 provides an overview of average amino acid composition of several pulses, while Table 10.4 outlines human amino acid requirements. In terms of essential amino acid composition, pulses have a balanced profile, but tend to be somewhat limited in the sulphur-based amino acids methionine and cysteine,[15] yet are rich in lysine and arginine. This is important because the other group of Roman staples, the cereals, have the opposite profile. Therefore pulses and cereals are nutritionally complementary and ensure a balanced amino acid intake (see Bahl, 1990). Co-consumption of pulses and cereals in a single meal as well as mixing them in a single dish are therefore beneficial practices. Finally, as with cereals, it is noteworthy that pulse amino acid quality may increase through traditional fermentation (cf. Steinkraus, 1994).

Anti-nutrients affecting macronutrients

In the discourse on Roman pulses, the presence of anti-nutrients and toxins has traditionally received much attention (cf. Garnsey, 1999; Flint-Hamilton, 1999). This has led to a somewhat negative image of pulses. Over the past decades our understanding of these anti-nutrients and toxins has much improved. In the current and following sections we will rectify the negative image of pulses by showing that recent research indicates that the anti-nutritional and toxic effects of pulses are less severe and would have been easily reduced or eliminated by traditional food preparation practices also used by the Romans.

Pulses may contain variable quantities of compounds that act as anti-nutrients for macronutrients: in other words they reduce the digestibility or metabolism of protein and carbohydrates. In this respect the oligosaccharides raffinose, stachyose and verbascose, types of plant storage carbohydrates the body cannot digest, are the least harmful. Humans do not possess the enzymes to break them down, although they are partially consumed by intestinal bacteria. This causes natural fermentation that produces gas and leads to flatulence (Wang et al., 2010).[16] While medically harmless, socially and culturally these aspects are not appreciated. Oligosaccharides (obtained from high pulse diets) have recently been observed to have a positive effect on the composition of the microflora in the intestine, and consequently on the digestive tract and overall health of individuals (De Filippo et al., 2010).

The effect of some anti-nutrient proteins in pulses can be more serious. Trypsin inhibitors, for instance, are a type of protease inhibiting proteins that bind and inactivate the digestive enzyme trypsin. Trypsin is responsible for hydrolysing (i.e., cutting) the bonds between protein

Table 10.3 Measurements of total amino acids composition (g/100 g protein) in modern pulses

AA	Bitter vetch[1]	Faba bean[2]	Lentil[3]	Chick pea[4]	Common pea[5]	Grass pea[6]	Vetchling[7]	Spanish vetchling[8]	White lupine[9]	Fenugreek[10]	Mung bean[11]
Arg	7.42	9.2	5.9–8.8	6.9	13.4	2.03±0.14	9.5±0.3	8.7±0.3	4.38 (W), 5.1 (D)	6.40 (UGS), 5.35 (GS)[10a]	4.51 (R), 4.44 (C)
His	2.76	2.8	2.1–3.4	2.3	2.7	0.52±0.01	2.7±0.1	2.5±0.2	1.19 (W), 1.28 (D)	1.67 (UGS), 2.17 (GS)[10a]	2.36 (R), 2.34 (C)
Ile	3.88	6.0	3.5–5.0	6.0	7.4	0.95±0.04	3.6±2	3.8±0.3	1.50 (W), 1.73 (D)	3.85[10], 3.40 (UGS), 1.19 (GS)[10a]	3.75 (R), 4.02 (C)
Leu	6.63	8.9	6.3–7.3	8.2	9.5	1.79±0.10	8.0±0.2	9.8±0.6	2.41 (W), 2.69 (D)	5.35[10], 5.22 (UGS), 5.46 (GS)[10a]	6.95 (R), 7.23 (C)
Lys	7.42	6.8	6.3–7.3	6.3	8.9	1.76±0.11	7.4±0.1	7.7±0.2	2.10 (W), 2.26 (D)	5.14[10], 4.36 (UGS), 4.17 (GS)[10a], 5.7[10b]	6.19 (R), 6.08 (C)
Met	1.11	1.0	0.6–1.0	1.2	1.3	0.19±0.01	0.7±0.2	0.7±0.1	0.43 (W), 0.50 (D)	0.56[10], 0.833 (UGS), 0.685 (GS)[10a], 1.2[10b]	N.D.
Phe	4.47	5.5	4.1–5.1	4.9	4.6	0.75±0.03	5.0±0.1	5.1±0.1	1.36 (W), 1.36 (D)	5.80[10], 3.13 (UGS), 3.83 (GS)[10a]	4.59 (R), 4.82 (C)
Thr	3.88	3.3	3.0–4.6	3.4	4.2	0.83±0.04	4.4±0.1	4.2±0.1	1.43 (W), 1.58 (D)	2.66[10], 1.30 (UGS), 3.00 (GS)[10a]	2.72 (R), 2.44 (C)
Trp	N.D.	1.0	0.7–0.9	0.8	0.7	N.D.	0.8±0.1	0.7±0.1	N.D.	1.18 (UGS), 1.25 (GS)[10a], 1.3[10b]	0.64 (R), 0.61 (C)
Val	3.97	5.4	4.0–5.4	5.5	6.5	1.13±0.06	4.4±0.2	4.6±0.2	1.44 (W), 1.61 (D)	3.15, 5.00, 2.84 (UGS), 3.27 (GS)[10a]	4.23 (R), 4.40 (C)

Measurements of Total Amino Acids composition (g/100 g protein). Arg: Arginine; His: Histidine; Ile: Isoleucine; Leu: Leucine; Lys: Lysine; Met: Methionine; Phe: Phenylanine; Thr: Threonine; Trp: Tryptophan; Val: Valine. W: Whole; D: Dehulled. N.D.: not determined. UGS: Ungerminated seed; GS: Germinated seed. R: Raw. C: Cooked. 1. Sadeghi et al., 2009. 2. Bahl, 1990. 3. Bhatty, 1988. 4. Bahl, 1990. 5. Bahl, 1990. 6. Tamburino et al., 2012. 7. Pastor-Cavada et al., 2011. 8. Pastor-Cavada et al., 2011. 9. Pisarikova et al., 2008. 10. Nour and Magboul, 1986. 10a. El-Mahdy and El-Sebaiy, 1985. 10b. Rao and Sharma, 1987. 11. El-Moniem, 1999.

Table 10.4 Daily amino acid and protein requirements from the FAO 1985 and 2007 reports for various age groups

AA	Infants (3–4 months) mg/kg	Infants (6 months) mg/kg	Children (2 years) mg/kg	Children (2 years) mg/g	Children (1–2 years) mg/kg	Children (1–2 years) mg/g	Schoolboys (10–12 years) mg/kg	Schoolboys (10–12 years) mg/kg	Adolescent boys and girls (11–14 years) mg/kg	Adolescent boys and girls (15–18 years) mg/kg	Adolescent boys and girls (x>18 years) mg/kg	Adults mg/kg	Adults mg/g	Adults mg/kg	Adults mg/g
FAO Year	1985 ref. 12	2007	1985 ref. 82, 83	1985	2007 tab. 27, 36	2007	1985 ref. 12	1985 ref. 86	2007 tab. 36	2007 tab. 36	2007 tab. 36	1985, ref. 12	1985	2007, tab. 23	2007
Arg	N.D.	N.D.	N.D.	N.D.	N.D.	N.D.	N.D.	N.D.	N.D.	N.D.	N.D.	N.D.	N.D.	N.D.	N.D.
His	28	22	N.D.	N.D.	15	N.D.	N.D.	N.D.	12	11	10	8–12	15	10	15
Ile	70	36	31	28	27	31	30	28	22	21	20	10	15	20	30
Leu	161	73	73	66	54	63	45	44	44	42	39	14	21	39	59
Lys	103	64	64	58	45	52	60	44	35	33	30	12	18	30	45
Met + Cys or SAA	58	31	27	25	22	26	27	22	17	16	15	13	20	15	22
Met	N.D.	N.D.	N.D.	N.D.	N.D.	N.D.	N.D.	N.D.	N.D.	N.D.	N.D.	N.D.	N.D.	10	16
Cys	N.D.	N.D.	N.D.	N.D.	N.D.	N.D.	N.D.	N.D.	N.D.	N.D.	N.D.	N.D.	N.D.	4	6
Phe + Tyr or AAA	125	59	69	63	40	46	27	22	30	28	25	14	21	25	38
Phe	N.D.	N.D.	N.D.	N.D.	N.D.	N.D.	N.D.	N.D.	N.D.	N.D.	N.D.	N.D.	N.D.	N.D.	N.D.
Thr	87	34	37	34	23	27	35	28	18	17	15	7	11	15	23
Trp	17	9.5	12.5	11	6.4	7.4	4	3.3	4.8	4.5	4.0	3.5	5	4	6
Val	93	49	38	35	36	42	33	25	29	28	26	10	15	26	39

mg per kg of body weight per day — mg/g protein per day

peptides to reduce them to their constituent amino acids. This process is called proteolysis and is necessary to allow proteins to be taken up by the body (Wang et al., 2010). Trypsin inhibitors therefore hinder the metabolism and uptake of protein from food. Lectins are a group of carbohydrate-binding proteins occurring in many cereals, nuts and pulses. They reduce carbohydrate uptake and damage the function of the intestine and cause vomiting and diarrhoea. Very high lectin content, however, is only associated with the American *Phaseolus* species and Far Eastern soybean and would not have caused problems in the Roman context. Lastly, tannins are a non-protein group of biomolecules that occur in many plant families. Their function is to regulate growth and protect seeds and other tissues from animal predation because of their bitterness. Depending on type and content, they may act as an anti-nutrient that precipitates (i.e. binds) proteins and prevents the body from taking them up. Pulse cultivars with a darker colour contain more tannins (cf. Akroyd et al., 1982).

More recently advances in biochemistry have shown that the effect of these anti-nutrients may be greatly reduced through traditional preparation practices, which are now advocated by nutritionists (Curiel et al., 2015). While tannins can only be leached through soaking (and partially removed through dehulling dark-coloured cultivars), the other anti-nutrients are heat sensitive and are best removed through a combination of soaking and roasting, baking or boiling, although overcooking may lead to protein loss (Wang et al., 2010). Traditional lactic acid bacteria (e.g., sourdough) fermentation reduces the above anti-nutritional factors (Curiel et al., 2015; cf. Heinrich this volume on Roman fermentation). The Romans used at least some of these methods consciously (e.g. dough fermentation) or accidentally (storing liquid foods unrefrigerated, reheating them repeatedly and general non-sterile conditions during soaking and food preparation). Therefore, the effect of the anti-nutrients discussed here would have been considerably reduced.

Micronutrients

In terms of micronutrients, pulses share some characteristics with cereals, such as being devoid of vitamin D, but they are richer in B-complex vitamins, and do contain vitamins A and C. When pulses are eaten fresh from the pod, or as leguminous vegetables, they contain small amounts of vitamin A and C. The same is the case for germinated pulses (i.e., bean sprouts). Fresh pulses would have been a valuable seasonal addition to the diet. Of the other grain crops only chestnuts also contain vitamin C. Like cereals, pulses also contain trace elements such as iron (Fe), zinc (Zn), magnesium (Mg), copper (Cu) and especially calcium (Ca). Calcium content is of particular interest because cereals are often believed to be deficient in it (cf. Garnsey, 1999). In pulses most micronutrients are concentrated in the seed, while in cereals they are concentrated in the outer layers (in cereals the aleurone layer). Therefore, dehulling does not reduce the nutritional value of pulses as much as removing the 'bran' of cereals would.

The bioavailability of trace elements in pulses may be reduced by the anti-nutrient phytate, which also occurs in cereals. Phytate is an acid that plants use to store phosphorus (P), but that also chelates (i.e. binds) the trace elements above. In pulses, unlike cereals, phytate is not concentrated in the outer layers, but occurs throughout the seed. While phytate is not heat sensitive, enzymatic hydrolysis of phytate by naturally occurring phytase during soaking, fermentation or germination will increase the bioavailability of trace elements by several factors (Hamad and Fields, 1979). The Romans used these methods and Roman pulse cultivars probably contained less phytate than modern cultivars. Modern pulse cultivars have been modified since the decades following the initial Green Revolution with the primary objective to increase their yield. The phosphorus stored in the phytate supports and increases seed germination and thus yield; therefore high phytate content was a desirable trait in modern cultivars. As an additional consequence, as with cereals (see Heinrich, this volume), the focus on yield has also decreased the nutritional value of modern cultivars. Scientists are now trying to reduce phytate levels in high yield varieties to restore the nutritional value of pulses (Dahiya et al., 2013). Roman pulses would not have suffered from such modifications and nutrient content may have been higher on average and also more varied.

Toxicity

Several pulses contain (mildly) toxic compounds that may cause severe maladies or even death if consumed in large quantities without detoxification.[17] Lupine contains poisonous alkaloids such as lupinine, anagyrine and spartaine, which may cause convulsions, respiratory problems, paralysis, coma and death. However, its toxicity is easily reduced or eliminated by soaking and boiling (cf. Pisarikova et al., 2008). Today lupine seeds, pickled in brine like olives, are still a popular snack in the wider Mediterranean; it would seem the advantage of their extremely high protein content and high oil content outweighs the cost of detoxifying them.

Neurolathyrism is a neurological disease that causes paralysis of the legs and follows the prolonged overconsumption of grass pea (*Lathyrus sativus*), vetchling (*Lathyrus circea*) or Spanish vetchling (*Lathyrus clymenum*). It is caused by the presence of the neurotoxin 3-(N-oxalyl)-L-2,3-diamino propionic acid (ODAP), the quantity of which is somewhat reduced by the practice of boiling (Hanbury et al., 2000). If moderate, consumption is safe – as in present-day Italy and Spain, where these crops feature in several traditional dishes. Adverse health consequences, particularly in young men, arise only if consumption is excessive (a third to half of the daily food intake) for a prolonged period of time (3–6 months) (Akroyd et al., 1982). This may happen in a drought-induced famine as the very drought-resistant *Lathyrus* species often served as insurance crops. Famine related outbreaks were common in Europe into the twentieth century and still occur in the developing world, especially Ethiopia and India (Hanbury et al., 2000). For the Roman period a similar situation can be expected: the Romans were familiar with the relationship between lathyrism and the consumption of crops from the genus *Lathyrus* and would under normal conditions have limited their intake, although outbreaks during famine are recorded and would have been common.[18]

Favism is a severe, often lethal, type of hemolysis that occurs after faba bean consumption in individuals that suffer from a genetic deficiency in glucose-6-phosphate dehydrogenase (G6PD) production.[19] The condition is more common in men than in women and there is no treatment, although blood transfusion may help. Faba beans contain large amounts of non-toxic vicine and convicine that are converted into toxic divicine and isouramil by the enzyme beta-glucosidase, which occurs naturally in faba beans. Divicine and isouramil, in association with ascorbic acid (vitamin C), oxidize glutathione in red blood cells causing them to be seen as foreign by the immune system, leading to the destruction of 80% of the red blood cells within one day. In most individuals G6PD rapidly regenerates oxidized glutathione and there are no adverse consequences (see Crépon et al., 2010; Arese et al., 2005). It should be noted that dried and properly boiled faba beans are not toxic to healthy adult individuals who suffer from G6PD-deficiency, as drying, boiling and the acid gastric juice in the stomach destroy beta-glucosidase before harm is done. Young children with less acid gastric juice remain susceptible, as well as individuals who (accidentally) eat uncooked or insufficiently cooked faba beans. There is no reason to assume a greater occurrence of favism in antiquity than today. Today the low estimate of individuals with G6PD deficiency is 400 million (Crépon et al., 2010). The genes that are responsible for this deficiency appear to also provide better resistance against malaria; this is now seen as the explanation for its prevalence in human populations (Greene, 1993; Arese et al., 2005; Crépon et al., 2010; cf. Flint-Hamilton, 1999).[20]

Conclusion

In this chapter we reviewed the range of pulses known to the Romans, their importance in the diet, and their respective consumption modes. We established that although pulses were not perceived as a preferred good in Roman society, their consumption was ubiquitous and, as biochemical data suggest, nutritionally of tremendous importance in balancing the diet. The importance of anti-nutrients and toxins in pulses should not be overemphasized, especially because traditional preparation methods under normal circumstances negate much of their effect. Moreover, Roman pulses on average contained fewer anti-nutrients and more micronutrients than modified modern cultivars, although they were less productive. Currently, the nutritional sciences are increasingly arguing against the sub-recent marginalization of pulses and instead argue in favour of their dietary and health benefits for both the developed and developing world. With respect to the ancient diet, we perhaps should take pulses more into account, since they were not only agriculturally versatile crops, but also important staples and invaluable dietary components.

Notes

1 This chapter is intended as a diptych with Chapter 9 in this volume on cereals by Heinrich.
2 Both *Phaseolus vulgaris* and *Arachis hypogaea* are New World crops unavailable to the Romans that here just serve as examples.
3 Its etymology is uncertain, although *legere*, 'to gather' (supposedly the pods) has been suggested (cf. Akryod et al., 1982).
4 See below, cf. Heinrich this volume. This also goes for the species we use primarily as oil crops; for example, 'Flaxseed' porridge, hemp gruel or sesame paste (*tahini*) and porridge (*heukimjajuk*) (cf. Deitch, 2003).
5 Latin *puls* (or general 'porridge', *pultes*), from which our word pulse is derived, comes from Greek πόλτος, meaning porridge.
6 Cf. Wilkins and Hill, 2006.
7 See Kron, 2004a, for a list of archaeobotanical finds of legumes (between 1981 and 2004) at Roman sites.
8 For an overview see Heinrich and Wilkins, 2014.
9 Here we will discuss the processes; the (anti)nutritional details are discussed below.
10 Archaeobotanical analyses may in the future enable us to recognize processes such as soaking, dehulling and splitting in archaeobotanical material; see Valamoti et al., 2011.
11 There are also exceptions; in China the soybean was highly esteemed and in Indian society pulses were a preferred good and were consumed in greater amounts by more affluent individuals (Akroyd et al., 1982).
12 Interestingly, a positive correlation between urbanization and reduced pulse consumption was noted for the twentieth-century developing world (Akroyd et al., 1982), which was explained through the constraint 'fuel price'. A similar model, pertaining to the choice between (cereal) porridge and bread consumption in the Roman urban context has been made by Heinrich, 2017.
13 In fact, in recognition of this the FAO made 2016 'The International Year of Pulses'.
14 For a general introduction to these topics we refer to Heinrich, this volume.
15 It has been suggested that sulphur content in the soil may negate this deficiency, see Pastor-Cavada et al., 2011.
16 Cf. Hippocrates, *Regimen* II, XLV.
17 We should be cautious not to overemphasize the mild toxicity of foodstuffs. Under normal conditions the human body is perfectly able to deal with a moderate, continuous influx of toxins (Akroyd et al.,

1982). Following the principle of hormesis this may even be beneficial (for an overview see Mattson and Calabrese, 2009).

18 See Hippocrates, *Epidemics*, IV, case 47 on an outbreak of lathyrism in Ainos.

19 Favism has been associated with the Pythagorean aversion of beans (cf. Flint-Hamilton, 1999; Worm, 1696).

20 Another example is the protection provided by genes causing gluten allergy/Celiac disease against the Black Death and bacterial infections, as was suggested by Zhernakova et al., 2010.

11

OLIVES AND OLIVE OIL

Erica Rowan

Introduction

Almost every article, chapter and book on Roman food contains the overarching statement that the components of the Mediterranean triad, olive oil, wine and cereals, were the staple foods of the traditional Roman diet (Jasny, 1950, 228–229; Garnsey, 1999, 13; Mattingly and Aldrete, 2000, 143; Aldrete, 2004, 111; Thurmond, 2006, 13; Bowman and Wilson, 2013, 23). On a basic nutritional level, these staples acted as vital sources of calories and/or good sources of nutrients. While the precise degree of reliance on each of the three products can be debated, as can the term 'traditional Roman diet', there can be no denying that olive oil played a crucial dietary and nutritional role for many of the people living within the Roman Empire. The literary and archaeological evidence for the trade and consumption of table olives and olive oil, the two main products derived from the fruit of the olive tree (*Olea europaea* L.) is extensive (Mattingly, 1988a; 1988b; 1988c; Blázquez, 1992; Funari, 1996; Rodríguez, 1998; Dalby, 2003, 238–240; Hitchner, 2002; Brun, 2003; 2004b; Flohr et al., 2013; Lewit, 2011; Marzano, 2013a; Rowan, 2015). The quantity of contemporary data on both the immediate and long-term nutritional benefits of the olive is similarly extensive (Harwood and Yaqoob, 2002; Stark and Madar, 2002; Wahle et al., 2004; Beauchamp et al., 2005; Bendini et al., 2007; Preedy and Watson, 2010; Süntar et al., 2010; Ghanbari et al., 2012; Hashmi et al., 2015). Consequently, it is now possible, with a high degree of precision and nuance, to understand from a nutritional perspective exactly how and why olives and olive oil were such vitally important foods. This chapter will examine the nutritional properties of table olives and olive oil in relation to levels of consumption and accessibility.

There are 30 species within the genus *Olea*, but only the species *Olea europaea* produces edible fruits. Olive trees are slow-growing evergreens that reach heights of approximately 10 m (Hashmi et al. 2015, 2). They are long-lived and can produce fruit for hundreds and sometimes thousands of years (Fernández et al., 1997, 10). Each tree, however, will not produce fruit for roughly the first eight years, and afterwards, only every second year will it generate enough fruit to harvest (von Reden, 2007, 392; Therios, 2009, 20). The trees grow best on deep sandy loam soils but can tolerate nutrient poor, dry calcareous and gravelly soil. They can also survive in dry areas with little water (Mattingly, 1988b, 23; Therios, 2009, 52). Olive trees have specific temperature requirements and only produce fruit in climates that have dry hot summers and mild winters; between 30°–45° latitude north. Regions with mean annual temperatures of

15–20°C, where temperatures do not go below −7°C or above 40°C are best (Therios, 2009, 51–53). These climatic criteria describe much of the Mediterranean basin and olives grow on the coastal areas of the eastern Mediterranean basin, the coastal areas of southeastern Europe, northern Iran, western Asia and North Africa (Hashmi et al., 2015, 2) (see Figure 11.1).

Olive trees, however, do not grow well above 800 m as they are ill equipped to handle frost, nor can they survive temperatures below −12°C (von Reden, 2007, 391; Therios, 2009, 51). Consequently, olives are not found in the areas of higher elevation in Greece and Italy, nor anywhere in central or northern Europe. While olive cultivation has recently been introduced into Australia and California, the Mediterranean region still produces 98% of the world's olive oil (Ghanbari et al., 2012, 3293).

The olive fruit is a drupe (stone fruit) and formed of four layers: the epicarp (skin), mesocarp (flesh), endocarp (stone) and embryo (seed) (Cappers and Neef, 2012, 241). Fresh olives are composed of 50% water, 1.6% protein, 22% oil, 19.1% carbohydrates, 5.8% cellulose, 1.5% inorganic substances and 1–3% phenolic compounds (Ghanbari et al., 2012, 3297). There are 2,500 different olive cultivars in existence today with 250 cultivars utilized for commercial purposes. Those with less than 12% oil are used to make table olives while those with greater oil contents (c. 20%) are used for oil production (Ghanbari et al., 2012, 3294).

The Romans had access to a narrower range of cultivars (Cato, *Agr.* 6–7). The ancient sources make it clear that there was a distinction between olives suited for the table and those for oil. The general rule was that small varieties were better suited for oil production while the larger varieties were best for consumption (Columella, *Rust.* 5.8.5). Much like today, there were also noted differences in the quality; olives and oils from particular regions being favoured for their flavour, volume of output or shelf life. Columella (*Rust.* 5.8.3) names ten different

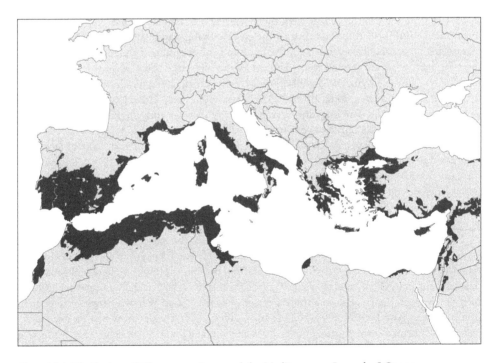

Figure 11.1 Distribution of *Olea europaea* L. around the Mediterranean (image by J.Oteros, © J.Oteros and WikiCommons).

cultivars, claiming that the Posia, Royal, Orchite and Shuttle-olive were good for
Posia olives could also be made into oil but the oil would go rancid within a year. .
to Columella (*Rust.* 5.8.3.3), Pliny (*HN* 15.3) and Juvenal (5.86–89), Licinian olives
Venafrum region in Campania made the highest quality oil, while the Sergian oliv
most prolific cultivar. Oil from Spain was highly regarded, while African olive oil was considered
by Juvenal (5.86–89) to be of a far inferior quality (Martial, 12.63; Pliny, *HN* 15.23).

Chemically, table olives are dissimilar to most other fruits consumed as part of the Roman
diet. They have a very low sugar content (2–5%) compared to many other drupes such as
apricots or cherries (12%) (Fernández et al., 1997, 12). Instead, they are high in oleuropein, a
compound that makes the fruit extremely bitter and inedible (Pereira et al., 2006, 8427). Unlike
apples, peaches, berries and grapes that can be eaten straight off the tree, shrub or vine, table
olives must first be processed to remove the oleuropein before they can be consumed. The
production of olive oil is a more simple process as the oleuropein is contained within the flesh,
not the oil itself. Nevertheless, steps must be taken to ensure that the oil does not go rancid.
Fortunately for modern scholars, the ancient agronomists, in particular Cato (*Agr.* 64–69;
117–119) and Columella (*Rust.* 12.49–52), left detailed accounts of the processing methods for
olive oil and table olives.

Roman processing methods

Olive oil

Until the mid-twentieth century, all olive oil was produced using traditional methods that had
changed little since antiquity.[1] The basic process involved four stages: harvesting, crushing,
pressing and separation. Olives were collected, in antiquity entirely by hand, and then washed
to remove dirt, twigs and leaves. They were then crushed using a *trapetum* type rotary mill,
although simpler methods such as mortar and pestle, stone basin and roller, and trampling were
also used (Warnock, 2007, 72–75). Once a paste had been obtained, it was placed in round
woven baskets and the baskets were stacked on the press bed. When enough baskets were in
place the paste was compressed using either a lever or screw press. The oil ran out of the
baskets, into the shallow groove of the press bed and into a collection tank.

Columella describes three pressings taking place for each batch of olives. He emphasizes the
importance of not mixing the final two pressings with the first as the quality of the oil in the
first pressing is considered far superior to the other two (*Rust.* 12.52.11). Since he describes
superior (first pressing) and ordinary eating-oil (first and/or second pressing), it is probable that
the oil from the third pressing was considered suitable only for non-comestible purposes
(Columella *Rust.* 12.52.22). Today oil extracted from the pomace (the remaining paste in the
baskets) after pressing is used to make goods such as soap and in antiquity would have been
used as lamp fuel (Gomes et al., 2010, 140). In preparation for the third pressing, the paste was
first washed with hot water as the water helped to separate the oil from the paste. After settling
in the tank, the oil was either skimmed off the top or the water was removed by opening a
plug at the bottom of the tank (Foxhall, 2007, 133–138).

Table olives

Table olives are a variable food, ranging considerably in colour, flavour, texture, and taste. The
different end products, as well as the processing methods, have also not changed considerably
since antiquity (see Table 11.1). Green, turning colour, and black table olives were produced
in the Graeco-Roman world as were ancient versions of tapenade and dried olives.

Table 11.1 Olive colours and ripeness

Name	Ripeness	Colours
Green	Picked during ripening period prior to colouring	Straw yellow to green
Turning colour	Harvest before complete ripeness	Pink to rose wine to brown
Black	Fully ripe or just prior	Reddish black, violet black, deep violet, greenish black, deep chestnut

(Rejano et al., 2010, 5)

There were three primary ways of converting fresh olives into edible table olives in the ancient world. The first, and by far the most common method, was through pickling; what today are called natural or Greek style olives (Rejano et al., 2010, 12).[2] After washing, the olives are placed directly into a brine (8–10% salt) and left for several days. Columella (*Rust.* 12.50) recommends 30–40 days. The diffusion of the salt through the fruit's epidermis and the leeching of the oleuropein, called *amurca* by the Romans, are slow processes. Once the oleuropein has been removed the olives can be consumed or stored in barrels (or amphorae) in a less concentrated solution of brine and consumed at a later date (Columella, *Rust.* 12.49.11; Rejano et al., 2010, 12;). Columella (*Rust.* 12.49-51) suggests using this method, with some minor variations, on olives of all degree of ripeness. In some of his recipes he recommends crushing or cutting the olives prior to submerging them in the brine (Columella, *Rust.* 12.50.5). Breaking the skin allows the salt to soak in faster (Thurmond, 2006, 180). Cato (*Agr.* 117) suggests breaking the olives and then soaking them in water to release the *amurca*. Afterwards he places the olives into a mixture of vinegar, olive oil and salt to create a sort of tapenade (Thurmond 2006: 178). In many of the Roman recipes, fennel and mastic are added to the brining solutions and on occasion parsley, rue and bay to create additional flavour (Cato, *Agr.* 117, 119; Columella, *Rust.* 12.49-51). Olives were often stored in a mixture of brine and vinegar, although some of Columella's recipes suggest storing them in a solution of must or honey water to give the olives a sweet and sour taste (*Rust.* 12.50.3).

A second and faster processing method is to soak the olives in a solution of lye before brining. The alkaline lye quickly penetrates the skin and flesh of the olive, facilitating the removal of the oleuropein (Rejano et al., 2010, 7). Afterwards, the olives are placed in water that is changed frequently and once all the lye has been removed the olives are put in brine to ferment (Rejano et al., 2010, 9). Although the Romans knew about lye and used it to make soap, it is unclear if it was ever used on olives (Toedt et al., 2005, 5).

The final processing method results in the creation of cured or dried black olives. Very ripe black olives are washed and placed in baskets with alternating layers of salt and olives. They are left for several days and once the oleuropein has leeched out, the olives are wiped off to remove any excess salt. They are then ready for storage or consumption (Rejano et al., 2010, 12). The recipe given by Columella is almost identical to the recipe described above (*Rust.* 12.50).

Accessibility of consumption

Today, olives are not just considered healthy but they have been elevated to the level of a functional food (Stark and Madar, 2002, 170). Functional foods, when of a sufficient quality, and when consumed in a sufficient quantity, provide clinically proven health benefits (Wildman, 2007, 2). In attempting to understand the dietary and nutritional role that olives played in the

Roman world, it is first necessary to determine who would have consumed enough olive products to receive the benefits. In the introduction, the validity of the term 'traditional Roman diet' was questioned. Geographical, climatic and cultural variability within the Roman Empire make it impossible to assume that all people consumed cereals, wine and olive oil as their staple foods. Based on this variability, the following section will use the literary material, in association with the vast quantities of archaeological material, to establish groups of olive consumers.

The strict climatic conditions required for olive tree growth, particularly with respect to temperature, means that we have a precise knowledge of the geographical spread of olive production in the Roman world. The extensive survey work done in Libya and Tunisia have shown that olive cultivation was pushed to the limits of the trees' water requirements (Mattingly, 1988b; 1988c; Barker, 1996; Hitchner, 2002; Ahmed, 2010). Some areas, such as Tripolitania and Baetica, produced vast quantities of oil for export. Other regions, for example Var in the south of France with its small number of presses, were only making enough oil for local consumption (Mattingly, 1988b; 1988c; Brun et al., 1989; Rodríguez, 1998; Brun, 2003). Pressing equipment such as *trapetum*, press beds, press uprights and settling tanks, have been found in all climatically suitable olive oil growing regions of the Roman world (Flohr et al., 2013; Rowan, 2015). These finds indicate that olive oil and table olives were produced wherever it was possible, and no region was left entirely unexploited.[3] Consequently, we may assume that in all regions suitable for olive cultivation, olives and olive oil were eaten in sufficient quantities by the majority of the population to ensure nutritional benefit (see Figure 11.1).[4]

Rome was located within a highly suitable olive-growing region but its population of roughly one million inhabitants meant that it was too large to be supplied exclusively by its hinterland. In practice, a larger range of oils and oil substitutes could have been utilized to feed the population. Radish, sesame, nut and castor oil as well as bacon fat are recorded in the sources as goods that played a similar role to olive oil (Pliny, *HN* 15.7; Davies, 1989, 191, 202; Brun, 2003, 179). Olive oil, however, was of great cultural importance. The evidence from sites such as Monte Testaccio indicate that olive oil, more so than any other fat source, was imported into Rome in vast quantities. The formation of this 35 m high mound of amphorae sherds began during the reign of Augustus and continued until the Severan period (Rodríguez, 1998, 194; Mattingly and Aldrete, 2000, 148; Funari, 2001, 586). In total, it represents the waste of over 53 million amphora with 83.1% (primarily Dressel 20) coming from Baetica and 16.8% from North Africa (Mattingly and Aldrete, 2000, 148; Funari, 2001, 586). Olive oil was officially added to the *annona* by Septimius Severus (SHA, *Septimius Severus* 18.3), but even prior to that date, the import of roughly 6,277,000 litres per annum (enough to supply the entire population with 6.27 litres per person/year), demonstrates that its constant supply was a high priority (Funari, 2001, 587).[5] Thus all people in Rome, with the exclusion of the destitute, regularly consumed olive oil.

Once we move outside the region of olive cultivation, determining who consumed sufficient quantities of olive oil becomes more difficult. Finds of one or two amphora may represent an imported luxury; a good that was consumed infrequently and only by the wealthy. The oil may also have been used for personal hygiene or as lamp fuel. Olive oil amphorae have been recovered in large quantities from some military and urban sites in central and northern Europe such as Nimegen and Cologne (Remesal Rodríguez, 1986; Martin-Kilcher, 1987).[6] However, outside of these major centres olive oil amphorae are not usually recovered in a high enough quantity to suggest regular consumption by the majority of the population (Blázquez, 1992, 174; Funari, 1996; 2002; Monfort, 2002, 81–87; Erdkamp, 2007, 67–68; Derreumaux et al., 2008, 62; Le Bohec, 2015, 329). Similarly, in areas such as Roman Britain, Dressel 20 amphorae are rarely recovered from rural sites (Cool, 2006, 123). Archaeobotanical finds of carbonized or waterlogged olives stones can indicate the consumption of table olives (Van der Veen, 2007, Lodwick, 2014, 544–545; Rowan, 2015). Even then, however, the variability in the preservation and subsequent recovery of these finds means that it is extremely difficult to determine the number of olives consumed within a site. Therefore, in areas outside of the olive-growing region, consumption of both olive oil and table olives must be assessed on a site by site basis. For the purposes of this chapter, in assessing the nutritional impact of olive oil, it will be assumed that the majority of people living outside the olive-growing region, except those in large urban centres or military sites, did not consume enough olive oil to obtain any nutritional benefits.

It is through the survival of papyri recording military diet and indirect references in the ancient sources, that the army is the one group for which we can say something about olive oil consumption regardless of their geographical location. Appian, when describing the Romans laying siege to the city of Intercatia in Spain, states that the troops had run out of wine, salt, sour wine and oil (Appian *Iberica* 54; Davies, 1989, 189). His comment suggests that olive oil was a normal part of the military diet. The recovery of hundreds of Dressel 20 amphorae from military sites in Roman Britain and the northwestern provinces supports this statement and indicates that soldiers were supplied with olive oil even when beyond the olive-growing regions (Blázquez, 1992, 174–176; Funari, 1996; Monfort, 2002). The distribution of food rations for foot soldiers and mounted troops are identical when the horses and servants are taken into account. The similarity in rations, regardless of pay, has led to the hypothesis that all troops received identical rations and higher paid individuals could supplement their diet with their additional income (Erdkamp, 2007, 102). A papyrus, dating to 564, describing military food rations is one of the only documents to specify the quantity of goods received by soldiers. It states that each day a soldier received three pounds of bread, two pounds of meat, two pints of wine and one-eighth of a pint of oil (*P. Oxy.* 2046; Davies, 1989, 283).[7] Davies (1989, 283) reasons that rations were similar during the Principate, although Jones (1964, 629) believes that these figures are too large to be representative of the Roman army more generally. Nevertheless, as part of the daily ration, all soldiers, irrespective of rank and pay, consumed at least some quantity of olive oil.[8]

In sum, it may be assumed that all those but the very destitute who lived in the olive-producing regions of the Roman Empire consumed an adequate quantity of oil with sufficient frequency to be of nutritional benefit. Many wealthy individuals living in large urban centres outside of the olive oil region probably did as well. In addition, all military personnel and all those living in Rome, except for the very poor, consumed nutritionally significant quantities of olive oil. Outside of the olive-growing areas, the consumption of oil depended upon wealth, personal taste, proximity to military sites, proximity to large urban centres and accessibility to trade routes. Table olives were probably consumed in sufficient quantities by those who lived in the olive regions and in Rome. Since table olives were not part of the standard military diet, the consumption of this good depended upon a soldier's geographical location, access to trade routes and personal wealth. The situation was similar for those living outside of the olive-producing areas.

Volume of consumption

Ancient historians and scientists alike are interested in understanding the relationship between volumes of consumption and human health. For ancient historians the quantity of an item consumed is usually converted into an intake of calories and subsequently into an assessment of overall health and survival (Foxhall and Forbes, 1982). For scientists and nutritionists the goal is often to find the minimal level of consumption at which the nutritional benefits become apparent so that this information can be passed on to the general public (Buckland and Gonzáles,

2010; López-López et al., 2010; Ghanbari et al., 2012, 3305). By combining the estimates provided by ancient historians with the knowledge obtained through modern scientific research, we can assess the major dietary benefits gained by the Romans through the consumption of olive oil and table olives.

Using ethnographic comparisons, particularly from modern Greece, scholars have come up with a range of estimates for Roman olive oil consumption. Amouretti posited that each person (who falls into the category of olive oil consumer described above) consumed 20 litres of olive oil per annum and this is the most commonly repeated figure (Amouretti, 1986, 183; Mattingly, 1988b, 22; 1988c, 34; Harris, 2007, 531; Jongman, 2007a, 603; Kron, 2008b, 86). Currently, the average annual per capita consumption of olive oil in 15 Mediterranean countries is six litres although the averages for Greece (23.7 litres), Spain (13.62 litres) and Italy (12.35 litres) are much higher (*California*, 2004).

Other scholars have used documentary evidence to suggest volumes of consumption. Allen (2009, 341) has suggested the much lower quantity of five litres per year. Using Diocletian's Price Edict, his estimate is based on the salary of an unskilled free labourer working 250 days per year earning 25 *denarii* per day and purchasing food at the subsistence level (Allen, 2009). According to Cato (*Agr.* 58), farm slaves should receive one *sextarius* a month or 6.47 litres per annum. A papyrus dating to the reign of Diocletian states that soldiers received 4 *librae* of olive oil a month, or roughly 16.73 litres per year (Roth, 1999, 35).[9] Based on a sixth-century document, Le Roux has suggested a slightly higher military consumption of 2.5 ounces per day or approximately 27.88 litres per year for each soldier (1995, 409). Thus the majority of the estimates fall into the range of 15–30 litres per year and following the general trend, the average quantity of 20 litres per year will be used in the upcoming discussion.

The United States Food and Drug Administration (FDA) recommends eating two tablespoons or 23 grams of olive oil per day in order to receive the nutritional benefits (FDA, 2004). This quantity equates to an annual consumption of 9.05 litres, well below the estimated average of 20 litres consumed per capita during the Roman period and well below modern levels of consumption in Greece, Spain and Italy. Therefore, those who consumed olive oil regularly in the Roman period, even if consuming only half the estimated intake, were eating enough oil to have a nutritional impact by today's standards. There are no recommendations for the consumption of table olives, although 15 g is considered a single serving size (FDA, 2014).

Macronutrient and micronutrient properties of table olives and olive oil

Olive oil

The modern-day Mediterranean diet is often lauded for its health benefits. It has been found to generate long life expectancies and people who adhere to the diet have very low incidences of heart disease, cancer and rheumatoid arthritis (De Lorgeril et al., 1998; Harwood and Yaqoob, 2002; Visioli et al., 2002; Wahle et al., 2004; Colomer and Menéndez, 2006; Shen et al., 2015; Martínez-González et al., 2015[10]). Although the Mediterranean diet varies somewhat between countries, the standard characteristics are that it is high in vegetables, fruits, legumes, grains and olive oil. The diet is also low in meat (especially red meat) with a moderate consumption of dairy products other than cheese and a moderate alcohol intake (Wahle et al., 2004, 1223; Buckland and Gonzáles, 2010, 689). The Italian version of the Mediterranean diet is higher in cereals compared to the Greek version which is higher in fat (Harwood and Yaqoob, 2002, 685). The high intake of olive oil within the diet serves two functions. First, it acts as a crucial source of fat and calories, making up to 85% of the fat content of the diet (Kalogeropoulos and

Chiou, 2010, 755). Second, olive oil provides significant quantities of vitamin E and potassium as well as protective antioxidants (Bendini, 2007, 1684; López-López et al., 2010, 713).

Based on literary, archaeobotanical and isotopic data, it appears that the ancient Roman diet, within the olive-growing regions was similar to the modern Mediterranean diet with respect to the balance of fats and calories (White, 1976, 190; Foxhall and Forbes, 1982; Davies, 1989, 283; Garnsey, 1999, 12; Mattingly and Aldrete, 2000, 154–155; Prowse et al., 2005; Craig et al., 2009; 2013; Murphy et al., 2013; Killgrove and Tykot, 2013; Rowan, 2014b; Robinson and Rowan, 2015).[11] The Italian version of the diet is especially applicable due to its high cereal intake. The Roman diet consisted of large quantities of cereals, frequent alcohol intake (although usually watered down), animal protein derived primarily from pork and fish, and a high level of olive oil consumption (Foxhall and Forbes, 1982; MacKinnon, 2001; 2004, 78, 90–91; Prowse et al., 2005; Killgrove and Tykot, 2013; Rowan, 2014b). Fruits and vegetables were consumed but it is difficult to assess the quantities. Thus olive oil within the Roman diet served the same two functions as it does in the modern Mediterranean diet.

Olive oil is high in calories and fat, where 100 g of olive oil provides almost 1,000 calories (Thurmond, 2006, 74). It has sometimes been suggested that olive oil could have represented up to 1/3 of an individual's calorific intake in the Roman period, but this figure is too high (Thurmond, 2006, 74). Ethnographic work has shown that olive oil provided one-third of the calories present in the traditional peasant diets of Greece, Crete and Italy, but those individuals consumed 50 litres of oil per year (Foxhall and Forbes, 1982; Mattingly, 1988a, 34). For moderately active men and women,[12] the USDA recommends eating 2,600–2,800 and 2,000–2,200 calories per day respectively (Table 11.2). Calorific requirements were probably at the upper end of these estimates for people in antiquity as they participated in more labour-intensive activities than most people living in the Western world today. The consumption of 20 litres is equivalent to eating 50.84 g per day which provides 449 calories; roughly one-sixth and one-fifth of the total number of recommended calories. The 23 g recommended by the FDA supplies 203 calories per day. If we assume the higher consumption rate of 20 litres per year then at roughly 450 calories a day, olive oil played an important role in the acquisition of sufficient energy sources.

It was not the calories, but the quantity of fat in the oil that was its most important feature. Similar to the modern Mediterranean diet, there were few sources of inexpensive fat in the Roman diet. The other staple foods, cereals and wine, are low in fat, as are pulses, fruits and vegetables (USDA, 2011b). The zooarchaeological data support the notion that in the southern provinces people did not consume much red meat and, aside from olive oil, the most readily available sources of fats would have been nuts and oily fish such as sardines and anchovies (MacKinnon, 2001; 2004, 78, 90–91; Prowse et al., 2005; Thurmond, 2006, 191; Le Bohec, 2015, 611). The USDA recommends a daily intake of 20–35 g of fat for moderately active adults (USDA 2011a). As Table 11.3 indicates, the daily consumption of 23–50 g of oil would have provided more than enough fat.

Finally, olive oil was a crucial source of vitamin E and a good source of vitamin K (see Table 11.3). Based on a nutritional assessment of more than 114 foodstuffs, remains of which were attested in the Cardo V sewer in Herculaneum, only olive oil and hazelnuts have nutritionally significant levels of vitamin E. Sardines, land snails and mint have moderate amounts, as do leafy green vegetables. The frequent consumption of olive oil meant it was the primary source of this vitamin. Similarly there were few foods from Herculaneum that had large quantities of vitamin K. However, the foods that did contain low levels of vitamin K were those frequently eaten and easily accessible, including wheat, dried figs, grapes, hazelnuts and blackberries, so the vitamin K derived from olive oil would not have been as essential (USDA 2011b; Rowan, 2014b; Robinson and Rowan 2015).

Table 11.2 Dietary reference intakes (DRI) for major macronutrients, vitamins and minerals found in olive oil and table olives

Life stage group	Energy (kcal/d)	Total Fat (g/d)	Total fibre (g/d)	Vitamin A (µg/d)	Vitamin E (mg/d)	Vitamin K (µg/d)	Ca (mg/d)	Fe (mg/d)	K (g/d)	Na (g/d)
Male 19–30y	Moderately active – 2,600–2,800 Active – 3,000	20–35	38	900	15	120	1,000	8	4.7	1.5
Female 19–30y	Moderately active – 2,000–2,200 Active – 2,400	20–35	25	700	15	90	1,000	18	4.7	1.5

(USDA, 2010, 78; 2011a)

Table 11.3 Nutrient quantities of olive oil and table olives based on different daily consumption estimates

	DRI for men/women	Olive oil 23 g	Olive oil 50.8 g	Table olives[13] 30 g
Energy (kcal)	2600–2800/ 2000–2200	203	449	44
Total Fat (g)	20–35	23	50.8	4.6
Total Fiber (g)	38/25	0	0	1
Vitamin A (IU)	900/700	0	0	118
Vitamin E (mg)	15	3.30	7.29	1.14
Vitamin K (µg)	120/90	13.8	30.6	0.4
Calcium, Ca (mg)	1,000	0	1	16
Iron, Fe (mg)	8/18	0.13	0.28	0.15
Potassium, K (µg)	4.7	0	1	13
Sodium, Na (mg)	1.5	0	1	467

(USDA, 2011b)

Table olives

The quantities of macro and micronutrients differ considerably between table olives and olive oil. Table olives are much lower in calories per unit weight and consequently their nutritional function within the Roman diet was based on their high levels of fat and particular vitamins and minerals (Table 11.3). A 30 g serving of table olives (approximately 11 olives) provides only 44 calories but 4.60 g of fat (USDA, 2014). Both natural directly brined olives and those treated with lye are good sources of vitamin E, vitamin A and sodium (López-López et al., 2010, 712; USDA, 2014). The vitamin E in table olives would have been important for the same reasons mentioned above. The Roman diet contained several other readily available sources of vitamin A, such as figs, plums, blackberries, eggs, fish and shellfish. Similarly, sodium, in the form of salt, could be found in *garum*, salted meat and fish, other brined foods and shellfish (Rowan, 2014b). While table olives did provide essential nutrients, their consumption was not as critically important to the maintenance of overall health and energy levels as olive oil.

Conclusions

For many individuals living within the Roman Empire, olive oil was a staple food. This chapter has established the regions and population groups where olive oil was consumed frequently and in high quantities. The geographical limits of olive tree growth put restrictions on availability and those living outside that region, with the exclusion of the army and those living in large urban centres, could only consume what olive oil they could access and afford. The vast quantities of archaeological evidence for olive pressing within the productive regions suggests that the majority of the population in those areas had readily available access to what must have been a relatively inexpensive good.[14] Similarly, table olives would have been eaten by those in the productive regions and by those who could afford to import them.

The Romans were unaware that out of all the sources of oils and fats available in the ancient world, olive oil would provide them with the greatest dietary and nutritional advantages. In other words, it was the best possible choice. As a staple food, it was an important source of calories. Based on the traditional estimate of 20 litres per person per annum, and the USDA's calorific intake estimates, olive oil would have provided roughly one-fifth to one-sixth of an individual's calories. In addition, the oil acted as a crucial source of fat, particularly if there was little meat consumption. The high levels of vitamin E and K in oil as well as the vitamins A and E, and sodium in table olives helped people obtain sufficient quantities of these essential nutrients. The large quantity of oil remaining in table olives meant that people obtained the same fat benefits as oil consumption, although on a smaller scale.

The study of nutrition in the Roman world, and of olive oil in particular, is cyclical. It is clear from the vast quantities of olive oil produced and traded around the Roman Empire that it was a highly valued good. As an item eaten in large quantities, it is important to examine the nutritional benefits the Romans received. This examination, however, is only possible because of our own modern health concerns. Hundreds of studies and millions of dollars have been spent discovering the health benefits associated with frequent olive oil consumption. In turn, we now know that the consumption of olive oil as a staple food by the Romans meant that many people were provided on a daily basis with crucial calories, fats and vitamins. The other chapters in this book are similarly part of this cycle and future research will no doubt reveal the full dietary benefits and nutritional strength of the Roman diet.

Notes

1 There are still areas in Turkey and Morocco where olive oil is produced using traditional methods (Doymaz et al., 2004, 214; Sassi et al., 2006, 75)
2 Kalamata olives are prepared in this way.
3 In areas where production was low, oil could be imported, as for example happened at Pompeii (De Sena and Ikäheimo, 2003).
4 Due to fluctuations in the olive harvest, prices would have varied. During some years the low supply would have driven up the cost, and for short periods of time people may have struggled to afford it.
5 Monte Testaccio does not represent all the olive oil imported into Rome, so the overall volume of import would have been much larger (Funari, 2001, 588). Quantities of oil in the review provided in kilograms, which has been converted here into litres using the conversion of 1 L of oil = 0.92 kg.
6 For example, thousands of amphorae have been recovered from Cologne and it is probable that at least some of the inhabitants consumed olive oil on a daily basis. As Remesal Rodriguez notes, however, it does appear that the distribution of Dressel 20 amphorae in Gaul and Germania relates primarily to military consumption (2002, 301).
7 Since the rations are for soldiers in Egypt, it is possible that the text refers to radish oil instead of olive oil (Hickey, 2012, 32).
8 At least until the time of Septimius Severus who substituted olive oil with bacon-fat (*laridum*) when the oil was too difficult to transport (Davies, 1989, 188; Monfort, 2002, 87).
9 4 *librae* is equal to 1.5 ounces per day. Ounces of olive oil converted to litres done using http://convert-to.com/549/cold-pressed-extra-virgin-olive-oil-with-nutrients-amounts-conversion.html.
10 This list is by no means complete and hundreds of studies have been conducted.
11 It is not similar in the range of foods consumed as many ingredients in the modern Mediterranean diet are new world foods (i.e., tomato, potato, corn, coffee) (Pellegrini et al., 2003; Wilkins and Hill, 2006, 2).
12 The USDA calculates the 'average' man to be 177 cm tall and weigh 70 kg while the average woman is 163 cm tall and weighs 57 kg. Moderate activity is defined as walking 1.5-3 miles per day at 3 to 4 miles per hour in addition to the activity associated with daily life (USDA, 2011a; 2011b; USDA and US Department of Health and Human Services, 2010).
13 The table olives are green olives that have been heat treated and are stored in salt brine (USDA, 2011b).
14 According to the Diocletian's Price Edict, second quality oil (pressed from ripe olives), cost a maximum of 12 *denarii* per pint (546 ml) (*DE* III, 3; Frank, 1940, 323). At the consumption rate of 50.84 ml per day (20 L per annum), this quantity would last for roughly 11 days. Thus for the unskilled labourer described above, who would have made 25 *denarii* a day, 11 days' worth of oil cost less than half a day's wage. If he lived just above subsistence, and consumed only 5 L of oil per annum, a single pint would last for 40 days.

12

WINE AND OTHER BEVERAGES

Wim Broekaert

Introduction

The ancient world knew a wide variety of beverages, but the iconic drink of the Roman Empire is without doubt wine. Wine drinking was attractive because of its tastiness and the ring of elite culture attached to it. The consumption of wine (but always in moderation and mixed with water!) was an essential part of the Mediterranean diet and remained throughout antiquity one of the main markers of a cultivated lifestyle, of true belonging to the Greco-Roman civilized world. People drank wine at dinner, in taverns, during festivities and when taking part in food distributions by civic benefactors. Wine was available at room temperature, cooled with ice or snow, or heated (Dunbabin, 1993; Curtis, 2001, 374). Vintages from all over the Mediterranean world reached Italy, leaving the more well-to-do consumer with the difficult choice of what to drink. Trimalchio certainly articulated the common perception of wine being consumed by everyone at all times, when stating that wine was life itself (Petron., *Sat.* 34). Yet, despite wine being considered the normal drink in the Roman Empire, it was neither produced nor consumed everywhere. The attention given to wine drinking in classical texts and in contemporary research often makes us underestimate the existence of countless other beverages. The nature of our evidence invariably turns the focus towards consumption of wines by the literate elite and, to a lesser extent, middling groups living in an urban context, while patterns of consumption in rural communities or by the urban poor remain virtually invisible. Similarly, archaeological evidence favours the analysis of wine production at villa sites and consumption in cities over other beverages, mainly through the remarkable amounts of presses, storage vats, amphorae and drinking vessels discovered there. The result is a complete mismatch between the amount of information on patterns of wine consumption and the part of the Roman population able to afford these often expensive vintages. This chapter will try to integrate the isolated and fragmentary information on beverages other than wine into a single description of drinking habits in the Roman world.[1]

Diet

Classical sources may give an indication of the omnipresence of wine and the different vintages produced, but they are far less clear as to who had access to wine, to what kind of wine and how often. There is little interesting in stories of wealthy gourmands like Trimalchio drinking considerable quantities of the best wines with every meal (Petron., *Sat.* 34), if the consumption patterns of the (far more numerous) lower classes completely escape us. Therefore, in order to give wine its due place among other drinks available to Romans, I will first isolate a number of closely intertwined factors affecting consumption patterns (von Reden, 2007, 385).

Location, location, location

The most important factor for drinking patterns is the productive capacity of the region. The apparent homogeneity of the Mediterranean might be misleading when discussing the role of beverages in diet and nutrition, because although some crops (including vines) were largely ubiquitous, local variations in ecology, climate and geology resulted in large differences in production and the development of various consumption patterns (Horden and Purcell, 2000; Morley, 2007, 22). Microclimates and regional variety can be found between mountain and plain or between coastal region and hinterland. The result of this wide range of environmental factors was, for instance, a remarkable diversity in flavour and alcohol percentage of wines and different acquired tastes: most people only drank local vintages, because due to high transport costs, wine-producing regions only imported wines during severe shortages or to meet the elite demand for exotic, luxurious wine.

Large parts of the Roman Empire, however, were not suited for viticulture or had never grown wine before the arrival of the Romans. People there had developed other alcoholic drinks, including beer, mead and cider (Tchernia, 1986, 11–19; Columella, *Rust.* 12.12; Plin., *HN* 14.102–104 and 113), or simply drank milk and water. Even though the Roman elite scorned the consumption of milk and beer as typical for barbaric nomads, pastoral mountaineers and societies on the (both cultural and geographical) perimeter of civilization (Shaw, 1982–1983; Garnsey, 1999, 66–68; Nelson, 2003), these beverages continued to play a considerable role in Italian and provincial diets. Fresh milk was drunk throughout antiquity wherever available (Columella, *Rust.* 7.6.4), and Pliny offers a long list of animals whose milk could be consumed (Plin., *HN* 28.123–124.). Beer on the other hand found few enthusiasts in Italy (except in Liguria, according to Strabo 4.6.2), but was highly appreciated in Celtic societies, Egypt and Mesopotamia. Despite the fact that it met with increasing competition from more prestigious wine consumption, in particular in response to indigenous elite demand and after the introduction of local viticulture, it remained a common drink in the provinces throughout the early Empire, only to slowly decline from the third century onwards (Drexhage, 1997; Ruffing, 2001). Nevertheless, people who could not afford to buy wine continued to drink beer (Ath. 4.152c; Amm. Marc. 26.8.2).

Often absent in studies of Roman consumption patterns is water (apart from that used to mix with wine), perhaps for fear of stating the obvious or because water consumption has been considered low due to the risks of infection (but wine was not always a particularly safe and healthy alternative, as additives included chalk, marble dust and ash (Ruffing, 1997)!). Nevertheless, classical authors were perfectly aware of the necessary attributes of good drinking water, the challenges of keeping it clean and the danger of consuming putrefied water (Alcock, 2006, 92; Plin., *HN* 31.16 and 31–72). In his attack on drunkenness, Pliny reproaches mankind with his longing for extravagancies in the consumption of wine, 'as if nature had not provided us with water as a beverage, the one, in fact, all other animals drink' (Plin., *HN* 14.28). Similar, Augustus referred people to the water supplied by the aqueducts when wine had become scarce and expensive (Suet., *Aug.* 42.1). A trustworthy supply of water was indispensable for Roman villas, villages and towns (Marzano, 2007, 165–171; Plin., *Ep.* 2.17). Most settlements relied on natural supply systems (wells, rain water and, if present in the vicinity, rivers and lakes), but

Romans also went to great lengths to improve the urban water supply through the construction of delivery and storage infrastructure (aqueducts, distribution towers, fountain houses, cisterns and tanks to collect rain and spring water) (Bruun, 1991; Hodge, 1992). Our best information on the infrastructure and organization of urban water supply systems evidently comes from Pompeii (De Haan and Jansen, 1996). The major challenge was to prevent water from becoming polluted, contaminated or warmed up. Most citizens therefore used wells, because the water, covered from the sun, is in constant agitation and filtered by the earth (Plin., *HN* 31.38. Schmölder-Veit, 2009; Richard, 2012). How important water was in the Roman diet is impossible to establish. Even if we could approach the average per capita consumption of water provided by the aqueducts (which seems hardly feasible, as most water may have run through unused), we would still be unable to distinguish between the usage for cooking, washing, cleaning and drinking. To elites, the habit of drinking water was so peculiar that it could be turned into a rhetorical invective ([Plut], *Par.* 19; Dem. 6.30), but for the urban poor, water was the cheapest solution to quench one's thirst (1 *Tim.* 5.23).

Distribution

In Rome, only a limited amount of beverages was fit to be transported over long distances. Beer, for instance, was produced without hops, resulting in an ale with considerable residue, which easily went off (Drexhage, 1997; Laubenheimer et al., 2003; Alcock, 2006, 90–91). This is why military settlements along the northern frontier (a prime market for beer), such as the Batavian auxiliaries in Vindolanda, probably had their own regimental brewers who purchased the ingredients on the local market (Birley, 1997). Milk was consumed primarily in the countryside, in the vicinity of the herds, because without refrigeration milk can only be kept fresh for a very limited period. Small quantities appear to have been available in cities: a Pompeian terracotta shop sign showing a goat might have indicated a bar where milk was sold (Mau, 1899, 379), but prices were probably high (see below). The only drink that could be shipped over considerable distances was wine and a number of by-products of viticulture, such as must, often boiled down to sweet syrups (*defrutum* and *sapa*; Plin., *HN* 14.83–85; Beltrán Lloris, 2000) and vinegar, which, mixed with water and herbs, was a typical drink for Roman soldiers, but also for rural slaves and the urban poor (Marlière and Torres Costa, 2005; Alcock, 2006, 91; Plaut., *Mil.* 836). Powerful drivers for the Roman wine trade were the military supply system, particular tastes and conspicuous consumption (such as the Roman elite's preference for high quality Greek vintages), but above all the increasing urban demand as a consequence of population growth and urbanization. A major part of the wine trade was aimed at supplying the capital with cheap wine from the Italian hinterland and the provinces (De Sena, 2005). Until Aurelian in the 270s decided to include wine distributions in the urban supply system, most citizens of Rome purchased their drinks on the market, in bars and taverns (SHA, *Aur.* 35.2, 48.1). Some people also received wine rations via non-market exchange. Elites sent each other amphorae as gifts (Cic., 2*Verr.* 4.62) and fed their household from the wine produced on their estates (Whittaker, 1985; Tchernia, 1987). The conquest of the Mediterranean had made the top tier of Rome immensely rich, and some of this wealth trickled down to their clients, freedmen and slaves.

Purchasing power and social inequality

Patterns of consumption are intimately related to spending power, in particular when the consumer can practically choose from a large diversity of beverages, ranging from free drinks (water and sometimes milk) to expensive alternatives. For Rome, per capita income has been estimated at somewhere between one and a half and two times subsistence on average (Hopkins, 2002, 197–203).[2] This leaves little room for luxurious spending or even occasional treats. Recent discussions of wages and income distribution confirm that for the majority of the Roman population, living standards were very modest and consumption was limited to the bare essentials for survival (Allen, 2009; Scheidel and Friesen, 2009; Scheidel, 2010). Using the notion of consumption baskets to approach Roman living standards, Allen and Scheidel have shown that a respectability basket (that of skilled labourers) could include an annual consumption of 68.25 litres of wine (or 0.18 litre per day), but that this basket was largely unaffordable for unskilled wage labourers. A bare bones subsistence basket, which was more in line with the wages earned, excludes wine altogether. Life was probably not much different in the countryside: occasional bad harvests could force farmers to sell all wine produced on their plot of land to raise money for taxation and other costs and made them turn to water and milk instead (Wilkins and Hill, 2006, 39, 52). Although these guesstimates entail a substantial degree of uncertainty and sometimes underestimate contributions to the family budget by other relatives, the conclusion must be that wine was not always nor for everyone affordable (see below). A list of purchases (if that really is the purpose of the inscription) made by a Pompeian citizen during eight days and recording day by day the food items and the price paid (*CIL* 4.5380), points in the same direction: wine was bought on three days only, in small quantities and for a total sum of 23 asses (compare with 66 asses for bread and porridge). The frustrating problem is that we have no idea about the spending power of the writer or the number of people to be fed with the shopping. Additional circumstantial evidence for rather limited levels of wine consumption can perhaps be found in the organization of the supply system. If wine really was being drunk in such huge quantities by the urban masses as is sometimes claimed, it is remarkable that the Roman supply system only started with wine distributions late in the third century (contrary to grain and oil) (Chastagnol, 1950; Cracco Ruggini, 1988; Lo Cascio, 1999). Are we to assume that until then the market was perfectly capable of supplying Rome without imperial support, or that consumption in reality was not as high as some authors argue, and that intervention was only required when in the turmoil of the third century the private market apparently failed to bring sufficient quantities to the capital?

In response to the limited spending power of the majority of the population, most bars mainly served low quality vintages, although some innkeepers may have stored a small selection of better quality vintages for the more demanding customer (Tchernia, 2000; Cic., *Pis.* 27). The famous notice written at the entrance of a Pompeian bar for instance lists three different wines: cheap wine for one as, better wine for two asses and Falernian for four (*CIL* 4.1679). More famous wines, especially those imported from the provinces, evidently only reached the tables of the rich. An exception should perhaps be made for Rome, where recipients of grain and later oil distributions could spend a larger share of their income on better drinks than cheap plonk, if only occasionally and in limited quantities (Morley, 1996, 57).

Ideology and taste

Because the quality of beverages was reflected in price levels, it is evident that people tried to articulate their identity and standing through consumption. First, the civic hierarchy in Roman society resulted in distinctive drinking patterns. Different beverages filled the cups of master and slave. The large variety of local and imported wines available on the urban market allowed wine consumption in particular to mirror wealth and prestige (Tchernia, 1986, 28–37). Martial wittily recommends not to touch wine of inferior quality, but to give it to one's freedman

(13.121), and Plutarch reports that only Cato's renowned penchant for simplicity could explain why he transgressed the socially accepted forms of behaviour by drinking of the same wine as his slaves (*Vit. Cat. Mai.* 3.1 and 4.3). Second, within the Roman Empire consumption preferences changed through the process of Romanization. The conquest of the Mediterranean and the arrival of foreign settlers with different tastes went hand in hand with the spread of wine drinking, initially by importing Italian wines for the elites, and later with the development of local viticulture (Los, 1997 for Crete; Pena and Barreda, 1997 for Spain). Egypt, for instance, started to intensify its grape cultivation from the Alexandrian conquest onwards, but production and consumption intensified especially under Roman rule (Clarysse and Vandorpe, 1997; Ruffing, 2001). Gallic tribal chiefs famously developed a considerable appetite for wine in the early days of the conquest of Gaul, which ultimately stimulated the introduction of local viticulture (Diod. Sic. 5.26.3). By the third century most provinces had eventually more or less adapted to Roman drinking patterns and local viticulture then catered for the demand (Morley, 2007, 98).

Nutrition

The four factors described above lead to the conclusion that not every Roman drank wine at all occasions and that one's prestige and above all purchasing power determined when and what kind of wine could be consumed. This may seem a disappointing truism, but it has major consequences for the nutritional contributions wine and other beverages could make to the Roman diet. It is generally assumed that wine played a considerable role in satisfying nutritional requirements, because it was one of the main supplements in the Mediterranean cereal-dominated diet (Foxhall and Forbes, 1982). Some additives to wine, such as honey and herbs, could further increase calorie intake. Nevertheless, trying to assess the proportionate consumption levels of wine and other beverages and their caloric values remains extremely hazardous.

First of all, we have very little and controversial evidence to measure the annual consumption levels of wine. Horace recommends half a litre to accompany one's dinner (*Sat.* 1.1.74), but is this the amount of wine appropriate for the elite and perhaps difficult to afford by ordinary citizens? Association members in Rome received 1.6 litre at common meals and festivities (*CIL* 6.10234), but this figure has little to say about daily rations when members did not meet. Equally unhelpful is the total annual wine consumption for slaves suggested by Cato (around 260 litres or approximately 0.71 litre a day), as this only applies to adult male slaves engaged in heavy physical labour (*Agr.* 57; Etienne, 1981). Manual workers required a special diet to fuel their hard labour (Wilkins and Hill, 2006, 61), and it is no coincidence that for grain, Cato recommends that slave workers should receive larger rations than the overseer (*Agr.* 56). It is also important to stress that Cato's slaves were working on a wine-producing estate, which may have been the most important reason for their considerable wine consumption. Horace's lands were not suited for viticulture, and consequently his bailiff did not drink wine (Hor., *Epist.* 1.14; Tchernia, 1986, 20). This begs the question whether people who did not receive wine from a master or patron, but had to purchase their drinks on the market, would also arrive at a similarly large consumption. Finally, and perhaps most importantly, we can never be certain whether or not the figures cited refer to unmixed or diluted wine. Most guesstimates therefore confront the ancient evidence with comparative data from medieval and early modern Italy, which, however, only suggest that consumption was probably well above contemporary levels, but also fluctuated heavily over time (Tchernia, 1986, 21–27). The result is a particularly wide spectrum of estimates, ranging from zero litres in the bare bones consumption basket to 182 litres for adult males in the city of Rome (Tchernia, 1986, 26). A consensus seems to exist for an annual consumption level of approximately 100 litres for the population at large (Purcell, 1985; Jongman, 2007a), but given the more recent evidence of the role of wine in premodern consumption baskets, this figure now seems overstated.

Second, calorie intake varies considerably depending on the particular vintage consumed. It has been argued recently that a consumption of 100 litres of wine would provide adults with no less than 25 per cent of the annual calorie intake (Jongman, 2007a, 603). However, to arrive at this high figure, only the consumption of sweet, white wines has been taken into account, because apparently these wines were favoured by Roman customers. It is true that the high sugar content in these wines results in a higher calorie intake per unit, and a preference for sweet, white wines can indeed be culled from the literary sources, but they only describe the elite consumption of expensive and often imported grands crus, which are without exception white and sweet (Tchernia, 1986, 109, 204–205, 342–357). Jongman duly recognizes that red or dry white wines offer far fewer calories. The nutrient database of the United States Department of Agriculture helps to illustrate the considerable differences in the caloric and nutritional value of beverages (http://ndb.nal.usda.gov/ndb/search [accessed 17 March 2015]). Table 12.1 shows, first, that in the countryside caloric requirements could more easily be met through the consumption of milk, rather than wine. Additionally, milk also has a considerably higher nutritional value than wine, providing high quantities of lipids, vitamins and minerals. In regions with intensive cattle raising and easy access to milk, only the tastiness of wine but above all the better opportunities for preservation must have induced people to consume wine. Second, the figures indicate that sweet dessert and raisin wines indeed contain 50% more calories than common table wines and could provide a major supplement to the Roman cereal diet. The question remains how often ordinary citizens would have been able to consume these high-calorie wines.

First, the literary sources clearly suggest that the urban poor consumed rather sour, red wines such as those produced in Veii (Mart. 1.103.9), or even 'wine substitutes'. According to Pliny, lower classes drank beverages made from pressed and soaked grape skins (*lora*) or from the dregs of wine pressing (*faecatum*) and called these (perhaps out of wishful thinking) 'workmen's wine' (*vinum operarium*) (Plin., *HN* 14.86; Columella, *Rust.* 12.40). Cato and Varro also mention that *lora* instead of wine could be issued to labourers and farm hands (Cato, *Agr.* 25; Varro, *Rust.* 1.54). Pliny elsewhere elaborates on the Roman (elite?) taste for sweet, raisin wine, which is preferred to all other vintages, but at the same time twice notes that a second quality version is produced by diluting the raisin wine (perhaps destined for the masses?) (Plin., *HN* 14.81–82). It seems that for the majority of the population, a big gap must have existed between personal preferences and actual purchasing power.

Table 12.1 Beverages and calories, based on the nutrient database of the USDA

Beverage	kcal per fl oz (=29.57 ml)
sweet dessert wine	47
table wine (late harvest)	34
milk (sheep)	31
table wine (red)	25
table wine (white)	24
milk (goat)	21
beer (regular)	13
water	0

A second approach, based on archaeological excavations in Rome and Ostia and an assessment of the productive capacity of the Italian hinterland, tends to corroborate this conclusion. The model of wine imports in the capital in the early second century, developed by De Sena, clearly illustrates the role of cheap wine from the provinces in urban consumption (De Sena, 2005; see Table 12.2): Gallic and Spanish red, low-quality wines outnumber the sweet wines from the Greek isles (Tchernia, 1986, 179–184; Mart. 1.26). Recent archaeological surveys have confirmed that Roman villas in the central part of the Rhône valley were equipped for mass production of cheap wine and show a clear peak in production infrastructure during the first two centuries AD (Jung et al., 2001). Africa also produced a very sweet raisin wine, but it was distributed in small quantities only, judging by the size of the amphorae and their rare occurrence in the archaeological records (Plin., *HN* 14.81; Lequément, 1980).

The nature of the Italian wines reaching the taverns of Rome is more difficult to establish, but it is possible that the import of low quality wine from the provinces encouraged local production of similar vintages, for production in the vicinity of the market was definitely cheaper than import (Purcell, 1985). Moreover, sweet raisin wines give low yields and require considerable labour investments, resulting in high prices and a limited clientele. Italian viticulture seems to have adapted to the increasing demand for cheaper wines and gradually moved towards the production of light, dry wines (Tchernia, 1986, 208). Tchernia, Patterson and Marzano, for instance, see a connection between the introduction of a smaller Italian wine amphora type (the Spello form), made from the mid-first century until the late second century, and the increasing production of low quality wine for Rome, because this wine easily spoiled and was only fit for immediate consumption (Tchernia, 1986, 253–256; Patterson, 2006, 63; Marzano, 2007, 165–166, n. 42). Morley also points out that the agriculturists' concern over viticulture shows a remarkable shift in focus: whereas Cato and Varro tried to find the best vine for the estate's soil, Columella, writing during the first century, also encourages the cultivation of high-yield vines of inferior quality for mass consumption (Morley, 1996, 118). Archaeology has shown that the increasing demand for cheap wine during the late Republican and Julio-Claudian period is also reflected in the construction of new agricultural estates and the installation of more presses (Marzano, 2013a).

Another, although circumstantial, indicator of the prevalence of low quality vintages in Italian distribution and consumption is the considerable attention devoted by Roman jurists to wine's tendency to go off (Frier, 1983). Sweet, white wines with a high sugar and alcohol percentage are more resilient to contamination and can easily age in the amphorae they had been stored in. The frequent references in the literary sources to the aging of wine therefore only describe what was stored in the wine cellars of the elite, rather than suggest the wide availability and consumption of high quality wines (Galen, *De Ant.* 14.15 and 25–26; Plin., *HN* 14.6.55-57; Mart. 8.15). The wine amphora assemblages studied during the DAI-AAR excavations in Ostia present a similar picture (Martin, 2008), even though a few caveats apply for the evolution into late antiquity. The table for Ostia represents in the first place a decline in wine amphora use in Italy and Gaul, in favour of bulk transport in barrels and container ships, rather than a reduced consumption of wines from these regions (Marlière, 2002; Heslin, 2011; see Table 12.3). The high quality wines from the eastern Mediterranean, however, continued to be imported in smaller quantities and thus in amphorae. As far as we know, the wines from the Eastern Mediterranean have never been shipped in barrels, container ships or hides, so they tend to be overrepresented in the ceramic assemblages compared to the actual consumption (Lemaître, 1998). This bias in the archaeological record also explains the remarkable amount of Greek wine amphorae in Pompeii compared to Italian containers. Frescoes, how-ever, show how local wines arrived in the city in large hides (Kneissl, 1981). Furthermore, the

Table 12.2 Wine imports in Rome (De Sena, 2005)

Origin	Litres and percentages
Sicily	800,000 (0.47%)
North-Africa	700,000 (0.41%)
Crete	3,500,000 (2.09%)
Rhodes	2,700,000 (1.61%)
Anatolia	3,700,000 (2.21%)
Egypt	200,000 (0.11%)
Tarraconensis	3,500,000 (2.09%)
Narbonensis	19,700,000 (11.78%)
Total provinces	*34,800,000 (20.81%)*
Etruria-Umbria	43,800,000 (26.19%)
Adriatic	10,200,000 (6.10%)
Phlegrean-Naples	3,500,000 (2.09%)
Roman hinterland	54,000,000 (32.29%)
Total Italy	*111,500,000 (66.68%)*
Unknown	*20,900,000 (12.5%)*

Table 12.3 Wine imports in Ostia (Martin, 2008)

Origin	50–100	100–150	280–350
Italy	58%	61%	22%
Southern Gaul	28%	21%	14%
Eastern Mediterranean	7%	15%	64%
Iberia	7%	2%	0%
North Africa	0%	1%	0%

imports in Ostia do not necessarily mirror the consumption in Rome: a large part of the wine consumed in the capital had been transported from the hinterland in containers no longer visible, and part of the imports in Ostia would be exported to other port cities.

Finally, the consumption of sweet wines by the urban masses can be approached through their price levels in relation to the ordinary citizens' spending power. Diocletian's Price Edict offers a good starting point to compare relative prices for beverages (*Ed.* 2.1–12; 6.95). Sweet, flavoured or even decent quality wine appears to be at least twice, but more often thrice, as expensive as ordinary table wine (see Table 12.4). It seems highly unlikely that ordinary citizens, even when being able to afford a respectability basket with wine included, would prefer to spend the share of their income reserved for wine purchases on high quality wine, instead of buying a larger quantity of ordinary wine. Only one of Martial's epigrams could point to lower price levels for sweet Cretan wines, as he calls them 'the honeyed wine of the poor' (13.106). This is quite remarkable, because Pliny considers Cretan raisin wine the best one available in Italy (*HN* 14.81). Whether or not his judgement is trustworthy (Martial seems to have a predilection for home-grown Italian wines), the price of some Cretan vintages on the Roman market may have been less expensive than expected, because the isle was located on the supply route followed by the

Table 12.4 Beverages in Diocletian's Price Edict

Beverage	Price (*in* denarii communes *per* sextarius, *approximately half a litre*)
high quality wine	30
must boiled down (*caroenum*)	30
Attic wine	24
spiced, honeyed wine (*conditum*)	24
aged wine, first quality	24
must boiled down (*defrutum*)	20
wine mixed with absinth	20
rose wine	20
aged wine, second quality	16
must boiled down (*decoctum*)	16
ordinary wine	8
sheep's milk	8
beer	4
Egyptian beer	2

grain freighters sailing from Alexandria, which could have taken aboard wine amphorae as a supplementary cargo and thus indirectly subsidized transport costs. Moreover, Augustus had donated land in the vicinity of Cnossos to the city of Capua and Italian settlers in Crete are known to have engaged in wine production and export, which again could have increased the number of amphorae exported and resulted in lower price levels (Chaniotis, 1988). Nevertheless, confronted with the otherwise overwhelming evidence showing that imported sweet wines were quite expensive, it seems better not to put too much weight on Martial's derisory remark. This is not to say that urban masses never found an opportunity to taste sweet wine. Occasional purchases to celebrate special events were probably affordable for people with a respectability basket. Middling groups able to meet the expenses of joining religious and occupational associations perhaps drank sweet wines during festivities, provided this is meant by the guild law requiring new members to donate an "amphora of good wine" (*CIL* 14.2112). That the magistrates expected wine of decent quality, might suggest that the association members were more accustomed to drink cheap, common wine. The poor on the other hand had the best chance of receiving honeyed wine during the occasional distributions by benefactors, who thus found an opportunity to translate wine surpluses into social prestige and recognition (Patterson, 2006, 172–173; *CIL* 9.2226; 10.4727; 11.2911). However, as munificence was an urban phenomenon, people in the countryside were less often treated with these distributions.

Conclusion

Real income sets the limits for spending and consumption patterns, which in turn determine people's living standards, caloric and nutritional intake and ultimately health. This is why historians have always been very keen on reconstructing wages, price levels and diets. Ancient historians face a difficult challenge, because our evidence rarely offers us more than a glimpse of common living standards. Literary sources are hopelessly biased towards elite preferences and consumption patterns and virtually ignore the eating and drinking habits of ordinary Romans. In this chapter, I have argued that as a result of this bias, consumption levels of wine by non-elites may have been overstated. An approach based on incomes, purchasing power and consumption baskets appears more promising. It seems that a considerable share of the urban masses could only afford wine occasionally and in small quantities. In the respectability basket, which was largely unaffordable for unskilled wage labourers, people consumed only 0.18 litre of wine per day. Some may have received additional quantities of wine during occasional redistributions by their patrons or civic benefactors, or shared a cup of decent wine during the festivities of associations. Equally important when discussing diet and nutrition is the kind of wine people tended to drink, especially when trying to assess the contribution of beverages to the daily calorie intake and nutrition. Despite many uncertainties and sometimes conflicting evidence, most of the wine consumed was cheap table wine, providing only a limited amount of calories and nutrition. Red table wine guarantees 25 calories per 29.57 ml or 845.45 calories per litre. With a consumption of 0.18 litre per day, drinking wine resulted in 152.18 calories. Whether one takes into account the total amount of calories the consumption basket could buy (1,940: Allen, 2009) or the daily requirements for moderately or very active males (2,852 and 3,337: Foxhall and Forbes, 1982), wine was responsible for respectively 7.8%, 5.3% or 4.5% of the daily intake. Many difficulties remain, but for the majority of the Romans, wine must only have been an occasional supplement to the cereal-based diet, and nothing more. That wine consumption nevertheless features so prominently in our sources, can ultimately be related to the elite nature of literary texts, limited preservation techniques for other beverages and the cultural value of wine in the Mediterranean identity.

Notes

1 Medicinal uses of beverages will not be discussed. See Wilkins and Hill, 2006, 213–244.
2 I am rather sceptical about some of the evidence (including wages for municipal scribes and annuities left to freedmen and foster children in legal sources) adduced by Jongman (2007a, 601), to argue in favour of wages well above subsistence level (nearly four to eight times subsistence), as these sources may only capture income levels of socially and economically superior groups.

13

MEAT AND OTHER ANIMAL PRODUCTS

Michael MacKinnon

Given our biological need for food, any reconstruction of this basic necessity for past societies must consider the range of materials available to, and exploited by humans. Although vegetarian resources arguably comprised the bulk of the ancient Roman diet across the empire, meat and other animal products, including fat, milk, cheese, and eggs, were also consumed. Moreover, as with many foodstuffs, their contribution fluctuated temporally, geographically, environmentally and socioculturally. A wider appreciation of the types of animal resources available, the variation among scales of production in raising, herding, manipulating, and using these animals, and the host of techniques involved in the acquisition, preparation, and consumption of edible products from these animals helps provide a more nuanced reconstruction of the ancient Roman diet across time and space.

Historians and archaeologists predominantly reconstruct patterns of animal consumption through several means. First, ancient textual and epigraphic evidence, in the form of recipes, menus, price lists, descriptions of meals, and tales about banquets, feasts, sacrifices and other events involving foodstuffs, provide pertinent information.[1] Second, images of animals, as livestock, butchered carcasses, or prepared cuts of meat, survive in ancient visual culture. Finally, analyses of recovered faunal remains from Roman archaeological sites yield evidence about the contribution of animals and their resources to ancient life.[2] Each source contains various strengths and biases, thus enforcing the need to successfully contextualize these data, in light of the assorted factors that created or shaped each component. In extracting meaning from Roman texts and iconography, for example, one must engage with issues such as (i) the intended audience, (ii) the skill set or acumen of the author/artist, (iii) the degree to which the work is original, copied, accurate, reliable, imagined, embellished or otherwise, and (iv) associated temporal, regional and cultural biases that underscore the creation, practice and purpose of textual and visual media. Similarly, faunal remains must be assessed within frameworks that consider the range of cultural and natural depositional and post-depositional factors impinging upon the creation, transformation and collection of archaeological materials. Although challenges surround the use of each dataset – bones, texts, art – interdisciplinary exploration ultimately affords a more holistic assessment. Drawing upon each, but with particular attention to the ancient textual and zooarchaeological records,[3] this chapter seeks to provide an overview of our understanding of the contribution of meat and other animal products in the ancient Roman diet. What animals were eaten, and in what proportions? What products were used and how did their exploitation vary over time, across space, and among cultural groups? How were animal resources acquired, processed, preserved, prepared, and ultimately consumed? And how might such actions inform us about social and cultural aspects such as identity, ethnicity, religion, and status? Such questions form the basis of analysis.

Meat and other animal products as referenced in the ancient sources

Discussion of the contribution of meat and other animal products in the Roman diet requires, as a foundation, some context about Roman meals.[4] Among the Roman system, cheese, and to some degree eggs, could register within the menu of various meals (i.e., breakfast, lunch, dinner – *ientaculum*, *prandium* and *cena*, respectively), and seem to have been available more broadly to a greater span of social classes. Meat was generally absent from the breakfast menu, regardless of social class, but could, for those who could afford it, form part of the lunch menu (as a type of cold cut, perhaps), or register as a central component of dinner. Doubtless, many poorer households could not acquire meat on a regular basis, while many individuals likely subsisted near the poverty line, perhaps only consuming one meal a day, with little, if any, meat factoring (Plaut., *Men.* 3.1.457–458; [Verg.], *Mor.* 55–59).

The Romans graded foodstuffs in terms of nourishment and digestibility, and strove to maintain some dietary balance, where possible. Celsus, the Roman encyclopaedist, known for his medical treatise *De medicina* (first century AD) rates meat of all domestic quadrupeds and all large game (such as deer, wild boar, and wild goat) among 'the strongest' (i.e., more nutritious) of foodstuffs (Celsus, *Med.* 2.18.2). Subcategories are identified. Beef, for example, ranks higher than pork; larger wild animals surpass their smaller equivalents; younger animals score less than adult ones; wild animals rate lower than their domestic counterparts (Celsus, *Med.* 2.18.7–8, 2.19.7). Fat content was particularly prized. Fat meat contained more nutriment than lean meat, and parts of the animal carcass were scored accordingly (Celsus, *Med.* 2.18.8-10). Less fatty sections such as the feet and heads of pigs and lambs are rated less nutritious than other parts of these animals (Celsus, *Med.* 2.18.8). Fresh meat ranked superior to salted and stale meat, while stewed meat was believed to be better than roasted, with boiled meat at the bottom (Celsus, *Med.* 2.19.10). As regards other animal resources, cheese ranks as importantly as meat among 'strong' foodstuffs, while milk was regarded as one of the most nutritious liquids (Celsus, *Med.* 2.18.11).

If the Romans followed Celsus' scheme dutifully, then those who had access to animal products and desired optimum nutrition might be expected to consume freshly stewed, fairly fat, selected pieces of meat from domestic animals. Cheese would also be regularly eaten; milk less so, unless it could be preserved somehow. Nevertheless, Celsus' system says little about the taste of meat or animal products, and nothing of the expense involved in acquiring and preparing such materials. A survey of the wider body of ancient texts provides further details. Important sources in this regard include the culinary recipes collated within the 'cookbook' (*De re coquinaria*) of Apicius, and descriptions of assorted foodstuffs recounted in examples of dinner parties or similar venues (be these real or fictional) within Roman texts. Price lists (such as Diocletian's Price Edict of AD 301) and comparable records linked to transactions, supply networks, taxation accounts, etc., yield further data on costs of various animals, meat cuts, and products.

Overall, available textual sources provide minimal information about consumption of beef, veal, and other cattle products for Roman antiquity. Apicius (5.1–4) lists several recipes for veal, fewer for beef. The latter appears to have been relatively inexpensive; Diocletian's Price Edict documents beef at only 8 *denarii* per pound, while most other meats sold for at least

12 *denarii* per pound (*Ed. Diocl.* 4.2). Cow's milk and cheese seem to comprise only a small proportion of the overall diet across the wider Mediterranean region, but with isolated mention of more regular consumption in select regions of Greece (e.g., Arcadia) and northern regions of the empire (Apic. 4.1.1–3). Columella alludes to reserving cow's milk for calves (Col. 6.24.4–5).

As regards sheep and goats, Apicius (8.6.1–11) lists eleven recipes for lamb or kid, one for mutton, but none for adult goat. Clearly a dietary preference for younger sheep and goats registers, reflected within pricing as well. Mutton and goat's meat cost 8 *denarii* per pound; lamb and kid fetched 12 *denarii* per pound (*Ed. Diocl.* 4.3, 4.47–48). Although Varro (*Rust.* 2.11.1, 3) rates goat's milk (and cheese) as less nourishing than that of sheep, the capacity of the goat to provide abundant milk is noted among several ancient authors (Plin., *HN* 8.76.202; Verg., *Ed.* 7.34, *G.* 3.308–310; Hor., *Epist.* 16.49–50). Presumably, large quantities of sheep and goat milk were converted to cheese, where prices of up to 8 *denarii* per pound for fresh cheese and 12 *denarii* per pound for dried cheese are recorded (*Ed. Diocl.* 5.11, 6.95–96).

Pigs were popularly consumed in Roman antiquity, especially in Italy. 'Who of our people runs a farm without keeping swine?' rhetorically asks the agricultural writer Varro (*Rust.* 2.4.3). Practically all Roman farmers, it seems, from small-scale peasants to wealthy agriculturalists and herders, kept pigs. The animal may also have been raised, to some degree, in urban settings, in backyard pens or even rummaging the streets consuming garbage (MacKinnon, 2001). The assortment of parts eaten, from head to foot, coupled with the diversity in preparing, seasoning and presenting dishes involving pork products validates its importance. Indeed, among livestock exploited in antiquity, literary evidence notes that only pigs were deliberately reared for the table. Apicius lists more recipes involving pig products than any other animal. Pliny (*HN* 8.77.209) comments that no other animal provides a larger number of materials for the diet. Such a role certainly affected husbandry operations. To accommodate demands, the Romans enhanced pig production to exploit schemes of raising and marketing them exclusively for consumption across the empire. By contrast, cattle, sheep, and goats were principally exploited for their secondary resources, such as traction, wool, and milk; most were consumed as older unproductive animals, after they had contributed in other economic capacities.[5]

Poultry birds, dominated largely by domestic fowl, were also popular commodities in Roman antiquity both as a source of meat and as a supplier of eggs. The ancient sources, particularly the agricultural writers, document tactics to maximize breeding, combat disease, and incubate eggs, among a host of particulars involved in raising and maintaining wild and domestic barnyard fowl (Kron, 2014a, 119).

Scarce ancient textual evidence exists to suggest that ancient Romans consumed other domestic animals beyond cattle, sheep, goat, pig, and fowl. No explicit mention of specifically Roman populations consuming dogs or cats occurs among the Latin texts, although this need not imply that other cultural groups refrained from eating these species, particularly dog, during antiquity.[6] Donkeys and mules were typically not eaten, but exceptions do register in the occasional delicacy involving either taxon (Plin., *HN* 8.69.170–174; Mart. 13.97). Horses were generally not deemed edible, at least among Roman cultures,[7] but could be consumed if famine circumstances warranted, notably among armies in battle (Tac., *Hist.* 4.60).

Among wild game eaten, a range of types is noted. While hunting them in person held prestige (especially for larger animals), game could also be purchased at the urban markets, if desired and when supplied (MacKinnon, 2004, 212–215). Nonetheless, it was relatively expensive. Prices for meat from wild boar, red deer, roe deer, and wild goat ranged from 12–16 *denarii* per pound; rabbit and hare were costly at up to 150 *denarii* (amounts unspecified), while dormice fetched up to 4 *denarii* apiece (*Ed. Diocl.* 4.32–33, 38, 43–45).

Clearly, the Romans placed great pride in presenting and consuming meat and other animal products among menu items, and established systems by which commodities were priced and ranked according to relative worth, taste, nutrient value, and accessibility, among other criteria. Nonetheless, while ancient texts provide a list of different types of animals consumed and parts that were edible, they supply no explicit details about how much and what types of meat, milk, cheese, eggs and other animal resources were eaten, or how contributions varied culturally and temporally. For that we must turn to zooarchaeological evidence.

Meat and other animal products in the zooarchaeological record

Zooarchaeological data provide perhaps our best measure with which to quantify what was being consumed in Roman antiquity, and to examine temporal and regional patterns across the empire. Mammals, birds, and fish typically comprise the bulk of faunal assemblages from ancient sites. Variations exist in proportions of each category, however, depending on aspects such as type of site (e.g., rural/urban, rich/poor, Roman/non-Roman, etc.), timeframe of investigation (e.g., domestic fowl tend to be more common among Roman sites than pre-Roman sites), and geographic location (e.g., sites near the coast tend to have higher relative frequencies of fish).[8] Even if meat comprised only a small part of the popular diet, zooarchaeological data highlight predominance of domestic taxa, and especially domestic livestock (i.e., cattle, sheep/goat, pig, and domestic fowl) among meats more commonly and universally consumed. Although wild game was eaten, this practice tends to signify elite consumption in Roman antiquity. Fish, and especially fresh fish, are also generally connected with higher status diets.[9] On average, wild game and fish normally account for less than 5% of the identified bones from zooarchaeological assemblages from Roman sites empire-wide; in many instances their values are much lower than this baseline.[10]

Figure 13.1 provides mean NISP frequency values of cattle, sheep/goat, and pig as recorded across sites among broad geographic regions of the ancient Roman world between generalized 'Pre-Roman/Iron Age' and 'Roman' temporal periods.[11] Typically, these taxa dominate faunal assemblages among most Roman sites, and their relative contributions provide a good measure to assess temporal and regional variation in animal husbandry schemes that affect (and in turn are affected by) dietary and cultural frameworks in the transition to Roman times. Patterns fluctuate, and each region and timeframe contains examples where individual sites, for a variety of reasons, may counter overall trends.

Certainly, at one level, regional climates and topographies assume roles in the representation of taxa over time and space. Cattle, for example, thrive in European lowlands, a condition that typically accounts for their relatively higher frequencies among ancient sites in northern regions. Roman occupation in these regions seems to augment this production to some degree, with the relative frequency of cattle increasing, on average, among all types of sites. Similarly, drier conditions, coupled with its critical importance as a cereal-producing zone – an agricultural scheme in which cattle would compete directly with available arable land – combined to limit, or restrict many large-scale cattle herding ventures in Mediterranean areas. Sheep are better suited to North African and Near Eastern scrublands, an environmental compatibility no doubt favouring their exploitation in those areas. Again, Roman presence in eastern regions of the empire acted to promote sheep/goat pastoralism (i.e., a strategy that was better suited to local environmental conditions) to a greater degree, largely at the expense of cattle in these cases. Nevertheless, while environments certainly affect animal ecologies, it is important to recognize that husbandry patterns and human diets are not determined exclusively by such agents; cultures shape these too. This interaction of nature and culture registers well as regards pigs during

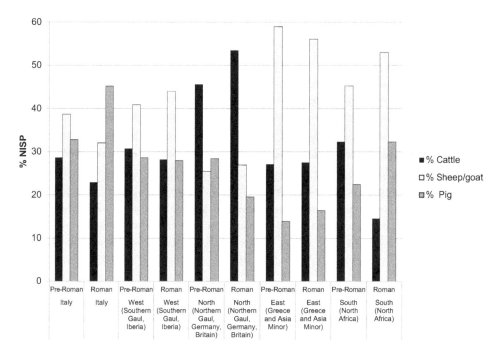

Figure 13.1 NISP frequency of cattle, sheep/goat and pig among geographic regions between 'Pre-Roman' and 'Roman' temporal frameworks.

Roman times. Pork was a popular meat for Romans in many areas, arguably helping to connect, bind, or otherwise shape identities and social networks. Exploitation and promotion of dietary pork, however, varied across regions and among cultural groups. While increased pork consumption often coincided with what might be categorized as 'Romanization' or 'acculturation' throughout the empire, regional and temporal variation existed over and above this aspect to present no strict universal pattern for pig exploitation. In regions such as Italy and coastal North Africa, the increase in the frequency of pigs during Roman times is often sizeable, and comes largely at the expense of cattle, whose frequency values drop concomitantly. In northern and western sections of the empire, only sites of strong Mediterranean orientation display the pattern; most typically these are urban centres, areas where Roman citizens, wealth, and Roman dietary preferences, such as pork consumption, might likely congregate. Basically, the pork-rich diet of Rome was often emulated within other high-status, 'Romanized' provincial sites, especially urban ones, but only where this could be successfully achieved within the constraints of local and regional environmental conditions (King, 1999, 188–189).

The Roman military also affect dietary change across the empire, but again in varying ways. Roman soldiers enjoyed a privileged diet of sorts, of which meat, typically beef and pork, was a component (Davies, 1971, 138). Armies could also supplement these meats with wild game they may have hunted or otherwise acquired. Nonetheless, while sheep and goat bones typically dominate zooarchaeological assemblages across all types of sites (e.g., military, urban, settlement, rural) in eastern regions of the Roman world, and remains of cattle factor more commonly in northern provinces, military sites across the empire often register relatively more pig bones than their local non-military counterparts, suggesting perhaps some overall army preference for pork, where of course this could be supplied (King, 1999, 189–190). Still, local environments set limits on outputs of pigs. Predominantly, this is less a factor of reduced cultural preference or desire for pork by the military, but rather constraints of drier conditions and scrubbier landscapes in some eastern and southern regions of the Roman Mediterranean that placed environmental and climatic restrictions on pig production. Consequently, the frequency of pigs among eastern 'Romanized' sites never increases as dramatically as it might elsewhere, such as Italy, as a consequence of Roman presence and influence. Cultural patterns in meat diets during Roman times, therefore, involve complex interweaving of numerous factors, including identity, location, environment, wealth, supply, demand, and convenience.

Although cattle, sheep/goat, and pig typically dominate zooarchaeological assemblages among Roman sites, and the husbandry operations involved with these taxa certainly shaped significant components of ancient life, it is important to acknowledge the role of domestic fowl as well, even if this taxon, by NISP counts, often registers much smaller figures than its mammalian counterparts. The contribution of domestic fowl as a meat source and provider of eggs should not be underplayed. Available zooarchaeological evidence indicates a general Mediterranean introduction of domestic fowl around the eighth century BC, but it is not until Roman imperial times that larger ventures to raise, breed, and manipulate poultry birds first occur. Bone metric data show great range, suggestive of various types; not surprisingly such variation proliferates across sites in more heavily populated urban areas at this time, places with correspondingly the biggest markets for poultry. While fowl were certainly raised on rural and suburban farms, with schemes for their care and production outlined by agricultural writers such as Columella and Palladius, it appears far more likely that they were kept and raised at the household level in Roman cities and villages, as judged by the ubiquity of their bones and the consistency in age and sex parameters for them, across such locations. Moreover, fowl figure somewhat regularly across different status and ethnic categories among sites. This key concept of urban production in domestic fowl, and their consumption among multifarious social classes, is important to stress in our reconstruction of ancient Roman diets and economics (MacKinnon, 2014b).

Meat and social status in antiquity

Zooarchaeological evidence indicates that meat was often considered a status item among many ancient cultures (MacKinnon, 2004). It was generally costly to produce, and, in the days before refrigeration, would not keep unless preserved through salting, smoking, or drying – procedures adding further time and expense (Garnsey, 1999, 222). Most people likely did not eat meat often or regularly during antiquity, save perhaps the wealthy; presumably, for the majority of the population, meat largely factored as part of some religious event and other special occasion, when indeed it was consumed. Nonetheless, although meat remained largely a luxury food within the Roman world, available literary and zooarchaeological data suggest it was consumed in greater quantities than among earlier Greek cultures, with a far greater percentage of it arguably deriving from non-ritual contexts (MacKinnon, 2004). Expense and availability of meat undoubtedly influenced its role among social classes in Roman antiquity, for which the ancient texts offer some details. For the elite, dietary diversity and ostentation could register. Martial notes that elite countrymen had much easier access to wild animals, which could be hunted more readily and cheaply (Mart. 4.66). Juvenal outlines the possibility of buying wild game at the market (Juv. 6.38–40). Numerous literary references allude to the range of exotic foodstuffs available and displayed by Roman elite. The lavish dining events of Trimalchio, as described in Petronius' *Satryicon*, yield one extreme. Such items are also displayed in scenes of Roman markets or butchery operations (complete in some cases with images of hanging carcasses or meat cuts of domestic and wild animals), as well as among visuals of Roman food-stuffs and meals.[12]

The ancient sources provide fewer clues about the role of meat and other animal products in the diet of the Roman poor. Meat is not specifically referenced among common items available to the Roman rural poor, but could have factored occasionally. It is not listed among food rations delivered to slaves and workers at a Roman villa, as delivered by the agricultural writer Cato. Milk and cheese, however, factor among resources perhaps more commonly consumed by rural poor.[13] Overall, it is likely that rural peasants operating a subsistence-level farm fed predominantly on staple cereals, supplemented, where possible, with some cheese and other foodstuffs (such as wild plants, and perhaps some small wild game or birds) that could be gathered at no extra cost. Shepherds presumably had greater access to milk and cheese products, but also may have eaten meat from ill, feeble, and unproductive elderly members of the flock that they might otherwise have had difficulties selling or trading (MacKinnon, 2004, 226).

The urban poor likely had fewer culinary choices available to them than their rural counterparts. Presumably cheaper varieties of cheese as well as eggs were more commonly available and affordable, but meat surely was a very infrequent addition. Sausages and other cheap snacks sold in cookshops could be purchased. Romans viewed sausage sellers as the lowest form of cook (Dohm, 1964, 31–35); at 10 *denarii* per pound, beef sausages were half the price of other prepared or specialty meats (*Ed. Diocl.* 4.14). Lower-rate and 'bland' cuts of meat, such as the brains, heads, feet, and minced products, might also have been acquired on occasion (MacKinnon, 2004, 209; Cels. 2.22.1–2). Some urban poorer classes may also have received meat that was left over from animal sacrifices[14] or which was made available to them from government or private distribution schemes, but such provisions were neither regular nor universal.[15]

To understand more about the social role of meat in antiquity it is important to consider how fat content in animal products influenced tastes, values, and choices in consumption. There are arguably cultural preferences and initiatives in Roman antiquity not simply to breed, or at least prioritize fatty animals and meat cuts for consumption, but also to maintain, enhance, or add fat while cooking and processing the animals. The ancient sources contain numerous supporting references, from Columella's (7.9.4) recommendation for castrating male pigs at six months of age, so they might grow fat, to Pliny's (*HN* 10.39–40) advice on how to fatten poultry, to culinary references in Apicius' cookbook that advocate preference for fatty cuts of meat, not to mention multiple means by which to cook or flavour foodstuffs with fat. Ham, lard, and grease are among the more expensive consumed animal products listed in Diocletian's price edict; pork was also costly among meats. Lard and grease, for example, both at 12 *denarii* per pound were more expensive than comparable weights of many meats (*Ed. Diocl.* 4.10). Fattened poultry birds sold for double the price of unfattened equivalents (*Ed. Diocl.* 4.17–23). Clearly, when it came to dietary meat, fat was preferred over lean (Varro, *Rust.*, 2.4.4, 2.4.12; Juv. 13.117–118; Prop. 4.1.a.21–24; Macr. *Sat.* 5.11.23), and pigs exemplified a peak resource among fatty, prolific animals.

Beyond the fact that wealthier Romans consumed relatively more meat and a greater variety of foodstuffs (including wild and exotic resources) than did poorer individuals, the basic differences that set apart the meat diet of Roman elite from poorer versions, as regards the contribution of domestic taxa (i.e., cattle, sheep, goat, pig, and domestic fowl), chiefly relate to preparation and presentation of the dish, selection of age categories within each domesticate, and quality (which included fat content) of meat cut. Poorer classes may have supplemented their predominantly grain-based diet with cheese, eggs, and cheaper and tougher cuts of meat, often from older animals, as well as with common poultry birds, especially chickens. By contrast, wealthy Romans could afford not simply more meat and animal products overall, but also more expensive, fatty, and succulent cuts, such as those from younger livestock. To help examine such practices we must return to the zooarchaeological evidence.

Zooarchaeological data largely confirm this cultural preference for fatty animals and cuts of meat along several lines. First, the predominance of pigs among many Roman sites suggests selective pressures. Their higher incidence, especially within the Mediterranean region, coincides with what appears to be broader, more popular, perhaps more secularized, engagement of meat in the diet, with the choice being pig—not surprisingly the animal that tends towards tenderer and fattier tissues within its body. Pigs represented good value for meat, and tasty meat as well.[16]

A second factor to consider in arguing a Roman preference for fatty animals and cuts of meat relates to breeding tactics. Although a general increase in size registers across all livestock taxa throughout antiquity, implying some morphological manipulation and selective breeding of animals, available zooarchaeological data suggest urban areas received bigger pigs, on average, than those consumed at rural sites.[17] Furthermore, urban sites typically seem to register a preponderance of pigs at maximum weights, around two to three years of age, as though a larger measure to control size ranges for pigs existed within the general urban market (MacKinnon, 2004, 216). Evidence, moreover, helps confirm the existence and promotion of a second, larger variety of pig at this time: a smoother skinned, fat-bellied, and shorter-legged type (MacKinnon, 2001). This 'breed,' alluded to among ancient sources and shown in some depictions, more likely allies with a stall-fed type that could be fattened easily under more controlled environments. However, it is not just pigs that see breed manipulation during Roman antiquity presumably coincident with exploitation of meat and fat; types of cattle and sheep also undergo variable morphological and metrical transformations through localized cultural and environmental selective pressures. Regarding cattle, many such changes might be linked with a need for stronger, powerful traction animals (MacKinnon, 2010b), but this does not preclude manipulation for larger, meat-producing animals by default in such ventures.

Finally, skeletal part data among zooarchaeological assemblages, at least from Roman sites in Italy, reveal a bias wherein bones associated with fattier areas of the skeleton, or what might be termed 'primary cuts' of meat (i.e., sections surrounding the ribs, vertebrae, shoulder, and pelvis area; bacon, a naturally fatty cut, derives from this zone as well), register with greater frequency among urban sites and in more elite settings (MacKinnon, 2004, 197–204). The impression is that augmented demand, shaped here by greater volume and costs, created differential social access to higher-grade (i.e., fattier and more tender) cuts of meat. Cities drew in more animals for consumption, and seem to have requested a greater proportion of more succulent types and cuts of meat. Nonetheless, an important issue to stress in seeking to determine status differences in zooarchaeological evidence for Roman antiquity is that relative frequencies of NISP counts for various animal taxa among 'elite' or 'peasant' deposits may show little variation. Consequently, percentage figures for contributions of cattle, sheep/goat, and pig may register similar values between what might otherwise be classified as 'rich' or 'poor' assemblages/sites on the basis of other archaeological evidence. For example, NISP relative frequency counts for cattle, sheep/goat, and pig among Augustan-period deposits in Pompeii yield nearly identical values (c. 5% cattle, 20% sheep/goat, 75% pig) regardless of context, be this elite household (e.g., Houses of Marcus Lucretius, Postumii, etc.) or more 'lower-class' neighbourhoods, such as excavations in the southern end of the city near the Porta Stabia (see Figure 13.2).[18] Deeper investigation, however, reveals greater variation within age categories and skeletal parts among these taxa, with those associated with elite settings registering greater

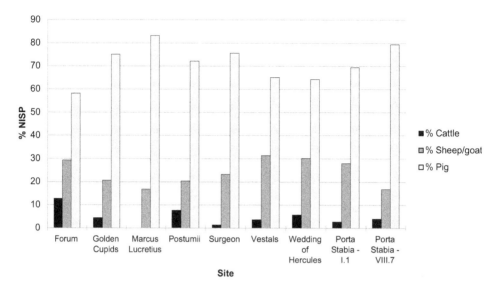

Figure 13.2 NISP relative frequency values for cattle, sheep/goat and pig among sites in Pompeii for the Augustan period (c. first century BC–first century AD).

frequencies both for younger animals (especially pigs), and for choicer cuts of meat, including those from the central section of the animal.

A similar situation registers among what might be termed rural villa (arguably elite complexes) and smaller-scale rural 'peasant' sites. The zooarchaeological database for the former category is much more extensive among Roman sites, but recent work is adding to our knowledge of the latter.[19] Whereas zooarchaeological data among Roman rural villa sites variously show evidence of components including specialization, dietary diversity and wealth, import of some exotic foodstuffs, higher frequencies of younger animals, and increased consumption of wild game, arguably 'less-elite' rural sites typically do not contain such markers. Such smaller-scale/peasant complexes tend to maintain some manner of self-sufficiency in all aspects of animal production and consumption. Animals seem to have been raised and herded, for the most part, more locally (as opposed to any larger, mobile, transhumant operations as registers at various rural villa sites). Slaughter, butchery, processing, and consumption also were localized. There appears to be little connection of these smaller-scale sites to larger marketing schemes, specialized butchery, or extensive trade and transport in animals or animal products. Available faunal data thus suggest small-scale, mixed husbandry ventures, presumably operated under the domain of a working-class/peasant rural household.[20]

Preservation techniques for meat in Roman antiquity

Although efforts were probably taken to consume perishable animal products like meat and milk quickly after retrieval or slaughter,[21] various forms of preservation were also practised during Roman antiquity. Moreover, methods chosen could affect the taste of the product, which itself could variously hold social or cultural significance. References to dried and/or smoked meat occur periodically within the ancient texts,[22] but are far less numerous than those for salted meat, by comparison.[23] Nevertheless, explicit details about the equipment and procedures required are rather scant. Depictions of racks, hooks, and hanging carcasses or meat cuts do appear in ancient art, all of which can connect with smoking or drying meat, although it is difficult to determine exactly where, and on what scale this operated.[24] Procedures for salting meat are better outlined in the ancient sources, through Columella, Cato, Macrobius, and Apicius (Col. 12.55.1–4; Cato, *Agr.* 162.1–3; Macrob., *Sat.* 7.12; Apic. 1.8–10). Tactics such as pressing strips of meat and salt between boards, layering meat and salt inside large tubs, jars or pots, as well as soaking pieces in brine solutions are outlined. Other mixtures might also be employed in preservation. Apicius provides a procedure for pickling meats, through some solution of salt and vinegar (Apic. 1.7.1–2), and coating meat with honey was also performed.

Zooarchaeological evidence to support or augment our understanding of meat preservation schemes in antiquity is sparse. Examples of pierced scapula (i.e., shoulder blade) bones from pigs and cattle are recorded, perhaps suggestive of hanging sections of meat for smoking or drying (Schmid, 1972), but this is not an exclusive method. Indeed, it seems probable that filleted strips of meat were preserved more often than sections with the bone still attached. Unfortunately, it is very difficult to determine how much meat was filleted from the bone on the basis of zooarchaeological data alone, given that the procedure may leave few, if any, traces on the bones themselves, especially among skilled butchers who are adept at not nicking the bones during such practices (MacKinnon, 2004, 185).

Although various options were available in antiquity to preserve meat, given its representational bias it is likely that salting predominated. Several reasons promote this. First, the process is relatively easy and less dangerous, especially in relation to smoking meat, where hazards of fire and smoke inhalation may ensue. Second, one can conduct salting in relatively large or small batches more effectively than among other techniques. There is more flexibility with it, one might argue. Finally, and perhaps most importantly, salting can disguise any rot or decay in the meat, and thus help extend its 'shelf-life', while at the same time administering a somewhat tempting, perhaps addictive, taste and flavour.

Cooking techniques and meat consumption in antiquity

The ancient Romans cooked meat in five basic ways: boiling/stewing, roasting, frying, grilling, and baking (as in a casserole). Boiling/stewing and roasting predominate, in some cases even mandated as the exclusive techniques for the Roman army (App., *Hisp.* 85; Frontin., *Str.* 41.1–2; Polyaenus, *Strat.* 8.16.2). Celsus (*Med.* 1.2.8; 1.3.24) notes that roasted or boiled meat is best in its ease for digestion. He recommends some seasonal variation – more boiling/stewing during winter months, and roasting/grilling in summer (Cels., *Med.* 1.3.34–35, 1.6.2). Apicius lists more than 50 recipes that require boiled/stewed meat (some of which relate to sauces to accompany or flavour such dishes), and 40 recipes involving roasted meat; frying, grilling and baking appear less than ten times apiece.

Roasting helps caramelize meat, melting fats and adding succulence and taste, additionally through the input of smoky flavours from cooking fires. Moreover, roasting may arguably entail great spectacle in engaging a communal, festival occasion, especially if larger cuts of meat, or whole animals, are being cooked.

Stewing, by contrast, allows meats to cook down within their juices, thus preserving all the fat, moistness, and consequent flavour and tenderness. The importance of fat to culinary tastes during Roman antiquity has already been addressed. But extended stewing also ensures thorough cooking, as opposed to grilled meat that might be perceived as half-raw if it is not otherwise charred right through.

Boiled/stewed meat can also be a rather versatile ingredient in Roman cuisine. Soaking preserved meat in water, and then boiling it, could help remove any potentially overpowering salty tastes, and rejuvenate the meat for subsequent flavouring. Adding broths, spices, and sauces, many of which include highly acidic or pungent fish sauces[25] would render a range of tastes for the meat.

Lastly, considerations surrounding the convenience of boiled/stewed meat surely also promoted its popularity. Essentially, these were 'one-pot' meals, ideal for feeding various scales from households to a larger crowd.

Zooarchaeological data help confirm cooking methods. The relatively low frequency of charred bones, even charred ends of bones that might be exposed to flames, suggests that roasting meat, at least meat with bones still attached, was not a common practice.[26] By contrast, a high incidence of spirally fractured bone pieces implies deliberate breakage of fresh bones, a convenient method both to extract marrow, and to rapidly portion meat cuts for stewing. The wide degree of variation in butchery marks noted from the zooarchaeological record – in some instances indicative of somewhat haphazard cutting and chopping – would be less problematic if materials were to be boiled/stewed in a pot, where splintering would not be a hazard. Moreover, such methods would preserve all meat as it slipped easily from the bone during cooking.

Conclusions

To conclude, a critical message to draw from this overview is that the ancient Roman diet was not exclusively vegetarian, even perhaps among the poorest of social classes. Indeed, meat and other animal products variously contributed to the ancient Roman diet, in whatever forms such a diet manifested itself in relation to aspects such as geographic region, timeframe, cultural group, and social class. Ancient texts comment on the range of commodities that can be procured from animals, and grade or rank their worth as regards nutriment, price, ubiquity, access, and popularity to some degree. Procedures and techniques involved in preserving, and cooking or otherwise preparing meat and other products find reference among the ancient sources, with particular attention devoted to salting and smoking cuts of meat (as key means of preservation), and stewing (as an effective and popular method of cooking). The importance of fat, as an element that augmented taste in meats (and consequently could hold value in marking status), and as a substance that could assist with preservation is noted in the ancient sources, and supported through zooarchaeological findings of husbandry techniques promoting seemingly larger, fattier animals, notably pigs. Faunal data also confirm the importance of domestic cattle, sheep, goat, pig, and fowl as providers of meat to the Roman diet, but highlight the dynamic interplay of environmental and social-cultural factors that shaped the contributions provided by various taxa. Pigs surface as a central animal marketed to a significant degree across the wider Roman world in light of augmented demands for meat among various cultural groups, many of which appear increasingly 'Romanized,' be this through emulation of elites and/or armies—social groups that often desired more meat, and notably pork, in their menus. Zooarchaeological evidence further shows wild animals factor more rarely in Roman diets, even among wealthier contexts, a finding that helps temper their more frequent representation in such settings as noted in the ancient texts.

Notes

1 Beerden in this volume discusses the textual evidence in greater detail.
2 See Halstead in this volume for an overview of zooarchaeological techniques and inputs.

3 This is not meant to diminish the role iconography plays in cultural reconstructions, but reflects the relatively smaller pool of images available from Roman antiquity that specifically portray meat, milk, and other animal foodstuffs *per se* (although there are multiple images of animals themselves, which can be helpful in understanding husbandry patterns and breeds of livestock).

4 See Donahue in this volume.

5 Certainly variation exists in this regard; specialization in supplying younger cattle, sheep, and goats for various urban dietary demands, including the animal sacrifice market, does register, but generally the data denote predominance for older individuals and exploitation of secondary resources.

6 Roy, 2007, reviews the archaeological and ancient literary evidence for the consumption of dog meat (in non-ritual contexts) in Greece from the Archaic period to Roman imperial times. He concludes that although available faunal data are currently too disparate to afford any reliable estimate of the significance of dog meat in the classical Greek diet, he nonetheless thinks that the practice did indeed continue in these periods, but on a very minor scale compared with the consumption of other species.

7 Although horse consumption may factor more regularly among some northern (and presumably non-Roman) cultural groups, its overall contribution in relation to other livestock is likely minimal. See Lauwerier, 1999, for a broader case study from the Roman Netherlands.

8 Considerable scholarship exists for these topics. See MacKinnon, 2007, for an overview of wider themes in osteological research in classical archaeology and a more extensive bibliography of related discussions, examples and case studies.

9 See Marzano in this volume for further details about consumption of fish in antiquity.

10 Certainly there is some regional variation among these figures (i.e., more fish at coastal sites, more wild animals among rural sites in forested zones, more wild animals among some sites in Iberia, where game was rather plentiful). Nevertheless, among the wider Mediterranean Roman world, game accounts for only a very minor portion of the meat diet.

11 NISP = number of identified specimens, a common zooarchaeological quantifier. Data for these calculations derive largely from King, 1999; MacKinnon, 2004; 2010a; and sources listed in MacKinnon, 2007. The temporal distinctions identified are meant as general guides only: c. 1000–c. 100 BC for 'Pre-Roman/Iron Age' and c. 100 BC–c. AD 400 for 'Roman'.

12 Chioffi, 1999, includes a wide assortment from Roman markets.

13 Col. 7.2.1. Virgil ([Verg]. *Mor.*) provides a recipe for 'moretum' a type of cheese and herb paste.

14 Was all of the meat consumed by the Romans sacrificed? Scheid, 2007; 2012, argues that this seems to be the case, stating that slaughter was a ritual act, even if its ultimate intention was for sustenance. While a provocative premise – which may be extended given that some ritualized aspect (e.g., a prayer, offering, or simply a patterned behaviour) might underscore various acts of slaughter, butchery, and/or consumption – to hinge such a broad proposal on several disparate textual references (Scheid offers quotations from the Elder Pliny, St. Paul, and Varro) seems rather tenuous, especially when details contextualizing each reference are debatable. Belayche, 2007 adds further dimensions to this issue, asking: What role did religion play in meat production and consumption? The answer is unclear. Christian and late pagan texts, sources one might expect to be lucid about alternative views relating to animal sacrifice, both entail discourse about the shifting and elusive nature of ritual acts. Belayche discusses that hunted animals were not typically considered as sacrificed, but documents conflict and there is flexibility in this viewpoint as regards animals hunted in the amphitheater. Both Scheid and Belayche acknowledge the limitations, ambiguities and frustrations of the textual sources in answering questions about the relationship between the religious sphere and the consumption of meat of any origin, whether from butchery shops or from domestic slaughtering. Neither incorporates the zooarchaeological evidence in their respective arguments, for which a rich collection exists across all types of Roman sites, and which challenge such a strict division among concepts (see MacKinnon, 2014a). Indeed, the dividing line between 'ritual' and 'profane' is not fixed. In some cases, things can have both meanings simultaneously, depending on which part of the animal is being considered. Alternatively, an animal (or its parts again) can transition between these seemingly opposing ends. Meanings, moreover, become further blurred when linking these concepts to 'public' and 'private' contexts. Scheid and Belayche concentrate on animal sacrifice and consumption in public, urban settings, which begs the question of similar views of meat as 'ritualized' in alternate settings, such as rural households. Acquisition and consumption of meat by other means, for example, from taxation in kind or from army expropriation, begs similar investigation.

15 Sirks, 1991, provides further discussion of meat provisions among imperial-regulated food distribution schemes.

16 Of course such is relative; for pork taboos see Harris, 1985, 73–86. Some Semitic groups avoided pork, but wider Roman cultures presumably did not.

17 This pattern is most pronounced for imperial contexts in central Italy; see MacKinnon, 2004, 155 for more details.

18 Zooarchaeological data derive from King, 2002 (Forum); Richardson et al., 1997 (Surgeon, Vestals, Wedding of Hercules); MacKinnon (remaining sites – currently in study).

19 A key venture here is the Roman Peasant Project: www.sas.upenn.edu/romanpeasants

20 See the 'Peasant Project' preliminary faunal report at www.sas.upenn.edu/romanpeasants/reports.html

21 Unsalted meat could only be kept for a few days in the summertime, according to Apicius 1.7.1.

22 E.g., Macrob., *Sat.* 3.17.9 (dried meat); Pers. 6.69–73 (smoked pig's cheek); *Ed. Diocl.* 4.15–16 (smoked sausages). Curtis, 2001, provides further comment.

23 A small sample of such references includes: Cato, *Agr.* 162.1-3; Col. 12.55.1–4; Mart. 1.4; Macrob., *Sat.* 3.17.9, 7.12; Strab. 3.4.11, 4.3.2, 4.4.3; *Ed. Diocl.* 4.7; among numerous times in Apicius.

24 Some examples are shown in Corbier, 1989b, and Toynbee, 1973.

25 Apic. 7.6.1–14 lists a number of such sauces.

26 Here excluding deliberately burnt sacrificial materials, as in some ritual practices.

14

FISH AND SEAFOOD

Annalisa Marzano

Introduction[1]

'At Rome a fish sells for more than a cow!' These were the words that, according to Plutarch (*Quaest. Conv.* 4.4.2.9), Cato the Elder (234–149 BC) uttered in condemning the excessive luxury of his own times. Indeed, from references in literary works, such as the comedies of Plautus and Terence, and other available historical information, it is clear that by the mid-Republican period increasing demand for fish and seafood, and the appreciation of the culinary qualities of different kinds of fish, were well established in Rome. The city had acquired a dedicated fish market, the Forum Piscatorium, sometime before 210 BC, when the historian Livy reports the destruction by a fire of this market and other buildings in the Forum area (26.27.2–3). Molluscs are listed alongside other gastronomic delicacies (dormice and exotic birds) in the Lex Aemilia, a sumptuary law, probably dating to 115 BC, attempting to ban certain luxury foods from banquets (Plin., *HN* 8.57.223; André, 1961, 109).

In the case of seafood, a clear hierarchy of the desirability of various foods developed over time, as it did for a variety of foodstuffs and drinks. As early as the third/early second century BC the poet Ennius wrote a sort of gastronomic catalogue praising various kinds of fish from different geographic areas, an adaptation of earlier Greek literary works, which offered a qualitative hierarchy of seafood. Rankings such as these had at the top the most desirable types of fish and shellfish, which not only expressed gourmet appreciation for certain tastes and products, but were status symbols of one's success. In the Roman world, both public and private banquets were, above all, occasions in which social order and social standing were visually expressed. While commensality indicated membership into a specific group, it also set out hierarchies within the group itself. Seating arrangements, type, quality, and quantity of food served to individual guests could all clearly mark out one's social standing within the group. Literary sources contain many references to fish and seafood served at the banquets of the elite, often marking, together with other foods, such as peacocks and flamingos, the extravagance and expenditure of the wealthy. Some anecdotes single out certain difficult-to-obtain fish sold at auction and reaching very high prices. For instance, under emperor Tiberius, three large red mullets – a fish that could not be farmed in artificial enclosures – were sold in Rome for 30,000 sesterces, prompting imperial intervention to regulate such excessive prices (Sen., *Ep. Mor.* 9.42; Suet., *Tib.* 34). However, with the exception of some satirical poems, literary works contain scarce references to what kind of fish and seafood, if any, the ordinary people and lower strata of society ate. In this case, one needs to turn to the archaeological and, to an extent, documentary evidence for clues.

Fish consumption in antiquity, particularly of fresh fish, varied greatly according to geographic locations, epochs, and social strata, but certain kinds of fish certainly appeared regularly in the diet of ordinary people. In general, fresh marine fish of the kinds still appreciated nowadays (e.g., sea bass, sea bream, gilthead), especially if the specimens were of large size, was a food for the wealthy. A few selected freshwater fish were part of the foods sought by the upper classes, together with oysters, scallops, and murices among the molluscs, although, as discussed below, there was considerable regional diversity, and something that was reserved to the rich in Roman Italy could be common food in other areas of the empire. The ordinary people could afford and ate small fresh marine fish such as anchovies and fry, and some freshwater fish. Preserved fish (salted, smoked or dried) and fish sauces and pastes came in a range of quality, and hence prices, and are discussed in a separate section.

The upper classes

Taste and culinary fashion are not the same among different societies and cultures and even within the same culture they tend to change over time. A type of food that is appreciated as a delicacy at one time may not be held in the same regard in a different period and this applies to fish and seafood too (for discussion of concepts of 'affluence' and 'luxury' in diet see Ervynck et al., 2003; Van der Veen, 2003). Take the case of the sturgeon (Lat. *acipenser*); this fish was appreciated because of its rarity, since it was not found in the Mediterranean and could not be farmed, and we find literary references to its desirability and social value from the time of Plautus to the late Republic (Dalby, 2003, 312–314. Plaut. *apud* Macrob. 3.16.5–7; Lael. *apud* Cic., *de Fin.* 2.24, 2.91; *Tusc. Disp.* 3.43). The sturgeon then appears to have gone out of fashion for a time, as according to Pliny this fish was not popular in his own time (*HN* 9.60), but some years later Martial does mention it as a fish worthy of an emperor (*Xenia* 13.91).

By the late Republic Roman wealthy upper classes (and those who aspired to be part of this group) showed a marked preference for certain types of fresh marine fish (gilthead, sea bream, and bass; Lat. *aurata*, *dentex*, and *lupus*) over freshwater fish. A case in point in the shift of tastes from freshwater to marine fish concerns the bass itself. The bass is a fish that can easily adapt to live in rivers and lakes and that normally spends part of its life cycle migrating between sea and coastal lagoons. According to the first-century AD writer Columella, in earlier times the bass had been commonly farmed in the lakes of Etruria and Latium, but by the late Republic gourmands were spurning freshwater bass, preferring instead those from the sea, on account of the difference in taste (*Rust.* 8.16.1–4). The only exceptions were the bass fished 'between the bridges' of the Tiber (*infra pontes*: Hor., *Sat.* 2.2.31–33; Juv. 5.104–106), which maintained their renown as a delicacy at least until the late first century AD. The second-century AD physician Galen, who lived in Rome from the 160s AD, comments in one of his works that the fish caught in the Tiber in Rome tasted very different from those fished at the river mouth, because it was contaminated by pollutants such as sewage and the waste of the fullers' workshops (*On the Properties of Foodstuffs* 3.29.721–722 = 6.721–722 Kühn). For this reason, Galen advises against consuming fish from 'between the bridges', because it could have negative effects on health. His observations in all likelihood reflect the fact that compared to the Republican times, when the bass from the Tiber had acquired its reputation, imperial Rome had grown in population to be a metropolis of around one million inhabitants, with all the connected consequences in terms of fluvial pollution.

Elite fondness for fresh marine fish, and the extent to which fresh fish could have social clout, is also clearly indicated by the keen interest Roman upper-class members of the first century BC had in marine intensive fish farming in artificial fishponds (*piscinae*). In fact, while farming of freshwater fish dates back to Egyptian and Mesopotamian civilizations and was practised by the Greeks, the Romans seem to have been the first to perfect intensive marine fish farming, introducing important technical innovations, such as the mixing of seawater with freshwater in order to increase oxygen content in the tanks (Marzano and Brizzi, 2009; Marzano, 2013b, 210–226). Equipping luxury maritime villas with large marine fishponds, such as the one at Torre Astura, south of Antium, which housed the largest known fishpond in the Roman world, measuring around 15,000 m^2, was part of the competitive display members of the elite engaged in (Higginbotham, 1997), but also a form of investment to provide fresh, quality food for the wealthy in large urban markets such as Rome and the densely inhabited Bay of Naples area (Marzano and Brizzi, 2009). Farming of marine fish is, in fact, included among the *villaticae pastiones*, or villa productions, by both Varro and Columella (Varro, *Rust.* 3.17.1–10; see also 3.2.12–13, 3.3.1–10. Columella, *Rust.* 8.16–17).

The moneyed elites had access to a wide range of foods and aimed at impressing their guests with the rarity or the elaborate preparation of the dishes served at banquets. Seafood was not excluded from these forms of display and figured prominently on the tables of the wealthy, even in the case of feasts organized on a vast scale. When Julius Caesar staged a grand triumphal banquet in Rome in 46 BC, entertaining around 198,000 people, a range of foods and wines were served, according to the level of social distinction of the participants; the menu included also about 6,000 eels supplied by a fish farmer (or moray eels; the Latin texts give the word *muraena*: on the translation of the term see Higginbotham, 1997, 43–46; Varro, *Rust.* 3.17.3).

Among the molluscs, oysters and scallops, especially oysters fattened in the Lucrine Lake in Campania, were highly appreciated. Romans practised oyster farming, of which Sergius Orata, who developed this activity in the Lucrine lake, is an example, but also exploited natural oyster beds where these were present (e.g., Britain, south of France). Roman gourmands claimed to be able to immediately identify, from the taste of a fish or oyster, from where it had originated. Differentiation of the key characteristics, and hence flavours, of molluscs and fish was so much a topic of interest that qualitative classifications, according to geographic regions, were created. For instance, at the time of the emperor Nero, Licinius Mucianus had developed a full qualitative hierarchy of oysters, singling out as the best those from Cyzicus, on the southern coast of the Marmara Sea (*apud* Plin., *HN* 32.21).

The rich could afford to get the food they wanted, even if logistically this might have been a challenge. Excavations at the grand Roman villa of Montmaurin, located at the foot of the Pyrenees and several hundred kilometres away from both the Mediterranean and the Bay of Biscay, have unearthed large quantities of oyster shells, thus proving that the transport of live oysters over long distances took place (Marzano, 2013b, 189–192). If one believes the anecdote reported in Athenaeus, while Trajan was campaigning in Parthia, Apicius devised a way to pack and send the emperor fresh oysters from the coast, to ensure Trajan could dine in style (Ath. 1.7d).

Iconographic evidence – the mosaics and wall paintings that decorated fine villas and urban houses – also give an idea of the types of seafood that were appreciated. The species that are depicted most often, either as still life or in marine scenes, are bass, red mullet, moray eel, lobster, and octopus.

The ordinary Romans

In wanting to assess the role fish and seafood had in the diet of ordinary people in antiquity, the literary record, written by the educated upper class for their peers, is of limited use. Latin satirical authors such as Martial do comment on the different quality foods served at banquets to the host and important guests and to the clients (in one poem oysters and turbot are contrasted with cheap molluscs and brill: Mart. 3.60), or on the attempts on the part of individuals of modest means to give the impression of a higher social standing by sending as gift expensive oysters and mullet while forced to dine at home on cabbage (Mart. 7.78). However, these poems hardly account for the reality of the diet of ordinary people in the Roman world. Documentary evidence and archaeological data (e.g., remains of food consumption, such as fish bone assemblages; evidence for the containers used to transport salted fish and fish sauces; scientific analysis of human remains in order to determine type of diet) can reveal important information to fill these lacunae in our knowledge, but these data are fragmentary due to survival rates and methodological approaches followed in excavation projects.

To recover in excavation zooarchaeological taxa such as fish bones, wet sieving is needed, but not all excavation projects have in the past applied the technique regularly, developed appropriate sampling strategies, or followed a universal method so that results from different projects can be compared meaningfully. Just to give a simple example, the mesh size used when sieving will determine whether smaller fish bones can be recovered and apparent absence of certain specimens at one site compared to another one could, in fact, be simply the result of the recovery strategy employed, not of what people actually ate or did not eat in antiquity. Because of these issues, often the picture of food consumption at a given site has been skewed towards more easily recoverable taxa, such as mammal bones (on zooarchaeological evidence see Halstead in this volume). However, when sieving has been regularly applied in excavations, fish assemblages discovered at places such as Pompeii or sites in Greece indicate consumption of a notable variety of fish, molluscs, and crustaceans (Mylona, 2008). For example, excavation of a Roman villa at Mytilene has revealed consumption of congridae, mullidae, crabs, lobsters, sea urchins, and shellfish (Mylona, 2008), whereas a Roman butcher's shop excavated near the theatre in Corinth, which also sold cooked food, seemed to have served fish too (Mylona, 2008, 38–43, table 5.1c; Halstead in this volume, p. 70 for fish remains from a Roman tavern at Lattes, France). Results from the study of the sediments accumulated before the eruption of AD 79 in the Cardo V sewer in Herculaneum, located in the northeast corner of the site, beneath the *insula orientalis* II, have also shown that the inhabitants of that neighbourhood consumed a remarkable array of seafood (Rowan, 2014a). This neighbourhood, adjacent to the *palaestra* complex, consisted of a combination of commercial (e.g., bakery, wine shop) and domestic units (apartments above the shops), but did not comprise large urban houses of the upper strata of society, although it did comprise some apartments larger than others. The study indicated that particular species of fish – sea breams (*Diplodus* sp.), damsel fish (*Chromis chromis* L.), picarels (*Spicara* sp.), and Pandora (*Pagellus* sp.) – were eaten regularly and in notable quantities. Other species identified include mackerel, greater weaver, anchovies, sea bass, and eel (Rowan, 2014a, 67 for the table of identified taxa). In the two latter cases these fishes did not seem to have been commonly consumed, confirming the picture that emerges from the documentary and literary sources: ordinary people ate mostly fry and small fish, whereas fish that can grow to a large size and that are not caught in schools during migrations cost more. Some of the taxa identified from the sewer deposit as belonging to small-sized fish were probably consumed as fish pastes (e.g., *allec*). For larger specimens, the absence of certain fish bones does not exclude the consumption of the fish, especially of dried or salted fish, as some or all of the bones were removed during processing (particularly in the salting process; drying or smoking could leave the fish whole, after it had been gutted).

The archaeozoological results of the Herculaneum study match nicely the information offered by a second-century inscription discovered in another Mediterranean city, Pergamun in Asia Minor. The text is an imperial letter, probably to be dated to Hadrian's reign, concerned with abuses on the part of money changers (e.g., imposing a surcharge for worn coins), which seems to have affected the sellers of fish in particular (*OGIS* 484 = *IGR* 4.352, see ll. 26–27). The interest of this text is that it gives an idea of fish prices in second-century Pergamum and of what common people bought: 1 *denarius* worth of small fish consisted of enough fish to be divided among several individuals, who pooled together to make the purchase, so that they could pay in silver *denarii* rather than in the smaller local bronze denominations. In addition, the inscription also indicates that the local authority intervened in regulating the price of small fish only, possibly in order to control at least the price of fish that people with limited means could hope to buy (Lytle, 2010, 288–289; Marzano, 2013b, 282).

The price of fish, as in the case of other goods, was primarily determined by availability (regional, but also seasonal availability) and demand (culinary fashion, local traditions, etc.), and, in the case of fresh fish, being a highly perishable item, by when in the day one was buying it. It is probable that, just as happens nowadays at the market, the sellers started reducing the price of the food items left towards the end of the day in order to sell as much as possible.

Inscriptions like the text referring to the religious association for the worship of Diana and Antinous from Lanuvium, around 30 km southeast of Rome (*ILS* 7212, dated to AD 136), indicating that the *magistri cenarum* (officers in charge of the dinner preparations) had to contribute to the regular dinners of the association an amphora of good wine, four sardines, and bread, or the price for an otherwise unidentified black fish from the Nile (called *korakinos* in Greek = the 'raven') listed in a first-century AD account of expenditure from Tebtynis in Roman Egypt (*P. Mich.* 2.123) demonstrate that fresh small fish and fry was not expensive and would have been within the economic means of ordinary people living in coastal locations or by rivers. The price for the *korakinos* in the Tebtynis account varies between 1 to 2 obols per fish (probably depending on the size of the fish); the same document gives as 2 obols the price of two loaves of bread or six eggs. Diocletian's Price Edict (*Edictum de pretiis rerum venalium*, AD 301), an attempt by the authority at regulating the maximum price one could charge in the empire for certain goods and services, contains some entries on seafood. The edict makes a distinction between marine and freshwater fish, and then between first and second quality: 1 Italic pound (327.45 g) of marine fish 'from rocky bottoms' is priced at 24 *denarii*, while 1 pound of 'second-quality marine fish', costs 16 *denarii*. Freshwater fish is cheaper: 1 pound of first quality fish costs 12 *denarii* and second-quality 8 *denarii*. Sardines are listed separately with a price of 16 *denarii* for 1 pound. The edict mentions also: salted fish (6 *denarii* for 1 pound); oysters (100 *denarii* for 100 oysters); sea urchins (50 *denarii* for 100); salted sea urchins (50 *denarii* for 1 *sextarius Italicus* = 0.547 l); and *spondyli*, a term probably here indicating the thorny oyster, the *Spondylus gaederopus* (50 *denarii* for 100).

One finds evidence for consumption of fish, both preserved and fresh, even in the desert. The wealth of written documents and zooarchaeological taxa discovered in excavation at various Roman sites in the Egyptian eastern desert has revealed that workers at the quarries and soldiers stationed in the area consumed different kinds of fish. Zooarchaeological data from the excavations at the quarries of Mons Claudianus and Mons Porphyrites have revealed the consumption of fish from the Red Sea (mostly groupers, snappers, emperors, sea breams, wrasse, mullet, and parrot fish, but other species are attested too: Hamilton-Dyer, 1990, 76–77), whereas documents have shown that soldiers placed orders for fresh fish to be bought at locations on the Red Sea and sent to them where they were stationed. The fresh fish mentioned in the texts include parrot fish, mullet, and red mullet (*O. Max.* 707, 793, 869, 1300; *O. Krok* 1; 63; Bülow-Jacobsen, 2003). However, this varied diet including preserved and fresh fish was not accessible to all the personnel serving at these forts in the desert and certainly the fresh fish was not part of the standard food rations given to the military. These were extras and the price paid for the fresh fish had to include the transport cost from the Red Sea over a minimum of 70 km of desert (Marzano, 2013b, 289–290).

Some scholars believe that in the first two centuries of the Roman Empire there was, on average, an improvement in standards of living. Better diet, for instance increased meat consumption, would have resulted in an increase in the average height of individuals (Jongman, 2007a; MacKinnon, 2004; Killgrove in this volume on using skeletal analysis to understand human health). Scientific research in recent years has focused on trying to determine the role of fish proteins in the diet of ordinary people, because it has been assumed that preserved fish provided a good proportion of the population who could not afford meat with access to protein. By conducting stable isotope analysis on human bones or teeth enamel recovered at some Roman sites, scientists have tried to assess the protein contribution of fish in the diet of the ordinary Romans (see Bourbou in this volume for an explanation of stable isotope analysis). Results have not been so clear cut, however, even when the study involved coastal settlements, where one would expect that the sea and its resources had a major role in the diet of the local inhabitants. One such case is the town of Veleia, to the south of Salerno in Italy, the object of a study involving isotope analysis on human remains from the necropolis (Craig et al., 2009). According to the first-century AD writer Strabo, the inhabitants of Veleia were 'compelled, on account of the poverty of their soil, to busy themselves mostly with the sea and to establish factories for the salting of fish, and other such industries' (*Geogr.* 6.1.1), so one would have expected to see a marked contribution of fish in the diet of the local inhabitants. The results, however, did not show signs of considerable consumption of fish. However, these results do not necessarily mean that fish and seafood had a minor role in the diet of these individuals. It is necessary to have a basic understanding of how the stable isotope method works. First, to determine how much human diet diverges from a diet based exclusively on plants, scientists need to establish a comparison and control line by using the bones of herbivores found at the same site, or at least in the general area, for the same chronological period of the human bones. Isotope values of foods can vary due to climate or agricultural practices and this means that 'isotope data from human consumers, when compared directly, may appear to vary between populations, even though the diets were essentially the same' (Müldner, 2013, 139), so the establishment of secure baselines is important.

Second, the isotopes used as markers leave a much clearer trace in human bones in the case of marine fish and fish that is higher up the food chain (so larger species). This means that the bones/teeth of individuals regularly eating freshwater fish or small marine fish (fry, anchovies, sardines, picarels) or regularly consuming fish pastes/sauces such as *allec*, which were made by using these species, would not necessarily show a high contribution of fish to protein intake.[2] Finally, when scientists determine whether consumption of fish protein by the ancient individuals studied equated to a low or high consumption of fish, they use as comparison tables containing modern data on the consumption of fish in countries such as Japan, Iceland, and Scandinavia, where fish, compared with other foods, plays a dominant role in the diet. There are no similar tables for modern Italy, Spain, and Greece, which would be more appropriate comparisons for the ancient data, since ancient and modern diet in these regions (with due differences for modernization) rested on a more varied range of foods: legumes – an important source of protein – dairy products, and vegetables. Since from what one can gather from the literary, documentary (and ethnographic) record, ordinary people would have eaten fry and small fish and some freshwater species, the results of isotopic studies such as the one conducted at Velia are not surprising.

Another study that employed isotopic analysis on human bones from the Roman town of Leptiminus in Tunisia has identified evidence for a diet heavily reliant on terrestrial plant food, but also for a significant amount of dietary protein derived from marine resources (Keenleyside et al., 2009, 59). The specific values of the analysis led the authors to suggest the consumption of higher trophic level species, such as sea bream. Other scientific studies using isotope analysis to look at the diet of ancient individuals have, overall, started to stress the degree of variation that occurred in the diet, even among settlements not too far from each other and within groups broadly similar from a social point of view. Killgrove and Tykot (2013) have analysed bones from two imperial cemeteries in Rome, one periurban (Casal Bertone) and one suburban (Castellaccio Europarco), and concluded that the two groups of people were utilizing different food resources. The consumption of some aquatic foods (from freshwater and/or saltwater protein sources) was confirmed only for the individuals who lived closer to the city of Rome, perhaps reflecting the larger choice in terms of foodstuffs offered by the urban markets of the capital, whereas the suburban individuals appear to have made greater use of millet in their diet. For the later imperial period, a study of a selection of early Christians buried in the catacombs of St Callixtus in Rome (radio-carbon dated to the mid-third through early fifth century AD) has suggested regular consumption of freshwater fish, seen by the authors of the study as indicative of the individuals' relative lack of wealth rather than religiously motivated (Rutgers et al., 2009).

A wider region of the Roman Empire for which several studies have used isotope analysis in order to reconstruct the ancient diet is Roman Britain. Foodways identified in Britain before and after the Roman conquest in AD 43 show that changes occurred and from archaeobotanical and other archaeological data it is known that several new foods were introduced to Britain during the Roman period (the changes in diet are most visible in towns, military sites, and villas). A review of various isotopic studies has concluded that marine products, which were scarce in the diet of Iron-Age Britain, played a more important role in the Roman period. Although these changes in respect to consumption of marine products were not uniformly widespread (socially and geographically) and were restricted to parts of the population, the differences identified in the isotope signal of Iron-Age and Roman humans in Britain suggest that the dietary change that occurred was very significant (Müldner, 2013, 141). General trends identified show a link between higher social status and Roman-style burials with marine food consumption (Müldner, 2013, 143). This rise in marine foods consumption has been observed also in the zooarchaeological record (Locker, 2007).

Preserved fish and fish sauces

While almost everyone has heard of *garum*, this was not the only processed fish product consumed by the Romans. *Garum* was a fish sauce widely used in ancient cuisine (not just by the Romans, but by the Greeks and Phoenicians too) as a seasoning agent instead of salt. Contrary to popular belief, which imagines *garum* to have been a smelly sauce made of rotten fish guts, this was a 'fermented' fish sauce, similar in concept to the modern Italian *colatura di alici* (from Cetara) or Vietnamese *nam nuoc*, produced by enzyme autolysis. When fish parts are left in contact with a great amount of salt for a long time, the proteolytic enzymes found in the muscle and gastrointestinal tract of fish cause almost complete degradation of fish material, resulting in a clear, yellow-amber coloured sauce, with a predominantly salty taste rather than a fishy one. *Garum* could be made out of large fish, using the guts and other parts of the fish or of medium-sized fish, such as mackerel. We know of a producer and trader in *garum* from Pompeii in the first century AD, Aulus Umbricius Scaurus. A product of his, advertised both on the painted inscriptions (*tituli picti*) on small terracotta containers known archaeologically and on the mosaic in the atrium of his house in Pompeii, was precisely made from mackerel and was marketed as 'the best *garum* from mackerel' (Curtis, 1988). What not everyone is aware of, however, is that *garum* manufacture was the by-product of fish salting. As clearly explained by Curtis (2001, 406–409), salt fish, fish paste, and fish sauce were integral parts of the same production process.

The need to preserve fish occurs when large quantities of fish are available for given periods of time, and Roman fish-salting factories are concentrated in those geographical areas affected by the seasonal passage of schools of fish, most notably the areas on both sides of the Strait of Gibraltar, coastal Morocco, Tunisia, and Sicily for the schools of tuna and mackerel entering the Mediterranean; Brittany for sardines, anchovies, and herring shoals moving between the North Sea and the Atlantic; and the Black Sea region and Sea of Marmara, affected by the transition from the Mediterranean to the Black Sea and vice versa, for different kinds of fish including, but not limited to, tuna, mackerel, sardines, and anchovies.

Sometimes in modern studies, when referring to imports of processed fish products as attested by amphora finds, references are made to *garum* only, but in most cases what the amphorae contained was salted fish. Of the amphora types known to have contained salted fish products (*salsamenta*), if the vessel had a large neck and mouth (see, for example, the Beltran II A type) it contained salted fish, not fish sauce. If the fish sauce was made with very small, whole fish (sardines and anchovies in the Mediterranean; juvenile herrings and sprats in the northern provinces) rather than fish guts of larger types of fish, the final product was called *hallec* or *allec* and it contained small fish bones and vertebrae, which can be found deposited at the bottom of transport amphorae or salting vats. *Garum* and *allec* were not the only processed fish products; *muria*, for instance, was a popular fish sauce made with the small sardines called *maenia* in Latin (Dalby, 2003, 259; see Curtis, 1991, especially 6–15 for discussion of the various processed fish products).

Salting was not the only preservation method used in antiquity. Drying and smoking were important too and we know that dried and/or smoked fish was produced and commercialized, but unlike Roman salting workshops/factories, which were equipped with batteries of masonry salting vats (so durable archaeological features), drying and smoking required only ephemeral structures, thus these activities are more difficult to identify in the archaeological record.

Papyri from Roman Egypt indicate that salted fish products were a staple in the diet of all classes, ordinary people and elite alike. Fish sauces and salted fish are frequently mentioned in private correspondence, and this seems to imply production in the domestic context alongside professional producers and sellers of salted fish products (Curtis, 1991, 134–136). Certainly salted fish products of very different quality existed on the market, to satisfy every purse. Some kinds of *garum* could be rather expensive and therefore their consumption was limited to the wealthy. The *garum sociorum* produced in Carthago Nova (Cartagena, Spain) was a very expensive kind of *garum* and cost, according to Pliny the Elder, 500 sesterces per one *congius* (Plin. *HN* 31.94; the *congius* was one-eighth of an amphora = 3.375 l.).

Fish sauces and pastes were not limited to products utilizing only one kind of fish or mollusc. Oysters could be combined with other seafood to make elaborate recipes, such as the *allec* sauce made with oysters, sea urchins, sea nettle (some kind of zoophyte), and livers of mullet mentioned by Pliny the Elder (*HN* 31.95). Some Republican amphorae with their palaeocontent still intact, excavated at the fish-salting site of Baelo Claudia in Spain, revealed the manufacture of preserves mixing seafood and terrestrial animals: the amphorae contained different combinations, including predominantly tuna meat together with smaller fish, young specimens of pigs, ovines, and also molluscs, including land snails (Bernal Casasola and Arévalo Gonzales, 2008, 21–24).

The vast majority of archaeological studies investigating production and trade of processed fish products in the Roman period has focused on the Iberian peninsula (in particular on the area of the Strait of Gibraltar) and on parts of North Africa. These were not the only regions of the ancient world where large-scale fishing, preservations, and trade of fish-based foodstuffs took place. The coastal settlements along the Black Sea shores, for example, were known to have produced and exported salted fish and fish sauces since the Greek Classical period. One of Demosthenes' speeches (*in Lacritos* 35.31–32, 34) mentions a landowner who bought salted fish from Panticapaeum, on the Black Sea, to feed the agricultural workers on his estate. However, while archaeological evidence for some fish-salting and smoking installations dating to the Roman period has been documented (Højte, 2005), the identification of the amphorae used to transport these products remains in part uncertain, so that distribution patterns and typology of the fish products produced cannot be fully reconstructed.

It is not easy to determine what kinds of salted fish ordinary people consumed the most, but Galen is an author that, because of his medical interests in the properties of various foods, includes several interesting observations in his writings about what ordinary people ate. He lists whale meat, together with dolphins, seals, dogfish, hammerhead sharks, and large tuna as species that were regularly salted because of their 'unwholesome flesh'. Among these, Galen singles out dogfish as a fish normally eaten, salted, by common people (Gal., *On the Properties of Food-stuffs* 3.30.728, 3.36.738 = 6.728, 738 Kühn). The example cited above concerning a landowner purchasing salted fish to feed his agricultural labourers and comparative evidence from later historical periods, such as eighteenth-century slave plantations in the British West Indies creating a large demand for pickled oysters produced in New York, which were purchased to feed the slaves with protein (Marzano, 2013b, 193), should make us aware that also in antiquity, when it was possible to acquire preserved fish or seafood products cheaply, these foods may have figured in the diet of manual labourers or slaves. Indeed in a letter the emperor Marcus Aurelius wrote to Fronto, the meal of the labourers engaged in the vintage on an imperial estate is described as having consisted of 'small dried fish, well-soaked' (Fronto, *Ep.* 4.6).

Like salted fish products, which were traded widely across the empire, dried fish was also exported. This type of trade was reconstructed in the case of the Nile carp and catfish *clarias gariepinus*, a fish from Egypt and Syria-Phoenicia. Bones of these two species of fish were found at various sites outside of Egypt, spanning from Lycia to Italy, largely in archaeological contexts dating to the Roman imperial and Byzantine periods (Van Neer et al., 2004; 2007; 2008). The fact that the fish bones were found shows that the fish must have been dried whole, because in the salting preservation method the fish is filleted before being salted. These finds attest to the commercialization of dried fish outside the region of origin of the fish, in all likelihood as goods accompanying other products which constituted the bulk of the commercial exchanges but that are no longer visible archaeologically, such as textiles. For this reason, faunal taxa for Nile carp and catfish have been used as a proxy to establish trade exchanges in a range of perishable goods mentioned as exported goods in the written sources.

Regional diversity

As the Roman Empire encompassed a vast geographic area, not only were there differences in diet among the social classes, as discussed above, but there were also regional differences based on culinary traditions and what fish and other seafood were naturally available in the area. To give an example, while *allec* produced in the Mediterranean was manufactured largely from anchovies and sardines, fish sauces produced by Roman workshops based in the northern Iberian Peninsula, in Brittany, and in other parts of the northern provinces utilized largely small clupeids such as herrings and sprats, which abound in the Bay of Biscay, the English Channel, and North Sea, sometimes in conjunction with small flatfish or sandeel as major ingredients (Van Neer et al., 2005; 2010). Since the Roman army units based in Britain and along the

German frontier were among the major consumers of these preserved fish products, salted fish and fish sauces imported from the Iberian Peninsula were supplemented by local productions. In some instances, the zooarchaeological taxa show a wide variety of species used in the manufacture of fish sauces, which together with the small size of the fish clearly indicates that they were fished from an estuary. An inscription from Beetgum, in the Netherlands, indeed seems to attest a contract to supply the army and/or the administration of the lower Rhine with preserved fish from the coastal lagoons of the area (*CIL* XIII.8830; Ørsted, 1998, 20–21).

A marked regional difference in consumption and attitude towards seafood can be observed in the case of oysters. As mentioned above, in Roman Italy oysters were considered a delicacy and their consumption was largely confined to the wealthy. In some of the provinces, however, particularly in Gaul and Britain, while great appreciation for oysters developed after the arrival of the Romans, their consumption was much more widespread among the various strata of society, largely because of the presence of rich natural oyster beds. It seems that the Romans introduced to Britain not only the taste for oysters, but also oyster farming. Excavations of Roman Londinium at Pudding Lane, on the London waterfront, have recovered well-developed oyster shells that grew attached to oyster, cockle, and mussel clutch, the material used to encourage the settling of oyster larvae during the spawning season. Although the oyster larvae must have come from natural beds, the use of clutch and the regular size of the shells, very different from the irregular shells found in the same excavation, but in an earlier chronological context, strongly suggest human intervention and control of the growing conditions (Milne, 1985, 93–95). In southern Gaul, in the area around the brackish coastal lakes between Marseilles and the mouth of the Rhône River, starting from the second century BC oysters replaced mussels (which in the earlier period had made a significant contribution to the local diet) at the various settlements in the area; by the first century BC oyster consumption became a province-wide phenomenon cutting across social strata (Hitchner, 1999). This phenomenon was a combination of the Roman presence in the area, following the establishment of veteran colonies in the late first century BC and early first century AD, which probably increased a demand for the 'prestige' food oyster, of local food traditions of eating molluscs, and of the environment of the coastal lagoons, very favourable to oyster farming.

Alongside oyster consumption, another change in food habits observed in southern Gaul in the Roman period concerns the types of fish consumed, which is also an indication of different fishing practices. The Roman period here is characterized by the consumption of additional kinds of fish compared to the pre-Roman period, indicating fishing for pelagic species in open waters. At Lattes (ancient Latera), fishing in open waters for mackerels, sardines, and other clupeids appears to have been introduced in the mid-first century BC (in earlier periods, fishing in the coastal lagoons was the norm) and the zooarchaeological finds indicate a marked preponderance of fish versus mammals in food consumption in the first century AD (Sternberg, 1998).

Oysters were a common food also among the Roman military. Oyster shells have been found in abundance at military settlements in Britain, together with the less frequent shells of mussels, cockles, and whelks, indicating the popularity of oysters (Alcock, 2001, 55, 156). One of the written documents recovered at Vindolanda, just south of Hadrian's Wall in Britain, mentions 50 oysters sent, presumably fresh, in order to aid someone's recovery from illness (*Tab. Vindol.* II 299). Indeed oysters – whether fresh or preserved in brine – had a general reputation as a food suitable for the ill. Consumption of preserved oysters at military hospitals appears to be attested by a painted inscription on an amphora from the hospital of the legionary base of Novaesium (Neuss), in Moesia. The inscription, in Greek, reads *almostra*, explained as the combination of the word *alme* (seawater or brine) and *ostrea* (oysters) (Bernal, 2011, 206), but it has to be said that the reading of this inscription is problematic. However, preservation of oysters in brine is suggested by archaeological finds. Large quantities of oyster shells were found in excavation at a Roman salting factory at Iulia Traducta (Algeciras, Spain); the shells were found discarded in late antique layers and with clear signs of forced opening, indicating that the molluscs were extracted to be preserved in some form, probably in brine (Bernal, 2011, 204).

To conclude, for the majority of the inhabitants of the Roman world, geographic location and purchasing power determined how much and what kind of fish they could consume. Since fishing in the sea and in public rivers and lakes could not be legally prohibited, people living by rivers and the sea could engage in occasional fishing. Certainly, subsistence farmers normally resorted to fowling and fishing to complement their diets. In the case of the wealthy, fish and seafood figured prominently in their diet; fresh fish and quality seafood also had a strong symbolic and social value and could be taken as synonymous of a good life. As declared in the funerary epitaph of a certain C. Domitius Primus (*CIL* XIV.914): 'I lived on Lucrine oysters, often drank Falernian wine. The pleasures of bathing, wine, and love aged with me over the years!'

Notes

1   This chapter was submitted for publication in 2015 and does not take into account any items published subsequently.
2   See Fuller et al., 2012 for research on carbon and nitrogen stable isotope ratios in fish bone collagen from a range of marine and freshwater fish from northern Europe in order to establish archaeological fish isotope datasets that can help in reconstructing more precisely the diet of ancient human populations.

PART III

Peoples and identities

15

WOMEN, CHILDREN AND FOOD

Christian Laes

Introduction

Asking about women, children and food in the Roman world means tackling an enormous research question. Indeed in most cultures, age and gender seem to have been key concepts to understand quite diverse issues concerning eating and drinking. Access to food (and consequently possible undernourishment, malnutrition or bad health) immediately comes to mind. Especially in the case of women and children such access often relates to ideas about upbringing and education, to religious and/or social taboos, to ethnicity, to social class, or to the urban or rural environment in which people lived. Indeed, food entitlement and deprivation are much more determined by sociocultural factors than by mere economic categories.[1]

Taking into account that the Roman Empire was a multicultural empire *par excellence* with a population of approximately 60 million people at its height spread over a territory going from present-day Britain to Iraq, and considering the important shift towards monotheism this empire witnessed from the fourth century on, it is clear that a comprehensive survey on food, women and children is an impossible task in the framework of one chapter. I will thus necessarily confine myself to painting with broad strokes, dealing with issues that must have been vital and relevant to most of the women and children in this vast area over a period of roughly five centuries.

I will first highlight the material conditions that made food a major concern for most of the population – a worry of the *longue durée*. After that, the nuclear family unit will be described as the place where and through which food was both acquired and distributed. This often required choices for which age categories and gender came in. Closely connected to this question is the socialising role of food and eating habits in the family: who was supposed to eat together with whom and from what age onwards? How were family members expected to behave at table, and in relation to visitors? Specific age- or gender-related food will be treated in the following section, dealing with topics such as milk, weaning and the feeding of babies, but also with the consumption of alcohol and topoi on children's preferences for sweets and cakes. The last section deals with the role of the state in taking care of children in need for food. Although in this chapter I will fully integrate the results of archaeological, osteological and demographic research, my focus will be on literary authors who may be expected to broadly reflect attitudes of the Graeco-Roman elite, and who were read and commented upon over centuries. Comparative and cross-cultural evidence from Jewish, Christian and Islamic sources will be adduced now and then, although other chapters in this volume will serve these more specific aims.

As a final introductory remark, it should be said that the standard surveys on women, children and youth in the Roman Empire only briefly mention the issue of regime and food. It is therefore to be hoped that this contribution will contribute to further research into a topic that is vital in more than one way.

A history of shortage and struggling for daily bread

In the Sermon on the Mount, Jesus goes deeply into the issue of worry about material provisions. He tells his followers not to be anxious about food, but to rely on God. Even the birds, who are worth far less than people, are fully provided for.

> See the birds of the sky, that they don't sow, neither do they reap, nor gather into barns. Your heavenly Father feeds them. Aren't you of much more value than they?
> *(Matthew 6: 26; transl.* World English Bible*)*

This verse has been much debated, but the overall meaning seems clear. Birds do not have the ability to do farming, to store food or to plan for the future. Despite the greater burden they have, they are not anxious about the future.[2] By emphasising the sorrows about having enough to eat and securing access to food, Jesus undoubtedly struck a familiar chord with much of his audience, for whom this search was indeed a daily burden and struggle (cf. 'give us our daily bread' in the Lord's Prayer). Also in the Old Testament, plenty of references are found to the daily trouble of securing food and income for the family.[3]

In contrast to Jesus, most Graeco-Roman elite writers were not at all concerned about the matter, though tellingly Galen acknowledges the enormous gap between eating habits of the persons mostly addressed in medical treatises, and the common people who were forced to eat almost anything available out of bare necessity.[4] Much more than literary snapshots, comparative historical evidence makes clear what such need for food could actually mean.

Earlier research had a tendency to offer a pessimistic view of the matter for much of the pre-industrial population. According to some estimates, before the French Revolution, about 20% of the French population were unable to work full days, due to the lack of sufficient proteins and calories.[5] There is, however, debate about these issues. While we may reject Geoffrey Kron's views on the ancient population as being the most well-nourished of all premodern societies as too optimistic, the historic truth probably lies somewhere between the two extremes. In particular Kristina Killgrove has offered a more balanced view and warned against the methodological shortcomings that distort the outcome of part of earlier research.[6] Still, the circumstances causing at least a part of the male adult population to be unfit for working and the ever-impending danger of shortage of food are basic facts to be taken into account when dealing with the ancient world.

Osteological finds throughout the empire again and again testify to scurvy and rickets, the former caused by vitamin C deficiency, the latter by vitamin D deficiency. Porotic hyperostosis and cribra orbitalia might be linked to iron deficiency and consequent anaemia. Also hypoplasia of the teeth occurs. These pathologies are found with both adults and children, and often go back to malnutrition in early childhood years. Soranus of Ephesus already remarked on the high frequency of malformation of the bones of children in the City of Rome (*Gyn.* 2.16 – possibly referring to rickets). Although his explanation (Roman mothers cared less for their children than their Greek counterparts) is remarkable to say the least, his observation remains interesting, as it probably refers to vitamin C deficient feeding habits in urban milieus and the consequences for children. And yet these women and children were often forced to take part in the labour process, since many adult men simply could only participate in an insufficient way.[7]

Early modern figures on consumption patterns in European cities indicate that about half to three-quarters of the income of the common people were spent on costs for daily sustenance.[8] Again, we can imagine urban families in antiquity depending on income to secure their livelihood and engaging both women and children to somehow secure their uncertain existence.

Also evidence from present day World Health Organization statistics on bodily appearance and the Body Mass Index may add to the picture. One can safely assume that the ancient world came closer to countries such as India, Pakistan and Ethiopia (with over 30% of underweight males, that is ≤18.5 BMI; and about 15% of moderate and severe thinness, namely ≤ 17 BMI for females and 13% for males for the first two countries) than to Western societies. In comparison, the underweight category for the United States only amounts to 2.4%.[9] It is thus safe to assume that, with present-day Western standards in mind, the presence of thin or even extremely thin women and children was an everyday occurrence in the ancient world. The somewhat corpulent and fleshy little children we find in art from the Hellenistic period onwards might point to opulence and a certain wealth, but they surely were not representations of everyday reality for the majority of the population.[10]

Admittedly, representing the Roman Empire as an environment with a considerable proportion of undernourished women and children, who were at the same time involved in the labour process, might strike the connoisseur of classic literature as odd or somewhat exaggerated. But nineteenth-century doctors, who for the first time performed state-regulated medical examinations in primary schools in the countryside or with children belonging to the labourers' class in France or other countries in western Europe discovered very much the same pattern.[11] And surely, all this does not imply a simplified dichotomy of rich versus poor in Roman society, not least because new analysis suggests a broader distribution of wealth across Roman society and therefore supports the hypothesis of the existence of 'middling' classes and of 'the poor', the latter constituting perhaps half of the population.[12] By modern standards, most people indeed lived a life of risk and survival, vexed by uncertainties such as famine caused by bad harvest or decreased income; this was very much the common fate of many women and children. Moreover, the situation could affect them more than others. The birth of yet another hungry mouth to feed could lead parents to the act of exposure or infanticide, perhaps even more so in the case of girls for whom a dowry had to be paid in the case of marriage. Due to the perils of giving birth frequently, combined with marriage at an early age and the pressure of performing corporal labour, women could indeed well turn out to be the weaker sex. In a way, the stereotypical image of the ancient medical writers became self-fulfilling.[13]

The family unit as the place to get food

For families of certain affluence, it was the wife in charge and/or the slave personnel who provided the family with the basic fare on a daily basis. For special occasions, a professional cook – usually a slave or a freedman – could be hired.[14] Theoretical works by Roman authors on the management of large country estates (*latifundia*) and legal sources testify to a role pattern that ascribes the tasks of preparing and administering food to women and children. Their remarks also apply to large households in the towns. Boys before the age of puberty are mentioned as the ideal kitchen help for women. Women and children belonged to the *instrumentum instrumenti*: staff responsible for the feeding, clothing and accommodation of the farmworkers and labour slaves who belonged to the *instrumentum*. Their typical tasks were bread baking and maintenance of the *villa*; typical professions that of kitchen maid, female weaver and cook.[15] In such large *familiae* there was no daily concern about having enough to eat – except perhaps for the slaves. Cato the Censor put his slaves on a special ration when they were ill, and it belonged to the power of the master to punish slaves with famine.[16]

For the largest part of the population, the daily search for food happened in the context of the family.

Due to the scarcity of the sources, we often tend to regard the peasantry in the Roman Empire as a uniform and undifferentiated class. The opposite was true: there were prosperous farmers who had close social ties with their poorer neighbours, who in turn could assist them whenever needed. Most of the peasants lived in family units. Anthropologically, in agricultural environments the responsibility of preparing the food and household chores has been a task for women and children in most cultures.[17] The few literary sources we have depict the countryside as a rustic idyll and confirm this role pattern. Thus, the famous poor farmer in pseudo-Virgil's Moretum lived together with his black African servant in a dwelling with a heap of grain on the floor. She is said to be his 'solitary housekeeper', as he summons her to lay upon the hearth some logs to feed the fire, and to boil some chilly water on the flame, while he continues to transfer the copious meal from the hearth into a sieve and shakes it. Pliny the Elder claims that since there were no bakers in Rome before the year 174 BC, women took care of baking the bread, 'as it still is nowadays with many people'. A similar idealised picture turns up with Juvenal, who reflects on the golden days of the Roman agrarian past. He describes a farmer going to work on the land and returning home in the evening, together with his elder sons. He is awaited by his wife, who took care of the household tasks and of the food, and by four children who are glad to join him at the table.[18] The most telling evidence comes from the story of the simple hunters in the wilds of Euboea, a discourse by Dio Chrysostom – a typical rhetorical piece of art proving the preferability of sober poverty above decadent wealth. Here, Dio describes the lives of two farmers, each one married to a sister of the other (*Or.* 7.10). Their fathers had been hired herdsmen, tending the cattle of a wealthy man. When the latter fell in disgrace, his stock was butchered and his land left alone. The herdsmen decided to stay in the place, and made their living by cultivating the land on the plots around their huts, and by hunting. They married their sons to wives, each giving his own daughter. Both men had died in old age, keeping their strong and vigorous bodies till the end (*Or.* 7.11–20). Now, both sons had children, sons and daughters. They lived in two pretty huts, and had a third one where the grain and the pelt were kept. There they surely managed to live in reasonable conditions: among their possessions were four deer pelts, smoked sides of bacon and venison, portions of wheat and barley. They maintained 22 vines producing fine-quality wine. Among their cattle were eight she-goats, and a cow with a calf. Also, they possessed some utensils (*Or.* 7.43–47). One daughter was married to a rich man living in a village, who got game, fruit and vegetables from them, while he in return helped them by borrowing wheat for seed (*Or.* 7.68). This is very much the kind of reciprocity by which peasants have been known to secure their lives in many cultures. When they received guests, a daughter of marriageable age served the food and poured the wine, and the boys prepared the meat and passed it around. Another youth already seems to be a good hunter, since he brought in a hare (*Or.* 7.67).

One wonders whether a similar role pattern existed with families of modest means in the cities. Archaeologists have recognised kitchens in various places throughout the Roman Empire, but they all belong to houses that show some affluence. Most inhabitants of apartments (*insulae*) would eat their meals cooked on braziers set up in the *medianum*, a corridor hall facing out onto a street or courtyard. Surely the cramped living space of the majority of the city population did not allow for any kitchen space. For a hot meal, standing at one of the many open bars with a hearth was the only option – not really a closed familial occasion.[19] Again, Dio Chrysostom hits the nail on the head when saying that contrary to the countryside in the city everything had to be paid for, except for the water in the basins (*Or.* 7.105–106). Surely very few families would have the luxury of possessing a small city garden where they could raise some crop.[20] As an alternative, families might go out fishing when the city was situated next to a river. However, due to the presence of sewers, waste and excrements, fishes from the streams of bigger cities were notoriously inferior in quality.[21] We can also imagine mothers doing their utmost to secure some food or income for their family, as did the fathers who went out working. When grain was distributed, it was most likely women who went to the big bakery ovens to have it made into bread, as implied by Pliny the Elder (see note 18). Attending the market could have been a typical female business. At the Roman fruit and vegetable market, the Forum Olitorium, there was a column called *columna lactaria* where infants could be fed with milk. Should we imagine this as a place where exposed little babies were picked up by passers-by? Or was it rather a market where mothers went to in order to secure their families fruit and vegetables, as well as fresh milk for their babies?[22]

However, crisis and hunger were an impending danger for most of the urban population. Poor harvest due to bad weather conditions might be an immediate reason for peasants to seek food and assistance in the towns. Of course, populous cities were themselves very dependent on food supply from the countryside and were subject to fluctuating prices of food. Ancient authors, surely but not exclusively in late antiquity, have gone to great lengths to describe the horrors of famine and pestilence (which were of course closely related). In their gruesome depictions, the fate of women and children turns up again and again.[23] In telling detail, Ammianus Marcellinus reports on the anxiety of the prefect Tertullus and the population of Rome in the year 359, when the ships transporting grain could not reach the harbour due to bad weather. In ultimate despair, Tertullus showed his little children to the angry crowd, suggesting that they sacrifice them if they thought that would resolve the situation. Ultimately, the crowd was deeply touched by his gesture, and decided to wait calmly for whatever the future would bring. When the winds finally lay down and the ships arrived, a crisis was overturned.[24] Other evidence comes to mind. A father had to decide which of his children to sell in order to secure some food for the others. Honourable ladies went into public markets to beg, constrained by want to throw away all shame and evidence of their formal liberal education. Some were eventually driven to suicide, like the father who leaped into the Tiber while his five hungry children witnessed his death.[25]

Peasant families could of course decide to stay in the countryside, but they were not always better off. Sheer necessity forced men in closed communities to put women and children to work on tasks that were normally meant to be performed by them. Established sociocultural values and role patterns could be trampled on in such communities.[26] In the Anthologia Palatina, we read about an impoverished elderly lady called Nico who, together with her daughters, was forced to glean corn-ears in order to escape starvation. The heat was unbearable. She died in the baking sun and was subsequently cremated on a pyre. This is as far as the empathy of ancient authors for countrywomen goes: they were seen to be poor, to age quickly and not to be able to cope with the heat of the sun.[27]

Dining habits and socialisation of women and children

It would be hard to deny the socialising effects of dining. The ancient writers were also very much aware that meals were occasions *par excellence* to focus on domesticity and family values.

Needless to say, their remarks on it very much relate to the higher class, as we know so little about the ways a 'proper' meal was held in the cramped spaces of the urban environment of the average city dweller, or in rural huts and houses. But also for the upper class, one should be aware that the dinners and feasts mentioned in the texts were primarily public affairs. Just eating together with the family was not socially meaningful at all, and the rules and habits for it are thus not mentioned in the sources. In any case, Roman aristocrats limiting themselves to dinners within their own families would isolate themselves as much as those preferring the solitary meal or *cena solitaria*.[28]

That meals should be sober and frugal is an ideal much cherished by the Epicureans. One will remember Epicurus' insistence on the simple pleasure of having bread and water, at best combined with a piece of cheese. The ideal family dinner should be similar. Hence the Stoic philosopher Posidonius pictures fathers or mothers asking their son which fruit he would like to have for dinner. After his meal consisting of fruit and water, the satisfied boy would go to sleep.[29]

Dinners also served to distinguish Roman habits from other customs. Cornelius Nepos was very much aware of this:

> There are numerous actions decent by our standards which are thought base by them (the Greeks). For what Roman is ashamed to take his wife to a dinner party? [. . .] This is all very different in Greece: she is only invited to dinners of the family.
>
> *Cornelius Nepos, praef. 7 (transl. K. Vössing)*

Also, Roman society distinguished itself from Etruscan culture, which unabashedly permitted men and women to recline together on dinner couches, even when they were not a married couple.[30] So, Roman women were presented at dinner parties, be it invited or at their own homes. But they usually sat on chairs, and surely did not lie on the same couch with their husbands, although Scintilla and Fortunata famously did so in Petronius' *Satyricon* (67.5). This of course testifies to the lack of class and manners of wealthy freedmen. Supposedly, reclining was seen as an unseemly position for women, although remarks by Valerius Maximus suggest that the custom had already changed in the first century AD.[31]

Also children were supposed to sit during dinner. Most probably, they were not meant to serve up dishes.[32] In the old fashion, children would sit beside their father on the lowest couch. In the first century, children and adolescents were seated at their own tables, where they had a banquet in which the rules were the same as those observed by the adult upper class.[33] There surely was an age of reclining, from which boys were allowed to fully participate and lie down at the banquets, but it is impossible to fix a precise age limit for this.[34] As to the presence of slave children hanging around the tables, serving and entertaining the guests with sometimes deliberately naughty behaviour, they added to the display of wealth and luxury that made the master and his guests happy. In this, a component of sexual entertainment was part of the picture, as was the animalisation of the slave boys concerned. After all, the citizens of luxurious Sybaris took delight only in Maltese puppy dogs, surely a worthy alternative.[35]

The appropriate food for the right gender and age

It was firmly rooted in ancient medical thought that the same food products were not fit for every single body. Humoral theory came in. Since babies were considered to be moist and hot, their food should be drying and cooling. Hot and dry young people should preferably receive cooling and moisturising substances. And surely young women should get substances that modified their sexual desire. Needless to say, these alimentary measures only applied to those who could afford the luxury of sticking to them.[36]

Both symbolically and in actual practice, milk was very much related to infants. According to medical writings, little children who were in need of strengthening were given a portion of asses' milk each day. Tepid milk with poppy juice was administered to little children before they went to bed. In Rome, offerings for infants were done next to the Ruminal fig tree. For such occasions, milk was used instead of wine to pour over the offerings.[37] For babies, mother's milk was in any case preferred. One wonders what happened on the occasion that an infant was not able to suck milk from the breast, a case reported by Caelius Aurelianus. In the life of Saint Theodorus, there is the remarkable instance of the father Erythrius who, after the death of the mother, fed the baby with wheat and barley porridge, by means of a feeding bottle made out of glass and having the shape of a female breast. Since the mother had died, he did not want to take the risk of hiring a nurse who by means of her milk could pass her pagan creeds and customs into the little child.[38] There has been little research on artificial milk feeding in antiquity, although both the archaeological and the iconographical record amply testify of this possibility.[39] Surely in the Mediterranean regions, goats' milk was much preferred over cows' milk. Due to storage issues in hot climates, yoghurt or cheese consumption prevailed over simple milk. Bioarchaeologists have linked porotic hyperorstosis in children's and adults' bones in Greece with goat milk's anaemia.[40]

There can be no doubt that the middle classes and the well-to-do preferred breastfeeding by a wet-nurse.[41] The insistence of some writers that it is much better to feed your child yourself actually proves that the opposite was common practice with their audience. Both the medical authors and the dossier of wet-nursing contracts preserved on papyri point to a rather extended period of breastfeeding, that is up to two or three years of age. Since prolonged breastfeeding is known to have contraceptive effects, there might be an important demographic consequence of this. Women from the higher classes possibly got pregnant more often, since they mostly abstained from the practice of breastfeeding.[42]

An inquiry of 113 non-industrial populations has observed the age of 5–6 months as the most common age for weaning. First supplementary foods invariably took the form of cereal-based gruels or porridge. Weaning is a gradual process, and the cessation of breastfeeding occurred between two and five years of age. Quite unsurprisingly, ancient medical authors confirm the pattern. Galen proposed the eruption of the first teeth as the appropriate time for introducing first solid food, Soranus mentions a bodily firmness that could scarcely be achieved before the age of six months and proposes a gradually taking off from the breast from approximately two years of age on.[43] Regional variation must have been an important factor throughout the Roman Empire. Stable isotope analysis has been applied to some bioarchaeological investigations of sites from the Roman period. While Isola Sacra (first–third century) reveals weaning taking place over a short period and commencing at an age of around 1.5 years, contemporary evidence from the city of Rome shows subadults being still nursed into their second and third year. Sites from London and Queenford Farm show weaning occurring gradually over an extended period, with a complete cessation of breastfeeding at an age of around 3–4 years. The same extended breastfeeding period appears in the Byzantine evidence.[44]

As for water, people were very much aware of the severe risks of pollution. The search for clean water is a constant concern up to early medieval hagiography.[45] In such situations, it does not come as a surprise that even little children were fed small quantities of wine. Galen was opposed to the administering of wine to children, but his mentioning of the practice seems to suggest that it was actually quite common. According to Aristotle, a two-year old child should be given lots of milk and little wine. Perhaps he referred to just a little drop of wine, just to prevent contamination?[46] In the Iliad, centuries of generations of (young) readers encountered the significant detail that as a little kid Achilles, sitting on Phoenix's knees, used to spit the wine he was offered on the chiton of his educator (Il. 9.488–491). Also note in the same context that, in medieval times, children were given beer, because water was often polluted. It is very difficult to find evidence for this in antiquity, although one papyrus text may refer to beer being bought for 'the children'.[47] Also, the low average height of Roman bars gave children the opportunity of attending them. Perhaps it was here that they gradually got accustomed to the do's and don'ts of consuming alcohol.[48]

Consumption of alcohol brings in other age- and gender-related questions. While ancient writers, especially moralists, were keen to condemn excessive drinking as damaging to the social order (surely in the case of rulers lacking self-restraint), ancient society undoubtedly condoned inebriation on certain occasions, such as the Saturnalia, *convivia*, or victories. For the upper-classes, drinking was very much a matter of etiquette and social decorum. It was also learned behaviour that teenagers would acquire in their peer group of *iuvenes*. Among the lower classes, too, there seems to be sufficient source evidence for heavy drinking and the outrageous conduct caused by it.[49]

As regards women and wine, it was only conservative writers who stressed the golden age when decent *matronae* were not even allowed to drink, and a violation of the rules on sobriety (often connected with adultery) might even lead to their being put to death by their husbands.[50] Drunken women were a favourite theme for satirists (famously Juvenal, *Sat.* 6.300–301) and Hellenistic sculptors. However, the grave inscription of a man actually praising his deceased wife for the fact that she liked to have fun and drink wine tells another story, as does all the information on the availability of wine and the possibility for women to enjoy it.[51]

Stereotypically, children were linked to cakes, sweets and sugary fruit. Cornelius Fronto mentions how his little grandson was absolutely fond of grapes, and he recalls himself as a child enjoying the same delights. The child with grapes is a favourite motive in Hellenistic art, and the image lasts till the fifth century depiction of Theodoret as a little child sitting on the knee of Peter the Galatian and enjoying bread and grapes.[52] Bioarchaeological investigations on teeth, however, do not demonstrate an overexposure of children to sweet substances and the consequences of it.[53]

Medical writers found that unmarried girls at the onset of menstruation were experiencing a troublesome period. They sometimes prescribed a strict regimen of diet. Rufus of Ephesus advised girls in puberty to moderate their intake of food, to avoid wine, and to spurn meat and other excessively nourishing food altogether.[54] Whether the emphasis on restraint in food and the cultural belief that young women must be given just what they needed led to ignoring the real nutritional needs of young women is a question not easily to be answered.[55]

In general, puberty was considered a crucial period for food for both males and females. After puberty some boys and girls who were previously thin put on weight and become healthier. By the discharge of sperm or menses, that which had been impeding their health and nutrition had been removed.[56]

Finally, the phase of youth needed special precautions. Overconsumption of seasonal fruit led to severe liver problems for Galen at the age of 19 years. At his father's advice, he then decided to consume grapes and figs only in moderation and to abandon all other fruit. Although this text belongs to the tradition of the stubborn son first not listening to the father's advice but finally yielding, it informs us again of special food precautions related to age. At least Galen believed that others were helped by the same diet.[57]

Did the state take care of hungry children?

After the quite worrying details on hungry children and the impending dangers of malnutrition, it may come as a relief to read that the Roman Empire actually had alimentation schemes for children (see Holleran in this volume). The emperor's euergetism is proudly presented in inscriptions. At least 49 towns in Italy, with a heavy concentration on central Italy, testify of *alimenta* for free citizen children: allowances in the form of cash distributions that were needed for securing food. Also private endowments schemes are attested. We may imagine the children congregating each month in the forum of the town, accompanied by their parents. In silver *denarii* they would then accept their allowance, which varied between ten and sixteen *sestertii* (1 *denarius* = 4 *sestertii*). A total of 192 *sestertii* per annum was quite a sum, enabling them to buy approximately 400 kg of wheat, the minimum subsistence being estimated at approximately 250 kg of wheat.[58] Some inscriptions also mention age limits: 14 years for boys and an unreadable age for girls in Florence (*CIL* 11.1602), 3–15 years for boys and 3–13 years for girls in Sicca Veneria in Africa Proconsularis (*CIL* 8.1641), 16 years for boys and 14 for girls in Tarracina (*CIL* 10.6328). A legal regulation defines 18 years of age as the upper limit for boys and 14 for girls, at the same time stressing that this is an unusually high limit that nevertheless had been settled as such only 'for the sake of piety' (*tamen pietatis intuitu*) and only in the case of the *alimenta* (*Dig.* 34.1.14.1). In Tarracina, 200 children, equally divided between boys and girls, were helped by the measure. Estimating the population of Tarracina in imperial times is an impossible task, but 8,000 inhabitants would be a rough educated guess. Taking into consideration the comparative demographic models, 2,640 of them would be below age 15. About 2,000 would belong to the category of being freeborn Roman citizens. The 200 who are helped were only a small part. What is more, as the *alimenta* were by no means a charitable institution, the well-off also had their children profit from the institution, by which children of the municipal aristocracy might confirm their dependence and loyalty towards their 'father', the emperor. In all, these *alimenta* were more beneficial symbols of the caring role of the emperor towards his citizens, who were somehow 'infantilised'.[59]

It is safe to assume that for the matter of charity and food, Christianity was a turning point (see Raga in this volume). Eusebius' testimony on the Christians' zeal and piety during the famine and pestilence which struck Palestine in the years 312–313 is a remarkable source for this. Here we notice a real difference between non-Christian euergetism and religiously inspired charity. As the pestilence struck on every house and family, Christians were there to help day and night, taking care of the burial of the dead and the distributing of bread to all.[60]

Conclusion

Readers acquainted with studies on food in modern and recent history will be struck by the absence of ego-documents in this chapter. For antiquity, there are no interviews of adults who as children survived a period of famine, or women who testify of a profound interiorisation of societally imposed tasks, like Valeria in twentieth-century Florence who severely criticises women who went out with their husbands and did not spend all their time on the education of their children. She herself proudly testified that she spared the food out of her own mouth just to be able to feed her children in a better way.[61] Apart from some letters on papyri, we do not hear ancient women or children making remarks on food (see Clarysse in this volume).

What we do have invariably stems from the male perspective. This evidence, combined with the broad comparative perspective, suggests that for sociocultural reasons women who are in fact the stronger sex from a biological point of view were reduced to become indeed the weaker gender. Compared to present-day Europe, Japan or the United States, which by law and regulations secure an even access to food, income and health care for men and women, life expectancy of women in antiquity would have been shorter.[62] For children, the situation could have been even harsher, since biology already makes them weaker. One wonders how the situation of being both female and a child could have aggravated the situation. Ancient authors are mostly silent on this, although a remark in Xenophon's *Oeconomicus* testifies of a young woman who had strictly interiorised societal rules. By her own mother, she was taught to strictly observe and control her appetites, and undoubtedly she would have given the same pattern to her daughters (Xenophon, *Oec.* 7.5). This is the closest one gets to Florentine Valentina who spared the food out of her own mouth.

However, this rather negative picture should by no means give way to a gruesome image of a society that did not care about its hungry or deficient women and children. Not only did the upper-classes and at least a part of the middling classes mostly manage quite well, when times were good, we may also imagine peasants, slaves and even poorer city folk getting along reasonably well, although danger was always imminent. It was the task of the family unit, and preferably of both parents, to secure food for their offspring (as it was in the Jewish tradition, see Kraemer in this volume). At least ideologically, there existed the image of the caring Emperor or municipal benefactor, who took care as a father by supplying fellow citizen children with food. Also, eating and dining served as important means for socialising and educating children. At least the medical writers showed concern about which food was appropriate for which age and gender.

Early Islam is surely a different tradition, but it also rose in the late Mediterranean world. When asked what was the greatest sin, Sahih al-Bukhari (9th century AD) replied that it consisted in ascribing divinity to someone other than Allah. The next sin, however, was to kill your child out of fear that it will share your food. Another saying states that no one earns his food better than the one who worked with his hands.[63] These are surely statements stemming from an agricultural environment – the kind of wisdom which for Graeco-Roman literature is mainly found in monks' sayings from late ancient Egypt. But undoubtedly, the large silent majority of people in the Roman Empire would have recognised itself in the second two sayings. As such, both care and concern co-existed with sociocultural and economic conditions that were unfavourable to the non-adult male part of the populace.

There is no need for moralising judgement on the subject of food, women and children. All the more, there is need for careful consideration of the many different aspects which shaped the lives of people in the past, and the present.

Notes

1 Sen, 1981.
2 See also Luke 12:23. Johnson, 2010 reads Jesus' words as a challenge to the traditional role pattern for women.
3 E.g. Job 7:1–7 on the dayworker always concerned about his income; Ps. 58:7 wishing for enemies that they would wander around the town and suffer famine like dogs.
4 Galen, *De aliment. fac.* 1.2 (6.488–489 Kühn).
5 For example, Fogel, 2004 and Clark, 2007. See Saller, 2012, 72 for the example of the French population.
6 Kron, 2005a and Killgrove, 2010a.
7 Fox, 2012 offers an excellent overview about undernourishment, labour and the bioarchaeological evidence.
8 Erdkamp, 2012c, 67.

9   World Health Organisation, Global Database on Body Mass Index (http://apps.who.int/bmi/index.jsp, accessed 9 September 2014).

10 Backe-Dahmen, 2006.

11 Rollet, 2001, 187–218.

12 Scheidel, 2006, on poverty and middling classes; Mayer, 2012, on urban middle classes.

13 Hin, 2012, 135–139 for an overview of the problem of female infanticide and women as the weaker sex.

14 Aristotle, *Pol.* 1323a4 (wife or personnel); Curtis, 2012 (cook).

15 Columella, *RR* 12.4.3 (boys in kitchen); *Dig.* 33.7.12.5 (*instrumentum instrumenti*); *Dig.* 33.7.12.6 (typical tasks). See Saller, 2003, 200–201 for implications on the status of slave women.

16 Cato, *De agricult.* 2; Lactantius, *De ira Dei* 5.12.

17 Whittaker, 2003, 104.

18 Virgil, *Mor.* 31–46; Pliny the Elder, *NH* 18.107; Juvenal, *Sat.* 14.166–171. Note that from Severan times, bread was distributed, which implied more regular distributions and did not involve women going to bakeries.

19 Curtis, 2012, 124–130.

20 Laes, 2015, 96, 101.

21 Galen, *De alimentarum facultatibus* 3.19 (6.702 Kühn); 3.25 (6.709 Kühn); 3.30 (6.722 Kühn).

22 Festus, s.v. Lactaria (p. 118 ed. Mueller). The suggestion of market place for fresh milk occurs in Baudrillart, 1900, 886.

23 Erdkamp, 1998; 2002; 2012a, 68–74.

24 Amm. Marc. 19.10.

25 Basil, *Hom. in illud Lucae destruam* 4 (PG 29.268–269) (father's decision); Eusebius, *Hist. Eccl.* 9.8.1–15 (on honourable ladies during the famine in Palestine of 312–313); Procopius, *Bell Goth.* 7.17 (Tiber suicide in Rome during the sieges of 545 and 546).

26 Scheidel, 1995, 210–213 on the (too) high costs of having house slaves and the reversed role pattern in isolated communities.

27 *Anth. Pal.* 9, 89.

28 Vössing, 2012, 143–144. One may note the amazement of the fourteenth-century traveller Ibn-Battuta when encountering the Samira people in the city of Djanani, who never eat with anyone, nor let themselves be observed while eating. See *The Travels of Ibn-Battuta AD 1325–1354. Translated by H.A.R. Gibb* (Cambridge, 1999) vol. 3, p. 597.

29 Diogenes Laertius, *Vita Phil.* 10.11; Seneca, *Epist.* 18.9 (Epicurus); Athenaeus, *Deipn.* 6.275a (Posidonius).

30 Athenaeus, *Deipn.* 12.517d–f (Etruscans).

31 Varro in Isidorus of Sevilla, *Et.* 20.11.9; Valerius Maximus 2.1.2.

32 As is implied by Varro in Nonius Marcellus, *De comp. doctr.* (ed. Lindsay) 229.15 (ed. Lindsay): *sic in privatis domibus pueri liberi et liberae ministrabant* (he explains why *puer* means both servant and child in Latin). The custom of higher class boys serving at official banquets is sometimes attested for the Middle Ages and the Modern Period.

33 Suetonius, *Aug.* 64.3; Tacitus, *Ann.* 13,16.1 (Prince Britannicus is not yet with his father Claudius at the same table).

34 Booth, 1991; Bradley, 1998; Sigismund Nielsen, 1998; Vössing, 2012, 138–143. Bradley, 1998, 40–47 has collected the few passages referring to children sitting at their own tables during banquets. Apart from the ones cited in footnote 33 these include Suetonius, *Claud.* 32 and Clement of Alexandria, *Protr.* 2.54.3.

35 Athenaeus, *Deipn.* 12.1519 on which see Vössing, 2012, 141. On slave boys at banquets, see D'Arms, 1991; Pollini, 2003.

36 Nadeau, 2012, 149–151.

37 Pliny the Elder, *NH* 28.33 (ass milk); Ovid, *Fast.* 4.347; Plutarch, *Quaest. Rom.* 57 (Ruminal).

38 Caelius Aurelianus, *Morb. ac.* 3.105; Herter, 1964 (on Theodorus).

39 See Jaeggi, Forthcoming. Apart from the literary testimony on Theodorus, there also is Soranus, *Gyn.* 2.17 and Mustio, *Gyn.* 1.131.

40 Fox, 2012, 419.

41 For Greek antiquity, starting from the archaic period, a considerable number of literary sources point to breastfeeding by the mother herself. See Marshall, 2017.

42 Parkin, 2012, 113.

43 Powell et al., 2014, 103; Galen, *Hyg.* 1.10 (first teeth); Soranus, *Gyn.* 2.46 (scarcely before six months); Gyn. 2.47 (gradual taking over).

44 Powell et al., 2014, 103–105; Bourbou and Garvie-Lok, 2009.

45 Urso, 1997, 10–11.

46 Galen, *De san. tuenda* 1.10–11 and 5.5 (6.47–54, 6.334 Kühn); Aristotle, *Pol.* 1336 a 2–24. Diluted wine: Hippocrates, *Salubr.* 6 (6.80–82 Littré); Galen, *In Hipp. vict. rat. in morb. acut. comment.* 3.24 (6.181–182 Kühn). See Hummel, 1999, 119–121.

47 On the Middle Ages, see Orme, 2001, 71–72. *Sel. Pap.* 1.186 mentions barley water (line 51) and beer (line 60). It is a shopping list, and shopping for children is included, but it does not explictly state that the barley water and the beer should be bought for the children. See Clarysse in this volume.

48 Laurence, 2017, 33–34.

49 D'Arms, 1995, 304–308 (drunkenness and *decorum*), 308–312 (drinking and childhood), 312–314 (socioeconomic aspects of drinking). Cf. Ammianus Marcellinus, 14.6.25 on 'bibulous Rome'.

50 Dionysius of Halicarnassus, *Ant. Rom.* 2.25.4–7; Valerius Maximus 6.3.9

51 Drunken women are famously satirised in Juvenal, *Sat.* 6.300-301. See *CIL* VI 19055 – second century AD, *Bacchoque madere*.

52 Fronto, *Ad amicos* 1.12 (178.11–179.3 van den Hout); Theodoretus, *Hist. rel.* 9.4.

53 Laurence, 2005.

54 Laes and Strubbe, 2014, 144. Rufus is cited by Oribasius, *Lib. inc.* 18.10.

55 Garnsey, 1991, 100–112 and Nadeau, 2012, 151.

56 Laes and Strubbe, 2014, 69 on Aristotle, *Hist. anim.* 581a13–582a33.

57 Laes and Strubbe, 2014, 66–67 on Galen, *De prob.* 1 (6.755–757 Kühn).

58 Jongman, 2002, 63, 74.

59 Note that I fully agree with the tenor of Jongman, 2002 (who uses the term 'infantilisation' to describe the relationship between the Emperor as a father and his citizens as sons and daughters), though I am less optimistic about the amount of young people who might profit from *alimenta*.

60 Eusebius, *Hist. eccl.* 9.8.1–15. See Erdkamp, 2012c, 68–72.

61 Counihan, 2004, 139–140.

62 Sen, 1990.

63 Sahih al-Bukhari, Book 86, Hadith 41, Chapter 20: I said, 'O Allah's Messenger! Which is the biggest sin?' He said, 'To set up rivals to Allah by worshipping others though He alone has created you.' I asked, 'What is next?' He said, 'To kill your child lest it should share your food.' Sahih al-Bukhari, Book 34, Hadith 25, Chapter 15: The Prophet said, 'Nobody has ever eaten a better meal than that which one has earned by working with one's own hands. The Prophet of Allah, David used to eat from the earnings of his manual labor.'

16

CENTRAL AND NORTHERN EUROPE

Tünde Kaszab-Olschewski

Introduction

This chapter focuses on the territory of Roman Britain, Gaul and Germania as far as the provinces of Raetia, Noricum and Pannonia during the first to the third centuries AD. This part of Europe is bordered by major rivers such as the Rhine and the Danube as well as the North Sea and the Atlantic Ocean, which configured the border (*limes* or *ripa*) of the Roman Empire. The landscape is strongly diversified, because every kind of geographical region from seashores through to fertile plains to mountain and alpine mountain ranges can be found here.

The majority of those living in this region belonged to the Celtic (or Gaulish) peoples. North or northeast of them on the right side of the Rhine (but also on the left), and north of the Danube lived mainly tribes who were known under the collective name Germans (so-called Rhein-Weser-Germans and the Elbgermans or Suebi). In addition, a variety of other ethnic groups could be found in the region, for example Sarmatians (Iazyges) or Dacians. Due to the size of the area considered here, only a brief overview can be offered, and the focus will be primarily on the German provinces, *inter alia*, because of their central location.

History and Romanization

The Roman conquest of the northwestern regions (Gaul, Germany, Britain) was initiated under Julius Caesar (100–44 BC) by the middle of the first century BC and was completed in the course of the next 200 years (Steidl, 2008, 45–46). The occupation up to the Danube region (Noricum and Pannonia) started with Augustus, while the border shifted towards the Danube in the 30 to 40 years following the start of his campaigns (Borhy, 2014, 46).

The Roman invaders came from the Italian Peninsula and from the western Mediterranean areas. The captured peoples, such as the tribe of the Belgii, were located originally in the northwestern regions, or they were forced by the Romans to move within the Gallic territory, such as the tribe of the Nervii or the Menapii (Deru, 2010, 15). On the other hand, as the case of the Germanic Batavians and Ubii shows, tribes settled from the right side of the Rhine in the occupied territory of the empire to the left side of the river (Eck, 2004, 46–55). We find here also a multiethnic and inhomogeneous group from immigrants to indigenous people.

All tribes were necessarily in close contact with the conquerors and consequently their interactions involved the exchange of material goods and of mutual cultural influence – the intensity of this process, however, turned out to be unequal. This resulted in the origin of a new culture. This process, continuing for several decades or centuries, is referred to as 'Romanization', the intensity of which differed from marginal to complete assimilation of 'Roman' culture by the peoples (Krausse, 2007, 16–17). Celtic sociopolitical structure and agriculture lent itself to relatively easy incorporation within the Roman Empire.

In Gallic society the existence of a privileged elite is detectable by princely residences and tombs (see below). This aristocracy participated more or less willingly in the adoption of new cultural practices: one could call it active self-Romanization. Germanic society was less structured; the members of the aristocracy were not so numerous. In this case, the change of habits came from outside, with Roman soldiers and other migrants helping directly or indirectly in the Romanization of more passive Germanic tribes. The concept of Romanization is a very complex one, encompassing numerous controversial elements, such as colonialism, imperialism or globalism (Woolf, 1998; Hingley, 2005; Versluys and Pitts, 2014). Debates about these topics are not the focus of this chapter, but nonetheless it is generally accepted that the Roman conquest had a deep impact on the object/material consumption and behaviour of nearly every single individual in the northwestern provinces. This included not only the acquisition of Mediterranean architecture or the association of Roman and local gods, but also changes in, for example, burial or in eating and drinking habits as an essential part of life.

The southerners brought their Mediterranean eating habits and taste preferences with them into the northwestern regions, and clung to them. According to the archaeological, botanical and zoological sources, the native inhabitants had found favour in the Mediterranean diet, because they adapted parts of it and they changed/transformed their food traditions consciously. Apart from the adoption of Mediterranean cooking utensils, such as the mortar (Baatz, 1977), or the construction of a bricked-up hearth, this also meant the introduction of new foodstuffs and foodways. The tangible and intangible elements of the dining and drinking culture, such as the food itself, the recipes, the place of food preparation, the cook/chef, the equipment, the sequence of the dinner from hand washing to *convivium*, including their rooms (*triclinium*), were transferred to the north (Meurers-Balke and Kaszab-Olschewski, 2010, 30–31; Kaszab-Olschewski and Meurers-Balke, 2014, 146–147). A new diet and nutrition system completely modified everyday life in central and northern Europe in a huge way.

Furthermore, a new Mediterranean structure of food production, including the baker's craft or trade was introduced into urban areas. For the local population, a mixed cuisine arose combining regional and Mediterranean elements that G.E. Thüry (2007, 11, 15) described as 'culinary acculturation', or as 'culinary Romanization'. How long-lasting the success of this food transfer was is shown by King Charlemagne (AD 747/8–814) about 400 years after the decline of the Roman Empire, who compiled a planting list for his gardens, with the majority of the plants having reached the north with the Romans (Wies, 1992; Strank and Meurers-Balke, 2008).

In considering the way that societies deal with the raw materials of nutrition, some differences can be found between the indigenous agriculture in the north and the monocultural cultivation of wheat, vines and olives in the countries around the Mediterranean Sea. Within the indigenous groups, the best possible utilization of local resources was high on the agenda, with a focus on the most basic goal of having enough to eat.

While the overwhelming majority of foodstuffs were locally produced, the leading Celtic social classes participated in long-distance importation of goods. The example of the Iron Age saline-settlement of Bad Nauheim (D[1]) shows the import of coriander and dried figs as well as plums, and from the late Hallstatt to the early La Tène period at Glauberg (D), a grapeseed is known that also must have been imported (Heiss and Kreuz, 2007; Kreuz, 2012a; 2012b).

During periods of peace the majority of the Celts worked in agriculture with farming and animal husbandry. Production beyond their own personal needs enabled them to feed members of other professional sectors, since many craftsmen and traders lived in major settlements such as the *oppida*. In the southern part of Germany and in northern France hundreds of late Celtic farms 'Viereckschanze' or 'ferme indigene' are known, whose structure shows many parallels with the Roman *villa rustica* (Wieland, 1999; Heimberg, 2002/2003, 62, 69). The farm was surrounded by ditches on four sides and separate buildings were used for residential and agricultural purpose. An architectural planning concept of the farm is also recognizable. This helped to advance the Romanization of agriculture; because the framework is pre-Roman even if the contents are Iron Age.

Among the Germans also a mixed economy based on the cultivation of oats, barley, and vegetables, and focused on animal husbandry is to be assumed (Kreuz, 2004; 2012a; Joachim, 2002). About or shortly after the birth of Christ neither Mediterranean food items or horticulture nor Roman table manners or dining habits were found in the early Germanic households (Kreuz, 2010; Schamuhn and Zerl, 2009). In this aspect the Germans apparently demarcated themselves against the Romans more or less consciously.

Soon after conquest, however, the transformation of agriculture began with the stimulation of local native farming by increased demand and the founding of a new farm type, the *villa rustica*, according to a Mediterranean model for market-oriented farming with surplus production. The natural conditions, however, could hardly be controlled: a look at the climate and soil map of Europe reveals that with increasing distance from the southern part of Europe the weather gets cooler and wetter. The predominant soil type in central and northern Europe is brown earth with Luvisols: This also includes fertile loess soil, which the Romans incorporated into the Roman-controlled territory whenever this was feasible (e.g., Picardie (F) or Wetterau (D)).

However, the growth of vegetation also depended on the altitude above sea level of the location. Only those plants whose fruits and seeds were able to ripen in a shorter growing season could thrive north of the Alps. This meant a smaller selection of plants for people to eat compared to the Mediterranean region. People also had to survive a growth-free period in the winter lasting several months, and to equalize the lack of calories with a substitute, perhaps with meat consumption. Ancient written sources such as the descriptions of Caesar or of Tacitus reflect precisely this concerning the Germans. Caesar (*BGall.* 6.22.1) wrote about them: 'They are not keen on cultivation of land and the greater part of their diet consists of milk, cheese and meat.' Next Tacitus (*Germ.* 23): 'The dishes are simple, wild-growing fruit, fresh game or curdled milk: Without special preparation, without spices they drive hunger away.'

The increased consumption of animal products may have helped during the winter. But these reports written by Caesar and Tacitus are to be partly rejected, at least for the area left of the Rhine in Cologne, as well as for the Gallic areas such as Picardie and Lorraine, as pollen diagrams convey in that time the image of a developed cultural landscape with fields, meadows and pastures, and several varieties of crops, including wheat species, especially emmer and spelt, barley, foxtail millet and proso millet, as well as lentils, broad beans and ervil (bitter vetch), flax, poppy and 'gold of pleasure' (*camelina*) (Kalis and Meurers-Balke, 2007; Deru, 2010, 61). Even the Rhine Delta, which was essentially just dry land, shows forms of arable farming (Kooistra, 2009).

Although it was evident to the Romans that they would be reliant upon establishing an adequate agrarian economy in the north, many foods fit for storage and transport were initially brought there: from basic foods such as cereals or occasionally meat (bacon), to items that are to be classified as luxury (or prestige) goods, such as wine, olive oil, fruits, vegetables or fish. Anyone who could or wanted to pay for it had easy access to Mediterranean products. Even in the remotest corners of the empire, traces of transport containers such as amphorae or wooden barrels were found (Schimmer, 2009; Ehmig, 2003; Tamerl, 2010).

For Britain, northern Gaul and Germany this mainly meant the supply of products from the Iberian Peninsula or south Gaul on the Rhone-Rhine waterway. But in the eastern Alps, in Noricum, or in Pannonia the supply of wine and oil was carried out, through the distribution of Adriatic and Black sea coast or Asia minor/Aegean amphorae, also from nearby sources (Ehmig, 2011/2012; Magyar-Hárshegyi, 2016). In the long run, all deliveries of more ordinary products would have not only failed to be secured militarily but were also uneconomical, which also spoke in favour of local cultivation. The procurement of locally available food was a difficult task. However, the army required food for humans and also feed for animals not only in time of war but also of peace (Junkelmann, 1997, 52–54). But Rome had something to offer: money for the products and know-how in the agricultural sector. Whether this was made use of on a voluntary basis or whether pressure was applied, cannot be determined on the basis of the available evidence.

The conquerors, with their developed agricultural technology, interfered consciously in the characteristics of animal breeds and plants. They changed a lot by their highly developed horticulture, ranging from grafting to fertilization (Stika, 2005). As can be seen in the archaeozoological evidence, the results were inevitable, because during the Roman period significant growth occurred, especially in oxen and bulls, due to crossbreeding and better feeding (Stephan, 2005); this was particularly evident in certain areas, such as the southern Rhineland (Becker, 2007). However, some things remained unchanged, because, for example, the sandy soils of the Lower Rhine area had, already in the Iron Age, been only suitable for the keeping of cattle (Brüggler, 2012; 2016; Becker, 2007). Here the pollen diagrams showed a continuous grassland management for cattle feed from the Iron Age to the Roman period (Kalis and Meurers-Balke, 2007).

Food and drink

But what was eaten and drunk by the people in the Roman culture of the north? Human food included first of all a lot of cereals as well as vegetables, fruits and several sorts of meat. Today we find at excavations only a very small part of all of them, in the form of dried seeds or carbonized plants or some animal bones. As they are organic material they were destroyed during the last 2,000 years by microorganisms. So we have a small foodstuff database and must be careful with historical analyses, social interpretation and dating of the find contexts (see Part II in this book).

A basic foodstuff: cereals

Let us start with a short overview about the cereals (see Table 16.1). In Europe they were already the most important basic food during the Iron Age and the Roman Period.

Up to the third or second century BC, the inhabitants of Italy themselves were considered to be porridge eaters (*pultiphagi*) (Plaut. *Mostell.* 828; Plin. *HN* 18.3), and so various cereals formed the base of their diet. The porridge, the so-called *puls*, was prepared from whole or coarsely ground grain together with flour and water or milk. Barley was also popular, although it had to be roasted before threshing (André, 1998, 46–47), and because of the low gluten/adhesive protein content, it was more difficult to use to bake bread. It was, therefore, replaced by bread wheat, which only had to be threshed like wheat, and so the custom changed towards the eating of bread. In bread preparation one must differentiate between flatbread (made of

Table 16.1 Type of cereals in the region

Cereals in the region	Origin	Using as human food mainly by	Regionally differentiated growing place
Millet	Local	Natives	All over
Oat	Local	Natives	All over
Emmer	Local	Natives	All over
Barley	Local	Natives	All over
Rye	Local	Natives	Near the Alps
Spelt wheat	Import, later local	Romans	In warm areas
Bread wheat	Import, later local	Romans	In warm areas
Rice	Only import	Romans	Not growing in the north

flour, water and salt) and species produced with the help of yeast leaven (*fermentum*). Light and dark bread was to be distinguished by the quality of the flour.

Both the Celts and the Germans also preferred cereals as their food. During the Iron Age they had millet and oats cooked as porridge (Ebel-Zepezauer, 2009, 78), since these cereals were not suited for baking bread. Several findings demonstrate the bread baking process: in Bad Nauheim (D), for example, a whole loaf of 'Celtic' bread made of milled and sieved flour fell victim to an Iron Age fire (Heiss and Kreuz, 2007). Millet can be considered as the favourite plant of the Celts, who hung on to it even in Roman times (Knörzer, 2007), as can be shown by two stores destroyed by fire with charred millet in the Roman settlements of Carnuntum and Mautern (A), inhabited among others by the Celtic Boii (Thanheiser and Heiss, 2014, 126). From the Germanic settlement Köln-Porz-Lind (D) from the La Tène period, on the other hand, several bread shovels originated which testify to the baking of cakes or pastries (Joachim, 2002). Another important plant was oat and it served the Germans as a food, but in Italy it was regarded as animal feed. In Pannonia the emmer preferred by the locals was replaced by the bread wheat that the Romans favoured after the early first century AD (Borhy, 2014, 78).

Rice was introduced only in small quantities from India or from the Middle East as an import, mainly for medical purposes, and a singular find of rice grains in the northwest provinces comes from the legionary fortress at Neuss (Knörzer, 1970, 43). We do not know about the consumption of rice in antiquity because we find it very seldom.

Cultivation and storage of cereals

In addition to the selection of grain, the Romans influenced the method of cultivation, harvesting, storage and processing. Improved metal appliances or metal-reinforced wood utensils were introduced for work in the fields. But Gallic technical innovations, such as the harvester – *vallus* – (Plin. *HN* 18.296; Palladius 7.2.2–4) or a plough with a wheel (Plin. *HN* 18.172), must not go unnoticed.

Concerning the storage of grain in the north, alongside the airtight vacuum functioning silos, free standing silos on stilts were also utilized. The Roman influence can be seen in the granaries (*horrea*), which were built with floating floors, first made of wood and later of stone, and were bigger than their Iron Age counterparts. Unambiguously Roman is the stockpiling in brick or stone cellars, which could be integrated into the house or be situated separately.

Processing of cereals

Even with grain processing things changed. While the native people smashed their grain between stones, crushed it on so-called Napoleon's hats (Holtmeyer-Wild, 2012) or shredded it in small hand-mills, the Romans launched technically improved (e.g., grooved ones) or powerful large devices that were operated by animal power (so-called Pompeian or donkey mills – *molae asinariae*). On the other hand, the latter were replaced by water mills (*mola aquaria*). Ausonius (*Mosella* 133) describes a water mill on the river Ruwer (D), and there is archaeological evidence for others at Montaigu-la-Brisette (F) or Munich-Perlach (D) (Ferdière, 2011, 86; Volpert, 1997). Hand- or donkey-driven mills and water mills have been used in Roman Britain (Upex, 2008). In Germany already during the Augustan occupation phase, the army, because they had high demand, exploited locally available stone material for their mills, which the explorers found in Mayen in the Eifel area (a low mountain range) (Hörter, 2000).

Archaeological remains of cereals and associated products

Mills were needed to make porridge, bread buns, and loaves of bread (*panis*) or pastries or cakes (*crustulum, liba*). Remnants of these were discovered in pre-Roman and Roman cremation burials (see Table 16.2).

We must also mention in this context the cake pans made of clay or bronze (*crustuli*) that reflect the Romans' preference for sweets. The bigger cakes moulded from these pans (the diameter is more than 20 cm) were distributed on imperial feast days, a means of imperial propaganda. Their moulded surface shows a recent picture message; perhaps for a special social group. For example, one cake pan from Aquincum, modern-day Budapest (H), from the second century AD shows emperor Marcus Aurelius' triumphal procession (Facsády, 1996, 24) (see Figure 16.1). The smaller ones show mythological or erotic scenes.

We have more cake pans from military and larger civilian contexts than from agricultural contexts (see Table 16.3). Already in the Iron Age honey was used to sweeten dishes and cakes, and later in the Roman Period fruit syrup (grape must, *defrutum*) was added.

Table 16.2 Remnants of food pieces

Food pieces	Find places/graves	Context	Dating	Author
Porridge and crumbs of bread	Wederath-Belginum (D)	Rural context with native people	pre-Roman and Roman	Cordie-Hackenberg et al., 1992, 111; Währen, 1990
Bread bun	Duppach-Weiermühle (D)	Rural context with Romanized people	Roman	Henrich, 2010, 90–91
Loaves/crumbs of bread	Saffig (D) and Büschdorf (D)	Rural context	Roman	Währen, 1983; 2000
Bread bun	Haus Bürgel/Monheim (D)	Military context with Romanized people	Roman	Schamuhn, 2010
Crumbs of bread or pastries or cakes	Vienna (A)	Urban or military context with Romanized people	Roman	Thüry and Walter, 2001, 21

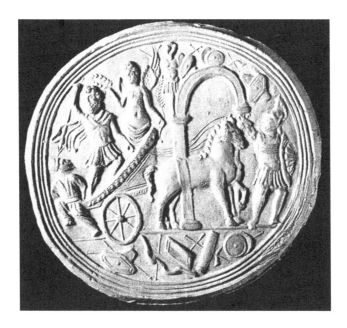

Figure 16.1 Cake pan from Aquincum with imperial triumphal procession (Facsády, 1996, Taf. 8,1; photo by Budapesti Történeti Muzeum).

Table 16.3 Cake pans and their contexts

Cake pans in military and/or urban context	Author	Cake pans in rural context	Author
Budapest (H)	Szirmai, 1997	Villa rustica Windenam See (A)	Thüry, 2007
Neuss (D)	Scholz and Pause, 2010	*Flavia Solva* by Leibnitz (A)	Wedenig, 2005

Legumes: peas, beans, lentils and chickpeas

Legumes were already the second most important basic food during the Iron Age. Later they lost nothing of their popularity, not only because they were a cheap and substantial locally grown product, but also because they delivered protein that was missing from a mostly vegetarian diet. They also improved the soil quality (Jacomet and Kreuz, 1999). The main legumes were eaten as a soup or stew; they were cooked as cereal porridge or dried and ground as flour. Remains of beans of the Roman era were found in southern Germany, in the Rhineland, in the Netherlands as well as in Britain. As grave goods, legumes were found at the Treveri territory (Cordie-Hackenberg et al., 1992). One legume, the chickpea, was certainly imported (Knörzer, 1970, 43).

Vegetables

The changes introduced by the Roman spice plants and other exotic imports (see Table 16.4) like garlic, pepper corns, coriander or dill, etc., led to a big leap in flavour variations. In Roman

Britain, coriander, poppy seed and celery were very common in both (military and civil) contexts (Cool, 2006, 65).

Leaf and root vegetables also had an important role to play: root vegetables have a relatively long durability if stored in cool and dark places, and locally grown edible weeds were eaten as a leaf vegetable. Because of their frequency in the find data, initial cultivation of carrots and

Table 16.4 Imported and local herbs and spices

Foodstuffs	Origin	Find place	Frequency	Site type	Author
Pepper corns	Import (India?)	Oberaden, Xanten, Cologne Hanau, London	rarely	Military and civil	Kučan, 1992 Knörzer, 2007; Kreuz, 2012b; Cool, 2006
Onion, leek, garlic	Import, later local	Baden-Baden Bad Wimpfen Gerlingen, Neuss	common	Military and civil	Küster, 1995 Knörzer, 2007
Fennel	Local	Rhineland	common	Military and civil	Knörzer, 2007
Coriander	Import	Passau Baden-Baden Rainau-Buch Rottweil Weisweiler Aachen Valkenburg Nantwich Lincoln, Etc.	very common	Military and civil	Küster, 1995 Knörzer, 2007
Dill	Import, later local	Carnuntum Straubing Köngen Welzheim Butzbach Neuss Alphen a. d. Rijn De Horden Weisweiler, Etc.	very common	Military and civil	Küster, 1995 Thanheiser/ Heiss, 2014
Celery	Local	Oberwinterthur Seebruck Ellingen Kallmünz Mainhardt Aachen Neuss Xanten Köln Oberaden, Etc.	very common	Military and civil	Küster, 1995

rocket salad can be assumed already during the Iron Age (Knörzer, 2007). Seeds of lettuce – probably a Roman import foodstuff – have been discovered for example in the *villa rustica* near Babstadt (D) (Stika, 2005). Wild sorrel, which contains vitamin C and grows well in cool temperatures, is versatile and can be used in salads, sauces, soups and vegetable dishes. It also played a role as a medicinal plant (Meurers-Balke and Kaszab-Olschewski, 2010, 84; Künzl, 2002, 30; Krause, 2009, 96–97).

Radish, which was first cultivated north of the Alps during the Iron Age, is also very tolerant of the colder climate. Radish seeds, for example, were discovered in Uitgeest (NL) (Meurers-Balke and Kaszab-Olschewski, 2010, 78). Even wild asparagus was 'en vogue' north of the Alps. The popularity is proven, *inter alia*, through knife handles, which were designed in the form of an asparagus (Faust and Schneider, 2013; Birkenhagen, 2013). The exclusive collecting of wild plants came to an end after the arrival of the Romans by the application of kitchen and herbal gardens but most of all through orchards. Celery was useful as a spice (Thanheiser and Heiss, 2014, 128; Thüry, 2007, 19; Körber-Grohne, 1995). The best *siser* (turnip?), according to Pliny (*HN* 19.27), grew in Germania at Gelduba, in the area of modern-day Krefeld on the Lower Rhine (D). Brassica may be deemed as one of the most popular vegetables during

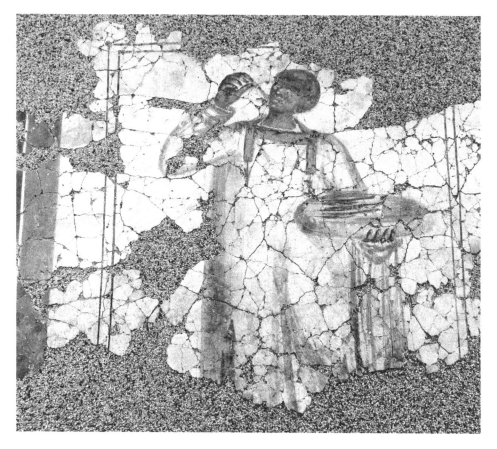

Figure 16.2 Wall painting from Brigetio showing vegetable consumption (photo by author; Courtesy of Klapka György Muzeum Komárom).

antiquity; it grew in nearly any climate and as food was easy to prepare in different ways. The word stems kol/kal, bresic and cape indicate that the Celts knew cabbage (Körber-Grohne, 1995).

Onion, leek and garlic must be counted as Roman naturalizations to the northwestern provinces. Apparently, vegetable-eating contests were used for popular amusement: on a wall painting in a private home in Brigetio, modern-day Komárom (H), the consumption of boiled or roasted spring onions or leeks was immortalized. On the wall, as graffiti, several strokes are to be found, perhaps indicating the number of eaten onions or leeks (Borhy and Számadó, 2010, 104–106) (see Figure 16.2).

Fruits and nuts

Wild-growing fruits like raspberries, blackberries, forest strawberries or elderberries were collected habitually in great numbers by the natives because of the sweet juices and healing properties. With the Romans a huge amount of import fruit and nuts reached the north (see Tables 16.5 and 16.6).

The oldest evidence of cultured fruits that came as merchandise could be detected in Germania only in Roman find layers. Several types of fruit could (because of climatic reasons) only be present in the north through importation. For example, during the Augustan occupation figs came with the solders dried and/or pickled (Thüry and Walter, 2001, 27–28; Knörzer, 2007, Meurers-Balke and Kaszab-Olschewski, 2010, 101). Even dates were part of the supplies

Table 16.5 Imported foodstuffs

Imported fruits and nuts	Frequency	Sites with imported fruits (reference see text)
FIGS	Very common	Oberaden, Neuss, Cologne (all D) and 30 others
DATES	Common	Avenches (CH), Petronell (A), Györ (H), Kempten, Haltern, Cologne (D) and some others
POMEGRANATES	Very rarely	Cologne (D)
TABLE OLIVES	Very common	All over
LEMONS	Very rarely	Salzburg (A)
ALMONDS	Rarely	Southwark (GB)

Table 16.6 Imported and local foodstuffs

Imported, later local fruits and nuts	Frequency (reference see text)
RAISINS	Very common
PLUMS	Very common
PEARS	Common
APRICOTS	Rarely
APPLES	Very common
CHERRIES	Very common
MELONS	Rarely
WALNUTS	Common
SWEET CHESTNUTS	Common
PEACHES	Rarely

of the soldiers, indicated by the fact that they were found largely in military places during the first century AD. They were not only a substantial delicacy but also an obligatory part of many sauces. Even Italy had to import the ripe fruits from North Africa or from the Levant. Date stones were detected in military locations in the Augustan period, such as Neuss or Haltern (Thüry and Walter, 2001, 27; Meurers-Balke and Kaszab-Olschewski, 2010, 102). Later the traders delivered dates in larger quantities and they were very popular under leading native groups maybe as a prestige good. It is noteworthy that here even in the second century AD dates are given as burial objects in the graves of the local native elite, as in the grave mound of Siesbach (D) (Cordie-Hackenberg et al., 1992) or in Southwark (GB) (Cool, 2006, 12). Pomegranates are known from Cologne (Knörzer, 2007). In addition, a few more imported dried fruits like raisins or plums have been detected in the Augustan military places such as Oberaden. The same could be determined for apples and olives in the Augustan settlement of Waldgirmes (all D) (Kučan, 1992; Kreuz, 2010).

Although the wild pear was more at home near the Alps, pear trees could continue to yield ripe crops further north. The somewhat delicate peaches were either pickled or cultivated in warm and wind sheltered locations (Meurers-Balke and Kaszab-Olschewski, 2010, 93). The apricot, however, was found in Roman areas in Linz (A) or in Budapest (H). The melon has been documented from Roman regions in the Wetterau region (D), from southwestern Germany and also from Carnuntum (A) (Meurers-Balke and Kaszab-Olschewski, 2010; Thanheiser and Heiss, 2014, 128). Differences in the fruit consumption between leger and smaller settlements (*coloniae* and *villae rusticate*) are to be accepted (Herchenbach and Meurers-Balke, Forthcoming).

The olive stones and the *tituli picti* on the amphorae reveal the fruits of the olive tree, which were imported from the south. Interestingly, the consumption of table olives in the area of Germania inferior ends with the departure of the Romans (Knörzer, 2007). Regarding a more classic southern fruit, the lemon, a mosaic representation from Salzburg (A), from the third century AD is remarkable (Thüry, 2007, 22). The depiction suggests that the fruit was so well-known at a place that does not belong to its natural growing region that the representation for the viewer was easily identifiable.

As a part of the Romanization of the agricultural sector, a large-scale cultivation of apples, cherries and plums can be assumed. There is evidence for the cultivation of wild species and the local cultivation of fruit (Thanheiser and Heiss, 2014, 128; Knörzer, 2007). Archaeological traces of gardens have been detected in the northern provinces, such as at Reims, in Caurel (Gallia Belgica) or in the Paris Basin (Deru, 2010, 61; Cribellier, 2014; Pilon et al., 2014).

A significant role in the diet of local native people – and not only in times of need – was played by freely collectable food such as mushrooms, herbs, sprouts, or hazelnuts or acorns (Cordie-Hackenberg et al., 1992). Other gathered goods were also almonds, pine kernel (Knörzer, 2007) or walnuts and sweet chestnuts, which not only were imported but had been cultivated since Roman times (Jacomet and Kreuz, 1999; Conedera et al., 2004).

Meat and other protein consumption: animal husbandry, hunting, fishing

Meat and fat

First of all, it should be emphasized that the majority of meals in Roman antiquity were vegetarian rather than meat-based (Päffgen, 2014). Meat or animal products – from wild or domesticated animals – were important to the diet of the northern provinces not only as a source of protein, but also as a source of fat. Apart from the oily seeds of flax, camelina or poppy, animal fats were particularly used here, rather than the Mediterranean olive oil (André, 1998, 159). Lard was preferred by the Gauls and butter by the Germans – as wooden churns at a settlement site of the Sugambrii in Köln-Porz-Lind (D) demonstrate (Joachim, 2002). Butter was used by the Romans at most as a healing ointment (Thüry and Walter, 2001, 24; Thüry, 2007, 34). With meat consumption, the mapping and evaluating of the archaeozoological bone material in the upscale living quarters in bigger urban settlements allows us to distinguish between the diets of rich or poor people and between ethnic groups, as well as between civilian or soldiers (see Table 16.7): see the inhabitant of the civil settlements from Augusta Raurica (CH) or soldiers in military camps; for example, Hofheim (D), Valkenburg or Velsen I (both NL) (after Peters, 1998; Schatzmann, 2013, 204).

The pigs – as lard suppliers – were partially kept indoors or in wooded areas (Upex, 2008). Pork was considered as a very popular good by the Romans, because the animals were kept only for their meat (André, 1998, 115, 117; Plin. *HN* 8.209) and not for other purposes, for example, as working animals or as suppliers of milk, wool or strong leather and bones etc. Meat from pork was more expensive than from cattle, sheep or goats (*Edictum Diocletiani*, 4). It seems, however, that the Gauls also liked to eat pork. The pork ham of the Menapii north of the Belgica, which was mentioned in a poem by Martial (13.54) and in the *Edictum Diocletiani* (4.8), was famous (Deru, 2010, 63). Pigs were often, but not exclusively, bred in rural areas at *villae rusticae*, apparently also in greater numbers. In the remains of a conflagration inside of a *villa rustica* in Baláca (H) (Pannonia inferior), the remnants of 28 piglets were discovered in one room (Vörös, 2000, 71–72).

In contrast to pig farming, cattle were kept longer, until their meat was almost too chewy for human consumption, because their working capacity had to be fully exploited first. They delivered milk and also a variety of other products, including leather, bones, horn, tendons, and animal glue. Cattle were housed in large numbers inside the same building as their inhabitants during pre-Roman times by the Germans in the so-called Wohnstallhaus, or they grazed outside all year, in open, unwooded areas. The numbers and importance of cattle in livestock increased towards the Lower Rhine, and its dominant position existed during the Iron Age and continued into the second and third centuries AD (Becker, 2007).

Milk consumption or processing in the north during the Roman period may point to cheese-making taking place, for example in the rural hinterland of Cologne. Mapping the find sites of the typical ceramic cheese forms leads to the assumption that cheese was here a regular part of the diet (Gaitzsch, 2010). Probably a special jug for milk or milk products was created near Cologne (Höpken, 2016, 102). From the territory of Gallia Belgica, the presence of colanders also attests to cheese production (Deru, 2010, 63) that can be considered, in addition to butter production, as a by-product of cattle farming. In free Germania the consumption of milk was part of the diet (Ebel-Zepezauer, 2009). Maybe it was a characteristic native habit (see above).

If feed for the livestock could not be secured for the winter, these farm animals were slaughtered in the autumn. The meat was made durable in larger quantities by smoking, drying

Table 16.7 Distinguishing between meat consumption

Most important meat for the higher society/ Romans and Gauls	*Most important meat for the lower society/ native inhabitants*
Pig	Cattle
Chicken	Horse
Game (hunted wild animals)	

on the air and/or salting. The technique of fumigation was important, especially in troubled times, like the military occupation or during late antiquity. Multiple smokehouses from the third century in Augusta Raurica indicate that smoking (or salting) meat served as a preserve (Schatzmann, 2013, 214). It was easily transported or hidden and helped people to survive in case of siege. Smoked, dried, or salted meat was ready-to-eat, if necessary without further preparation.

Moreover, the food range was added to by domesticated poultry such as chicken, duck, pigeon, and goose, which were partially kept indoors. Chicken was used for food (meat and eggs) in middle Europe since the Hallstatt-time, also by the early Celts, and from the fifth century BC was known by the Germans, as indicated by bone assemblages in Sünninghausen or Göttingen (D) (Nobis, 1973; Amberger, 1982). Later on, bones from chickens were found at nearly every Roman settlement apart from the Alps, where winters were perhaps too harsh. After the occupation, big specimens of Roman chickens were imported and we find them in military camps (e.g., Saalburg, Niederbieber) or in vici (e.g., Weißenburg) (Peters, 1998, 234). Pigeons and domestic ducks were brought to the north by the Romans, although it is unclear whether there were livestock breeding farms here, as there were in Italy (Stephan, 2005). Pigeon meat was considered a delicacy and was consumed in higher social circles (Peters, 1998).

Geese, however, were not only popular among the Romans, but also traditionally among the Germans, as in Germania libera (free Germania) and in the province Germania inferior (Ebel-Zepezauer, 2009, Peters, 1998, 232). Also, Pliny (*NH* 10.53) mentioned the high quality of white down feathers, which reached the Roman Empire as an export. From Roman Cologne (D), on the border with Germania libera, the place name of the new Geese-Market *ad gantunas novas* (*CIL* XIII 1015, 115a) survived, which could mean that the animals were regularly traded there in greater numbers. Painted geese eggs as grave goods in a woman's burial from the fourth century AD in Hürth, near Cologne, confirm the special status of the animals (Gottschalk, 2014). Similar finds were also observed in Worms (D). Moreover, chicken and chicken eggs were eaten often or used as grave goods, not only in the Rhine-Mosel region but also, if less so, in Germania libera (Pösche, 2010; Cordie-Hackenberg et al., 1992; Ebel-Zepezauer, 2009).

Meat could also be procured by hunting, which was regarded as a hobby, as well as by catching birds. The soldiers in the Odenwald (a low mountain range) along the Obergermanisch-Rätischer Limes (D) sometimes used hunting to catch and eat animals such as red deer, wild boar or hare (Becker, 2012). Bones of sheep (or goats) were discovered at several watchtowers along the borders of the Imperium Romanum (Obergermanisch-Rätische Limes and Hadrian's Wall). The animals obviously were not on the list of preferred suppliers of meat for soldiers, but they played an important role in keeping the border strip vegetation-free (Becker, 2012). Bones from oscine birds were found also in the kitchen of a *mansio* in Krefeld (D) near the Rhine (Reichmann, 2014).

Fish, seafood, amphibians, snails

Even the water offered food. Along the coastline (e.g., Aremorica, Brittany, F) fishing and fish farming took place (Ferdière, 2011, 87). When fishing, the same techniques were used as in the pre-Roman Iron Age, as demonstrated by the discovery of a net float from the Sugambri settlement in Köln-Porz-Lind (D) from the La Tène period (Joachim, 2002). However, the conquerors built installations, such as the embankments, at the hinterland villas of Pátka or of Balf (H) in Pannonia, indicating fish farming (Borhy, 2014, 78). The surplus beyond their own needs could then be sold at the market. Commercial fishing is probably indicated by some

Roman instruments, such as a fish trap of Ellewoutsdijk on the North Sea coast (NL) (Dütting and van Rijn, 2017, 37–59). Legacies of fish farming are suspected in Lynch Farm in Orton Waterville (Upex, 2008).

Furthermore, coast mussels were collected along the North Sea and transported as far as Xanten or Cologne (Päffgen, 2014, 33–34; Nehren and Strauch, 2012). Sweet-water oysters were a luxury product that could be found in surprisingly high numbers, as, for example, in Aachen (Inv. No. 2013/1034-2-78) or in Cologne in findlayers of the first century AD (Nehren and Strauch, 2012) (all D). The oysters in the studied area had been imported either from the Mediterranean/Adriatic Sea, or from the North Sea/Atlantic coast. This resulted in an internal boundary, because in the find material from Trier, oysters were found from the south and from the north, while in Cologne and Xanten only from the North Sea. Sites in present-day Austria and Switzerland indicate southern suppliers (Thüry, 2007, 29; Thüry and Walter, 2001, 25).

In addition, a particular culinary speciality since the pre-Roman Iron Age shall be mentioned, namely eating frogs' legs, which remained limited only to the Celtic territory, or maybe was introduced by Gallic immigrants to Cologne, because here also were found bones from grilled frogs' legs (Thüry and Walter, 2001, 25; Thüry, 2007, 35; Nehren and Strauch, 2012). Moreover, finds in the fully sedimented branch of the Rhine in Cologne suggest the consumption of snails (Nehren and Strauch, 2012).

Salt and fish sauce

Salt was, in all periods, the main flavouring agent and played also a fundamental role in preservation – because of this, the demand was high (Cool, 2006, 56). The supply of salt had to be ensured either through import or exploitation. By mining large amounts, for example, in Hallstatt (A) (Kern et al., 2008), salt had been exploited and traded and also 'briquetage' was used to obtain salt in the salines of Celtic Bad Nauheim (D). In coastal areas, salt was generated in facilities such as those in Zeebrugge or Leffinge (B) etc., where the brine was boiled and reduced from seawater. Salt production in the region of the Menapii and Morini on the North Coast is attested through inscriptions (Päffgen, 2014, 28; Deru, 2010, 66–67). Further information about *negotiatores salarii* (salt traders) is provided here from consecration altars in the Oosterschelde area (NL) (*AE* 1973, 0364; *AE* 1973, 0378) (Stuart and Bogaers, 1971, 62, 71; Stuart, 2013).

Fish sauce (*garum, liquamen*) was essential for flavouring and was an integral part of Roman cuisine. It is documented by amphora finds and epigraphic evidence on consecration stones, which occurred across the region (see, for example Ehmig, 2003; Päffgen, 2014, 38). Furthermore, even the production in Britain is assumed (Cool, 2006, 61).

Beverages

In terms of beverages, water, wine, vinegar, fruit juices, beer, mead and milk (all together NABs and ABs) were consumed, depending on the location (see Table 16.8).

Non-alcoholic beverages (NABs)

For the human organism daily water consumption is vital, therefore water supplies must be easily accessible. The Romans created their settlements according to this criterion. Not only do written sources note this, such as Vitruvius (*De arch.* 8.6.1–14, 10.4–7), but architectural evidences such as conduits, channels or wells can also be seen in each type of settlement (civil

Table 16.8 Type of beverages

Non-alcoholic beverages (NABs)	Origin of NABs	Alcoholic beverages (ABs)	Origin of ABs
1. Water	Naturally	1. Wine	Only human product
2. Milk	Nature product	2. Beer	Only human product
3. Fruit juices	Nature/human product	3. Mead	Only human product
4. Vinegar	Nature/human product		

and military), which ensured a high quality of drinking water (Grewe, 1986; 2010; Grewe and Knauff, 2012).

Alcoholic beverages (ABs): wine and beer

The consumption of alcoholic beverages played an important role in social as well as private life, and in cult practice.

Wine

Wine may be regarded as the preferred drink of the people during antiquity in each social group, with or without Mediterranean roots. At first a difference must be made between wines made from grapes or honey, so-called mead, because this was, according to the archaeological sources, very popular among the Celts (Rösch, 2014). The earliest evidence of the grapevine in the form of wine or raisins is found in an Iron Age context. They came as a trading good or prestige product from the south and so any royal residences or *oppida* knew wine consumption (Reuter, 2005; Ehmig, 2011/2012). Wine amphorae emerged from noble tombs in Göblingen (Goeblange)-Nospelt, Clemency or Ettelbrück (L) (Metzler and Gaeng, 2005, 152–167). Wine came in amphorae or packed in barrels as a Mediterranean import during the Iron Age and later.

Concerning wine cultivation in the provinces, its organizing was difficult at first, because Domitian (AD 81–96) interdicted by decree the new cultivation of vineyards and ordered at the same time to lay down the grape vines (Suet. *Dom.* 7.2). Archaeological and paleoethnobotanical research indicates that vineyards were unknown in the Germanic Provinces between the first and third century AD. The situation changed significantly in the third century AD during the reign of Probus (AD 276–282), who repealed the edict (Reuter, 2005; Weeber, 2013, 108). Despite this late date, however, a centre of wine production was established alongside the Mosel, which can be explained partly by the proximity of the imperial court in Trier. The poet Ausonius described in his poem the local vineyards (*Mosella* 20–22, 25, 152–156, 194–195). Today here several Roman wine presses, for example, in Piesport-Müstert, Erden or Brauneberg, are known (all D), which date from the third century AD onwards (Gilles, 1999).

As shown on stone reliefs, and even on terra sigillata (Samian ware), the wine merchants shipped their goods in wooden barrels (Bockius, 2008). Reliefs depicting attributes of Roman viniculture are also recorded from southwestern Germany (Ettlingen) (Reuter, 2005). But also in the area of Gallia Belgica (Valley of the Oise), in Gallia Lugdunensis (Rully, Gevrey-Chambertin), or Beaune-la-Rolande and Chateaubleau in the Paris Basin (Cribellier, 2014; Pilon et al., 2014), we have clear evidence of wine growing in the form of tools, winepresses, inscriptions and finds of grape seeds (Ferdière, 2011, 87; Deru, 2010, 61). Even from Britain there is evidence of viticulture, for example in Wollaston (Upex, 2008). In Pannonia also, finds including a wine press at the Villa in Winden (A) and a wineknife from the villas of Baláca or

Gyulafirátót (H) (Borhy, 2014, 78), provide evidence of wine production. Possibly in the homes, instead of winemaking, vinegar was sometimes inadvertently created.

Beer

In addition to wine, beer enjoyed great popularity among the natives of the northwestern regions of the empire. Beer was cheaper than wine and the price edict of Diocletian (AD 301) mentioned different beers that were called in Gaul, for example, *cervisia* or *curmi* (Konen, 2013; André, 1998, 155). The southerners did not drink beer for pleasure and their rejection of it was unmistakable (Höpken, 2015; Päffgen, 2014, 106). For example, the former governor of this province, Cassius Dio, complained about the Pannonian brewery (49. 36. 2):

> The Pannonians [. . .] lead the most miserable existence of all mankind. For they are not well off as regards either soil or climate; they cultivate no olives and produce no wine except to a very slight extent and a wretched quality at that, since the winter is very rigorous and occupies the greater part of their year, but drink as well as eat both barley and millet.

Both of these cereals were considered as an inferior foodstuff in Italy, where they were something for the slaves and the poor to eat. There, beer was used at most as a medicine and as a cough syrup (Thüry and Walter, 2001). Brewed beer for personal and for commercial purposes stored in amphorae could be sold by the *negotiator cervesarius* (*AE* 1941, 0168). However, beer has a short storage life and was transported regionally rather than over long distances. In the Upper Rhine area beer was probably transported in Dressel 20 *similis* amphorae, which were produced in Worms and in Rheinzabern (D). In the Lower Rhine area Scheldt-Valley amphorae from Dourges (F) could be used (Konen, 2013).

Beer production itself was evidently the task of women and in Trier, for example, an inscription records the occupation of one Hosidia Maternaus as a *cervesaria* (Höpken, 2015, 195). Besides Xanten, there is evidence of beer breweries or beer from Bonn, Regensburg, Krefeld, Alzey, Bad Dürkheim (all D), or Ronchinne and Anthée (F); from Eisenstadt and Göttlesbrunn (A) there are name designations on grave stones like *Curmisagus* or *Curmisagius* (Höpken, 2015; Päffgen, 2014, 32; Thüry, 2007, 33). In Carnuntum, a kiln that germinated barley and spelt wheat has been discovered (Thanheiser and Heiss, 2014, 127); there are also numerous threshing barns detectable, which are necessary for beer production (Höpken, 2015; Meurers-Balke and Kaszab-Olschewski, 2010, 152), as well as the special crops and the buckets or other containers. The native inhabitants of the British Isles liked to consume beer and used corn-driers for the production (Upex, 2008).

The kitchen and dining room

In all nations the hearth has always been the 'nerve centre' of family life in the house (Thüry, 2010; Cool, 2006, 51). It played a ritual role also as the religious centre of the house, and the gods were responsible for its protection. In the Germanic areas, in the 'Wohnstallhäuser', all room functions, as well as the kitchen, were united without separation in a single space under one roof. Living and cooking were similarly combined in the Celtic small house farms in so-called Neunpfostenbauten (Simons, 1989; De Boe et al., 1992, 488–490).

With the Romans, the idea of catering facilities built separately into the houses reached the north. Above all, the kitchens are adapted to the newly developed provincial Roman rural housing types, such as the portico villa with corner projections (Risalit-Villa). Inside the main building of the Rhenish estates, three different positions for the hearth can be observed: in a central location, in the corridor location or in a corner position. Of these, the central location of hearths in the majority of constructions indicates clearly the continuation of a regional tradition; with respect to the typology of stove, floor hearths and underpinned block hearths can be particularly distinguished here (Kaszab-Olschewski and Meurers-Balke, 2014, 139–145). In urban centres, such as Carnuntum (A), both in private and in public spaces, substantial hearths which were even equipped with smoke extraction could be found (Humer, 2014, 106). However, some sections of the population used their kitchen also for residential purposes, and in big cities they perhaps had no kitchen or hearth in tenements because of fire danger (Päffgen, 2014, 14).

The equipment of the kitchens and dining rooms demonstrates Mediterranean influence in the variation of vessels, such as cooking pots, bowls, baking sheets, plates, lids, strainers, funnels, saucepans, cups, etc. made of clay, metal or glass and – in case of the Alpine regions – made of steatite. Pokers, ladles, hatchets, knives, baskets, bags, etc., served as accessories and various trays or basins helped when serving. Probably some of the cooking, roasting and preservation techniques got a new impetus.

With regard to the culinary Romanization, dining rooms (*triclinia*) located separately in the houses constituted another important element. Due to the lack of characteristic features (*cline, mosaic*) their identification is sometimes difficult. A centrally located, representative dining room can be reconstructed, for example, in the Axialcourt-Type Villa of Blankenheim (D). Here, from the second phase, an axial reference to the (garden) landscape – can be recognized – a characteristic feature of Mediterranean rooms. But also the main building of the *villa rustica* of Neerharen (B) had a vestibule provided with a central area. The viewing guidance into the garden from this probable dining room, was apparently reinforced by tree plantations (Kaszab-Olschewski and Meurers-Balke, 2014, 146–147). Comparable systems are also known from elsewhere; for example, Little Weldon (GB) (Upex, 2008).

And who works in the kitchen?

It is rarely clear who used to cook or bake in the kitchens. The traditional daily work to be done for a woman of antiquity included heating the furnaces, grinding the grain and baking bread (Columella, *Rust.* 12. 4. 7). In commercial bakeries, which made the hard work of baking bread at home dispensable, only male workers were employed. The establishment of bakeries, as well as the butcheries, were concomitants of urban developments (Ferdière, 2011, 44). The emergence of an independent bakers' craft, split up in Rome from the profession of a chef, occurred at the end of the third or early second century BC and the collegium of the bakers was founded there in 168 BC (Päffgen, 2014, 9; André, 1998, 52–53).

The professional associations were formed quickly in the provinces. From Roman Cologne, a *collegium pisstricorum* (*CIL* XIII 8255) is recorded as a professional association of bakers, and there is also evidence for bakeries in Jülich (D) and Bliesbruck (F) (Rothenhöfer, 2005, 266–267; Deru, 2010, 60). Also from Cologne a wholesaler of flour and bakery products, designated as a *negotiator pistor[ic]i(us)* [*Terti*]*nius Secund(us)*, is attested by an inscription (*CIL* XIII 8338; Rothenhöfer, 2005, 182).

Despite the presence of *tabernae/cauponia* and cook shops in every settlement, cooking and baking for one's own family in the wider population was probably the job of the women who had also to care for the children at home – but we do not know exactly. However, Moselle or Rhenish grave monuments showed not one woman in the kitchen with cooking pots or other cooking utensils in their hands and it is unclear why. The representation of a domestic kitchen scene on the side of the Igel-Column (Pillar Tomb, D) represented only men (Ritter, 2002/2003,

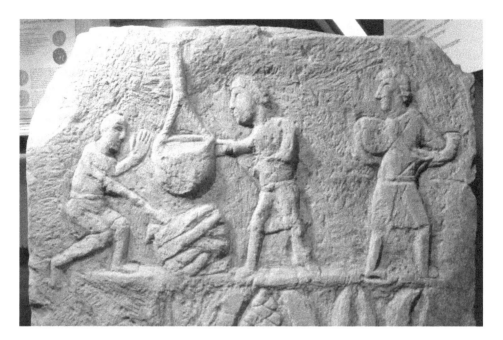

Figure 16.3 Kitchen scene with men cooking, maybe soldiers (photo by Gerald Volker Grimm; Courtesy of Römerausstellung im Bürgerhaus, Wörth am Main).

159). Another unique culinary scene has been recorded on the side of a Matron's altar from Bonn (D); here also a man wields the mixing spoon (Kaszab-Olschewski, 2015, 32). On a third relief with a cooking scene, from Wörth at the Main Limes (D), there are again men who are standing around the fire. However, they are possibly self-supporting soldiers (Schallmayer, 2010, 74) (see Figure 16.3). These reliefs could give the impression, that men were responsible for cooking. Maybe after 20–25 years of military service veteran soldiers continued to take part in cooking in private households? At burials, there are no grave goods, which would demonstrate gender-specific attention to cooking, so this question remains unsolved.

Conclusion

A part of the Celtic and Germanic tribes had abandoned their usual settlement area immediately before or during the Roman conquest. They were uprooted and possibly more receptive to a new, Roman-influenced identity. But why did the native peoples in central and northern Europe change or transform their diet and nutrition? Were they forced to do so, or did they choose to? And how long did this process go on for? Did it happen across the region? With the occupation, the Mediterranean diet and foodstuffs were brought together into the north. Quickly the supply of local products started for the conquerors, produced primarily by the *villa-rustica*-system. The natives learned – if they had not known it before – about the new food partially on the agricultural farms, or in the houses of a tribe's elite. But this does not necessarily mean that they all used these products also in their own kitchens. At first, their aristocracy, if it existed, adopted new food and foodways.

Many of the native men were obligated to do military service, where they inevitably ate imported Mediterranean food, so they had first to adapt their diet partially. In the *taberna* of a

Table 16.9 Phases of diet transformation

Phases	Groups	Using Roman diet (+ more/− less)
1ST PHASE	Romans	+++
	Native 1	+
	Native 2	−
	Native 3	−
2ND PHASE	Romans	+++
	Native 1	++
	Native 2	+
	Native 3	−
3RD PHASE	Romans	+++
	Native 1	+++
	Native 2	++
	Native 3	−

vicus militaris or *canabae legionis* also, a Roman-style diet was offered. When the soldiers were dismissed from military service, they took their eating habits with them. Whether their whole family at home got used to them is uncertain. The native women and children may well still have hung on to their own local eating habits. However, the success of Roman cuisine depended also on women's changing tastes. But they had every reason to change their habits, because the range of goods quadrupled with the arrival of the Romans and the new spices led to a veritable taste revolution. The transformation was perhaps linked to prestige and was considered as a demonstrative identification with the new Roman lifestyle.

During the period in which the diet was changing (first to second century AD), a period that can be divided into three phases (see Table 16.9), not all people in the north changed − or were able to change − all of their habits, or not simultaneously, or to the same intensity. The natives formed three groups in this respect. The first (mainly Celtic tribes) had experiences of Roman foodstuffs and dishes as well eating and drinking habits before the conquest, and by the end of the third phase, ate virtually identically to the Romans. The second group had no experience but was willing to change their diet (Germans, like Ubii), but in such a way that traces are still kept of their earlier food habits. The third group (mainly Germanic tribes in the Lower Rhine) had insufficient agrarian possibilities to change their diet fundamentally (Kooistra, 2009; Brüggler, 2016) and possibly refused Roman dishes altogether (like Cugernii?), perhaps as a mark of resistance. In short, no homogenous Romanized diet emerged but due to various influences regional differences and local nuances remained.

The highest level of Romanization, also regarding food and foodways, was in general reached at the beginning of the third century, with nearly the same appearance of cities in the north and in the Mediterranean heartlands, with forum, temple, baths, marcellum etc., with the same divinities, the Capitoline Triad (Iuppiter, Iuno and Minerva), with emperor or with the Mithras cult, etc., and with Caracalla's grant of universal citizenship to the free inhabitants of the Roman Empire in AD 212 (*Constitutio Antoniniana*) (Pferdehirt, 2012). In the third century, a new era began that inter alia saw the increasing influence of 'barbarian' cultures.

Note

1   Abbreviations here and following refer to modern country − with International Vehicle Registration Codes.

17

JEWS IN PALESTINE

David Kraemer

Jews were dispersed throughout various parts of the Roman world, predominantly in Palestine but also including important populations in Egypt, Syria, Asia Minor, and Rome itself. In each of these places, Jews were a noted, distinctive population, at least some of whom were set apart from their neighbours by various practices and beliefs. With respect to the diet of Jews, however, there is – beyond Palestine – little evidence, the documentary record being sparse and, in the matter of food, focused only on what would have struck observers as 'unusual' details.

Both the documentary corpus and archaeological record from Palestine in the Roman period are abundant. The writings of Palestinian Jews from this period, many of which include references to diet, include apocryphal or pseudepigraphical works, Dead Sea scrolls, books of the New Testament, the works of Josephus, and rabbinic compositions – the Mishnah (c. AD 200), various works of midrash (third–fifth centuries), and the Palestinian Talmud (fifth century). Many sites in Judea and the Galilee have been excavated, and animal bones from many of these sites have been examined. The remains of other organic materials have also been documented, helping to fill in the record as it pertains to food.

Outside of Palestine, only the Alexandrian Jewish community leaves us with a documentary record, which includes the writings of Philo and several apocryphal works. Archaeology outside of Palestine provides little evidence for Jewish diets, not because there were no Jews but because there are no sites where evidence of a Jewish diet – as opposed to the local diet more generally – can be isolated. For the wider Roman world, the only direct evidence we have of the Jewish diet comes from non-Jewish writers who notice Jewish dietary avoidances. This evidence allows us to say something about what at least some Jews would not eat, but nothing about what they would eat.

This does not, however, mean that there is nothing to say about the Jewish diet outside of Palestine. By virtue of the nature of food production and distribution in the ancient world, diets were primarily restricted to foods and ingredients that were produced locally. Local products were supplemented by others that could be shipped and effectively stored over longer periods. Of course, wealthier classes could also acquire and consume rarer, luxury items. But within classes, the market was, of necessity, relatively uniform, meaning that any given population, including Jews, ate what was available on the local market. If we know what the general population ate in a given locale, therefore, we know what Jews ate. Compared with the local diet, the Jewish diet will require only minor modifications.

The common Palestinian Jewish diet

Given the reality just described, any exploration of the Jewish diet in the Roman world must begin in Palestine. In view of the fact that the Palestinian Jewish diet privileged the 'Mediterranean triad', thus echoing the cultural prejudice of the broader Roman world north and east of the Mediterranean, what we note concerning this diet will inevitably be true for Jewish (as for other) diets in adjacent regions as well.

The culturally privileged foods of Jews in Palestine – echoing biblical[1] as well as Roman preference – were bread, wine, and olive oil. The privileged status of the first two is evident in the fact that they serve specialized ritual functions in both the early Christian-Jewish and rabbinic communities. In rabbinic ritual, bread and wine are the only two foods that attract unique rabbinic blessings (= the requirement to recite a formulaic blessing before enjoying a food); although they both 'belong' to other categories in rabbinic opinion (bread to 'the fruit of the ground' and wine to 'the fruit of the tree'), the blessing they demand is specific to them. Suffice to say that legal, narrative, and casual references to bread and wine are also widespread, leaving no doubt concerning the ubiquity of these foods in the Palestinian Jewish diet.

There is clear evidence that in the eyes of Palestinian Jews not all breads were alike. This is simply expressed in the early rabbinic composition, the Tosefta, in its elaboration of priority in the blessing of bread. The teaching is this:

> [When several kinds of bread are eaten at the same meal], we bless over the breadstuff that is of the best quality. How so? [If] a whole fine loaf and a whole homemade loaf [were to be eaten], he blesses over the whole fine loaf. [If] a piece of fine loaf and a whole homemade loaf [were to be eaten], he blesses over the whole homemade loaf. [If] a loaf [made] of wheat and a loaf [made] of barley [were to be eaten], he blesses over the one of wheat. [If] a piece [made] of wheat and a whole loaf [made] of barley [were to be eaten], he blesses over the piece [made] of wheat. [If] a loaf [made] of barley and a loaf [made] of spelt [were to be eaten], he blesses over the one of barley. But is not spelt superior to barley? Rather [it is because] barley is one of the seven kinds [of produce for which the Land of Israel is praised in Deut. 8:8] and spelt is not one of the seven kinds.
>
> *(Berakhot 4:15)*

The rabbinic blessing system, as reflected here, considers a variety of criteria, reflecting clear cultural preference in connection with bread: whole loaves are superior to partial loaves, fine flour is superior to courser flour, and wheat is superior to spelt, which is superior to barley (although, from the specific Jewish perspective, barley is preferable by virtue of its association with 'the Land of Israel').[2] Such privileging is of course connected with wealth and class differences, and may also reflect an adoption of Roman cultural preferences.[3]

Awareness of class distinctions and the privileging of certain breads above others are reflected in a rabbinic story regarding Jerusalem during the war with Rome. As recounted in the Babylonian Talmud (but fairly taken to represent Palestinian cultural preference), the story portrays Martha, the daughter of Boethus, one of 'the wealthy women of Jerusalem', during the siege and accompanying famine. The story proceeds simply but dramatically:

> She sent for her messenger and said to him, 'Go, bring me some fine flour'. By the time he went, it sold out. He came and said to her, 'There is no fine flour, but there is white flour'. She said to him, 'Go bring it to me'. By the time he went, it sold out.

He came and said to her, 'There is no white flour, but there is dark flour'. She said to him, 'Go bring it to me'. By the time he went, it sold out. He came and said to her, 'There is no dark flour, but there is barley flour'. She said to him, 'Go bring it to me'. By the time he went, it sold out. [In the meantime] she had taken off her shoes. She said, 'I'll go out and see whether I can find something to eat'. Some dung stuck to her foot and she died.

(Gittin 56a)

Beyond the fact that Martha is explicitly identified as being wealthy, the story also makes clear how 'delicate' she is, and her delicate quality is associated with her delicate appetite. So she, a representative of the wealthy class, prefers bread made from fine flour over that made from common white flour, white over dark, and wheat over barley. The culture's most powerfully symbolic food represents, in its symbolism, the status of the one it sustains.

Similar distinctions of quality, correlated with wealth and status, are evident in wines. Aged wine is superior to new wine (Mishnah Avot 4:20) and Italian wine is recognized as superior to other wine (Mishnah Sanhedrin 8:2). (Wine was produced locally in Palestine, of course, so this record speaks to the reality of international trade in – and local market demand for – 'fine wines'.) Moreover, it was not merely the *quality* of the wine that gave expression to the status of those partaking, but the way the wine was used. Ritual manipulation of the wine, in the fashion of the symposium, was deemed an elevated cultural act, to the extent that, in the opinion of one rabbi, if the wine was not mixed in a crater, it was not fit for the recitation of the blessing over wine (Tosefta Berakhot 4:3).

In the opinion of some rabbis, at least, consumption of wine also distinguished men from women. Famously, as part of the Passover evening table ritual (which closely reflected symposium rituals[4]), the rabbis required Jews to consume four cups of mixed wine. R. Judah, however, is reported to object that women and children should not consume wine but rather 'that which is fitting for them' (Tosefta Pesachim 10:4). The Palestinian Talmud adds that what is fitting for women is 'fine linen garments and belts', not (it implies) wine (Pesachim 10:1, 37b).

Beyond the Mediterranean triad (the other element of which, olive oil, was used primarily for dipping), other common foods included legumes (beans, lentils, chickpeas, and vetch), vegetables, and dairy (cheese and, less frequently, milk) (Rosenblum, 2010, 20–25, following Broshi, 2001, 121–143, and Dar, 1995, 327–332). Rounding out the common diet was a variety of local fruits, including figs, dates, carob, pomegranates, melons, and plums. Cisterns found throughout Palestine show that water was stored and used for drink, but, as indicated earlier, wine of various qualities, mixed with water, was the most important drink, and certainly a very common one (Broshi, 2001, 144–156, 162).

Fish was a common source of protein in the Palestinian Jewish diet. Whole, fresh fish preparations were certainly available, but most fish was probably preserved. Evidence for the latter claim is found in the common mention of 'fish hash' in rabbinic documents, while bone-remains uncovered at various sites testify to the general popularity of fish. In his review of the evidence, Justin Lev-Tov emphasizes the quantity of fish bones discovered at many sites, adding that they generally represent a small number of species: sea bream, tuna, and mackerel, groupers, and mullets (Lev-Tov, 2003, 435–436). In Lev-Tov's view, the fact that these are all Mediterranean species, and that they are all found even at in-land sites, is evidence of a well-organized fishing industry, responding to a healthy demand for fish on the market (437). Lev-Tov considers this appetite for fish a development of the Roman period (440) and suggests that what is uniquely *Roman* about the Palestinian diet is the increase of fish consumption.

Meat consumption in Palestine

Meat surely constituted a part of the Palestinian Jewish (and non-Jewish) diet, but to what extent and on what occasions is subject to considerable debate. Common wisdom, repeated by most who have written on the Palestinian diet of this period (Krauss, 1910, 108–110; Broshi, 2001, 132), suggests that, for all but the wealthy, meat was a relatively rare dietary item, consumed only on special occasions. This wisdom is supported by a simple economic logic: if live animals were productive resources, used for their labour and for the renewable products such as wool and dairy, then their owners would have hesitated to slaughter them before the end of their productive lives. Only the wealthy, therefore, could afford regularly to use animals for meat.

Literary references to meat consumption also seem to support this picture. For example, Tosefta Peah 4:10, instantiating the rabbinic requirement to support wealthy individuals who have fallen on hard times at the level of their former comforts, reports a case in which an 'extravagant' amount of meat is supplied; commenting on this teaching, the later Palestinian rabbinic composition (5th century), the Palestinian Talmud (Peah 8:8, 21a), expresses shock at the suggested quantity. Both individually and especially in combination, these two texts clearly imply that even the wealthy in Palestine consumed relatively small quantities of meat, while common persons consumed truly modest amounts. Jewish writings from outside of Palestine support the same picture. Philo, although living in the large, cosmopolitan, resource-rich city of Alexandria, suggests that meat-eating was not the first use for which animals would be considered. He writes of 'innumerable herds of cattle in every direction' that are milked daily because 'milk is the greatest source of profit to all breeders of stock, being partly used in a liquid state and partly allowed to coagulate and solidify, so as to make cheese' (*On the Virtues* 144). He testifies, then, that animals were raised for commercial purposes, and even for the food they produced. But despite the great quantity of edible animals he sees around him, he fails even to mention that they might be used for their meat. Since they obviously were sometimes used for this purpose, his comment must reflect a reality in which meat consumption, and therefore the market for meat, was secondary to other uses of animals.

Writing probably in the same context, the author of the Testament of Job makes the same assumption. The Job he represents (chapter 3) boasts about his support of the needy, speaking of his supplying bread to the many. His vast herds of sheep are used to supply clothing, his oxen for ploughing, his cows and ewes for dairy. He does speak of supplying small quantities of meat to widows and the poor, but this is clearly secondary and described as a burden (3:32–33). Meat is obviously not a staple. Similarly, in a clear statement of class associations of meat consumption, the author of Joseph and Asenath – again, probably from first-century Egypt[5] – says that 'fatted beasts' and fish and meat constitute a 'royal dinner' (10:14). If all of this was true in Alexandria and environs, there is no reason to imagine that the situation would be different in Palestine.

But the archaeological record, at least as interpreted by scholars who have studied it, challenges the conclusion just suggested. Anthony King (1999) offers a broad examination of the evidence throughout the Roman world, collating the finds from reports representing all regions. Overall, he reports, there is evidence that meat was widely consumed as a regular part of contemporary diets. With respect to the eastern Provinces, which concern us here, bone remains show that dietary meat was dominated by sheep and goat, while pig consumption was very low, usually under 15% (185). Some assemblages, he remarks, have no pig at all, including Jerusalem and other identifiably Jewish sites. This was not, however, the case throughout Palestine (see below for a more detailed discussion of pig avoidance and Jews). In King's view, this overall pattern can be considered the 'natural' one for an arid and semi-arid region (187).

Not surprisingly, there is evidence in Roman colonies and military sites of high consumption of pork, following Roman dietary preference. But this is nowhere common in the east outside of such colonies, meaning that the dietary influence of Rome was slight. Culturally speaking, according to King, outside influences in eastern provinces seem to have derived mainly from earlier Hellenistic patterns, which preferred sheep and goat meat. Speaking of the general picture, King comments that 'regional patterns retained their strength' (190).

Justin Lev-Tov offers a more detailed examination of the evidence from Palestine, resulting in important claims. Summarizing the evidence as a whole, he writes:

> Taken together, archaeological evidence from animal bones, human bone chemistry, agricultural economics, and even ceramic analysis strongly suggests that the Hellenistic and Roman period populations of Palestine ate meat on a regular basis. As Dar (1995: 332) suggests, it is time to rethink and re-examine the 'meat as luxury food in the ancient world' hypothesis, given the growing amount of archaeological evidence which contradicts this long-held view.
>
> *(Lev-Tov, 2003, 429)*

But while his general comments make broad claims supporting a meat-rich diet (on page 427 he writes, 'period diets included plenty of flesh, mainly from domestic animals raised in order to supply meat'), elsewhere his analysis reveals that the picture might not be quite so clear. So, while commenting on the 'large numbers of broken and butchered animal bones' found at various sites, he admits that 'we do not know how many meals, from how many people, over how much time, these piles of bones represent . . . At the very least, these animals were slaughtered for meat once they no longer generated an adequate quantity of wool, milk, or labour' (427–428). This is a much more balanced reading of the evidence. Returning to his claim for more abundant meat consumption, he remarks that 'the mortality profiles based on sheep/goat bones from late antique settlements . . . indicate that juveniles were often slaughtered and flocks often kept for both meat and milk production' (428). But one of the prime sources for such claims is discoveries at Tel Anafa, concerning which he remarks, 'the observed high mortality rates for domestic bovids (sheep, goats, and cattle) are inexplicable except as the product of a market system' (428). But he later admits that Tel Anafa 'has been understood by the excavators as having been occupied by cosmopolitan Hellenized Phoenicians' (429). This example, therefore, may prove little about the general Palestinian diet and actually reinforce the common wisdom that only upper social strata regularly ate meat (429). We might only add that a city colonized by Phoenicians would have little to tell us about the diets of common Jews.

The critique of the 'high quantity of meat' conclusion goes beyond individual sites. As Lev-Tov admits, it is difficult to fix a quantity of bones that would allow one to say that people ate meat 'on a regular basis'. We would have to ask about the chronological and demographic limits of any site (how many bones for what size population over what period of time?), and answers are often unclear or circular (does presence of pork really mean 'gentile' and its absence always mean 'Jewish?'). If our interest is the Jewish diet, we would have to know whether a location may be considered to be 'representative' of Jewish society as a whole or only of particular groups or social classes within it. Bone remains are suggestive and it is essential to consider them, but the questions are many and conclusions, therefore, must remain tentative.

The debate concerning the quantity of meat in the common Palestinian diet will surely continue, but one thing, at least, is clear: the evidence of bones that have been uncovered from local sites indicates that, as in earlier times, sheep and goats constituted the most widely consumed meats (Lev-Tov, 2003, 433), while beef was primarily restricted to the Carmel region, the only place where meat-producing herds could profitably be raised (cattle being ill-fitted for life on the rocky, sparse slopes of the mountainous Palestinian spine or the coastal region with its dry, hot summers).

When we ask about the overall balance of the Palestinian Jewish diet, there is one rabbinic text, in particular, we must consider. This text, Mishnah Ketubbot 5:8, has long been at the foundation of scholarly claims concerning the Palestinian Jewish 'food basket' and nutrition. The text lists a husband's obligations to his wife with respect to food, declaring that:

> One who provides his wife through an agent should not provide her with less than two *kabs* of wheat or [and?] four *kabs* of barley [for the six days of the week, the Sabbath being considered separately] . . . He gives her half a *kab* of legumes and half a *log* of [olive] oil and a *kab* of dried figs or a *maneh* of pressed figs, but if he doesn't have these, he assigns her other fruits in their place.

Helping to put this list into perspective is another text, roughly contemporaneous with this one, that describes what is to be supplied to a poor person:

> They do not give to a poor person going from place to place less than a loaf worth a dupondius [made from wheat costing at least] one sela for four seahs. If he stays overnight, we provide him with support for lodging, [namely] oil and legumes. If he spends the Sabbath, we give him food for three meals, [namely] oil, legumes, fish, and a vegetable.
>
> *(Tosefta Peah 4:8)*

According to Saul Lieberman's calculation, a dupondius would purchase half a kab (Lieberman, 1955, 183), meaning that what is provided to a woman and what is provided to a poor person (multiplying the daily allowance by six) are not all that different. Of course, there are obvious unknowns in this calculation (is the poor person to be given wheat or barley bread? What about fluctuations in the worth of currencies?), but even if we are able to make a rough comparison, we would still be left with many unanswerable questions: Are these lists meant to be generous or only basic? Are they meant to cover all of the nutritional needs of the needy party or only some of them? Do they reflect the conditions of years of plenty or of years of deprivation, or do they ignore such considerations altogether? In the end, what is perhaps most striking about these two lists is how similar they are, but we can't know whether that is because women are considered worthy of less food, like poor people (this would certainly reflect a common cultural prejudice of this as of other ages), or whether both correlate to some current notion of what is needed for survival.

Whatever the answers to these questions, it is important to emphasize that we can learn little about Palestinian Jewish nutrition from these lists. They are both prescriptive (as one would expect of rabbinic compositions), not descriptive, so we have no way of knowing how they compare with actual diets. In any case, it is safe to say that Jews consumed essentially the same diet as their neighbours (with possible exceptions to be discussed below), and their consumption would have fluctuated from year to year and from season to season, depending upon recent environmental conditions, the same as everyone else.

Jews participated in the market system for the trade and distribution of food and agricultural goods precisely as did their neighbours. Rabbinic literature testifies widely to the activities and mechanisms of the marketplace, often specifying the kinds of goods that were exchanged.

Exemplary is a discussion such as that found in Mishnah Baba Metziah, chapter 2, addressing the question of one's responsibilities when one finds lost items:

> 2:1 Which lost items are his [= the finder's], and which ones is he liable to proclaim? These lost items are his: [if] he found pieces of fruit scattered about, coins scattered about, small sheaves in the public domain, cakes of figs, bakers' loaves, strings of fish, pieces of meat, wool shearings [as they come] from the country [of origin], stalks of flax, or tongues of purple – lo, these are his, [these are] the words of R. Meir. R. Judah says, 'Anything which has an unusual trait is he liable to proclaim. How so? [If] he found a fig cake with a potsherd inside it, a loaf with coins in it'. R. Simeon b. Eleazar says, 'commercial merchandise he is not liable to proclaim'.

> 2:4 [If] he found [merchandise] in a store, lo, these are his. [If the merchandise was located] between the counter and the storekeeper, it belongs to the storekeeper. [If he found them] in front of the money changer, they are his. [If he found them] between the stool and the money changer, lo, these belong to the money changer.

Represented here is a world of traders, shop-keepers, money-changers, and (by implication) purchasers; that is, the world of the Palestinian market, as Jews and their neighbours knew it. The market is populated by bakers, butchers, fishmongers, and other food merchants, along with sellers of materials for clothing and other necessities. Crucially, the Mishnah distinguishes between commercial goods and home-made goods (in a section not quoted here) assuming that a baker's product, for example, will be generic, while a loaf baked by an individual will have distinguishing characteristics. 'Mass' production of foods and other goods, a part of this market system, leads to standardization.[6]

Jews and pork consumption

Perhaps the most important question pertaining to the Jewish diet in the Roman world, in Palestine and elsewhere, relates to the pig taboo; that is, the degree to which Jews were distinguished from their neighbours by their refusal to eat pork. In view of the fact that Jews overwhelmingly ate the same foods from the same markets and agricultural sources as their neighbours, this means that, if there was a distinct Jewish diet at all, it was the pigless diet. Among the questions that need to be clarified before suggesting conclusions in this matter are both whether and to what degree Jews avoided pork and whether their non-Jewish neighbours consumed pork with any regularity.

In his review of animal remains in sites throughout the empire, Anthony King notes that 'the pork-rich diet seems to have been a remarkably consistent dietary pattern that was normal and desirable in the region around Rome' (King, 1999, 171) meaning *only* around Rome, as well as in Roman colonies (177) and military encampments.[7] By contrast, even in the more immediate region of Rome, 'mountain areas tended to have more sheep and goats, because they were better adapted' (171), and, overall, 'strongly established regional characteristics' dominated other regions, where the 'Roman' fondness for pig gained little traction (178).

With respect to the Roman east, including Palestine, King writes that, based upon the evidence of bone remains, the meat diet was 'dominated by consumption of sheep and goat meat' (185). Throughout the region, pig consumption was evidently very low, with less than 15% of the bone remains being from pigs. He adds that some sites – Jewish sites, including Jerusalem – had no pig remains at all, but this was not the case throughout Palestine. King explains the general paucity of pig remains in this region by suggesting that it was a 'natural' product of ecological conditions, 'one that fits best with arid and semi-arid environmental constraints' (187). This would mean that Roman mocking of Jewish refusal to eat pork, found in contemporary writings cited below, represents a naïve, 'localized' Roman cultural prejudice.

Justin Lev-Tov builds upon King's observations, offering some important additions. He wisely remarks that 'dietary customs within the Jewish population of Palestine were probably more complex than has so far been acknowledged' (Lev-Tov, 2003, 432). How so? On the one hand, pig consumption was generally quite low, so it is difficult to state with confidence that the avoidance of pig boldly and obviously announced someone as a Jew. On the other hand, the bone remains show that 'pigs and other forbidden species dot the Jewish communities of Palestine'. Some have argued that such remains are evidence of the non-Jewish demographics of these cities, but this argument is almost always circular. Lev-Tov suggests, far more reasonably, that 'in reality, it may have been that Jews differed in regard to their observance of the dietary laws, with some being more Romanized (or Hellenized) than others' (432). Some Jews, like some of their neighbours, ate pig following Roman culinary fashion. Other Jews, also like some of their neighbours, didn't eat pig, because it was not a popular local food. Arguably, the 'Jewish' diet may have been little marked by the presence or absence of pig meat.

But other testimony, from a variety of times and locations, suggests powerfully that some Jews avoided pork *because* they were Jews and that their avoidance of pork marked them as Jews in the eyes of others. Among those who noticed the Jewish avoidance of pork were Apion (Egypt, first century), Petronius (Rome?, first century), Epictetus, (Rome and elsewhere, first–second century), Plutarch (Delphi, first–second century), Tacitus (Rome, early second century), Juvenal (Rome, second century), Sextus Empiricus (Egypt?, early second century), Porphyry (Tyre, third century), Julian (mid-fourth century), and Macrobius (fifth century). Plutarch also notices the Jewish avoidance of hare (Stern, 1976, 556), Porphyry adds that Jews are 'forbidden . . . unscaled fish . . . and also any uncloven animals' (Stern, 1980, 441), and Julian also remarks on the Jewish avoidance of blood (Stern, 1980, 552).

Of course, Jews who ate pork and other forbidden substances would not have been noticed by their neighbours for their avoidance. So we cannot conclude from this range of testimony that Jews all avoided pork. But we can learn that a sufficient number of Jews refused pork and other foods and that they were noticed. The chronological range of these testimonies (first–fifth centuries), along with the geographical range, shows that this was a persistent, widespread practice. It is notable that the recorded observations emerge predominantly either from Rome or from Roman authors, who, as pig eaters, would have noticed those who did not. It is also notable that some remarked upon other dietary avoidances, all of which are biblically based, suggesting that direct or indirect familiarity with Jewish scripture, and not necessarily observation, was the source of the author's knowledge (this is particularly suggested by Porphyry's language). In any case, it is fair to say that if there was an identifiably Jewish diet in the Roman world, even if it was not observed by all Jews, it was the one that excluded pork from the menu.

The rabbinic diet

The Palestinian rabbis who sought to provide a new and sustainable direction for Jewish practice after the destruction of the Temple and the failure of the Bar Kokhba revolt in AD 135 created a new eating regimen, later known as *kashrut*, that would one day be thought identical to *the* Jewish diet. Aside from the inherited biblical prohibitions, defining which living creatures are permissible as food and which not, the most outstanding – and innovative – element of the rabbinic diet is its prohibition of eating meat and dairy at the same meal. Did Jews beyond the circles of the rabbis observe this eating prohibition or didn't they? The answer lies in the fact that the Jewish dietary practices noticed by the observers listed above are all *biblical* prohibitions. Aside from the biblical food prohibitions, the one element of the 'Jewish' diet that might have been noticed by outsiders is the rabbis' prohibition of eating meat and dairy together. Of course, this prohibition would have been relatively inactive for those who ate little or no meat. But the evidence cited earlier suggests that meat consumption may not have been as rare as has been assumed, so if observers noticed the Jewish refusal to eat pork, they may well have noticed their refusal to eat permitted meats with dairy. The fact that they did not supports the conclusion that rabbinic authority or influence was slow to spread beyond rabbinic circles (a conclusion shared by most historians today[8]), even in Palestine, let alone beyond. Hence, it is fair to say that there was no rabbinic-Jewish diet current in Jewish populations in the Roman world outside of very small circles.

The Jewish diet beyond Palestine

As I wrote at the beginning of this chapter, the evidence for Jewish diets beyond Palestine is sparse. The testimonies cited earlier suggest that many Jews, throughout the Roman world, were known to avoid pork and other biblically forbidden substances. In our discussion of meat eating, we also saw that the literary evidence from Egypt corresponds with the literary evidence from Palestine, suggesting that consumption patterns were similar. Further, we have noted that, overall, it is fair to say that the diet of Jews in any locale would have been virtually identical to the general local diet (with the exception of specific avoidances), given that the local market supplied Jews and their neighbours alike.

Still, since we may locate small pockets of evidence pertaining to Jewish diets in the diaspora, it is worth surveying them here. As we saw, Philo suggests regarding the typical diet in Alexandria that it was not centrally comprised of meat. Animals would have been the source of dairy for food, but not typically more. *The Testament of Job* emphasizes the centrality of bread in the diet, while *Joseph and Asenath* (8:4–5), employing bread and wine metaphorically (much like the early church), suggests that at least the major constituents of the Mediterranean Triad were as dominant in Egypt as they were elsewhere.

A brief mention of the market supplying food to Jews in Sardis, part of a document quoted by Josephus (*AJ* 14. 261), suggests that at least some Jews there had particular Jewish dietary requirements, but no food or restriction is specified so we can say little more about what their diet may have been. In light of everything we have seen above, it is likely that the specific assurance refers to permissible meat.

Jews dining apart[9]

In the end what distinguished Jewish eating in the Roman world was, more than anything else, the refusal of at least some Jews to dine with their neighbours. Tacitus's statement that Jews 'sit [or "dine" = "epulis"] apart at meals' (*Historiae* 5.5.2; Stern, 1980, 26) is frequently cited. Even more explicit and extreme is Philostratus' report that Jews live 'a life apart and irreconcilable, that cannot share with the rest of mankind in the pleasures of the table' (*Via Apollonii* 5.33; Stern, 1980, 341). These observations can be said to reflect both the law and practice of some Jews, beginning in at least the second century BC, who forbade themselves the consumption of 'gentile foods'; that is, foods that were otherwise permitted but that had been prepared by gentiles. With respect to wine, which may encourage conviviality, the prohibition was even stronger: any wine that a gentile merely touched was prohibited by the rabbis and others for Jewish consumption.

Notes

1   Typical of the many references to this combination in the Bible is Hosea 2:8. For a broader discussion of the Mediterranean Triad in the Bible, see MacDonald, 2008, 19–24.

2   For a fuller discussion of the cultural privileging implied by the rabbinic blessings, see Kraemer, 2009, 77–86.

3   See Beer, 2010, who writes (p. 19) that 'the principal grain was barley in Greek territories, whereas there appears a marked preference within Roman culture for wheat'.

4   There is a longstanding scholarly debate whether or to what degree the Passover seder (a term not used for this meal-ritual until post-Talmudic times) is to be understood as a kind of symposium. For a cogent articulation of the negative position, see Bokser, 1984. Even for Bokser, the symposium ritual defines the terms of what must be negated.

5   Philonenko, 1968, 107, argues that the work originated in a rural setting in the environs of Alexandria. See also Sparks, 1984, 469–470.

6   For more on Palestinian markets during this period, see Rosenfeld and Menirav, 2005.

7   MacKinnon's detailed survey of the evidence in Italy shows that pig was consumed in notably lower quantities outside of central Italy – although consumption was higher in the north than in the south – and consumption in general rose during the imperial period (MacKinnon, 2004, 139–140, 153, 194).

8   See Schwartz, 2001, 175–176. Shaye J.D. Cohen confirms this judgement in personal correspondence, dated 18 March 2015.

9   For a full review of evidence pertaining to Jewish commensality with their neighbors, see Erdkamp, 2011.

18

EGYPT

Willy Clarysse

The sources

Our main source of information are papyri, thousands of which were found in houses, tombs and rubbish dumps, mainly in Middle Egypt, the Fayum and the Roman camps in the eastern desert. Information on eating and drinking is especially frequent in private letters and household and travelling accounts. Up to the late twentieth century, digging in Egypt was concentrated on finding papyri; other finds, such as bones or grains, were usually neglected. Recent excavations take account not only of animal and vegetal remains, but also of human bones, where the study of stable isotopes allows reconstruction of dietary patterns.[1] The archaeological record may be somewhat biased because most of it comes from desert sites, and reflects material imported from the Nile valley.

Basic foods

Cereals and pulses formed the basis of the ancient diet (σῖτος), providing up to 75 percent of the necessary calories (see Heinrich in this volume), to which protein supplements were added in the form of meat, fish, vegetables or fruit (ὄψα) (Wilkins and Hill, 2006, 114).

In pharaonic Egypt husked emmer (*Triticum dicoccon*, ὄλυρα) was the most common grain. It was still popular with the native population in the Ptolemaic period, for example in a temple environment (Thompson, 1995), but emmer gradually gave way to naked tetraploid wheat (*Triticum durum*, hard wheat, πυρός) (Boozer, 2015, #3045–3050). Per volume, emmer is less nutritious (because it has to be dehusked; see Heinrich, Chapter 9 in this volume) than *Triticum durum* (which has now been replaced by bread wheat (a subspecies of *Triticum aestivum*), but is still used for pasta and couscous). The change is clearly visible in the papyrological documentation, where the word ὄλυρα all but disappears in the first century AD (van Minnen 2001, 1271–1273).

In most excavations *Triticum durum* is the most common cereal, but barley (*Hordeum vulgare*, κριθή) and lentils (*Lens culinaris*, φακός) are also common (Leighty, 1933, 87–88; Maxfield and Peacock, 2001, 190–191; Cuvigny, 2011, 208; Peacock et al., 2011, 230). Barley was used as animal fodder and for brewing, but also for human consumption, even for second-rate bread (Cappers et al., 2014); lentils are in fact a pulse, but in the papyri they are often put on a par with grains; for example, in P. Petrie III 76 and 98. Rice is attested in Mysos Hormos and in

Berenike already in the first century AD, but it was not a staple food before the Arab period (Van der Veen, 2011, 46–48; Sidebotham, 2011, 79, 228; Peacock et al., 2011, 228–229).

Wheat, emmer, barley and even fenugreek were made into various breads (Bagnall, 2003, 26). The classical word ἄρτος is gradually superseded by modern Greek ψωμίον in the third century AD; emmer bread is called κύλληστις (Battaglia, 1989, 90–91). Breads usually take the form of flat round loaves, not unlike the present day *beledi* bread and often came in pairs ζεύγη)[2]. Bread-making took place in the courtyards of private houses, where many small bread ovens have been found. The dough adhered to the inner surface of the sides of the oven and curled up when baked; the loaves were then removed from the open top of the oven. Although there were also industrial bakeries, for instance in the temples and for the army, home-baked bread prevailed. The twins Taous and Thaues, who worked for the Memphite temple of Sarapis, received a monthly ration of 120 loaves (60 pairs), which amounted to 48 artabas (of emmer) a year. Demotic marriage contracts record annual figures of 36 and 60 artabas of emmer as a yearly allowance for the wife. This roughly amounts to yearly 500 kg unmilled *durum* for the twins, 360 and 613 kg of wheat (reckoning the artaba at 25 kg and the relation between wheat and emmer at 5:2). This is more than necessary for subsistence (c. 250–300 kg.), but these were relatively well-to-do families and the twins had to share their bread between the two of them (Thompson, 2012, 171–173). In P. Cairo dem. 30604 (Thissen, 1984) a nurse receives monthly 1 1/6 artabas of wheat, i.e., 350 kg. The monthly ration of wheat for soldiers in the Roman army was 1 artaba of wheat (Rathbone, 2009, 314; Cuvigny, 2014, 75–77).

A similar cereals could also be eaten as gruel (ἀθήρα, wheat flour mixed with milk), which was considered to be inferior to bread by some, although it appears several times on festive occasions (Perpillou-Thomas, 1992). Lentils were probably mostly eaten as gruel (like Indian dahl), to which oil was added (cf. O. Claud. 3, 44–45).

Bread came in different qualities. In the Zenon archive a distinction is made between fine flour (σεμίδαλις or καθαρός) and coarse flour (αὐτόπυρος), the former being reserved for more important individuals, the latter for the slaves (Battaglia, 1989, 81–83; Reekmans, 1996, 16–17). A similar distinction between fine and coarse bread (ψωμία καθαρά vs. κιβάρια) is found in the accounts of Theophanes in the early fourth century AD (Matthews 2006, p. 144). Perhaps this coarse bread was made from a mix of wheat and barley (Mayerson, 2002, 106–108). From the third century onwards first quality bread is also known by the Latin term σιλίγνιον (Battaglia, 1989, 93–95), which may be contrasted with ἀννωνικόν, ἄρτος or ψωμίον (CPR 7 41).

The two main meals were lunch (ἄριστον) and dinner (δεῖπνον), often mentioned side by side (see P. Wash. 98 introd. for references). Wine was available on both occasions. When breakfast was taken in the early morning (ἀκράτισμα), it was probably light; for example, some bread dipped in undiluted wine. The evening meal was the more important, including a choice of bread, cooked meat, fresh fish, cheese, eggs, vegetables and fruit (Matthews, 2006, 171),

Table 18.1 Annual allowances of cereals

	olyra (art.)	*durum (art.)*	*durum (kg.)*
twins	48 2/3	(20 art.)	500
marriage contract	36	(14.4 art.) (?)	360 (?)
marriage contract	60	(24 art.)	600
nurse contract	–	15 art.	370
Roman soldiers	–	12 art.	300

whereas lunch was usually cold. Formal invitations that survive are always for the evening meal (see most recently P. Oxy. 75 5056–5057, with further references), which could take place at home or in a restaurant (δειπνητήριον), and usually started at the ninth hour (i.e., around 2pm).

Basic drinks

The most common drink was of course water, which was sometimes sold in the cities and in the quarries (see SB 28 17099 and O. Claud. 1 134, where a further study is announced; Cuvigny, 2003, 332–333; the demotic ostraca of Cologne and Pisa, which deal with water supply in the western desert, probably date from the late Ptolemaic period, see Vleeming et al., 2005, 813).

There were two alcoholic beverages; beer and wine (see Broekaert in this volume; for wine in general, see now Dzierzbicka 2018). On the whole, Egyptians were beer drinkers and Greeks drank wine. Shops for beer were found in nearly every village, whereas wine-shops were concentrated in the major agglomerations, where no doubt most Greeks lived (Clarysse and Thompson, 2006). The gradual disappearance of beer in the Roman period, may have had several causes (van Minnen, 2001), but the changing foodways are certainly also a sign of dietary Hellenization. Thus in AD 10–12 a brewery is still founded inside the temple economy (I. Prose 51). Coptic literature often warns against wine, but hardly ever mentions beer (Clarysse, 2001). In the monasteries, wine was produced on a large scale even in the Arab period (P. Brux. Bawit, 85–86 and P. Mon. Apollo 45).

Beer and wine could be drunk at home or in a pub, but an important occasion for drinking (and eating) were the meetings of social clubs (Ascough, 2008 on different forms of commensality); rules of associations are preserved both in Greek (e.g., P. Mich. 5 243) and in demotic (Monson, 2006). One such text stipulates that "on the day of drinking members are allowed to bring two jars of wine. After having drunk their two jars, they should go." If anybody brings more than two jars, he has to pay a fine to the temple (P. Berl. dem. 3115 3.1–4). The rules also provide penalties for drunken misconduct (P. Mich. 5 243, introd. 92–93). Sometimes petitioners stress that their opponent in a quarrel was drunk, clearly as an aggravating circumstance (Clarysse, 2001, 163–165).

There is scarcely any textual information on the color of the wine, but the deceased represented on mummy portraits usually hold a cup of red wine in their hands (see, for example, Parlasca and Seemann, 1999, 294–295). The age-old Greek habit of mixing wine with water is nowhere attested in the papyri, and the rare κρατῆρες are probably not wine mixing bowls. This does not mean wine was now usually drunk pure: *posca*, the drink of the Roman soldiers, for instance, was a mixture of sour wine and water (*acetum*, ὄξος). Since wine jars were often coated with pitch in order to keep the wine drinkable for longer periods, ancient wine may have tasted somewhat like modern Greek retzina. Egyptian wines, however, were rarely kept for more than a few years (Ruffing, 1998, 22–24; Clarysse, 2009, 163–165). Unlike the case with beer, the texts often mention different brands and qualities of wine: sweet, fragrant (εὐώδης "with a good smell," Cuvigny, 2011, 213–216), coming from the Mareotis area or from Greece, old and new (Ruffing, 1998). Clearly fine-quality wine was sometimes imported from Greece in the Roman period (see, for example, Papathomas, 2006 and P. Bingen, 77). Wine making is not easy and often the wine turned sour, gradually becoming vinegar (ὄξος) or moldy (ὀζόμενος) (Kruit, 1992, 266–268).

Alongside grapes other fruit juices were sometimes also made into wine, but palm wine (σπαθίτης οἶνος) (P. Ross.-Georg. 3 9) or pomegranate wine (ῥοιτικός) (P. Mich. 11 619.10) are found only in a few papyri.

Oil

Olives form the third item in the "Mediterranean triad," alongside wheat and vines. As in modern Mediterranean cooking, oil is used to moisten bread and to prepare meat and vegetables. It contributed to a balanced diet by adding unsaturated fat.

In Egypt, as elsewhere in the Mediterranean, olive oil was considered the best (cf. Wittenburg, 1980, and P. Dublin 16.2 note), but vegetable oils were up to 30% cheaper (Drexhage, 1990a, 103). Because the terminology is fluid (ἔλαιον can be any kind of oil) it is unclear how far olive oil remained a luxury item for the better-off classes. In the Fayum, olive groves were certainly far more common in the Roman period than earlier. No less than 40 leases are preserved and about AD 100 the Roman veteran L. Bellienus Gemellus apparently specialized in olive cultivation (Ast and Azzarello, 2013; cf. also Strabo XVII.35). The Kellis oasis exported olive oil to the Nile valley (Bagnall, 2013, 35–36). Like vines, olives were grown on land that was artificially irrigated and therefore not suitable for grain and this may have contributed to a dietary change (van Minnen, 2001, 1276–1280). Bitter oil, made from green olives, was often designated as σπανέλαιον; the link with Spain was only indirect (Kramer, 1990).

In the Ptolemaic period the common oil for lamps was castor oil (κρότων, called κικι in Egyptian), for food it was sesame oil (Sandy, 1989, 35–71). In the Roman period, castor and sesame oil are replaced in the documents by radish oil (ῥαφάνινον ἔλαιον, Morelli, 2004). The servants of the Appianus estate in Euhemeria received a monthly ration of 1 artaba of wheat and 4 *kotylai* (about 1 L) of vegetable oil (Rathbone, 1991, 109–110). This is comparable to the allowance for members of the *familia* (the workforce) in Mons Claudianus one and a half centuries earlier: 0.73 L (3 *kotylai*) of oil, alongside 1 kg of grain and 3.9 L of lentils (O. Claud. 3, 44–46). In the Byzantine period, oil was used to pay wages (discussed by Morelli, 1996).

Meat and fish

In an average Egyptian family, meat was only consumed at religious and private festivals, such as birthdays (Perpillou-Thomas, 1993, 201–209). Usually the animal was slaughtered for the gods, but eaten by men. In ordinary household accounts meat appears only infrequently, but there are exceptions; such as SB 26 16577, where 14 dr. are spent on meat and fish in a two-week period, at a time when workmen earned no more than one drachma a day. In the daily account of a butcher (P. Homb. 42) meat is consumed on ten days of a one-month period, including three times for offering (θυσία) and twice "alongside the river," no doubt to celebrate the end of the flood (see the editor's note).

The most common meat was pork (e.g., P. Kellis IV, p.46; Boozer, 2015, #3029–3032), which becomes even more visible in papyri of the later period, when soldiers receive a regular meat allowance (Mitthof, 2001, 214–215; see also SB 26 16570, a report of a meat collection, both pork and veal, in several villages of the Oxyrynchite nome). In the eastern desert pork, usually from young animals, was often salted (Leguilloux, 2003, 550–558; 2011, 169–170; 2018, 18–21). All parts of the pig could be eaten, as appears in the cook's account P. Oxy. 1 108, mentioning breast, trotters, head, tongue, snout, and kidneys (liver is found in O. Claud. 1162 and 167, pig's trotters in O. Homb. 42 and SB 22 15302), but no doubt some parts were more choice (and more expensive) than others. In O. Claud. 2 307 a piglet is slaughtered and the meat is distributed among 23 men, usually at 1 or 2 mina (350 g or 700 g) a person, for a total of 12 kg; the head and the feet are treated separately.

Lesser quality meat could be processed in sausages (λουκανικά and ἰσίκια). Piglets (and even suckling pigs) were highly valued and often presented to important visitors or on festive occasions (Rathbone, 1991, 201 n.32). When the directing manager Alypios comes to visit one of his farms in Theadelpheia, he insists that a fine piglet should be killed and served the next day (P. Flor. 2 127.12); in fact the meat cannot have been really soft, just one day after the killing. Poultry (goose, chickens and pigeons) is also common, sheep and goats less frequent, and cow meat even rarer (in the Roman army in the west cow meat was more popular, see Junkelmann, 2006, 154–163). In the papyri veal is mainly attested through the certificates for sacrifice, whereby Egyptian priests guaranteed that the animal was pure and fit for offering (Reiter, 2004, 229–235).

Ancient religious taboos do not seem to have played a major role: pigs are offered also to Egyptian gods and at Mons Claudianus camel and donkey meat, usually of adult animals slaughtered on the spot, was eaten on a regular basis, as appears from the osteological remains (Leguilloux, 2003, 561; 2011, 171–175; 2018, 18–23). It was forbidden to catch (and eat) some kinds of sacred fishes in particular areas (PSI 8 901), but on the whole religious food restrictions were limited to certain areas and types of people (e.g., priests on duty in the temple; Palmyrean soldiers in the eastern desert, cf. Leguilloux 2018, 37–40). Perhaps of greater impact was the abstinence from meat during Lent in Christian times. In monastic ideology, as in Manicheïsm, food deprivation by fasting and abstinence plays a prominent role. In Shenute's monasteries, for instance, healthy monks receive only one meal a day and are not supposed to eat meat, fish or dairy products, nor to drink wine. They are, according to the rules, veganists (Layton, 2002, 44–45). Such extreme deprivation, however, could only be maintained with difficulty by strong social control at common meals. In the ostraca of the eremite Frange, for instance, there is more diversity, although meat and wine are also limited to the sick and for festivals (O. Frange, 20–21; for food in the monasteries, see now Mossakowska-Gaubert, 2015).

Whereas in Mons Claudianus and Myos Hormos most fish came from the nearby Red Sea (Van der Veen, 1998a, 104; O. Claud. 2 241), in Egypt fish was plentiful in the Nile, the canals and stagnant water after the flood. Shellfish is only rarely mentioned in the papyri – for example, κόχλια, perhaps snails (P. Mich. 619.7) and ὄστρεα (P. Oxy. 4 738.5, apparently a feast with dinners lasting several days; in the Zenon archive oysters are clearly a luxury, see Reekmans, 1996, 24) – but shells are found in Qusair. If we had more texts from Alexandria, oysters would probably figure more often on the menu. They were eaten raw, as appears from a Hellenistic riddle in verse form preserved on a Ptolemaic papyrus (Parsons, 1977).

Dairy products

With the exception of cheese (Drexhage, 1996), dairy products were not easy to preserve (butter, milk) or to transport (eggs). They therefore leave few traces in the archaeological remains, and are not mentioned in the papyri either, since they were produced and consumed within the household. Eggs are usually those from hens and in several instances one chicken is offered together with ten eggs (P. Oxy. 12 1568.2–3, for a birthday party; 16 1890.12, for a festival; P. Oxy. 42 3056; SB 10270 passim for visiting officials). In P. Wisc. 2 60 goose eggs are mentioned, but this is exceptional. Butter (βούτυρος) is found only rarely before the Arab period; milk (γάλα) and cheese (τύρος) are more common. Probably most milk came from sheep and goats (e.g. P. Wisc. 2 78 passim), but cows' milk is mentioned on a few occasions (CPR 10 53; Mitteis, Chrest. 104.17–18).

Vegetables and fruit

Below I present the papyrological documentation for the main vegetables and fruits in tabular form. Items attested fewer than ten times are not included, such as asparagus (ἀσπάραγος),

Table 18.2 Vegetables

	Greek term	translation	BC	AD Rom	AD Byz	total
1	ὄροβος	vetch	8	111	8	133
	ὀρόβιον		0	5	1	
2	κύαμος	beans	21	51	3	77
	κυάμιον		0	2	0	
3	φάσηλος	beans	29	11	30	70
	φασήλιον		1	3	6	
4	ἐρέβινθος	chick-pea	40	2	5	51
	ἐρεβίνθιον		0	2	2	
5	κράμβη	cabbage	25	16	0	41
	κραμβίον		1	4		
6	σκόρδον	garlic	19	11	2	34
	σκορδίον		0	2	0	
7	κρόμμυον	onion	14	9	3	32
	κρομμύδιον		0	4	2	
8	σεῦτλον	beet	7	12	2	31
	σευτλίον		6	3	1	
9	κολόκυνθα	gourd	8	10	5	31
	κολόκυνθος		1	4	3	
	κολοκύνθιον					
10	ῥάφανος	radish	10	6	2	27
	ῥαφάνιον		8	2	0	
11	θρίδαξ	lettuce	14	10	1	25
12	σίκυος	cucumber	6	5	3	21
	σικύδιον		0	7	0	
13	καυλίον	cabbage	1	12	1	14
14	πρᾶσον	leek	7	5	2	14
15	γογγύλη	turnip	0	2	2	14
	γογγυλίς		3	6	0	
	γογγυλίδιον		0	0	1	

1. Vetch is mentioned more than 80 times in the custom house receipts, as a product exported from the Fayum (Sijpesteijn, 1987, 66). It was mainly used as animal fodder, but ὀρόβιον was a gruel for human consumption (O.Did. 397).

2–3. Κύαμος and φάσηλος may be two kinds of beans, but the former word gradually disappears in the later period. Modern Greek uses only φάσηλος.

5 and 13. The term κράμβη for cabbage in the Ptolemaic period is gradually replaced by καυλίον from the second century onwards (cf. Cuvigny, 2007).

6. A new strain of garlic for the Greek market was introduced in the third cent. BC Fayum, with a center in the village of Oxyrhyncha (see Crawford, 1973).

9 and 12. For gourds and cucumbers, see Konen (1995). Gourds could be eaten raw, or cooked (as in P. Ryl. 629 l.326).

10. Radish was mainly grown for oil. There are no certain examples where it was eaten as a vegetable; it could also be cooked (P. Petrie III 140 d2).

13. For καυλίον, see Cuvigny (2007).

Table 18.3 Fruit

	Greek term	translation	BC	AD Rom	AD Byz	total
1	φοῖνιξ	date	17	196	20	256
	φοινίκιον		0	16	7	
2	ἐλαία	olive	8	61	9	82
	κολυμβάς		2	2		
3	σταφυλή	grape	10	13	17	74
	σταφύλιον		1	8	4	
	βότρυς		4	4	2	
	βοτρύδιον		0	2	0	
	τρώξιμον		5	1	3	
4	σῦκον	fig	23	17	3	49
	συκάριον		0	2	0	
	συκίον		0	2	0	
	συκίδιον		0	1	1	
5	κάρυον	nuts	18	10	0	35
	καρύδιον		0	2	5	
6	στρόβιλος	pine-cone	4	20	1	32
	στροβίλιον		1	2	4	
7	ῥοιά, ῥοά	pomegranate	15	9	2	26
8	μῆλον	apple	7	11	7	25
9	ἰσχάς	dried fig	12	5	6	25
	ἰσχάδιον		0	1	1	
10	θέρμος	lupine	1	9	6	16
11	δίζυφος,	jujube	0	5	7	14
	ζίζυφος ,		1	1	0	
	δίδυφον					
	παλίουρα					
12	περσικόν	peach	0	9	4	13
13	πέπων	melon	0	2	0	8
	πεπώνιον		0	1	5	
14	κίτριον	lemon	0	7	0	8
	κύθρον		0	1	0	

1. The figures for φοῖνιξ are problematic because the word indicates both the palm tree and its fruit. That dates were by far the most common fruit, however, is confirmed by the archaeological record (Van der Veen, 2011, 149–151; Peacock et al., 2011, 231; P. Kellis IV, 42). Dates were often exported from the Fayum (Sijpesteijn, 1987, 68–69). They could be eaten fresh (green dates, χλωροί), but were often dried (ξηρός). Two varieties of date are regularly mentioned in the texts: the juicy φοίνικες πατητοί (cf. Hohlwein, 1939, 18–22) and the nut-like φοίνικες καρυωτοί.

2. The figures for ἐλαία are problematic since the word indicates both the olive tree and its fruit; moreover the plural τὰ ἔλαια can also be used for olive oil. It is clear, however, that olives, both green and black, were not only used for oil, but also consumed as fruit. Olive stones are abundant in the archaeological finds (P. Kellis 4, 43). Olives could be cooked (P.Flor. 3 334) or pickled (P. Prag. 1 90; PSI 13 1313).

3. Except for the rare word (ἀ)σταφίς (e.g., in SB 14 11903 vo.9, "black raisins"), the texts do not distinguish between fresh grapes and dried raisins. Four different varieties of grapes are sent as a present in P. Fouad 77 (white, royal, Mareotic and smoke-colored).

4 and 9. The apparent disappearance of figs in the Byzantine period must be accidental, since dried figs (ἰσχάδες) continue to occur in the texts. Also in the archaeological remains whole figs and fig seeds are commonly found (P. Kellis 4, p.41). There are three different diminutives here, of which συκάριον in P. Flor. 2 176.9 clearly has a pejorative meaning.

continued . . .

Table 18.3 Continued

---

5. There are different kinds of nuts, walnuts (κάρυα Περσικά) and hazelnuts (κάρυα Ποντικά). Chestnuts (καρύα Εὐβοικά) are not explicitly mentioned in the papyri (Eideneier, 1971).

6. It is unclear whether pine-cones were eaten or rather burned on the altar. In P.Graux 2 10.12 and BGU 3 801.17 pine-cones go with *tragemata* [sweetmeats] but elsewhere with offerings of *artymata* [condiments] (P. Oxy. 9 1211; 2797; P.Petaus 33, 34 and 38; P.Strasb. 837). In P.Graux 2 10 and P.Mich. 2 123 verso v.21 the pine-cones are "for the children." Pine kernels and even pine cones are also found in Myos Hormos (Van der Veen, 2011, 156–157).

7. Pomegranates are twice given to children (P.Oxy 4 736.58 and P.Oxy. 58 3923).

8. Apples are rare in the papyri, and pears even rarer (cf. P. Col. 10 273.5 note).

10. Θέρμος is one of the rare Greek words which is also found in demotic and survives even in present-day Arabic, where the seeds are still sold by street vendors (Clarysse, 1987, 11; 2013, 17 no. 41).

11. Jujubes seem to have been popular in Kellis, where their stones were found in abundance (P.Kellis 4, 44). Except for BGU 4 1120 (Alexandria; 5 BC) all references date from the Roman period and later.

12. With the exception of P. Ross.-Georg. 2 19 (AD 141) peaches are not found before the third century AD (cf. P. Col. 10 273.5 note).

13. For melons, see Konen (1995). Seeds of water melons were found in large quantities in Myos Hormos and in Berenike (see Van der Veen, 2011, 155; Sidebotham, 2011, 79).

14. Lemon is not attested before the Roman period.

---

rocket (εὔζωμον), chicory (σέρις), and fennel (μαράθον). I have not taken into account general words like λάχανον (vegetable; more than 500 references; see Drexhage, 1990a) or ὄσπρια (pulse, but in the later period the word is used for all kinds of cereals, especially when mixed, cf. P. Mich. 15 732.39 note). The figures are not a direct reflection of what was eaten, but depend to a large measure on what was transported (custom house receipts playing a large role in the high figures for pulses and vetch), taxed and traded. The numerous letters from the eastern desert asking for or accompanying vegetables skew the numbers in favor of products that could be sent to the forts.

With the exception of ῥαφάνιον, neuter terms ending in -ιον turn up in the Roman and Byzantine period, indicating that the product was used or even prepared as food; for example, *orobos* is the plant, whereas *orobion* can also be a dish prepared with vetch, like present-day *foul*, a bean stew popular in Egypt (Cuvigny, 2007 and O. Did. 397 note).

Fruits that were easy to transport and to keep, such as dates, olives (sometimes pickled or sweetened; cf. Youtie, 1978), grapes (probably often raisins), figs and nuts come on the top of the list, whereas apples, pears or peaches are less likely to appear in the papyri.

Conservation techniques

In a hot climate many foodstuffs, like milk, meat and fish, can only be preserved for a longer period by processing them. In that way they remain available all year round and can be transported over long distances (Curtis, 2008, 372). Thus cheese is a way of preserving milk, wine preserves fruit juice thanks to fermentation, fruit can be dried, as is the case with raisins, plums, figs and dates (see, for example, Cappers, 2006, 148–151). Pulse (e.g. beans and peas) and nuts dry more or less naturally, dried (ξηρός) figs and dates can be more easily stocked and transported (Schnebel, 1925, 299). Dried fruit and nuts were often presented as desserts after dinner. Even vegetables could be preserved, like the λαψάναι συνθέται (prepared, i.e., pickled vegetables) put on the table by Pachomius on Easter Sunday, together with cheese, olives and some fresh vegetables (λεπτολάχανα) (Hist. Laus. 23, discussed by Draguet, 1945, 54–65).

Meat and fish could be eaten fresh, for instance at a festival with a sacrifice, but as soon as they were transported they had to be pickled (fish cannot be kept fresh for more than two days in the climate of Egypt). The same method was used for salting fish and for meat, layers of fish/meat alternating with layers of salt. The popular piquant fish sauce was a mixture of salt and small fish or fish innards, which ripened in the sun for a couple of months, until the top layer was a liquid (*garum*) and the bottom layer consisted of undissolved fish matter (Curtis, 2008, 386). In one instance the bottom layer of a jar is said to be superior to the top (P. Oxy. 33 2680. 22–25). *Garum* could be imported from the Mediterranean (sea fish), but also made locally with small Nile fish, as is the case of two jars found in Oxyrhynchus (Van Neer et al., 2015). *Garum* is a Latin loan-word and it is surprising that there are examples before the second century AD. It is not clear if consumption patterns for salted fish in Egypt changed under Roman influence as they did in northwest Europe (Broekaert, 2016). P. Herm. 23 distinguishes white and black, PUG 5 209 between first and second quality *garum*; red *garum* (αἱματίτης), the very best quality, is mentioned in SB 14 11340 (Drexhage, 1993).

Dried fruits of different kinds were called τραγήματα and often transported in baskets (cf. P. Sijpesteijn 59b.10 note). They included, for instance, nuts and dried figs (P. Oxy. 3 529; 42 3065) and were eaten as dessert and appetizers.

Sweeteners and spices

Among the papyri only a single cookery book has been preserved (Froschauer and Römer, 2006, 102). The following recipe, similar to those in Apicius, gives a good idea of the extensive use of flavors, which can otherwise only be seen in lists of spices with unknown purpose.

> Pickled meat or pieces of ham. The meat is raw but the pickled meat they cook first just to wash the salt off. Then put all in a frying-pan, 4 parts of wine, 2 parts of sweet wine, 1 part of vinegar. Roast dry coriander, thyme, anise and fennel, all together from the start. Add this and cook. When it is half-cooked, add honey and grounded cumin (others also add pepper). Then they throw the sauce in a hot vessel and add morsels of marrow (?) and hot bread.

The diversity of spices and flavorings is also shown in a declaration of prices by the condiment sellers guild of Oxyrhynchus, listing sesame, black cumin, dried coriander, oregano, mustard, and safflower (P. Oxy. 54 3761). Wines could also be spiced or sweetened in many different ways (Maravela-Solbakk, 2009; Dzierzbicka, 2018, 209–226).

Salt is a basic product that was added to most foods and was essential for preserving meat and fish (see above). When Pachomius wants to show his disciples how to live with the barest minimum of food, "he put some salt on his hand and he ate his bread with this" (Lefort, 1933, 5; 1943, 4).

Pepper comes to the fore in the Roman period thanks to the trade with India. In the texts it is not found before the third century AD, except for ostraca of the desert road in Didyme and Quseir. Black pepper is common from the first century AD onwards, in Myos Hormos and in Berenike, where one storage jar contained 7.55 kg (Cappers, 2006, 111–119; Sidebotham, 2011, 224–227, see also Peacock et al., 2011, 228; Van der Veen, 2011, 4–46).

Honey was the main sweetener in the classical world, with dates as a cheaper equivalent for the poor (sugar cane is not found before the Arab period). It was used in all kinds of dishes (as in the recipe above) and it was the main component in all kinds of sweet cakes; for example, πλακοῦντες (flat-cakes), ἴτρια (with sesame grains), πόπανα (offering cakes) or μελικηρίδες/μελιτώματα (honey cakes). Even olives could be sweetened as γλυκελαία (see P. Vindob. Worp 11.4 note). Sweet beer is mentioned once (O. Claud. 4 867). Water (ὑδρόμελι) or wine (οἰνόμελι, Latin *mulsum*) mixed with honey were popular drinks, also used in medicine (Chouliara-Raïos, 1989, 136–153).

Children did have a special menu, with milk of course and sweetmeats (τράγηματα, τραγημάτια; e.g. in P. Graux 2 1012), cakes, white bread and sweets (P. Oxy. 4 736.26, 48–49, 81–83). In P. Lond. 3 899.6–7 a dozen eggs are sent "for the little girl" (τῇ μικρᾷ). Another little girl received 12 salted fish (τάριχοι) and 22 sesame cakes (κοπταί), but they should be given to her one by one (δίδι αὐτῇ ἀνὰ ἓν P. Col. 8 215, 30–31). The child Paulina has offered ten grapes in a basket as a present for the writer in P. Mil. Vogl. 2 61.23–25. Five hundred nuts (κύαμοι) and 50 apples are sent for the children in P. Oxy. 2 298.40–44. No doubt the beans (ἀράκια) that the boy Theon received from his father and which he contemptuously rejects in his famous letter (P. Oxy. 1 119) were also some kind of snacks.

Luxury foods

Qualitative distinctions among different foods and drink often occur in the papyri (Reekmans, 1996, 20–42 offers a full survey for the Zenon archive; see also PUG 5 209 ii.1 note for the terms πρωτεῖος and δευτερεῖος, indicating first and second quality), and they are also taken into account in Diocletian's Price Edict. Thus white bread is preferred to brown bread (see above), fragrant wine to sour wine (e.g., P.L. Bat. 20 30), succulent meat to tough meat (cf. Alypios' complaint in P. Flor. 2 127.12–14 that the piglet should be καλὸν πάλιν (of good quality this time) and μὴ ὡς πρώην λεπτὸν καὶ ἄχρηστον (not miserable and unusable like last time), olive oil to radish oil, and within olive oils different categories may be distinguished (Wittenburg, 1980; Mayerson, 2002). There is no clear dividing line between excellent quality and luxury.

All cultures have prestige foods. These are usually protein, frequently of animal origin. Luxury foods offer a refinement or qualitative improvement over a basic food and a means of social distinction because they are not widely available. Such luxuries are reserved for the upper class, such as visiting officials (BGU 6 1495), or for special occasions, from small-scale family celebrations to large-scale feasts (Perpillou-Thomas, 1992, 203–209; Dunbabin, 2003). The status of luxury foods may disappear when the product becomes more widely available, thus pepper became a staple commodity in the Roman period. Often luxuries are imported from abroad, e.g. wines from Greece or Italy (Reekmans, 1996, 40–42; SB 12 10918). It is often impossible to distinguish imported products from types named after a foreign country (cf. our "Brussels sprouts"), but the import of wines is well attested by the stamped amphorae from Rhodos, Knidos and elsewhere.

In one case mullet is brought from the Red Sea overnight, probably, as suggested by the editor of the ostracon, for the table of the prefect, who was in Koptos at the time (O.Krok. 1, introd. 12–13). Another rare item are ostrich eggs, once mentioned in an early Christian private letter (SB 8 9746.21), and once as a gift at the royal court in a Zenon papyrus (P. Mich. Zen. 9.2). A kind of bird, called λευκομέτωπος "with white forehead", perhaps a coot, was considered a table delicacy in the Ptolemaic period (see, for example, P. Lond. 7 1998), but disappears from the menu later.

Meat being in itself a sign of the good life, luxury could be found in quantity and diversity; for example, half a porcelet, two chickens and two pigeons for dinner (P. Brem. 56 app.), or two chickens, two pigeons and a suckling pig for an absentee guest (SB 1 4630). In a list of cooked meat products, made up by a gymnasiarch, no doubt for a feast, peacock meat occurs alongside different parts of pork (SB 28 16881).

Notes

1　For a recent survey of work in this field, see Touzeau et al., 2014.
2　The "breads" found in Karanis, which figure, for example, in the handbook of Ellis, 1992, p.30 pl. 16, are in fact cakes of residue from an olive oil press (information by T. Wilfong).

19

THE IMPACT OF CHRISTIANITY

Emmanuelle Raga[1]

Why would Christianity have had an impact on the diet and nutrition of the people of the Ancient world? Food and diet were explicitly excluded from religious preoccupations in the Christian founding texts and were not supposed to be a matter of importance for the new religion, even though it was, of course, a debated issue.[2] Christians were invited neither to follow nor to replace the Jewish alimentary rules and to remember that it is not what is eaten that is pure or impure but rather the individuals themselves. However, in the process of the definition of what it meant to be Christian (and, more importantly, to become Christian), the question of the adequate diet was one of the aspects of everyday life that became a central part in the development of the new Christian ethos. Then, in a latter phase, the spread of asceticism[3] as the increasingly dominant interpretation of the best version of Christian life from the fourth century onwards had a radical impact on what was perceived as a good diet and good food.

The various early Christian discourses on food had actually more to do with the classical Greco-Roman discourse on food, health and morality than with anything related to early Christian theology. In both the classical Roman and the early Christian normative discourses, the necessity is for dietary guidelines on the three main usages of food: physiological, social and moral. Concretely, Roman literature provides dietetic guidelines 1) to maintain and restore health; 2) to master the rules of offering and sharing food (the banquet is the most fundamental social tool in Roman society, where social connexion and social status are created and expressed); and 3) to relate to food according to high moral standards. The Christian discourse about food can be divided into roughly the same three categories: 1) dietetic guidelines to maintain health, in accordance with specific Christian goals (as the control of sensual passions); 2) guidelines relative to the sharing and offerings of food; and 3) guidelines to relate to food in a way that pleases God (food and fasting were a central tool of mortification).

Christianity would thus naturally challenge and alter the ancient way of consuming food, for at least two reasons: first, because of its will to provide a new normative discourse on moral, social and physiological hygiene in contrast with the ancient way of life that would mark the act of conversion – even more so when it comes to a conversion to the ascetic life; second, because the developing of a specifically Christian discourse on food is part of a wider more theological discourse regarding the relationship between body and soul, which derives from a particular understanding of health, sickness and medical treatment.

Consequently, the question of how and how much Christianity has impacted on the perception of diet and nutrition, and thus potentially on the diet and food practices of the people of late antiquity, can be approached through the study of the shifts in the normative discourse about food in late antiquity.

It must, however, be kept in mind that when it comes to studying the influence of Christianity on the people of late antiquity, the written evidence available is over-representative of the ascetic trend. Ascetic Christianity, established as the most desirable form of Christian life after the fourth-century religious existential crisis (Markus, 1990; Leyser, 2000), must not be mistaken as an accurate representation of the way of life of the majority. Also, what people conceived as a healthy and morally or religiously adequate diet and the way in which they nourished themselves are two different things. Great energy and interest were mobilised in the search for the perfect diet, many predicators provided a plethora of dietetic advice, and it can be repeatedly seen that the act of conversion to a Christian life or to a better Christian life was always accompanied by a change in diet. However, to what extent the new diets were applied, for how long, and to what extent they did develop into a new permanent normative environment can be difficult to grasp. This is why besides looking at the normative discourse on food produced by Christian preachers we will also be looking at its reception. Through material written in different literary environments (aristocratic, ascetic, monastic, medical), we can see how the Christian normative discourse about food has been received and adapted by the public it was aimed at.

We will start by looking into the main features of the Roman classical normative discourse about food as it appears from the sources of western late antiquity. We will then focus on the construction of a specifically Christian set of norms surrounding food in late antiquity, its reception by the various forms of "Christianities", and the issues and tensions that were caused, particularly regarding sociability and the dilemma between active and contemplative life. Finally, we will address the specific case of meat in the early western coenobitic discourse as it illustrates how the influence of a new Christian discourse might have impacted on the dietetic and medical discourse itself.

Food for pleasure, food for health in Roman society

It must be remembered that food in the Roman world had two very distinctive uses and was subject to two separate sets of norms. On the one hand, food was consumed to restore the body and followed the recommendations of the physicians. On the other hand, food was shared to create or maintain social bonds and in this case it followed the rules of sociability and status distinction (see Scheid, 2005; Garnsey, 1999; Schmitt-Pantel, 1992; Tchernia, 2008). Nutrition could happen whenever and wherever the individual needed to eat, while commensality happened almost exclusively during the occasion of the very ritualised banquet (Dupont, 1999).

Food at the banquet was not consumed to nourish the bodies of the participants but to express and strengthen the social connections among them and to expose social distinctions and power. It did not abide by dietetic norms but was concerned more with taste, sophistication, pleasure, and beauty. The Roman banquet was in fact seen as a space of relaxed enjoyment of pleasures, through the food, through the comfort of the benches and of the fluid garments, and through the enjoyable lightness of the conversations (Cabouret, 2008; Romeri, 2002; Gowers, 1993).

Food at the banquet followed the recipes of the cooks (with Apicius and his book of recipes as the most legendary),[4] while food outside the banquet followed the recipes of the physicians. The former did not take health into consideration, and their recipes were actually regularly considered harmful to the bodies of the participants.[5] The later only marginally took taste and pleasure into account (but did not exclude them as we will see later on) to the point that a healthy diet was often associated with insipidity or even bad taste.[6]

The dichotomy between the social, pleasurable and lavish consumption at the banquet and the solitary, pragmatic and healthy consumption at any other time was one of the central structures of the Roman aristocratic life (Dupont, 1996; 1999) and was associated with the alternation between excessive banqueting developing into sickness and solitary dieting leading to the restoration of health. When Sidonius Apollinaris, a Gallo-Roman aristocrat of the fifth century (c. 430–c. 485 AD), is about to visit a friend after a weeklong debauchery at the country house of another friend, he writes: "I only hope that the completion of a week's interval will see the prompt restoration of that feeling of hunger for which I yearn: when the stomach is upset by a debauch, nothing repairs it so well as abstemiousness."[7]

It is in part this organisation of everyday (aristocratic at least) life balancing between austerity and excess, between practical and pleasurable, between necessary and superfluous, which will in itself be condemned by early Christian preachers. It is in fact partially through the promotion of an always austere and monotonous consumption that the Christian normative discourse will challenge a fundamental aspect of the ancient way of life.

Food and the Christian life

Although there is no dogmatic discourse on food in early Christianity – as food is not supposed to be a matter of dogma – food is central to the definition of a new Christian way of life. The question of what it meant to become Christian and how much of everyday life was to be transformed through conversion occupied a great portion of the Christian debate in the late Roman World (Markus, 1990). In this debate, food and diet became a central tool of religious expression, and the act of conversion to Christianity or to a higher form of Christianity was apparently systematically accompanied by a change of diet.

Early Christian authors such as Clement of Alexandria (c. 150–c. 215 AD) or Tertullian (c. 155–c. 240 AD) saw the importance of providing new norms surrounding food consumption to guide the new Christians in their everyday life. For both, the approach to food had more to do with the classical discourses on the "good life" than with anything specifically linked to the words of Christ, and for both, the dominant ideas are that food should be simple and limited to responding to physiological needs, while avoiding inducing pleasure (Leyerle, 1995; Grimm, 1996).

There was, however, no articulate consensus about what it meant to eat in a more Christian way. The various normative needs of the diverse "Christianities" (ascetic men and women, monastic men and women, high clergy figures, aristocratic men and women, kings and queens, etc.) have led to a profusion of discourse about food and diet in the Late Ancient written sources, which were inspired by the various contemporary ascetic discourses (Stoic, Cynic, Judaic, etc., see Finn, 2009; Elm, 1994). The result is an agglomeration of specifically Christian norms regarding nutrition and its relationship with pleasure, health, sin, sociability and contemplation. In general, a search for greater austerity, insipidity and scarcity have characterised the change in diet (Grimm, 1996; Shaw, 1998; McGowan, 1999; Effros, 2002). But the articulation and intensity of these three notions was relative to the cultural environment and to the type of Christian life one decided to embrace.

In addition, a particularity of the Christian discourse about food derives from a specific understanding of the relationship between body and soul. Contrary to the most diffused classical perception of a relationship between the soul as a benevolent master and the body as a thankful slave, Christianity has adopted a more martial and contentious perception of the relationship (Cooper, 2007; Baschet, 2000; Brown, 1988). From this perspective, the soul must use food as a tool in its fight against the constant threats and attacks from the body. Fasting to the point of underfeeding the body, depriving it from feeling replenished and never enabling it to relax in sensual pleasure and torpor is one of the most common strategies used by ascetics. And in fact, the written sources being over-representative of the ascetic trend, the Christian diet most documented consists of a food intake so limited it kept the ascetic at the brink of being underfed, and living on foods that were selected for their coarse or bad taste. On a pragmatic point of view, the avoidance of pleasure is often justified by a belief central to many ascetic traditions sustaining that sensual pleasure is the open door to all physiological and spiritual sins (Grimm, 1996; Brown, 1988). In particular, the pleasure drawn from the consumption of food, inevitable since it is necessary to survival, is often considered as a dangerous doorway to all the other vices. [8] But in addition to the pragmatic reading of the physiological consequences of pleasure, the sensation of pleasure itself is perceived as inappropriate to a life of compunction. Augustine himself interpreted the act of fasting as above all fasting from the food one loves.[9] Beyond the dietetic effect attributed to the experience of pleasure, it is the fact itself of drawing pleasure from food that should be avoided.

Establishing the Christian diet

Unsurprisingly, there is no consensus on the ideal Christian diet when it comes to the specifics. First of all, any food in excessive quantity was perceived as the real danger, rather than certain foods in particular.[10] A particular diffidence towards meat and wine can be found in the writings of many preachers, for various and not always clear reasons (for more details, see Raga, 2016; Scheid, 2007; Grottanelli, 1996; Corbier, 1989a). For one thing, meat and wine were two items traditionally consumed for the pleasure they provided, as well as the two central and indispensable commodities of the banquet. Also, meat was considered as a "heavy" food in the medical tradition, thus a food difficult to digest and that tended to burden the body if the consumer did not happen to be in very good shape. Actually, only athletes could and should consume meat in large quantities. Meat was thus considered as not only unhealthy but also unnecessary to someone choosing a rather static contemplative life. Finally, meat and wine were traditionally considered as not suitable to a life of contemplation in most normative discourses around the ancient world (see for example Goody, 1982, 113–117). Renouncing the consumption of meat and wine thus made sense on various levels when choosing to lead an ascetic life. However, Christian preachers were very conscious of the dangers of excessive stigmatisation to the point of declaring meat impure, which would be a sin (see for example Grimm, 1996). Even though the only exception Paul made about food was to suggest Christians should avoid eating sacrificial meat as much as possible, he did add that if a Christian happened to eat sacrificial meat to honour the rules of sociability with a pagan or simply because he was unaware of the fact the meat had been sacrificed, it would not matter to God.[11] Meat could thus be consumed and was consumed by most Christians but it was the first food to be removed from the diet of those aspiring to a "better" life.

The choice of what food to eat was more debated and was in fact determined by the diverse cultural conceptions of what made a diet adequate to a Christian life, and by the food locally available. Roots, herbs, and chickpeas were often associated with the perfect diet of the

Egyptian desert ascetics.[12] Figs and dates are found as emblematic of the eremitic diet in Jerome's writings. [13] Ashes were a classic of ascetic literature,[14] as well as millet[15] or barley, which could be considered as worse than fasting by Constance of Lyon when writing about the ascetic diet of Germain of Auxerre.[16]

Beyond the ideal diet suggested by the ascetic predicators, individuals choosing to lead a (more) Christian life made a variety of choices. For example, Sidonius Apollinaris, at that time still a young layman, describes an old aristocratic acquaintance who was now living a more rigorous Christian life:

> When I arrived he came himself to meet me, but the man who (as I had known him) had been erect in stature, brisk in step, bluff in voice, and beaming in countenance, now carried himself in anything but his old style: his dress, his step, his modest air, his colour and his talk, all had a religious suggestion; moreover, his hair was short, his beard long, three-legged stools served as seats, his door-ways had hangings of haircloth, his couch was devoid of down, his table of purple, and even his hospitality, though kindly, was frugal, with a greater abundance of vegetable than of meat—at least, if there was ever anything more dainty on the menu, he was making a concession to the guests, not to himself.[17]

In the eyes of these late Roman aristocrats, adopting a serious Christian life implied to adapt physical appearance, domestic comfort, and diet. In this case, the choice was to favour vegetables over meat and avoid rich and delicious preparations, even in the context of the hospitality of a social and aristocratic life.[18] The idea that vegetables were the perfect frugal counterpart of meat is a classical dichotomy often found in the Roman sources.[19] It is thus unsurprising that this aristocrat chose to limit meat and favour vegetables. This idea is, however, not as common in the contemporary ascetic discourse inspired by the Egyptian tradition and represented in the West by authors like Jerome (c. 347–420 AD) or Cassian (c. 360–c. 435 AD; see Goodrich, 2007). In this cultural environment, vegetables can be considered unsuitable to a proper ascetic diet while cereals are preferred:

> nor have we seen that anyone who has rejected this rule and given up the use of bread and taken to a diet of beans (*leguminum*) or vegetables (*holerum*) or fruits (*pomorum*), has been reckoned among the most esteemed, or even acquired the grace of knowledge and discretion.[20]

In sum, the specifics of the Christian diet varied according to the different geographical and cultural contexts where various actors were searching to incarnate the new religious perfection while experimenting with different diets.

Sociability in Christianity

Theoretically, the dominant understanding of a Christian life leaves no space for the consumption of delicious, sophisticated, and excessive food. All food consumption should ideally be limited to the intake strictly necessary to restore the body. In other words, it leaves no space for the classical banquet itself. Christians aspiring to perfection thus need solutions not only on what to eat to adequately nourish the body while not experiencing pleasure and achieving or maintaining control over bodily desires, but also on how to share food in the context of hospitality or communal life now that the traditional banquet is to be excluded. Both points are closely interrelated, as it is impossible to organise one's diet without taking into account the social duties. Sociability, in both classical Roman and Christian culture, is inseparable from the act of offering and sharing food. However, this fundamental rule materialises a profound dilemma in Christianity, which is the balancing, articulating and hierarchising of active and contemplative life. The old Greek debate is particularly problematic for the new religion[21] and is at the basis of the Christian difficulty in reconciling social and individual food practices: is either fasting or sharing a meal the most Christian thing to do?

In addition, the greater importance given to individuality and personal mortification in Christianity is accompanied by a greater focus on the uses of food for personal religiosity. The space now dedicated to personal aspirations was unthinkable under the weight of the absolute loyalty to family and network that characterised Ancient society (see Cooper, 2007). The ensuing conflict between individual ambitions and social responsibilities – or in other words, between fasting and sharing a meal – is one of the determinant features of the transition to a Christian social space in the late Roman world.

It is for that matter often in relation to the dilemma caused when individual mortification clashes with social responsibilities and hospitality that the written sources give us a more pragmatic kind of evidence on the dietary choices made by various individuals. In fact, the issue provides us with testimonies of the difficulties generated by the effective application of the radical and ideal diet promoted by various authors. Concretely, beyond the ideal model, these sources evoke the strategies put in place to be able to receive fellow Christians and exercise proper hospitality while still embracing a demanding Christian life.

Sidonius Apollinaris gives again a very valuable testimony on this subject. As a Christian aristocrat (who is to become bishop at the end of his career), he practiced intensive and excessive banqueting as we know from his correspondence (see also Raga, 2009; Shanzer, 2001). It is, however, also clear that he regularly encountered models of asceticism inside his own network. Sidonius is actually often seen confronted, like Ausonius of Bordeaux before him,[22] with the disruptive impact of asceticism on his aristocratic network. His encounter with this new social phenomenon of Christian asceticism leads him to promote his idea of how one should cope with the situation. In a series of letters across his correspondence, he praises the ones who keep on cultivating their social connections through attending the dinner parties of friends despite having chosen a clerical or a religious life. For example, of his friend Patiens, bishop of Lyon, he praises "the tact with which you combine the hospitable and the ascetic virtues, so that the king is never tired of praising your breakfasts and the queen your fasts".[23]

Patiens is admired for mastering the equilibrium between private piety (incarnated by the femininity of the queen), and public splendour represented by the male figure of the king (on asceticism and gender see Cooper, 2009; Wilkinson, 2015; Elm, 1994).

Elsewhere, Sidonius talks of a young priest, son of a friend, of whom he says:

> Fasts are a joy to him, yet he does not abjure the social board; the way of the cross keeps him faithful to the first, love of his kind inclines him sometimes to the last. In either case he uses the utmost moderation; when he dines, he mortifies his appetite; when he fasts, it is without vainglory.[24]

Another of Sidonius' acquaintances having chosen to become more religious is said to have continued to partake in a central aristocratic activity, the hunting party, but when attending the subsequent hunting banquet, he discreetly avoided consuming the meat: "Though he abstains from eating game, he indulges in the chase; to have the sport without the spoil accords with the secret delicacy of his religious feeling."[25]

The idea for these Christian aristocrats was thus, in a very classical tradition, to build individual ways of living the new faith while respecting the responsibilities of aristocratic life. The delicate combination between private mortification and social pleasurable relaxation is one of the strategies promoted to preserve the social ties and the classical networking structures. Such a promotion points at the fact that the appeal of asceticism would have had a negative impact on the way of life of these Christian aristocrats, in part because of the non-attendance at the social gatherings indispensable to the cohesion of the network. Banqueting was indispensable to the sociability of the elite (and bishops were part of the elite, as urban governors) and even figures of ascetic aristocrats such as Martin of Tours, the model of many future ascetic aristocrats, or Honoratus, the very ascetic bishop of Arles, are shown sharing banquets with local *potentes*.[26] The necessity to continue participating in aristocratic sociability is what leads Epiphanius, bishop of Pavia, to adapt his daily routine and to fast in the evening rather than during the day so that he can still receive his possible guests in midday banquets (in general, fasting in early Christianity consisted in having no food at all until the end of the day when the ascetic would break his fast with a light meal).[27]

Beyond the figure of the aristocratic Christian, the social dilemma posed by the social and contemplative aspirations of Christian life also concerned the monastic communities, as well as the proper ascetics and hermits. No one apparently could evade social responsibilities and it is obvious from the hagiographical sources that hermits and monastic communities received plenty of visits in their "desert", either proper or figurative. The question of how hermits and coenobitic communities should deal with the impromptu visit of guests is frequently addressed in early ascetic and monastic literature. The advice is, in the majority of the cases, for the monks and ascetics to break their fast and break the monotony of their diet to attend to the guests. In other words, the responsibilities of active life should overrule the rules of contemplative life, when confronted. As Julianus Pomerius puts it quite clearly in his *De Vita Contemplativa*: "It is often beneficial to place hospitality to visitors before fasting or abstinence."[28] And indeed, a passage from the Rule of the Four Fathers from the monastery of Lérins attests how receiving travelling monks implied theoretically the breaking of the fast for the whole community.[29] Elsewhere, a passage in the *Regula magistri* on the problems posed by the "gyrovagues", the fake wandering ascetics accused of taking advantage of monastic hospitality, suggests that monasteries were expected not only to offer and share food but to kill barnyard animals and serve them to the visitors: "They oblige their successive hosts, who rejoice at the arrival of a guest, to prepare choice dishes for them and to put the axe to poultry because of their coming – this, every day by different hosts."[30]

What this also suggests is that the serving of meat is associated with the expectation of visitors to be served "choice dishes", thus confirming that meat was still the obvious choice when looking to mark an occasion with a better tasting and more sophisticated meal, while in theory, the monks of the *Regula magistri* would have avoided the consumption of meat although it is not explicitly stated in this particular rule (see Raga, 2016).

Hermits were also regularly confronted with the rules of hospitality. The works by Cassian or the *Verba seniorum* on the desert fathers are full of stories of hermits adapting their routine to adequately receive visitors.[31] And the responsibility to conform to the rules of sociability also falls to the visitor himself.[32]

Also interesting in these sources regarding hermits and monastic communities is the fact that the issue of sociability versus private mortification also concerned the non-elite. Apparently any free (male) individual had the social responsibility of establishing and maintaining social connections and they were to do so by offering and sharing food.

Dietetics, medicine and Christianity

In some aspects, the essence of the ascetic Christian dietetic discourse can appear similar to the classical medical discourse. In accordance with it, the ascetic Christian diet will favour what looks like a classical regime for the sick, an austere diet made of insipid broths (liquids are considered easier to digest[33]), consumed in small quantities and made of "light" ingredients, avoiding anything rich, heavy or delicious, and in particular meat.[34] However, the motivations are obviously profoundly different.

First of all, while ancient physicians favour the liquid broths of plain foods because they believe they are easy to digest and can thus bring strength to the organism of the sick without loading the body with nutriments it would be too weak to process, the Christian authors who advise such light and simple broths do so for their belief that they will bring above all very little pleasure. For key figures as Clement of Alexandria, Tertullian, and later on Jerome and Cassian, a Christian diet is of course to be composed of food chosen for nutritive and pragmatic reasons like cost, availability, and efficiency in restoring the body but it is much more important that the foods should never respond to desire or pleasure. We have seen for instance in Sidonius' passage about the converted aristocrat that the change in diet aimed above all at reducing the sources of pleasure ("if there was ever anything more dainty on the menu, he was making a concession to the guests, not to himself"[35]). Also, the first thing that was important to Epiphanius of Pavia when he became bishop as regards to his diet was for his meals to be as bland and unsophisticated as possible.[36] As for Germain of Auxerre, he is said to have nourished himself with barley bread because the experience was even worse than fasting.[37] Cassian also tells of this ascetic tradition consisting of adding just one little drop of oil to the daily insipid broth of the ascetic so as not to be enough to actually make it taste better but still depriving the consumer of the pride of having eaten a perfectly ascetic meal.[38] The focus is thus not only on how to avoid pleasure because of the physiological consequences of the feeling, but also to seize every occasion to make a sacrifice – a preoccupation completely absent from the writing of classical physicians.

Second, even though the recipes of the physicians had to aim at health first and were generally less tasty, the classical medical discourse could associate good taste with health. For instance, if adding herbs, salt, and a bit of oil to the broth could make the dish taste better, it would also be easier to digest and thus more efficient in restoring the health of the sick. As Galen says:

> For we physicians aim at benefits from foods, not at pleasure. But since the unpleasantness of some foods contributes largely to poor concoction, in this regard it is better that they are moderately tasty.[39]

> For among things that are equally healthy, the more pleasant is better for concoction.[40]

Also, among similar foodstuffs, the tastier the healthier.[41] In sum, the question of pleasure in the classical diet did not submit to the dichotomy dividing food for sharing and food for nourishment. Pleasure was indeed absolutely indispensable at the banquet but it was not excluded from the healthy, physician-approved diet. Neither was it excluded from the preparations served to the sick. The most pleasant recipe between two equally healthy dishes was to be preferred as it was "better for concoction", more easily digested, and thus healthier.

In any case, contrary to the traditional medical discourse, the Christian normative discourse on food is much more radical in its stigmatisation of pleasure. There was theoretically no space at all for any form of sensual pleasure in the perfect Christian diet and this radicalism had an obvious and inevitable impact on the general approach to food, diet, and nutrition, but also on sociability and its articulation with everyday life, for the people of the new Christian Europe.

For one thing, the intolerance for pleasure would have had an effective impact on the perception of what constituted a healthy nutrition as it might have triggered conceptual shifts in the dietetic and medical discourses themselves. The case of meat is noteworthy for that matter, as we will now see.

Christian shifts of the dietetic discourse: the case of meat in early western monasticism

Meat was considered in the classical dietetic discourse as a heavy, strong, very nourishing food but, for that reason, it was only adequate for stomachs strong and healthy enough to digest it.[42] Meat was at the basis of the recommended diet of athletes but was to be consumed with care by everybody else.[43] If a man leading a normal life ate as much meat as an athlete, he would undoubtedly become sick.[44] Consequently, meat was radically excluded from the diet of the sick and weak. Meat was also the central and most indispensable element of the classical banquet and was considered a delicious and pleasurable food. For all these reasons combined, meat was naturally excluded from the ascetic diet.

However, an interesting development occurred with meat in the western coenobitic discourse: meat came to be excluded from the monastic diet *except* in the case of sickness. The following passages from the monastic rules of Caesarius of Arles, of Benedict of Nursia (the most influential early monastic rule by a long way) and of Leander of Seville, all written at the end of the sixth century, attest to this association between sickness and authorising meat:

> Caesarius of Arles, *Rule for the Virgins*, 71: Fowl will only be authorised for the sick. At the communal meal it will never be served. As of meat, no one will ever consume it. If a sick sister is in a desperate state, she will receive some if the abbess accepts and by herself.[45]

> Benedict of Nursia, *Rule*, 36: Sick monks will be permitted to have some meat for their recovery. But when they'll be better they will avoid it as everyone else.[46]

> Benedict of Nursia, *Rule*, 39: As for the meat of quadrupeds, all will avoid it, except the very weak sick.[47]

> Leandre of Seville, *Rule*, 15: I dare not authorise or forbid meat to you due to your weakness/illness (*infirmitas*).[48]

The idea of reintroducing meat in the monastic diet in case of illness goes against all logic from the point of view of classical medicine, since meat was precisely perceived as extremely heavy and thus advisable only to those with strong stomachs. It was certainly too heavy to be processed by a sick or dying individual and would only have made him weaker.

In addition, meat was the most strongly stigmatised foodstuff, the one to be most radically avoided for an aspirant ascetic and the first food to be retracted from a regular diet when choosing to live to higher religious standards. So if the issue was undernourishment and weakness, why not add more vegetables, cereals, fruit, and cheese to help restore health? Why reintroduce precisely meat, a food that was not traditionally considered restorative and was the least proper food for an ascetic diet?

Light can be shed on this contradiction if we take into consideration the following passages from John Cassian's and Augustine's works:

> John Cassian, *Instituta*, V, 7: Bodily weakness is no hindrance to purity of heart, if only so much food is taken as the bodily weakness requires, and not what pleasure asks for. [. . .] For bodily weakness has its glory of self-restraint, where though food is permitted to the failing body, a man deprives himself of his refreshment, although he needs it, and only indulges in just so much food as the strict judgment of temperance decides to be sufficient for the necessities of life, and not what the longing appetite asks for. The more delicate foods (*esculentiores cibi*), as they conduce to bodily health, so they need not destroy the purity of chastity, if they are taken in moderation. For whatever strength is gained by partaking of them is used up in the toil and waste of care. Wherefore as no state of life can be deprived of the virtue of abstinence, so to none is the crown of perfection denied.[49]

> Augustine, *Praeceptum* III, 5: Let the sick whose weak condition during illness obliges them to take less food be treated when their sickness is past in the way that will enable them most quickly to regain their strength even if they were formerly in the very lowest state of poverty; for then their recent illness gives them the same claim to lenient treatment as the habit of their former life gives to those who once were rich. But when their strength is restored let them return to that happier rule of abstinence which the servants of God ought to observe with greater strictness as their needs grow less; for they must not continue for mere pleasure (*voluptas*) what was begun for the requirements of health.[50]

What appears from these passages is an association made between a diet for the sick and pleasure. Cassian speaks of *esculentiores cibi*, more delicate foods, and Augustine of *voluptas*, pleasure, drawn from the exceptional diet granted to the sick. Augustine also makes a comparison between the treatment of the sick and the treatment of the monks from "delicate origin", meaning those coming from a higher class. This comment refers to Augustine's belief that monks should all be exposed to the same intensity of mortification, but that there should be differentiated treatment according to the relative comfort of previous life. In fact, Augustine believes that it is much easier for a monk from modest origin to adapt to the austerity of coenobitic life than it is for an aristocrat. Consequently, monks of "delicate origin" must be allowed more comfort in food and bed then their more modest brothers.[51] Thus, when Augustine associates the diet of the sick with the diet of the monks of delicate origin, it suggests that what determines the exceptionality of the diet of the sick is to be more delicate and more pleasurable.

Consequently, what these passages suggest is that the reintroduction of meat in the diet of the sick monk would not have been justified because it was the most nourishing or repairing food but because it was the most delicious. It is because meat provided pleasure but also because it was typical of the pleasurable life of the elite in contrast with which coenobitic life was built, that it made sense for these authors to reintroduce meat – and only meat – in the diet of the sick or dying monk. It is all about reintroducing pleasure in the diet, and meat was the most sought after food for pleasure.

The case of meat suggests thus that by revolving around the issue of pleasure, the late ancient ascetic discourse would have influenced the medical and dietetic logic produced in the coenobitic environment, twisting its own reasoning to now revolve around the experience of pleasure and the avoidance of it.

Concluding remarks

Two main conclusions can be drawn from this study. Firstly, a change in diet being part of the basics of conversion to Christianity or to a "higher" form of Christian life (meaning an ascetic one), the impact of Christianity on the food practices of the people of late antiquity was direct and deliberate. Written sources give explicit demonstration of the fact that food practices were now a central tool of religious expression and a central element used as a marker for conversion and religious "upgrading". Consequently, Christian preachers produced abundant discourses on food and diet, and flooded Late Ancient society with new norms articulating food, nutrition, sin and health.

Second, the ascetic obsession with pleasure appears to be the paradigm on which the ascetic Christian discourse on diet, nutrition, and health is built. This particular focus would have produced a specifically Christian dietetic discourse taking health and illness into consideration through the lenses of the absence and presence of pleasure, at least in the coenobitic sources. But more importantly, if the full impact of the ascetic Christian discourse was, of course, most relevant to the individuals aspiring to asceticism, while the greater part of society continued to engage in the shared consumption of delicious and abundant food as a social tool, it remains that the dominant discourse sustained that perfection was asceticism, and that living the monastic or eremitic life was the most direct (or even the only) path to salvation. The strong and growing voice of the ascetic way of life in late antiquity replaced as the dominant normative context a system for which the simplicity and austerity of everyday nutrition alternated with the legitimate delicious and delicate excesses of the banquets, by a system in which monotony and constant austerity are the ideal, and for which pleasure is systematically problematic and frowned upon. But then also, in an odd twist, potentially therapeutic.

Notes

1 Many thanks to Andrew Donnelly for the many stimulating discussions we had on this topic and for his assistance with this chapter.

2 Paul, *Rm* 14.17, *non est regnum Dei esca et potus*, "the reign of God is not about food and drink". See McGowan, 1999.

3 For what is meant by asceticism, I refer to the definition suggested by Ville Vuolanto: "a physically and mentally disciplined life, based on practices (or 'exercises', *askesis*) to contribute to the contemplative life, control of the passions, abstinence from physical comforts and pleasures, and the renunciation of worldly power and wealth." Vuolanto, 2005, 119, see also Vuolanto, 2015.

4 Apicius is a legendary cook who would have lived in the first century AD and to whom a fourth-century collection of recipes was attributed, the *De re coquinaria*.

5 Galen, *On the property of Foodstuffs*, II.51 "For we physicians aim at benefits from foods, not at pleasure. But since the unpleasantness of some foods contributes largely to poor concoction, in this regard it is better that they are moderately tasty. But for cooks, tastiness for the most part makes use of harmful seasoning, so that poor rather than good concoction accompanies them." Tr. Powell, 2002, 105.

6 See for example Plutarch, *De Tuenda Sanitate*, 3. "The second, I think, concerned the food which you people serve to the sick. For he urged that we should partake of it and taste it from time to time, and get ourselves used to it in time of health, and not abhor and detest such a regimen, like little children, but gradually make it familiar and congenial to our appetites, so that in sickness we may not be disaffected over our fare as if it were so much medicine, and may not show impatience at receiving something simple, unappetising, and savourless." Tr. Babbitt, Loeb 222, 1928, 220–221.

7 Sidonius Apollinaris, *Ep.* II.9, *modo nos quam primum hebdomadis exactae spatia completa votivae restituant esuritioni, quia disruptum ganea stomachum nulla sarcire res melius quam parsimonia solet.* Tr. Anderson, Loeb 296, 460–461.

8 Tertullian, *De ieiunio* 17; Cassian, *Inst.* V.6, among many others.

9 "I do not ask from what food you abstain but what food you choose. Tell what food you prefer so that I may approve your abstaining from that food," Augustine, *De utilitate jejunii*, v.

10 Cassian, *Instituta*, V.6, "For not only is drunkenness with wine wont to intoxicate the mind, but excess of all kinds of food makes it weak and uncertain, and robs it of all its power of pure and clear contemplation. The cause of the overthrow and wantonness of Sodom was not drunkenness through wine, but fulness of bread." *Non sola crapula uini mentem inebriare consueuit: cunctarum escarum nimietas uacillantem eam ac nutabundam reddit omnique integritatis ac puritatis contemplatione despoliat. Sodomitis cause subuersionis atque luxuriae non uini crapula, sed saturitas extitit panis.* Leander of Seville, *Regula* XV. *Fomenta vitiorum, esus carnium: nec solum carnium, sed et nimia satietas aliorum ciborum. Quoniam non culpatur escae qualitas, sed quantitas reputatur in vitio,* (*PL* 72, Caput XV. *De indulgentia et prohibitione carnium* (col 889)).

11 Paul, *Rm*, 14.1–23

12 Chickpeas are a classical staple for ascetics, see *Verba Seniorum, interprete Pelagio*, VIII.22; Cassian, *Conferences* VIII, Sulpicius Severus, *Vita Martini*

13 Jerome, *Vita Pauli*; *Vita Hilarii 3.1.*

14 Caesarius of Arles, Sermon 65; Constance of Lyon, *Vita Germani*, I.3.

15 Paulinus, *Letter* 23.

16 Constance of Lyon, *Vita Germani*, I.3.

17 Sidonius, *Ep.* IV.24.3, *ut veni, occurrit mihi ipse, quem noveram anterius corpore erectum gressu expeditum, voce liberum facie liberalem, multum ab antiquo dissimilis incessu. habitus viro, gradus pudor, color sermo religiosus, tum coma brevis barba prolixa, tripodes sellae, Cilicum vela foribus appensa, lectus nil habens plumae, mensa nil purpurae, humanitas ipsa sic benigna quod frugi, nec ita carnibus abundans ut leguminibus; certe, si quod in cibis unctius, non sibi sed hospitibus indulgens.* Tr. Anderson, Loeb 420, 158–161.

18 Sidonius was actually visiting the man in question to request a year delay in debt reimbursement for two brothers who had lost their father and had difficulties repaying the loan the family owed to the now very religious aristocrat.

19 See for example Juvenal, *Saturae*, XI, v.78 opposing the highly virtuous Curius and his taste for vegetables to the debauchery of slaves dreaming of a dish of sow's womb, a famous Roman delicacy. See also the *Historia Augusta*, X. Life of Septimus Severus, XIX.8, another model of virtue preferring vegetables to meat, among many others.

20 Cassian, *Instituta*, V.23.2, *nec eorum quempiam, qui hanc regulam declinantes praetermisso panis usu leguminum uel holerum seu pomorum refectionem sectati sunt, inter probatissimos habitum aliquando conspeximus, sed ne discretionis quidem aut scientiae gratiam consecutum.* See also Cassian, *Conf.*, II,19, "For in discussing the abstinence of some who supported their lives continually on nothing but beans (*leguminibus*) or only on vegetables (*holeribus*) and fruits (*pomis*), they proposed to all of them to partake of bread alone, the right measure of which they fixed at two biscuits, so small that they assuredly scarcely weighed a pound", *nam discutientes continentias diuersorum, qui uel solis leguminibus uel holeribus tantum uel pomis uitam iugiter exigebant, praeposuere cunctis illis refectionem solius panis, cuius aequissimum modum in duobus paxamatiis statuerunt, quos paruulos panes uix librae unius pondus habere certissimum est.* According to Aline Rousselle, in the desert ascetic tradition, there was a concern not only about frugality but also about moisture and taste. To some of them, vegetables are tasty and humid while cereals are better because dry and insipid (Rousselle, 1974).

21 Despite being addressed in the Gospels, it was not satisfactorily resolved, see Luke 10.38.

22 Ausonius, *Ep.* 20, 21, 22, to Paulinus of Nola, fellow aristocrat, friend and former student, who chose to sell all of his properties with his wife and to move to Spain to build a monastery and live as an ascetic, to the great sadness and incomprehension of Ausonius.

23 Sidonius, *Ep.* VI.12.3–4, *Omitto illa, quae cotidie propter defectionem ciuium pauperatorum inrequietis tolerasexcubiis precibus expensis. Omitto te tali semper agere temperamento, sic semper humanum, sic abstemium iudicar, ut constet indesinenter regem praesentem prandia tua, reginam laudare ieiunia*

24 Sidonius, *Ep.* VII.13.3, *Ieiuniis delectatur, edulibus adquiescit; illis adhaeret propter consuetudinem crucis, istis flectitur propter gratiam caritatis: summo utrumque moderamine quia comprimit, quotiens prandere statuit, gulam, quotiens abstinere, iactantiam.*

25 Sidonius, *Ep.* IV.9.3. *ferarum carnibus abstinet, cursibus adquiescit ; itaque occulte delicateque religiosus uenatu utitur nec utitur uenatione.* Tr. Dalton 1915.

26 Martin of Tours was invited to the table of the emperor Maximus as told by Sulpicius Severus in *Vita Martini* 20; Honoratus and his brother Venantius were said to be irreproachable in their asceticism as well as in their hospitality, to the point that the aristocrats and bishops invited at their table were inspired and humbled by their perfection, Hilarius of Arles, *Vita Honorati*, 9.3.

27 Ennodius of Pavia, *Vita of Epiphanius* 48, *deinde decreuerat numquam esse* *** *prandendum:* *** *sed ne propositi sententiam superuenientum uis ulla temeraret et aut iactantiae nebulis aut auaritiae fama laederetur, definiuit numquam sibi cenandum, ut commutatio horarum ac per hoc semel in die reficiendi tempus adferret.*

28 Julianus Pomerius, *De vita contemplativa* II.24. *Quam utile sit, jejunio vel abstinentiae, advenientium caritatem plerumque praeferre* (PL 59, Col.0470B; *Regula Magistri,* 72).

29 *Rule of the Four Fathers,* 2.36, *Qualiter peregrini hospites suscipiantur. Venientibus eis nullus nisi unus cui cura fuerit iniuncta occurrat ut responsum det uenienti. Non licebit ei orare nex pacem offerre, nisi primo uideatur ab eo qui praeest, et oratione simul peracta sequatur ordinem suum pacis officium. Nec licebit alicui cum superueniente sermocinari nisi soli qui praeest et quos ipse uoluerit. Venientibus uero ad refectionem, non licebit peregrino fratri cum fratribus manducare, nisi cum eo qui praeest, ut possit aedificari.*

30 *Reg. Mag.,* I.13–18, *et pro gaudio superuenientis exquisita sibi pulmentaria adparari et animantia pullorum sibi creant cottidie a diuersis hospitibus pro aduentu nouitatis sub inporuna caritate diuersos conant sibi praeparare diuersa.*

31 See, for example, Cassian, *Conferences,* I. Conference with Abba Moses; or *Verba seniorum,* XIII,1, *Quando ergo est praesentia fratrum, cum gaudio debemus suscipere eos; quando uero soli sumus, opus habemus lugere* (PL 73, c. 943). When confronted with the laws of sociability, strategies suggested to cope with the necessary transgression of one's private diet could then be, for example, to keep part of the daily food on the side in case someone showed up (Cassian, *Conf.* II.26.) or to fast more intensely afterwards in order to repay for the broken rule (Cassian, *Inst.*, V.26.).

32 A passage in the *Verba seniorum* tells the tale of a monk so ascetic he even abstained from bread. When he came to see a desert father, he found himself in the company of other visitors. The father served a modest soup to the joyous company but the young ascetic declined to share the food and started chewing one single boiled chickpea he carried in his pocket. After the meal, the father took the young ascetic aside and explained that when he was in company, it was inappropriate to make a demonstration of his way of life and that if he wanted to keep his asceticism, he should just stay in his cell and never have any company. *Verba Seniorum, interprete Pelagio,* VIII.22, *Erat quidam abstinens a cibis, et non manducans panem; uenit ad quemdam senem. Opportune autem illic etiam alii superuenerant peregrini, et fecit senex modicum pulmentum propter eos. Et cum sedissent manducare, frater ille abstinens posuit sibi soli cicer infusum, et manducabat. Et cum surrexissent a mensa, tulit eum senex secreto, et dixit ei: Frater, si uenis ad aliquem, non ostendas illi conuersationem tuam; si autem conuersationem tuam tenere uis, sede in cella tua, et nusquem exeas. Ille autem acquiescens uerbis senis, factus est communis uitae in id quod cum fratribus inuenisset.*

33 Galen, *De alim. fac.,* I.23; Oribasius *Coll. med.,* II.65; Anthimus, *De obs. cib.,* 75, 76.

34 See for example Gal., *De alim. fac.,* III.29; Oribasius, *Coll. Med.,* II.68.5; IV.11.

35 Sidonius, *Ep.* IV.24.3,

36 Ennodius of Pavia, *Vita Epiphanii,* 48, "He chose to like the most cheap foodstuffs and that nothing in the preparations could offend his sense of smell or taste, except what was seasoned with herbs", *Cibos iussit sibi placere uiliores nihilque in apparatione ferculorum nares saporemque suum posse offendere, nisi quod aromatibus condiretur.*

37 Constance of Lyon, *Vita Germani,* I.3.

38 Cassian, *Conferences,* VIII.1.1.

39 Galen, *On the property of Foodstuffs,* II.51.

40 Galen, *On the Properties of Foodstuffs,* II.27.

41 See Oribasius I.48 about apricots which are tastier than peaches and thus healthier.

42 See for example Oribasius, *Coll. Med.,* IV.11.

43 See for example Galen, *De alim. fac.* I.2.

44 Oribasius, *Coll. Med.,* IV.11.

45 Caesarius of Arles, *Reg. ad. Virg.,* 71, *Pulli uero infirmis tantum praebeantur: nam in congregatione numquam ministrentur. Carnes uero a nulla umquam penitus in cibo sumantur; si forte aliqua in desperata infirmitate fuerit, iubente et prouidente abbatissa accipiat.*

46 *Reg. Ben.,* 36, *Sed et carnium esus infirmis omnimo debilibus pro reparatione concedatur; at ubi meliorati fuerint, a carnibus more solito omnes abstineant.*

47 *Reg. Ben.,* 39, *Carnium vero quadrupedum omnimodo ab omnibus abstineatur comestio, praeter omnino debiles aegrotos.*

48 Leandre of Seville, *Regula, Caput XV. De indulgentia et prohibitione carnium. Esum carnium infirmitatis tuae obtentu nec prohibere tibi audeo nec permittere. Cui tamen suppetit virtus, a carnibus se abstineat.*

49 Cassian, *Instituta,* V.7 *How bodily weakness need not interfere with purity of heart. Habet etiam corporis inbecillitas suae continentiae palmam, dummodo escis defectioni carnis indultis adhuc indigentem se refectione*

241

defraudet tantumque esus indulgeat, quantum sufficere ad uiuendi usum temperantiae discretio rigida iudicarit, non quantum desiderii adpetitus exposcit. Esculentiores cibi ut procurant corpori sanitatem, ita castitatis non adimunt puritatem, si cum moderatione sumantur. Quidquid enim fortitudinis esu eorum percipitur, aegritudinis labore ac defectione consumitur.

50 Augustine, *Praeceptum* III.5, *Sane, quemadmodum aegrotantes necesse habent minus accipere ne graventur, ita et post aegritudinem sic tractandi sunt, ut citius recreentur, etiam si de humillima saeculi paupertate venerunt; tamquam hoc illis contulerit recentior aegritudo, quod diuitibus anterior consuetudo. (. . .) Nec ibi eos teneat voluptas iam vegetos, quo necessitas levarat infirmos.*

51 Augustine, *Praeceptum* III.3–4, *Qui infirmi sunt ex pristina consuetudine, si aliter tractantur in uictu, non debet aliis molestum esse nec iniustum uideri, quos facit alia consuetudo fortiores. nec illos feliciores putent, quia sumunt quod non sumunt ipsi, sed sibi potius gratulentur, quia ualent quod non ualent illi.*

PART IV

A forum on energy, malnutrition and stature

20

USING SKELETAL REMAINS AS A PROXY FOR ROMAN LIFESTYLES

The potential and problems with osteological reconstructions of health, diet, and stature in imperial Rome

Kristina Killgrove

Introduction

Analysis of human skeletal remains is becoming increasingly common in classical bioarchaeology, particularly because of the way historians and demographers have begun to pair osteological and biochemical data with evidence from archaeology, epigraphy, and historical records. The field of bioarchaeology has been practised since the 1970s in both the US and the UK, so some geographical and temporal areas have been well studied and methods have been honed in order to answer questions as fully as possible. This is not the case in classical bioarchaeology, where the application of skeletal analysis to answer questions about the Greco-Roman world is much more recent. Skeletons and cemeteries are largely being studied piecemeal owing to vagaries in collections, funding, and personnel available for these sorts of analyses.

While the US and UK benefit from published standards for data collection, making many data comparable across time and space, data collection is more haphazard in the Mediterranean. Some researchers use the US *Standards for Data Collection from Human Skeletal Remains* (Buikstra and Ubelaker, 1994), some researchers use the UK *Guidelines to the Standards for Recording Human Remains* (Brickley and McKinley, 2004), and others use methods drawn from one or more additional sources (e.g., Moore-Jansen et al., 1994, Steckel et al., 2005; see also individual countries in Márquez-Grant and Fibiger, 2011). The lack of standardization in data collection leads to problems in undertaking synthetic treatments of classical bioarchaeological data. This in turn means a difficulty in being able to marshal evidence to answer larger questions about complicated topics such as imperialism, migration, and health. No true synthetic treatments of classical bioarchaeological data yet exist, although several recent edited volumes have begun to bring together osteological, biochemical, and contextual data for the Greek (e.g., Schepartz et al., 2009) and the Roman world (e.g., Eckardt, 2010, Piccioli et al., 2015).

For the reconstruction of ancient lives, both individual and collective, this means that we often cannot be sure that data drawn from one cemetery are able to be extrapolated to larger questions about bigger populations. This is not exactly earthshattering news, as researchers have grappled with lacunae in the written and archaeological records for centuries. Skeletal data, however, have different strengths and drawbacks than historical records and archaeological remains, and care needs to be taken in attempting to synthesize these disparate lines of data (Perry, 2007), particularly since history and archaeology represent the elite segment of the Roman population far more than do skeletal remains.[1]

Skeletons do not usually tell us what people died from; rather, they frequently tell us about the diseases and conditions people lived with (Wood et al., 1992; Wright and Yoder, 2003). In reconstructing Roman health, we need to keep in mind that the relationship among biology, culture, and the environment is complex. No single metric will sufficiently express the range of health outcomes for the culturally and socioeconomically diverse populace of imperial Rome, but multivariable and wide-ranging synthetic research has the potential to add considerably to our knowledge of life in the ancient world.

This contribution therefore attempts to look at what we do and do not know about health in imperial Rome from the bioarchaeological data. The lack of standardization in data collection and lack of publication of data are the biggest barriers to this, however, precluding all but surface-deep analysis. To the extent possible in this small space, I synthesize osteological information from cemeteries in the *suburbium* in order to look at disease, diet, and stature, all of which have been used as proxies for Roman health and, by extension, economic wellbeing (e.g., Scheidel, 2012a).

Osteological proxies for Roman health

Three primary lines of evidence inform our basic understanding of Roman health from an osteological standpoint: palaeopathology, or the investigation of patterns of disease; biochemistry, which uses carbon and nitrogen isotopes to approximate overall diet; and postcranial morphology, which employs length of long bones to understand secular changes in stature (Steckel, 1995; Ortner, 2003; Katzenberg and Saunders, 2011; Martin et al., 2014; Larsen, 2015). Individually, each approach involves different data collection and different methodologies.

Pathological data, for example, are often recorded as either present or absent, although some may be further coded with respect to the part of the body that is affected (Ortner, 2003; Buikstra and Ubelaker, 1994). These data include evidence of infectious, metabolic, and degenerative diseases, as well as traumatic injuries. Generic measures of health are usually drawn from evidence of metabolic diseases like anaemia, in which frequencies of porotic hyperostosis and, sometimes, the severity of those lesions are recorded. Childhood stress is recoverable through evidence of dental enamel hypoplasias; their presence is often recorded, but their location on the tooth much less often.

Dental enamel caries and sometimes wear are used in conjunction with biochemical analyses to uncover the ancient diet (Larsen, 2015). Carious lesion presence, severity, and location are all generally recorded in order to facilitate population-based analysis (Buikstra and Ubelaker, 1994). Dental wear is much more rarely collected systematically and is usually consigned to qualitative reports on specific skeletons. Analyses of stable carbon and nitrogen isotopes are gaining in popularity, as they more directly reflect an individual's diet, and as a wider range of statistics can be done in order to investigate these data.

Postcranial morphology, or measurements of long bones, is primarily used to reconstruct stature (Steckel and Rose, 2002). While the raw data of long bone length are highly comparable across time and space (Steckel, 1995), almost no researchers have reported these data for imperial Rome. Rather, calculated stature based on published regression equations is typically listed in reports and articles, making it impossible to directly compare the information across populations, particularly when the stature equation used is not provided or when only average stature is reported.

These sets of information that help create our proxies of health include both discrete and continuous data, which involve different statistics, reporting standards, and interpretive potential. In the remainder of this section, I summarize the published, verifiable information from the osteology of imperial Rome, with the aim of demonstrating what we know and where we need to go with this research.

Palaeopathology and health

As I note more fully in a different publication (Killgrove, 2017), among imperial Roman skeletons, the most commonly recorded pathological conditions are porotic hyperostosis and dental enamel hypoplasia. Porotic hyperostosis, which appears as holes in the eye orbits (*cribra orbitalia*) or cranial vault (*cribra cranii*), is a non-specific indicator of health, as it results from chronic anaemia (Goodman and Martin, 2002) that can be caused by diet, genetic conditions, and/or parasites. Dental enamel hypoplasias are lines or pits that form when enamel production is disrupted during childhood because of a prolonged episode of stress, such as weaning or illness, so it is also seen as a general, non-specific health indicator (Goodman and Rose, 1990; H. King, 2005). Owing to the interest in malaria in imperial Rome over the past several decades (e.g., Angel, 1966; Sallares, 2002), porotic hyperostosis in particular has been of palaeo-pathological interest.

Of the cemeteries excavated within the *suburbium* of Rome (here defined as roughly a 12 km radius from the walls, or about the extent of the contemporary Grande Raccordo Anulare), three have been relatively well published in terms of pathological data: a large sample from Basiliano/Collatina (Buccellato et al., 2003; 2008), Vallerano (Cucina et al., 2006; Ricci et al., 1997), and Osteria del Curato II (Catalano, 2001; Catalano and Di Bernardini, 2001; Egidi et al., 2003) (see Table 20.1). Together, they total 239 individuals. To this can be added my work at Casal Bertone and Castellaccio Europarco (Killgrove, 2010a), for an additional 186 imperial-era skeletons from Rome. Inferences into Roman health are therefore being made primarily on the basis of 425 skeletons, although the number of skeletons that have been excavated but have not been studied or fully published is much larger.[2]

A few recent attempts at synthesis of pathology data have been made by historians (Pilkington, 2013; Scheidel, 2013) and bioarchaeologists (Gowland and Garnsey, 2010; Minozzi et al., 2013; Piccioli et al., 2015), with the result being a suggestion that diseases such as malaria were problematic in imperial Rome but also with an admission that more data are needed to better understand the complexity of the question of Roman health.

Metabolic disease and childhood stress

In an article specifically addressing porotic hyperostosis and dental enamel hypoplasia (Killgrove, 2017) in imperial Rome, I found that the two sites that I investigated, Casal Bertone and Castellaccio Europarco, were statistically similar to one another in terms of frequencies of these conditions. These frequencies, however, are lower than those of Basiliano/Collatina, Osteria del Curato II, Vallerano, and the rural Lucus Feroniae (Salvadei et al., 2001; Sperduti, 1997; Manzi et al., 1999), and yet comparable to the reported frequencies at Gabii, Quadraro, and

San Vittorino (Ottini et al., 2001; Catalano et al., 2001c). More importantly, the frequencies of porotic hyperostosis vary widely throughout the *suburbium* and into the more rural areas of Latium (see Table 20.1). Similarly, frequencies of dental enamel hypoplasia were significantly lower at the two sites I studied than at any other site.[3]

Various reasons can be put forward to explain the differences in frequencies of these metabolic and stress-related issues. One is that inter-observer differences or variation in recording practices biased the data collection. Another is that factors such as nutrition, water sources, or disease ecology affected the health of people living in and near Rome differently. To further investigate these factors, I looked at where people came from and at potential comorbid conditions (Killgrove, 2017). In correlating oxygen isotopes with porotic hyperostosis, it seems that the people who came to Rome from warmer, drier areas were more likely to have anaemia. There may therefore be a relationship between parasitic infection or malaria and migration. I also noted a correlation between people with porotic hyperostosis and with high levels of lead in their dental enamel. As heavy metal poisoning can result in anaemia, this association points to a potential cause or to comorbid conditions.

As the question of malaria specifically and health generally continues to be of interest to many classical scholars (Sallares, 2002), there is hope in the form of a new biochemical test that can reveal malaria in ancient skeletal remains. Although the test, developed by Yale University scientist Jamie Inwood, was just reported in March of 2015, it has purportedly been tested on sixth century AD remains excavated by David Soren at Lugnano (Shelton, 2015). A test for the polymer hemozoin, which the malaria parasite produces, provides a much clearer way of

Table 20.1 Individuals affected and crude/true prevalence rates (CPR/TPR) for porotic hyperostosis and dental enamel hypoplasia among comparative imperial Roman populations

	km from Rome	Cribra Orbitalia		Cribra Cranii		Dental Enamel Hypoplasia	
		CPR	(n/N)	CPR	(n/N)	TPR	(n/N)
Casal Bertone	2	15.9%	(10/63)	1.2%	(1/83)	2.2%	(52/1962)
Basiliano/ Collatina[1]	4	*ca.* 65%	—	50%	—	42.0%	—
Quadraro[2]	4	8%	—	—	—	—	—
Osteria del Curato II[3]	11	79.2%	—	53.6%	—	—	—
Castellaccio Europarco	12	13.6%	(3/22)	15.6%	(5/32)	2.5%	(14/563)
Vallerano[4]	12	69.2%	(18/26)	26.8%	—	63.5%	(502/790)
Isola Sacra[6]	25	—	—	—	—	35.5%	(281/791)
Lucus Feroniae[5]	30	49.5%	(46/93)	10.7%	(14/131)	—	—
San Vittorino[2]	30	0%	—	—	—	—	—

[1] Buccellato et al. (2003); [2] Ottini et al. (2001); [3] Egidi et al. (2003); [4] Ricci et al. (1997); Cucina et al. (2006); [5] Salvadei et al. (2001); [6] Manzi et al. (1999). This table reflects data from Tables 3 and 5 in Killgrove 2017.

investigating malaria in an ancient population than does the presence of porotic hyperostosis, whose etiology is less specific.

In addition to better understanding malaria, biochemical DNA testing of skeletons could reveal inherited anaemias that may have been present in the Roman population, with the most common in the Mediterranean being thalassemia and G6PD (Crandall and Martin, 2012; Oxenham and Cavill, 2010). To add to our understanding of childhood stress, researchers may also want to look at Harris lines, or lines of growth arrest of long bones (e.g., Mays, 1995). This evidence can be coupled with studies that track vitamin D and vitamin C deficiencies (e.g., Brickley and Ives, 2008), to provide a more well-rounded picture of children's health in imperial Rome.

Reconstructing health in imperial Rome from osteological data

The data briefly presented above illustrate the drawbacks in using osteological data to reconstruct the health of the population of imperial Rome and, in particular, the problems with using just one proxy measure of health to do so. While the pathological conditions with the most data points, porotic hyperostosis and dental enamel hypoplasia, reveal the presence of anaemia and childhood stress in imperial Rome, the distribution of these data among cemeteries and age and sex cohorts is variable, and statistical analysis does not reveal any particular patterns. There is additionally no systematically collected, comparative data for trauma or for infectious or degenerative diseases in imperial Rome (but see Killgrove, 2015, for data, and Killgrove, 2010a, for interpretations). Given the data that can be compared, there is wide variation in frequencies of pathological conditions in Rome, which is not surprising given the diversity of the population.

Biochemistry and diet

The ancient Roman diet came from a variety of sources, mainly foodstuffs containing protein and carbohydrates (Garnsey, 1999; Prowse, 2001; Alcock, 2006; Cool, 2006). Stable isotope analyses of carbon and nitrogen have been used for decades to characterize human diets in the past because they provide a way to generalize the types and amounts of proteins and plant matter in an individual's diet (Krueger and Sullivan, 1984; Katzenberg, 2008; Kellner and Schoeninger, 2007; Schoeninger et al., 1983). Measuring carbon and nitrogen isotopes within the skeletal population of imperial Rome can therefore provide general information about subsistence practices, which may differ based on inclusion in different sex and age cohorts, based on status and occupation, or based on the location in which people were living (Beer, 2010; Garnsey, 1999; Purcell, 2003; Wilkins and Hill, 2006).

At the time of writing, the most recent biochemical study of the diet of individuals from imperial Rome was published in 2013 by me and Robert Tykot. Using samples I took from first–third century AD Casal Bertone and Castellaccio Europarco, Tykot analysed their carbon and nitrogen isotope values. We found using this technique that the individuals we sampled were all eating a diet based largely on plants such as wheat and barley, terrestrial meat such as pork, and some aquatic resources and millet. These findings are, of course, in line with our understanding of the ancient Roman diet, particularly considering that the dole in the late imperial period included both wheat and pork (Garnsey, 1991).

Further, we compared the results from Casal Bertone and Castellaccio Europarco with other data sets from imperial-era Italy (Killgrove and Tykot, 2013, 32–33) (see Figure 20.1). These two Rome-area samples were statistically different from Velia, an imperial necropolis 400 km south of Rome on the Tyrrhenian Sea, in both carbon and nitrogen, meaning differences in consumption of grain and aquatic resources (Craig et al., 2009). The distance between the sites speaks more to differences in ecology, however, than dietary preferences *per se*. The two Rome sites were also compared to St Callixtus (Rutgers et al., 2009), a late imperial burial location in Rome reported to contain early Christian ascetics, and a statistical difference was found in carbon values, possibly related to freshwater fish consumption at St Callixtus. In comparing Casal Bertone and Castellaccio to the Isola Sacra sample from Portus Romae (Prowse, 2001; Prowse et al., 2004; 2005; 2008), differences were again seen in both carbon and nitrogen, with the people from Portus eating more aquatic resources than the inland Romans. While most people in imperial Italy appear to have been eating wheat or barley, the variation in dietary protein sources is more dramatic.[4] Food choices likely varied based on age, sex, geography, socioeconomic status, and religious background, but not all of these are recoverable osteologically.

The question of millet consumption has been raised recently, particularly in regard to Bronze Age sites in Italy (e.g., Tafuri et al., 2009), in which people living in northern Italy were found to have eaten more millet than people in southern Italy. One individual from Castellaccio was shown to have eaten a diet composed of a significant amount of millet, but there is also a more subtle difference between Castellaccio as a whole and Casal Bertone, showing that the people from the site closer to Rome were eating less millet than were the

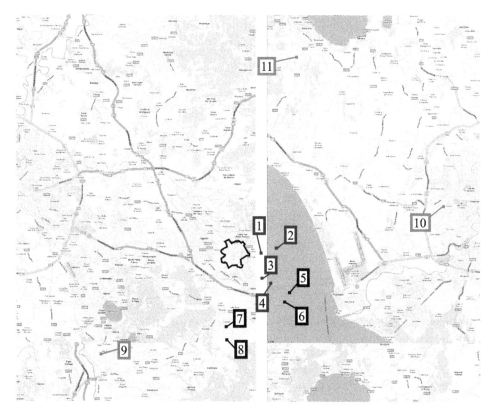

Figure 20.1 Map of imperial skeletal samples from Rome and its *suburbium*.
  Legend: 1 – Casal Bertone; 2 – Basiliano/Serenissima/Collatina; 3 – Quadraro; 4 – Tomba Barberini; 5 – Casal Ferranti; 6 – Osteria del Curato; 7 – Castellaccio Europarco; 8 – Vallerano; 9 – Isola Sacra; 10 – San Vittorino; 11 – Lucus Feroniae.

people living in the suburbs. There may be a relationship between social status and millet consumption, or it may be that people living further from the city simply had greater access to millet while those living near the city and potentially participating in the dole had greater access to wheat.

Dental pathology data can be used in correlation with carbon and nitrogen isotopes as a proxy for the ancient diet. For example, carious lesion and dental calculus frequencies are generally higher in populations engaging in agriculture than in hunter-gatherer groups (Larsen, 2015) because of easier access to sticky carbohydrates that, combined with lack of oral hygiene, give bacteria in the mouth free reign to produce cavities and plaque.

Frequencies of dental pathologies at Casal Bertone and Castellaccio Europarco (Killgrove, 2010a, 121–134 ff.) reveal that both conditions were more plentiful at Castellaccio than at Casal Bertone (see Table 20.2), which could be the result of differences in diet or differences in dental hygiene. The Isola Sacra sample from Portus Romae (Prowse, 2001), on the other hand, has a statistically higher calculus frequency than either Rome-area site. In her dissertation, Prowse (2001, 251–252) looked at correlations between dental disease data and stable isotopic measures of diet. While she found a positive correlation between isotope values and dental wear, suggesting that people who were eating more marine foods had more worn teeth, she did not find much of a correlation between carbohydrate consumption in the form of carbon isotopes and frequency of dental caries.

Future work on Roman diet may do well to correlate biochemical and pathological data to a greater extent than has been done so far. Although there is no evidence from imperial Rome that an over-reliance on a particular food led to dietary anaemia, this potential correlation has not been fully investigated. In research on ancient Native American populations, bio-archaeologists used to look to diet as the primary explanation for porotic hyperostosis frequencies, as consumption of too much maize can lead to a lack of bioavailable iron, contributing to iron-deficiency anaemia (Walker et al., 2009; Waldron, 2009). While dietary anaemia is not the only cause of porotic hyperostosis lesions, it may be worth investigating imperial Roman populations further to see if overconsumption of foods high in phytates, such as wheat bran, can be seen in the biochemical and palaeopathological data (on cereal consumption and phytates, see Heinrich in this volume).

Another largely unexplored topic is fluorine in the Roman water supply. An analysis of fluorine concentrations in dental enamel of skeletons from Herculaneum found much higher than normal values (Torino et al., 1995). Since this skeletal population also has high frequencies of dental enamel hypoplasias and much lower frequencies of carious lesions than expected, Torino and colleagues suspect endemic dental fluorosis. Volcanic activity can lead to high levels of fluorine in the environment (D'Alessandro, 2006), and Rome is situated between two dormant volcanic complexes, so it is not unreasonable to ask whether there is natural fluorine in the groundwater around Rome or in the water that was imported via aqueducts.

Table 20.2 Dental pathology frequencies in four imperial-era populations

	Caries Freq.	Caries TPR	Calculus Freq.	Calculus TPR
Casal Bertone	4.9%	93/1917	35.3%	515/1459
Castellaccio	8.3%	52/625	51.8%	260/502
Vallerano[1]	2.5%	35/1408	—	—
Isola Sacra[2]	5.4%	297/5548	72.9%	4004/5495

[1] Cucina et al. 2006. [2] Prowse 2001.

Clearly, variation existed in the diet of the Roman people and of the people of the Roman Empire writ large, so talking about the singular Roman diet is fraught with complications. Until we can produce more data, particularly taking into consideration the possibility of importation of foreign foodstuffs, the correlation with disease, and environmental and ecological variations, the dietary conclusions we have reached are in general agreement with the historical record but are population- and site-specific.

Postcranial morphology and stature

Because adult stature is influenced by both genetic and environmental factors, calculation of height has been used in osteological investigations around the world to answer questions of status and health (e.g., Steckel, 1995; 2009). If a child is sufficiently well-nourished and does not suffer from disease or a heavy workload, that child is likely to reach his or her genetic potential in terms of adult height. Stature is therefore considered a broad, non-specific indicator of the relationship between humans and their social, economic, and cultural contexts (Larsen, 2002), much like porotic hyperostosis is. Body height is useful in comparisons between populations as well as through time in order to view secular changes brought about by better or worse living conditions (Moore and Ross, 2013).

Stature data have been collected from Italian skeletal samples for at least half a century, but methodological problems with stature reconstruction began to be identified in the 1980s (e.g., Formicola, 1983; 1993). Researchers such as Becker (1999) and Giannecchini and Moggi-Cecchi (2008) have attempted to find the most accurate stature regression equation that can be applied to long bone lengths in order to reconstruct Roman height, and they settled on Trotter and Gleser's (1952; 1977) formulae for African-Americans from the early twentieth century. While some researchers in Italy use these formulae, others prefer the White formulae, and still others use different equations entirely. The choice of equation is not always referenced when stature estimations are presented.

More recent work by Klein Goldewijk and Jacobs (2013), however, questions the very utility of stature reconstruction of past populations. Using a database with long bone measurements from more than 10,000 individuals throughout the Roman Empire, Klein Goldewijk and Jacobs discovered that none of the commonly employed stature reconstruction formulae was internally consistent in the Roman data. 'Within a single population, long bone length varies more than stature does,' they write, which 'suggests that long bone length has gone up more than total body length, and that long bone length is a more sensitive indicator of change in living standards' (2013, 12). Rather than including lengthy discussions about the most appropriate equation to use for reporting reconstructed stature, researchers should instead simply report raw data for long bone lengths. In this way, comparisons across populations can be made more easily and more accurately, and body length can be tested as a proxy for health, diet, and socioeconomic status.

The Roman Empire database that Klein Goldewijk and Jacobs' report references is unfortunately unpublished, and Giannecchini and Moggi-Cecchi (2008) also do not appear to have published raw data from samples around Italy. This lack of publication of data should soon be changing as bioarchaeologists are increasingly being required by government and granting organizations to place their raw data into open-access repositories. (On the way that geography plays into comparisons of stature, see Flohr in this volume.)

The importance of Klein Goldewijk and Jacobs' work, however, cannot be overstated. In discovering inconsistencies in all stature reconstruction formulae, they essentially found that reports that provide only calculated Roman stature are unusable. In terms of imperial Rome, although reconstructed stature data are reported for Basiliano/Collatina (Buccellato et al., 2003), Tomba Barberini and Quadraro (Catalano et al. 2001a; 2001b), Vallerano (Ricci et al., 1997; Catalano et al., 2001a; 2001b; Cucina et al., 2006), Casal Ferranti (Catalano et al., 2001a), and Osteria del Curato (Catalano et al., 2001a; 2001b; Egidi et al., 2003), these data are presented in the aggregate. While it is possible to look at these data broadly and say that both suburban males and females are generally taller than their urban counterparts in imperial Rome (Killgrove, 2010a, 95), statistical analysis of trends is severely limited by the lack of raw data available.

To remedy the unavailability of long bone lengths, my own data from Casal Bertone and Castellaccio Europarco can be found online (Killgrove, 2015), in a relational database linking them to all other osteological and biochemical data I collected from the skeletons at these two imperial-era cemeteries in Rome. Although I could find no raw data from sites in imperial Rome with which to compare them, the data can be investigated statistically in terms of differences between the more urban site (Casal Bertone) and the more suburban site (Castellaccio Europarco), as well as in terms of differences through time between the Republican and imperial phases of Castellaccio.

Case study: long bone lengths from imperial Rome

In 2007, I collected a wealth of osteological data from two skeletal collections housed at the Soprintendenza Archeologica di Roma. The cemetery of Casal Bertone was found during construction activity in 2000 not far from the Aurelian walls of Rome. It is dated to the second to third centuries AD and includes both a simple necropolis and a slightly later mausoleum component (Nanni and Maffei, 2004; Musco et al., 2008). The cemetery of Castellaccio Europarco was also discovered during construction in 2003 about 12 km south of Rome. It has three different temporal components: two Republican-era phases of burial dating to the fourth to third and the second to first centuries BC, and one imperial-era phase dating to the first to second centuries AD (Buccellato, 2007; Buccellato et al., 2008).

In order to facilitate answering complicated questions about migration and urbanism, I performed a typical osteological analysis on each skeleton using *Standards* (Buikstra and Ubelaker, 1994) as a reference, including estimating demographic data; taking measurements; recording dental wear, dental and skeletal pathologies, and nonmetric cranial traits; and taking samples of bone and enamel for biochemical analysis (Killgrove, 2010a). A variety of publications have come out reporting biochemistry data and interpretations (Killgrove, 2010b; 2013; Montgomery et al., 2010; Killgrove and Tykot, 2013; Killgrove and Montgomery, 2016), as well as pathology data (Killgrove, 2017). Neither stature measurement data nor dental wear and pathology data have been published fully, however. Here I present results of a basic statistical analysis of the long bone measurement data.

Comparing stature between urban and suburban cemeteries

Owing to the small sample sizes of a data set that was already restricted to adults and had to be separated by sex, potential differences in populations were assessed using t- and Mann-Whitney U tests (see Tables 20.3 and 20.4). Maximum lengths of individual long bones[5] were compared between males and females from Casal Bertone and males and females from Castellaccio Europarco to investigate whether assumed differences in urban versus suburban lifestyles may have contributed to differences in stature.

Average length of the male long bones is consistently higher in the suburban population from Castellaccio Europarco. These differences, however, do not rise to the level of statistical

Table 20.3 Imperial Roman male long bone lengths

Site	Bone	Avg (mm)	Stdev	N	t-test (two-tailed)			Mann-Whitney U test	
					t	p	se	U	p
CB	Femur	438.41	16.51	17	0.1108	0.91	5.91	125	0.93
CE		439.06	16.89	15					
CB	Humerus	313.22	13.99	18	0.3092	0.76	5.52	118	0.76
CE		314.93	17.25	14					
CB	Radius	232.9	8.21	21	1.1099	0.27	3.90	133	0.28
CE		237.19	15.02	16					
CB	Ulna	253.57	8.12	14	0.7785	0.44	5.35	88	0.47
CE		257.73	18.38	15					
CB	Fibula	348.13	15.85	16	0.1082	0.91	8.08	54	0.89
CE		349.0	22.04	7					
CB	Tibia	365.35	15.82	23	0.1280	0.90	7.05	155.5	0.86
CE		366.25	25.97	12					

Table 20.4 Imperial Roman female long bone lengths

Site	Bone	Avg (mm)	Stdev	N	t-test (two-tailed)			Mann-Whitney U test	
					t	p	se	U	p
CB	Femur	414.5	17.74	6	2.1254	0.06	14.66	30	0.055
CE		383.33	31.23	6					
CB	Humerus	292.6	9.71	10	2.8063	0.01	6.57	50	0.03
CE		274.17	16.83	6					
CB	Radius	210.71	14.33	7	1.0576	0.32	10.13	17.5	0.51
CE		200.0	19.32	4					
CB	Ulna	231.7	16.0	10	1.2762	0.23	11.52	21	0.31
CE		217	23.07	3					
CB	Fibula	326	18.57	4	0.982	0.38	14.26	6	0.36
CE		312	7.7	2					
CB	Tibia	332.89	17.59	9	1.7438	0.11	11.12	33	0.07
CE		313.5	20.74	4					

significance in any of the bones. Suburban living may have been better for imperial-era males, but more data will be needed.

The opposite pattern is seen in the female samples. Average long bone length is consistently higher in the urban population, reaching statistical significance in the length of the femur, humerus, and tibia. Urban living may have been better for imperial-era females, but again, more data will be needed.

Comparing stature through time

Castellaccio Europarco presents three different phases in which burials occurred. The two earlier Republican phases have few burials, so for the purposes of this case study, those data are collapsed into one sample and compared with the imperial data to examine whether long bone length changed through time at this suburban site (see Tables 20.5 and 20.6).

The imperial-era male skeletons from Castellaccio have, overall, longer leg bones than do the earlier Republican-era skeletons. Only the tibia, however, reveals a statistically significant difference, and it is a weak significance. Interestingly, the Republican-era male skeletons have longer average forearm bones, although not significantly so. It is possible that these small samples demonstrate a change in body size from Republican to imperial times owing to better access to nutrition and medicine, but it could just as easily mean a change in activity patterns, particularly since the arms and legs show different size patterns.

There were far fewer female skeletons than male,[6] and not enough data points to compare tibiae or fibulae statistically. Republican-era female long bones are larger than imperial-era ones, although the only statistically significant difference is in the length of the humerus.

The arm bones of both male and female skeletons from the earlier Republican periods of Castellaccio Europarco are larger than the arm bones, particularly the lower arm bones, from the imperial period. This could be a spurious result from small sample size, or it could indicate a change in behaviour or environment between these two temporal periods.

Table 20.5 Male long bone lengths from Castellaccio Europarco

Site	Bone	Avg (mm)	Stdev	N	t-test (two-tailed)			Mann-Whitney U test	
					t	p	se	U	p
Rep	Femur	431.0	21.07	6	0.9233	0.37	8.74	29.5	0.23
Imp		439.07	16.89	15					
Rep	Humerus	312.4	22.57	5	0.2604	0.80	9.71	32	0.78
Imp		314.93	17.25	14					
Rep	Radius	239.75	13.05	4	0.3116	0.76	8.22	36	0.71
Imp		237.19	15.02	16					
Rep	Ulna	259.0	16.64	3	0.1102	0.91	11.49	26	0.68
Imp		257.73	18.38	15					
Rep	Fibula	340.6	14.12	5	0.7447	0.47	11.28	15	0.69
Imp		349.0	22.04	7					
Rep	Tibia	344.5	4.72	6	2.0052	0.06	10.85	21	0.159
Imp		313.5	20.74	4					

Table 20.6 Female long bone lengths from Castellaccio Europarco

Site	Bone	Avg (mm)	Stdev	N	t-test (two-tailed)			Mann-Whitney U test	
					t	p	se	U	p
Rep	Femur	393.0	15.12	4	0.5679	0.59	17.02	15	0.52
Imp		383.33	31.23	6					
Rep	Humerus	312.4	22.57	5	3.223	0.01	11.86	7	0.74
Imp		274.17	16.83	6					
Rep	Radius	207.75	6.4	4	0.7616	0.48	10.18	9	0.77
Imp		200.0	19.32	4					
Rep	Ulna	223.0	9.9	2	0.334	0.76	17.97	4	0.56
Imp		217	23.07	3					

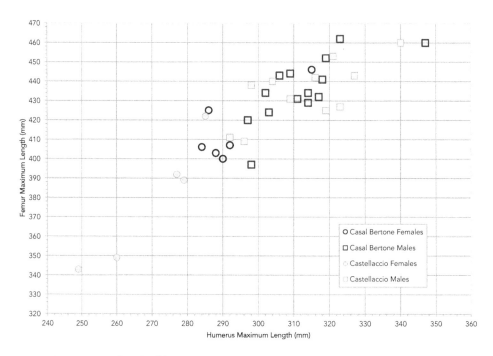

Figure 20.2 Maximum length of femur versus humerus in two imperial-era cemeteries.

Graphing the longest leg bone versus the longest arm bone provides a rough visualization of the trends in body size at imperial-era Casal Bertone and Castellaccio Europarco (see Figure 20.2). Males, of course, have larger bones on average than do females, but it is clear that Casal Bertone females are taller than their equivalent at Castellaccio. One Casal Bertone female, individual F11A, falls within the male range. Pelvic and cranial morphology for this individual were both clearly female. She was buried in the mausoleum component of the site and, as such, may have been of higher status than most women buried in this cemetery.

Stature difficulties

In general, this case study would appear to show that in the imperial period, suburban males were healthier than urban males, and that urban females were healthier than suburban females. But in looking at the Republican versus imperial periods at one site, earlier males and females had larger arm bones while later males had larger leg bones. Very few statistically significant differences were found, however.

Although all individuals examined were measured using standard protocols by one researcher, this data collection was not specifically set up for a study of stature. The resulting small number of individuals whose long bone lengths could be used in this case study likely presents a problem of bias of both the sample and the statistics. This method, however, does represent an advancement over typical data presentation of averages alone and demonstrates that using differences in body size to answer questions about past lifestyles is possible but needs to be undertaken systematically.

Conclusion: Roman bioarchaeology needs a multivariable and interdisciplinary approach to health and lifestyles

Several different metrics can be calculated to investigate the health of the imperial Roman people buried at Casal Bertone and Castellaccio Europarco. The more suburban sample had a statistically higher frequency of the *cribra cranii* form of porotic hyperostosis compared to the more urban sample, but both have much lower frequencies of porotic hyperostosis and dental enamel hypoplasia than other published samples from imperial Rome (Killgrove, 2017). In looking at stable isotopes, the people from Casal Bertone were eating less millet than the sample from Castellaccio Europarco, possibly indicating the latter people were of lower social status (Killgrove and Tykot, 2013), and Castellaccio also has a higher frequency of dental caries (Killgrove, 2010a). Both samples add to a growing data set of palaeodiet results and show that imperial Romans were not eating a single diet. In examining long bone lengths, however, the suburban males have the largest bones while urban females have longer bones than their suburban counterparts. These individual proxies for health are therefore inconsistent, with two suggesting the urban population was healthier and one suggesting the suburban one was. In addition, both populations are quite different in palaeopathology and diet than other published sites.

Clearly, no single metric alone will sufficiently explain Roman health, which means that researchers need to use data with caution but also with an eye towards complementarity. For example, if we agree that stature can be affected by diet, we can test for correlations in long bone length and carbon and nitrogen isotopes as both change through time or across populations (e.g., Arcini et al., 2014). If we agree that porotic hyperostosis can result from malaria but also from a host of other conditions, we can attempt to tease out an etiology using oxygen isotope and lead concentration data (e.g., Killgrove, 2017). If we agree that occupation might be identifiable based on skeletal remains, we can use data collected systematically on musculoskeletal stress markers[7] and osteoarthritis to find patterns of body movement.

Bioarchaeology has enjoyed an increase recently in methods used to extract information from the skeleton. Isotope analyses of C, N, Sr, O, and Pb are already being done, and will likely continue as they decrease in cost and difficulty. The potential of ancient DNA analysis has not been fully felt in Roman bioarchaeology, however, although researchers are certainly breaking ground around the empire. For example, Prowse and colleagues (2010) used DNA to investigate population origins at Vagnari, and Gasbarrini and colleagues (2012) used genetic evidence to back up a diagnosis of celiac disease at Cosa (Scorrano et al., 2014). DNA can reveal information on ancestry, population movement, and even pathologies that people inherited or acquired. Ensuring that this genetic work is done within an appropriate historical and archaeological context is perhaps the biggest challenge Roman bioarchaeologists face in moving forward.

As a field, bioarchaeology has also recently become more informed by social theory, which has allowed us to generate new questions and to examine data in a different way. Most prominently, life course analysis has been adopted as a reminder that what we see in the skeleton is an accumulation of life experiences (Agarwal and Glencross, 2011). Although an individual died at a specific point in time, at a specific age in his or her life, different osteological and biochemical indicators provide windows into different points in that person's life. Teeth in particular form at various times, so analysis of multiple teeth means looking at age ranges in that person's life. This perspective has been used by Tracy Prowse in her work on diet and dental health (Prowse, 2011) as well as immigration at Isola Sacra (Prowse et al., 2007), and I have incorporated sociological discussions of transnationalism into my study of immigrants to

Rome (Killgrove, 2010a; 2010b). Skeletons themselves may be static in the archaeological record, but osteological analysis of them is not. While we cannot recover every activity, illness, or event that happened during a particular person's life course, the fact that we can get glimpses of a lived life means osteological data are quite different than but also informed by historical or archaeological records. The monstrous corpus of the Roman past is challenging to wrangle, but collaborative work between anthropologists, archaeologists, demographers, and historians should produce well-rounded, synthetic treatments of this complex ancient society.

This chapter has outlined some of the issues with the premature use of bioarchaeological data for extrapolation to larger research questions. The practice of bioarchaeology in the classical world has progressed quickly and has produced groundbreaking results, particularly in regard to the lower-class individuals whose lives did not merit inclusion in historical records and who are archaeologically invisible. Combining osteological and biochemical data with archaeological information, historical context, and social theory holds outstanding potential in the Roman Empire. The major barrier to these more complicated studies, however, is in the collection and dissemination of data. If more researchers systematically collect and share their data in a form easily accessible to others, we stand to gain great insights into the population of ancient Rome.

Acknowledgements

Data collection at Casal Bertone and Castellaccio Europarco (2007) was funded by an NSF Doctoral Dissertation Improvement Grant (BCS-0622452). Permission to study the materials from these two sites was granted by Paola Catalano of the Servizio di Antropologia of the Soprintendenza Speciale per i Beni Archeologici di Roma. For inviting me to contribute to this volume, I thank Claire Holleran and Paul Erdkamp, and for helpful comments at various stages of this article, I thank Marshall Becker and Chryssa Bourbou. Any errors, of course, remain my own.

Notes

1 During the imperial period, inhumation and cremation co-existed. While cremation was the preferred rite for many elite Romans, inhumation in simple graves likely represents the remains of the lower classes (Toynbee, 1971). Cremation graves have been excavated in Rome dating to the imperial period, as at Castellaccio Europarco (Buccellato et al., 2007), but there has been no systematic study of these burials. This paper therefore addresses only the skeletal data from inhumations.

2 Some pathology data can be found in the aggregate in other publications (Catalano, 2001; Catalano and Di Bernardini, 2001; Ottini et al., 2001; Catalano et al., 2012), and further from Rome are well-published samples like Isola Sacra (Prowse, 2001; Prowse et al., 2004; 2005; 2007; Manzi et al., 1991), San Vittorino (Ottini et al., 2001; Catalano et al., 2001b, 2001c), and Lucus Feroniae (Salvadei et al., 2001; Sperduti, 1997; Manzi et al., 1999).

3 Killgrove (2010a, 132–135; 2015) reports all the dental enamel hypoplasia data from Casal Bertone and Castellaccio Europarco, in addition to the measurements of those enamel insults. Using regression equations, the location of the enamel insult can be employed to calculate the time at which it occurred. This in turn can provide information on potential systemic issues, such as weaning, that can be further investigated through such lines of evidence as nitrogen isotope analysis.

4 Nitrogen, which represents the dietary protein component, varies much more widely than does carbon across all of ancient Italy (Tykot, 2014).

5 Measurement standards for long bone maximum length from Buikstra and Ubelaker (1994) were used.

6 Potential reasons for the gender bias in these two cemeteries are outlined in Killgrove (2010a, 80, 86).

7 MSM data are not systematically recorded in the osteological literature of imperial Rome. I have been collecting these data at Gabii, although they are as yet unpublished.

21

COMPARATIVE PERSPECTIVES ON NUTRITION AND SOCIAL INEQUALITY IN THE ROMAN WORLD

Geoffrey Kron

Introduction

Until relatively recently, most studies of Greco-Roman diet and nutrition have tended to be largely descriptive and to focus primarily on the rich and sophisticated diet of the wealthy, which is very well attested by a range of literary sources.[1] The diet of the mass of the population has been largely neglected, or has traditionally been assumed to have been very poor and limited, much like the overwhelmingly cereal diet of the eighteenth- and nineteenth-century European working classes.[2] Although brilliant analyses of archaeological material and documentary and papyrological evidence had questioned this pessimistic view of the diet of ordinary Romans,[3] understanding the varying diets and levels of nutrition of different regions of the Roman Empire, and its many social classes demands a much more sophisticated investigation. A proper study needs to rely on comparative evidence from better-documented medieval and early Modern societies, as well as the full range of ancient evidence, most notably a systematic anthropometric study of skeletal remains (a critical issue to which we shall return in greater depth below). Modern historians have made great use of anthropometric evidence in tracing the biological standard of living of the populations past and present, much as Eveleth and Tanner did in a groundbreaking World Health Organization study of poverty and malnutrition throughout the world, relying primarily on human growth and mean final height as an index of the extent of under-nutrition and disease load among contemporary developed and developing societies.[4] A thorough analysis of skeletal material from throughout the Roman Empire, carefully chosen to be representative of both genders, and a range of regions, ages, social classes, and chronological periods would offer invaluable evidence with which to assess mass nutrition. Nevertheless, for some time we will likely have to be circumspect about the sort of conclusions which can be drawn from the osteological studies completed so far, even once Klein-Goldewijk's much anticipated thesis collecting this material is completed and we can better assess what is known, since far too little attention, and very few resources have been devoted to studying skeletal material from the Greco-Roman world by either archaeologists or physical anthropologists.[5]

Of course, even if we had complete anthropometric data, laying out to what extent protein or calorie under-nutrition may have undermined the ability of each class in society to reach their full growth potential and biological standard of living, we would still wish to know the nature of their diet, its cost, economic value, the methods of farming, distribution, processing and cooking employed, and for this we would have to go well beyond simply studying the effect of nutrition and health stresses on the bodies of the population using skeletal data. Roman diet and nutrition is an important aspect of the social and economic history of the population, and demands a thorough understanding of the agrarian economy and social structure of the empire. On the supply side, it requires some understanding of Roman agricultural productivity and innovation, and the impact of cultural preferences, demand, and the trade and distribution system on the products farmers were called upon to produce, and of the impact of land tenure and urbanization on the proportion of the population that the farmers would have had to feed. No less importantly, on the demand side, we would need to understand the distribution and level of income of the Roman population, both rural and urban, and the importance they placed on food in their household budgets. Nutrition would also depend upon social attitudes towards the entitlement of the poor to adequate wages and a healthy diet, and governmental provisions for social welfare and food supply. Moreover, non-nutritional stresses, such as disease, contamination of the water supply, and demographic pressures might also factor in to some extent in reducing the apparent nutrition and biological standard of living of the population. Although I cannot offer a comprehensive discussion here, particularly since our evidence is so lacunose and controversial on so many of these points and needs to be assessed very carefully and imaginatively, I will try to update and contextualize my thinking on Roman nutrition. In responding to a number of objections to previous work, which are of prime importance for our understanding of Roman nutrition, I will highlight some of my own recent research exploring important issues, which are too often ignored in this discussion, most notably agricultural productivity, trade and demand, and income inequality.[6]

Controversies in the anthropometry of Roman nutrition

In a 2005 article on Greco-Roman anthropometry, I offered an estimate of the likely mean height of adult males in Roman Italy of 168.3 cm, based on two separate calculations: 1) a survey of anthropological studies in Italy, recalculated to use either the Trotter and Gleser formula for 'whites' or the Olivier method; and 2) a calculation of mean height, using the Olivier method, based on average long bone lengths from Italian sites dated between 500 BC and AD 500, as compiled by the Italian physical anthropologists Mazzotta and Borgognini Tarli.[7] While my survey was by no means complete, and further studies have likely been accumulated by Klein-Goldewijk, or have been completed since, my tentative estimate has been very strongly corroborated by one of the most thorough recent studies of Roman skeletal material, a large scale investigation by physical anthropologists and archaeologists from Cambridge, the École Française de Rome, and the Servizio di Antrolopogia della Soprintendenza Archeologica di Roma of *necropoleis* throughout Rome and its suburbs, most dating to the early empire, which revealed a mean height of 168.1 cm.[8] Walter Scheidel has maintained, however, that a mean height of 164 cm for males in Roman Italy is preferable,[9] presumably basing his lower estimate on the claims of Gianecchini and Moggi-Cecchi, who have attempted to defend the practice of many Italian physical anthropologists of the 1970s and even 1980s of using the nineteenth-century Pearson and Manouvrier equations for calculating height from long bone lengths.[10] As I alluded in my 2005 article, and reiterated briefly in my 2013 chapter,[11] these very early regression equations were based on relatively small samples of individuals whose growth was stunted by under-nutrition, drawn from European populations whose mean heights were in the low 160 cm range, and have been shown to significantly underestimate the heights of taller populations by 3–4 cm or more.[12]

While these equations may have been tolerably accurate for many nineteenth-century working-class populations, and for the very short individuals in some of the earliest agricultural societies, with largely cereal diets,[13] studies of fully articulated medieval and ancient Roman skeletons, whose heights can be accurately measured *in situ* or calculated by the Fully-Pineau anatomical method,[14] seem to demonstrate that the Pearson and Manouvrier equations underestimate these heights, and that the Trotter and Gleser equations, which were based on a much larger sample providing a much larger range of heights, or other recent regression equation methods, produce much more accurate results for Roman Italy.[15]

Although the sort of detailed study and attention to *in situ* or anatomical measurements undertaken by Becker, both in his dedicated study and subsequent reports, are still too rare, there are a number of reliable height measurements of Greek or Roman skeletal remains that confirm that they were indeed significantly taller than the nineteenth-century working-class populations, which were stunted enough that they might be accurately estimated using the Manouvrier or Pearson methods, as in, to cite just one example, Breitinger's *in situ* measurement of the Spartan soldiers buried in the Kerameikos, which showed heights averaging 170 cm, and revealed individuals as tall as 178 cm, 181 cm and 185 cm.[16] Further confirmation comes from the information on the minimum height requirements for the Roman military, as explained by Vegetius, who gives six Roman feet (177.1 cm) for the cavalry and five Roman feet ten inches (172 cm) for the first cohort of the legions. It is only after the collapse of the Roman Empire, that the Theodosian Code permitted the recruitment of men only five Roman feet seven inches tall (164.5 cm) into the Roman army as an emergency measure.[17] The significance of these figures becomes clear when they are compared with the 149 cm minimum height requirement imposed for Napoleon's army in Italy,[18] or the minimum height requirements for the British military in the nineteenth century, which were consistently 4–5 cm less stringent than those of the Romans, a height gap that is broadly consistent with the height advantage of Roman males over their nineteenth-century English counterparts as revealed by the anthropometric evidence already noted.[19]

Of course, any remaining doubts about the reliability of this contrast between Roman and nineteenth-century European heights can be easily be dispelled by considering the work of Hasbach, Eden, Davies, and many more,[20] who demonstrated in great detail that the vast majority of the rural population in nineteenth-century England were landless labourers, forced to work long hours, six days a week, at wages that were generally barely adequate to cover the cost of sufficient bread, and little more than a pound of bacon a week for a family of four. The wages of the rural labourers of the Italian Mezzogiorno were generally even lower, typically around 830 g of wheat a day and a small jug of olive oil a month, significantly inferior to the base rations granted by the notoriously stingy Cato to his slave workforce.[21]

Scheidel has also questioned the significance of this height evidence by highlighting other potential indicators of nutritional stress among the Romans, such as cribra orbitalia and linear enamel hypoplasia (LEH) or Harris lines,[22] but the value of these conditions as indices of nutrition or mortality is far from clear, certainly inferior to height or body mass index,[23] and objective comparisons of their incidence with nineteenth- or early twentieth-century populations, actually serve to corroborate the anthropometric evidence of a better biological standard of living for the ancients.[24]

Physical anthropologists are making increasing use of additional scientific techniques, which have considerable potential to deepen our understanding of the Roman diet, such as studies of stable isotopes of nitrogen and carbon, which can trace the amount of protein in the diet, as well as some of its sources, whether meat, legumes, fresh-water or marine fish and seafood, as well as distinguishing cereals and certain types of C_4 plants like millet.[25] Although such studies are still relatively few in number, and are not normally designed to test nutritional levels for different social classes, those that have been carried out have shown relatively high trophic levels of nitrogen in a number of Greek and Roman populations, as well as a significant role for marine fish in the diet, certainly significantly higher than we typically find for the nineteenth-century working classes, and even many medieval populations.[26] One of the more interesting recent developments is the application of isotope studies to study animal nutrition and fodder sources, and even manuring and farming practices.[27]

Nutrition, wages and income inequality

The good nutrition of the Romans compared to the nineteenth-century working classes is not only clear from the skeletal remains, it can also be corroborated by a comparison of the distribution of income, and of the wages and living standards of the poor and the middle classes in the two societies. Most economic historians who have analysed Roman GDP,[28] have tended to rely heavily upon conjecture and a number of conventional assumptions about the structure of Roman Society. They have assumed that Rome was a highly inegalitarian agrarian civilization, comparable to western Europe under the *ancien régime* of the long eighteenth century, with at least 90% of the population (surely a vast exaggeration)[29] rural peasants, often assumed to be living, as the landless labourers of England or southern Italy did in the early nineteenth century, at a very low subsistence, with a scanty cereal diet. Those who have examined this traditional reconstruction of Roman GDP, most notably Lo Cascio and Malanima,[30] have noted a series of significant problems and internal contradictions in the model, without, however, abandoning it entirely. Scheidel and Friesen have argued pointedly that it is unlikely that there is no meaningful middle income group in Roman society. They point out that even our scanty direct evidence makes it clear that extremely high incomes were achieved by the equestrian and senatorial elite, incomes that are in fact very difficult to reconcile with the core assumptions about the poverty of the mass of the population,[31] or, for that matter, with the considerable wealth of the decurions and wealthy freedmen of the towns. Yet their own model, while slightly more realistic, remains essentially hypothetical, and is very pessimistic, unrealistically so in my view, of the size of the Roman middle classes.

I have recently argued in favour of using actual archaeological data, modelling income distribution in Roman society, as has been done successfully in other pre-industrial societies, using evidence for the likely rental values of housing or the distribution of housing space.[32] Although I have concentrated on well-known urban populations, such as those of small cities like Pompeii, it is clear that the distribution of income must have been radically different from the highly inegalitarian societies of nineteenth-century southern Italy or England, in which only 6% and 9–17% respectively of the population enjoy incomes significantly above the simple subsistence level of the typical landless labourer. In Pompeii, 60–70% of households were able to afford to rent or own small houses large enough to distinguish them from the poorest 20–30% of the population living in small apartments or *pergolae* over shops, who presumably lived much closer to subsistence, and nearly 20% of the population lived in lavish houses of 600 m² or more.

As Emanuel Mayer,[33] among others, have provocatively argued, there seems to have been a substantial Roman middle class, in broad social and economic terms, and, in fact, as I believe is clear from our housing evidence, a substantially larger one than the very modest upper middle class posited by Scheidel and Friesen. Roman society was certainly more inegalitarian than classical Greek society, which enjoyed high real incomes, several times subsistence,[34] greater mean heights,[35] a relatively even distribution of wealth, at least at classical Athens, comparable to mid-twentieth-century democratic welfare states,[36] and a lower level of housing – and therefore income – inequality, albeit one that would slowly but consistently increase, from the classical through the Hellenistic and Roman periods.[37] Nevertheless, a careful examination of the income distribution shows that the differences between the Greeks and Romans are relatively modest compared to the dramatic difference between these societies and highly inegalitarian ones like nineteenth-century England, for example, which has a similar Gini co-efficient, but for which housing standards are dramatically lower overall. Among the English, there is a vast difference in income between the wealthiest 1%, the very small middle class of perhaps 15% of the population, and the working classes, the poorest 85%.[38]

A comparison of Greco-Roman income distribution with the changes in Europe and North America from the eighteenth century through to the present day, as recently mapped out in great detail by Piketty, corroborates the impression, based on the secular increases of mean height since the mid- to late nineteenth century,[39] that the modern working classes would not enjoy diets or overall levels of social equality comparable to the Greeks or Romans until the social transformation ushered in by World War II.[40] The prosperity and social importance of this broad middle class in Roman Italy was also buttressed by a range of social welfare policies, many focused on maintaining low prices of agricultural commodities and freeing up incomes for the poor to buy luxuries,[41] or distributing free bread, and eventually wine, pork and olive oil to the urban *plebs*,[42] as well as a long tradition of elite patronage and euergetism, generally obligatory for the politically ambitious, and related *munera*.[43]

The remarkably high standard of housing, and the relative social equality that goes with it, which clearly distinguished Roman Italy, can probably be applied to most of the Hellenized or Romanized regions of eastern Spain, Gallia Narbonensis, North Africa and Greece, but it is not necessarily characteristic of many of the less Romanized regions of the empire, particularly Gaul and Egypt. Standards of nutrition among the Gallo-Romans seem to have been relatively good, at least in terms of heights and access to protein, which is not surprising given the fact that the Gauls were slow to take to urban residence and most lived in small rural villages or scattered farmsteads,[44] and so had ready access to livestock, and so to meat, milk, butter and cheese.[45] This does not mean, however, that their diet, while rich in protein, was necessarily varied or extensive, as is clear from the conservative Celtic diet of the British, which offered little of the fruit, nuts, vegetables, spices, fish, seafood, poultry and game which the Romans prized.[46] Nor were the northern provinces more egalitarian than Roman Italy, since Gallo-Roman chieftains could afford to build some of the most massive villas of the empire within the first generation of the conquest, while the common people would long live in tiny wattle and daub thatched cottages.[47]

Egypt deserves particular attention, since Scheidel's low estimates of Roman living standards are based primarily on calculations of the real wages of rural day labourers in Roman Egypt.[48] Pharoanic, and presumably Achaemenid, Egypt was a deeply inegalitarian society with an income distribution not dissimilar to nineteenth-century England, or to a number of other early or middle Bronze Age monarchical societies,[49] as we can see by using housing as a proxy for income and studying the distribution of housing space in fully excavated towns, such as Middle Kingdom Kahun or New Kingdom Amarna.[50] The vast majority of the population lived in small mud-brick houses with a median size around 50 m^2, while the houses of high-ranking priests, scribes and officials, who lived in barely 8–10% of the dwellings, ranged from 150 m^2 or 200 m^2 up to 750 m^2 or even 2,500 m^2. For Amarna, we have a Gini co-efficient of 0.48, and for Kahun 0.71, significantly higher even than England in 1831. Similar levels of poverty and social inequality seem to have persisted for much of Egyptian society into the Hellenistic period, as we see from the houses of the embalmers of Ptolemaic Memphis, who were surely more privileged than most of the Egyptian peasantry or *laoi basilikoi*, and range from 14.2 m^2 to 138.9 m^2, but with a mode of only 19–22 m^2.[51] While the Greek and Macedonian population of Alexandria likely enjoyed relatively good housing, and a few *metropoleis*, particularly in the regions with the strongest Greco-Roman influence, such as the Fayum, show distinctly larger houses, with an average of approximately 90 m^2 for Karanis, and reasonably secure estimates of 60 m^2 for the other Fayum towns,[52] even these houses are still distinctly smaller than in Roman Italy, comparable to the more modest third quartile of Wallace-Hadrill's Pompeiian population.

This impression of a highly unequal agrarian society is also suggested by the simple traditional diet of the Egyptian peasantry, heavily based on cereals and a few simple vegetables, which seems likewise to have persisted among a significant proportion of the population through the Hellenistic period,[53] and certainly presents a marked contrast to the relative luxury of the Greco-Roman diet in Egypt.[54] While there is some evidence for improvements in stature and nutrition in the Greco-Roman period, occasionally significant improvements,[55] among much of the population the poverty of the traditional Egyptian peasant diet seems to have improved relatively little,[56] with some heights, as at the Dakhleh oasis,[57] as low as those found in the Old and Middle Kingdom.[58] The Roman policy of transforming the *metropoleis* into *municipia*, and their encouragement of the upper classes to provide traditional Roman patronage and to pay *munera* and support public services,[59] most notably the introduction of the sale of bread at a subsidized, low price,[60] may well have improved the nutrition of a significant number of ordinary Egyptians, in a way that the Hellenistic rulers generally failed to do, with their concessions to the Egyptian priestly elite and the temples, but the effect of such changes is likely to have been limited, and it is, on the whole, very dangerous to use the Egyptian evidence, notwithstanding its exceptional richness, as a reliable index of real wages, or the standard of living or of nutrition, in Roman Italy.

Moreover, Scheidel reads too much into the significance or representativeness, even for Egypt, of some of the low wages he relies upon. In an agrarian society in which most of the rural population enjoyed relatively secure tenure of agricultural land, cash employment is likely to be relatively casual and to be a supplement to income from farming, as Rathbone consistently finds in his investigation of day labourers on the estates of Aurelius Isidorus,[61] very different from the cash wages of English or southern Italian rural labourers of the nineteenth century, for example, who had no other source of income or of subsistence. Moreover, the wages studied are the lowest on offer, for unskilled labourers, and will not reflect the incomes of more highly skilled workers, to say nothing of the incomes that independent craftsmen and small farmers could earn, who constituted a very large percentage of the Roman, if not the nineteenth-century, urban and rural population.[62]

The case of the workers at Mons Claudianus is particularly instructive, particularly for our purpose, as it is a settlement made up almost entirely of relatively low-paid quarry workers, and we know a great deal about their diet, as well as much more about their wages than any other comparable group in the Roman Empire, from a substantial series of documents studied by Hélène Cuvigny.[63] The cash wages of these workers, ranging from 28 dr. to 47 dr. per month, or approximately 600 HS per year, were about half of a legionary infantryman's pay, but, as Cuvigny points out, these wages, unlike those of the legionaries, were supplemented with 1 artaba (39.5 litres) of wheat per month as well as wine,[64] a wheat ration five times the amount needed for an adult male's subsistence.[65] Moreover, their wages were similar to those of workers in the *metalla* at Alburnus Minor in Dacia, dated to AD 163–164,[66] a possible indication that these wages are set by the imperial government, rather than reflecting the probably rather depressed local market for labour in Egypt.[67] The cash wages of the Mons Claudianus workers would buy 6.5 litres of wheat per day, and 8 litres, if one includes the wheat given in kind, well above the typical range of 3.5 to 6.5 litres of wheat, which Scheidel has calculated for the wages in a wide range of pre-industrial societies.[68] These quarry workers' wages are certainly a great deal higher than Scheidel's estimate of only 3 litres per day for the wages of unskilled labourers in Egypt, which he uses as a proxy for the empire as a whole. It is perhaps not so surprising, therefore, that archaeobotanical and archaeozoological research into the diet of these workers at Mons Claudianus,[69] shows that, despite their low social status (mine or quarry work was often used as a harsh punishment for criminals, after all), and isolation from arable land or markets, enjoyed a relatively rich diet. They ate meat, more than two dozen species of fish, including cuttlefish, groupers, bream, parrotfish, wrasses, grey mullets, snappers, emperors, and barracuda from the Red Sea,[70] and a wide array of fruits and vegetables, enlivened with a full range of spices and condiments.[71]

As I argue in greater depth elsewhere,[72] despite the paltriness of our documentary evidence for Roman wages, what we do know suggests, like our anthropometric and housing evidence, and the mine and quarry workers studied by Cuvigny and Van der Veen, that Roman wages tended to be relatively generous, particularly compared to those in nineteenth-century Europe, with ordinary Romans afforded many opportunities to improve their lot, rather than being constrained to work at a very meagre subsistence. The most striking contrast is between the pay of English soldiers and of Roman legionaries, who were recruited from the rural poor and hardly indulged, yet whose base pay, only 10–20% of which, as Duncan-Jones noted,[73] would easily buy all the wheat necessary for subsistence, allowing them to enjoy, as is very well documented,[74] a relatively rich diet. More importantly, legionaries could earn double or triple their base pay, up to 36,000 HS, and, if promoted to the rank of centurion, would earn from 18,000 HS to 72,000 HS per year, while English soldiers could earn no more than 38% over their base salary after 25 years of impeccable service.[75]

Agricultural productivity and innovation in the Roman diet

Although André and Dalby had amply documented the richness of the Roman diet, scholars debating the quality of the diet of the ordinary Roman have tended to pay far too little attention to the high levels of agricultural productivity achieved by Roman farmers, allowing them to produce large surpluses of a wide range of agricultural produce, and of their many innovations in introducing new types of fruits, vegetables, wines, meat and seafood to satisfy the increasingly sophisticated tastes of demanding urban markets of prosperous consumers. The Roman agronomic literature, utilizing comparative evidence and a wide range of archaeozoological and archaeobotanical studies can convincingly show that the Greeks and Romans had anticipated, and on occasion surpassed, most of the critical innovations of the agricultural revolutions of the medieval Low Countries and eighteenth-century England. Ancient agronomic innovations included convertible husbandry, improved manure and fodder management, sophisticated animal breeding, stabling and veterinary care, scientific methods of viticulture, oleiculture, and innovative approaches to the grafting and/or cross-breeding of a wide range of fruits, nuts and garden vegetables.[76]

Demand, however, is at least as important a factor in increased agricultural productivity as technical innovation, and it is the relatively high living standards of a broad Roman middle class, their high levels of urbanization, and the rapid democratization of tastes for once luxurious foods that helps to explain the rapid development of the Roman diet and of agriculture. Most inegalitarian societies restrict the diet of the poor to low cost staples and cereals, with meat, but also fish, poultry, game, fresh fruits, nuts and vegetables, with their higher price elasticity, effectively beyond the means of all but a privileged minority. While this was clearly the case in most of eighteenth- and nineteenth-century Europe, meat was an important part of the diet of ordinary Romans,[77] much as it was in medieval Germany or Renaissance Italy, if not more so, and this meat was derived, not only from common domestic animals, particularly pigs, and, to a lesser extent, cattle and sheep,[78] but also, as the result of *pastio villatica* and intensive fish farming, from game meat, poultry, game birds, fish, shellfish, snails and even dormice.[79] The importance of meat in the diet can be most reliably inferred not only from the abundance of animal bones, including more expensive fish and game, in archaeological contexts reflecting a wide array of social strata,[80] but from the very sophisticated animal husbandry strategies developed, including the application of convertible husbandry,[81] and improved fodder management and selective breeding,[82] leading to significantly increased withers heights and weights for livestock, reaching levels only rarely found in nineteenth-century Europe, as well as greater fecundity and better breeds.[83] As well as significantly improving both the quantity and quality of the traditional domestic livestock breeds, sheep, pigs and cattle, we see much more emphasis on breeding livestock specifically for meat, particularly encouraging intensive production of lamb[84] and pigs,[85] as well as some very sophisticated dairy farming.[86] The most impressive proof of the great demand for new and more luxurious types of meat, however, comes from the development of game and fish farming, which succeeded in reducing the cost of many once rare game birds and animals to prices little higher than pork, lamb or kid by the time of Diocletian's price edict, and saw them very widely consumed on sites reflecting a very wide range of social statuses.[87] We find, for example, a terracotta pot with 28 thrush breasts preserved in honey in a Batavian legionary camp,[88] and a farm raising and smoking chickens and venison for preservation, packaging and export.[89] The quest to perfect the game farming of new and more exotic species, and to bring their consumption within the means of the mass of the population, continued into late antiquity with the successful farming of the pheasant, still very expensive in Diocletian's time, carefully explained by Palladius in the fifth century AD.[90]

These increasing standards of nutrition and this democratization of luxury foods was not confined to meat, fish and game, however, even if animals and even birds and fish are more likely to leave archaeological remains, which are much easier and cheaper to collect and analyse, than other types of food. Wine was available to a mass market,[91] while simultaneously being produced from an ever expanding range of grape varieties and *terroirs*,[92] and the massive deposit of oil amphorae which formed Monte Testaccio allowed Hesnard to conservatively estimate olive oil consumption from these state imports alone at 17–19 kg per capita in the city of Rome, which should be compared to modern Italian consumption, which reached 8.8 kg per capita in the 1870s only to decline to around 6 kg from the 1880s through the Second World War.[93]

Alongside greater meat consumption, income growth among the Romans is most evident from the great variety of fruits, nuts, vegetables, spices and condiments, which were incorporated into the diet of the Romans. Diocletian's price edict listed maximum prices for ninety three types of fruits and vegetables,[94] and archaeobotanical work in the Roman provinces, which has been pursued assiduously for decades now and has been collected in several important recent syntheses, shows a dramatic contrast between the many exotic and rare fruits and vegetables in the Roman diet, compared to the relatively limited numbers of varieties attested for the Celts and Germans.[95] Moreover, most of these fruits and vegetables seem to have gone out of use with the fall of the Roman Empire, with many not reintroduced until the eighteenth or nineteenth century. For example, the peach, which was introduced to Rome in the first century AD[96] and cultivated extensively and to a high standard, with finds of peach pits showing that the fruit were highly standardized and uniform in size and very large,[97] disappeared from northern Europe until the eighteenth century, and even rather prosaic fruits like the plum and apricot were not reintroduced until the end of the seventeenth and the mid-eighteenth centuries, respectively.[98] The Romans cultivated a huge range of fruits, creating many different cultivars, many named for the Romans of equestrian or senatorial rank, who helped to create or popularize them,[99] including the apple, pear, pomegranate, nectarine, quince,[100] cherry, sorb apple, carob, damson, lemon (once thought to have been introduced only by the Arabs),[101] watermelon,[102] and such imported fruits as dates and coconuts.[103] Market gardening was likewise very highly developed in the Roman world, with a large range of vegetables introduced from all over the Mediterranean and grown to a very high standard, with careful irrigation, drainage, manuring, weeding and soil contouring, even using greenhouses furnished with double-glazed glass and heated in the winter.[104] There was also a very large market for spices and condiments,[105] and even wild plants, like capers and wild asparagus.[106]

Notes

1   André, 1981, and the work of Dalby stands out, most notably Dalby, 2003.
2   See Foxhall & Forbes, 1982, and, in particular, the very influential work of Garnsey, 1999.
3   Davies, 1971 is one of the first and best such studies, and still a model for the range of evidence that ought to be investigated, but Van der Veen, 1998a; 1998b; 2001 is also significant for isolati the evidence for the surprisingly varied diet of a community made up of relatively poor and isolated quarry workers.
4   See Eveleth and Tanner, 1990. For an introduction to the modern literature on using anthropometric evidence to assess the biological standard of living in a society, and my first attempt to assess our Roman anthropometric evidence, arguing that it demonstrates a significantly superior standard of mass diet than that which prevailed in eighteenth and nineteenth century Europe, see Kron, 2005a. For the importance of anthropometry, nutrition, and hygiene in assessments of ancient health and life expectancy, with references to comparative evidence and the scientific literature, see Kron, 2012c. For the relationship between health and social class, even in societies with adequate nutrition, see Wilkinson and Pickett, 2011 and Lahelma et al., 2015.
5   For the failure of classical archaeologists to put emphasis on osteological studies, see Morris, 1992, 101–102, and for a sobering assessment of the lost opportunities in studying the material potentially available in Sicily, see Becker, 2000. For a recent bibliography to osteological studies for Greco-Roman antiquity, see MacKinnon, 2007.
6   I apologize in advance for relying heavily on citing my own work, but I have been making the case for the high standard of living of the Roman middle and lower classes in a range of specialized publications, and this brief contribution allows me to bring the pieces of the argument together here, and these publications permit surveys of recent scholarship in much more detail than can be offered here otherwise.
7   See Kron, 2005a, and Borgognini Tarli and Mazzotta, 1986.
8   See Catalano et al., 2001d.
9   See Scheidel, 2012b, 327.
10   See Giannecchini and Moggi-Cecchi, 2008, and especially the low estimates in Giannecchini and Moggi-Cecchi, 2008, 290 table 6, effectively reviving the use of the Pearson and Manouvrier equations.
11   Kron, 2005a, 79–81; 2013, 58.
12   For bibliography on the methodological problems stemming from the Pearson and Manouvrier methods, see Becker, 1999, 226, in addition to his own analysis, of course. Controversy regarding the appropriate regression equations to use to calculate stature for our Greco-Roman samples have led some scholars to advocate using femur length rather than a calculation based on all long bone lengths to estimate changes in height, but while the femur is arguably the single most helpful long bone in estimating height, and is robust and tends to be fairly well preserved, this is not an adequate solution to the problem. Not only do accurate height estimates require a regression equation based on all long bone lengths, femur length alone is not only inadequate to reconstruct height, it is not

necessarily even adequate as a basis for height comparisons, since under-nutrition tends to lead to disproportionate reductions in the lengths of certain long bones, with the tibia, for example, declining in length at a faster rate than the femur. In the absence of large samples of fully articulated skeletons or burials allowing *in situ* measurements, we cannot avoid the methodological problem of choosing one or more regression equations. While I believe, and have and will argue, that the Olivier or Trotter and Gleser methods for 'whites' have been fairly clearly shown to give accurate results for Greco-Roman individuals, some uncertainty about the most accurate equations will remain until a satisfactory study is carried out to calculate regression equations based on a large sample of Greco-Roman skeletal remains, including enough fully articulated skeletons to allow accurate height calculations.

13 A more methodologically advanced alternative to the Pearson and Manouvrier methods when studying stunted populations, based on a much larger sample, are provided by Trotter and Gleser's regression equations for African Americans, based on the rich data compiled from World War II recruits, who grew up at a time when intense Jim Crow segregation, poverty, and incomes at least 50–60% lower than for the 'white' majority had created a significant height difference. See Myrdal, 1944, 230–250, 364–379, 1079–1124 for full contemporary data on the health and wage gap. The low heights calculated for the skeletal remains from Herculaneum offered by Capasso, 2001, which differ from those for Herculaneum and Pompeii calculated by Sara Bisel and Estelle Lazer, respectively, and have been questioned by Becker, 2003 and Lazer, 2009, 182–183, were presumably compiled using these equations. For the difference of 4 cm in the estimates derived from using the two different sets of Trotter and Gleser equations, see Lazer, 2009, 182 table 8.1.

14 Fully and Pineau, 1960.

15 See Bolsden, 1984; Formicola, 1993; Becker, 1999.

16 See Breitinger, 1937, 202–203.

17 See Shelton, 1998, 262–263 (no. 307–308).

18 Kron, 2005a, 75. Although it is possible that this relaxation of the height requirement was driven by an actual decline in Roman heights, rather than just difficulties in recruiting, a number of studies from late antique and Proto-Byzantine Greece seem to suggest little decline, with mean heights of 169 cm at Eleutherna (n=52); 170 cm at Messene (n=23); 173 cm at Gortyn (n=18); 168 cm at Abdera (n=17); and 170 cm at Soutara (n=27). See Bourbou and Tsilipakou, 2009, Table 8.4. See also Wittwer-Backofen & Kiesewetter, 1997.

19 At the beginning of the nineteenth century, the Heavy Cavalry were required to be 172.7 cm tall, and the Light Cavalry 170.2–175.3 cm tall, the Infantry of the Line 167.6 cm tall, and the general service Infantry 165.1 cm (Floud et al., 1990, 114). Although many potential recruits did not present themselves for service, knowing they were too short, a large proportion did so, and failed to meet even the lowest threshold, never less than 28.1% and as many as 45.9% in 1888 (Floud et al., 1990, 62, Table 2.4). For the complex problem of calculating likely mean heights from the heights of individuals who volunteered for military service and met the minimum height thresholds, see the detailed analysis in Floud et al., 1990.

20 See Davies, 1795; Eden, 1797; Hasbach, 1908; for a broader synthesis, see Burnett, 1979. For a detailed interdisciplinary treatment of English under-nutrition in the eighteenth and nineteenth centuries, drawing on detailed anthropometric evidence, and fleshing out the regional and diachronic trends, see Floud et al., 1990. While Davies and Eden highlight the plight of landless labourers in southern England, in a period of high grain prices, during the Napoleonic War, whose situation was admittedly more dire than among the rural poor in northern England or Scotland, where a significant number were able to retain their status as peasants or tenant farmers rather than landless labourers (see note 45), the poverty and under-nutrition of the rural population is well-documented throughout the United Kingdom, and continued through most of the nineteenth and early twentieth centuries.

21 See the brief discussion in Kron, 2008a, 79–86 and 2014c, 126–128 for references. The contemporary work of Cagnazzi, 1849 is of particular interest.

22 See, for example, Scheidel, 2012a, 273–275.

23 See Kron, 2013, 59–62. Note especially the thorough and all too rare methodology of actually measuring the incidence and severity of LEH and cribra orbitalia notable in the work of Fox, 2005, which shows how low the incidence of these syndromes was among the Hellenistic populations studied, and Dobney and Goodman, 1991, which reminds us that Harris lines or LEH were relatively common among working classes in Mexico and much of England as late as the 1980s. Unfortunately, although BMI can be of significant value in determining health and mortality for

historical populations, skeletal data rarely gives any indication of BMI, with the exception of relatively extreme cases of obesity or low body weight leading to noticeable skeletal abnormalities, as has occasionally been observed in skeletal remains from burials of privileged individuals in eighteenth- or nineteenth-century England, for example. Bisel's use of the robusticity and pelvic brim indices for her analysis of the skeletal remains from Herculaneum tends to suggest many of her subjects had healthy body weights and some had well developed musculatures, but analysis of this sort is rarely carried out with any consistency on our Greco-Roman skeletal remains.

24   See Vanna, 2007. Another intriguing study of children in Pharaonic Egypt showed that they experienced faster childhood growth and lower infant mortality than children in early twentieth-century Bologna, suggesting that notwithstanding the relative poverty and social inequality of ancient Egyptian society, the poor still enjoyed a better standard of nutrition than many nineteenth- and early twentieth-century Europeans. See Boccone et al., 2010, 343–344.

25   See Morris 1992, 100–101; Kron, 2013, 64. Many studies could be cited, but see Killgrove, 2013; Killgrove & Tykot, 2013 for recent discussions of work in Roman Italy. For similar work in Greece, see Papathanasiou et al., 2015.

26   To choose just one recent example, Killgrove and Tykot 2013 surveys several sites in the Roman *suburbium*, showing fairly high levels of protein, with most of it coming from fish and meat rather than legumes. These sites do provide rather less evidence of marine fish or seafood of the highest trophic levels than at the coastal site of Isola Sacra (Prowse et al., 2004), however.

27   See Fraser et al., 2011; Aguilera et al., 2016.

28   See Scheidel, 2014, 209 n. 1 for a bibliography of estimates of Roman GDP, to which one must add Lo Cascio and Malanima, 2014 with further, updated references.

29   This is a very important point for the question of overall economic growth (Lo Cascio, 2009) and especially demand for agricultural produce (Kron, 2012a), which we only treat quickly here. Among the Greeks, it is clear from Hansen, 2006; 2008; Bintliff et al., 2007, 22, that the population of early Hellenistic Greece had already reached urbanization rates of over 50%, and even in Egypt, urbanization rates of 20–30% are secure (see Tacoma, 2008). While it has been suggested that Roman urbanization rates may have been significantly lower than among the Greeks (as suggested by several of the authors in Bowman and Wilson, 2011), given the explosive growth of Rome, it is likely that Roman Italy as a whole had begun to achieve levels of urbanization not seen in modern Italy until the twentieth century. See Kron, 2017a.

30   See Lo Cascio and Malanima, 2009; 2014.

31   As was also noticed and argued by Milanovic et al., 2007.

32   See Kron, 2014c.

33   See Mayer, 2012; Forthcoming; Courrier, 2014.

34   See Scheidel, 2010; 2014, 212 n.14.

35   Typically 170 cm in the classical and 171.9 cm in the Hellenistic period compared to the approximately 168 cm heights that are attested for Roman Italy, as laid out in Kron, 2005a. The Etruscans, like the Greeks, seem to have slightly greater heights than the Romans (Kron, 2013, 62–63), and there is some good evidence from housing data and land tenure patterns suggested by rural surveys documenting a significant and prosperous Etruscan middle class, similar socially as well as culturally to Greece (see Kron, 2013, 64–66), which might explain this phenomenon. Scheidel, 2012a, 273–274, makes a great deal of the slight decline in Roman heights compared to the early Iron Age and the early medieval period, explaining it as a Malthusian effect, but as the heights of the classical and Hellenistic Greeks and the Etruscans, highly urbanized populations with very high population densities, in the case of the Greeks, much more so than at any time before the late twentieth century (Hansen, 2006; 2008), clearly refute this explanation.

36   See Kron, 2011. At Athens the richest 1% of the population owned just around 30% of the wealth of the society, far less than the 67% possessed by the richest 1% in 1911 England, a level eventually reached by American society in its gilded age at the turn of the twentieth century (see Williamson and Lindert, 1980).

37   See Kron, 2014a, 129, Table 2.

38   Despite the increased Gini co-efficient among the Romans, there is a still a substantial and very prosperous middle class, as among the Greeks, but there is a considerable appreciation of wealth among the richest 2–5% and a much richer upper middle class of the wealthiest 20%, while the poorest 20–30% seem to be disadvantaged vis-à-vis comparable social groups in Hellenistic Greece. See Kron, 2014c, 135, fig. 4.

39 In Kron, 2005a.

40 For the vicissitudes of modern social inequality, which broadly track secular changes in mean heights, most notably the consolidation of extreme inequality in the nineteenth century, its gradual relaxation, and the social democratic revolution of the post-World War II era, as well as the dramatic decline of equality in the United States since the 1980s, see Piketty and Saez, 2004; Piketty, 2005; 2014.

41 See, in particular, Prell, 1997, and Cao, 2010 on the *alimenta*. For the interest of the Roman government in ensuring the food supply, see Erdkamp, 2005.

42 See Lo Cascio, 1999.

43 See, for example, the recent study for northern Italy of Goffin, 2002.

44 See Pounds, 1969, fig. 3.6; Woolf, 1998, 106–141.

45 For a comparable situation, see Floud et al., 1990, 201, Figure 5.3, showing that in 1815 army recruits drawn from the Scottish rural population were 1.47 cm taller than the English, and the Irish 1.143 cm taller. This reflects a diet slightly richer in protein, based on potatoes or oatmeal rather than purchased wheat bread, and greater access to fresh milk from the cows kept by many small tenant farmers, a luxury rarely open to English rural labourers, whose employers denied them the opportunity to rent small plots of land near their cottages for growing garden vegetables or keeping chickens, cows or pigs (see Kron, 2008a, 93–94).

46 See the excellent monograph of Cool, 2006, and the discussion below.

47 For the massive villas of the Gallo-Roman chieftains, see the aerial photographs of Agache and Bréart, 1975. For the housing of the common people in Gaul, see in particular Audouze and Büchsenschütz, 1992. For the persistence of traditional dwellings in regions of the Loire valley not in the cultural and economic influence of the large Roman *coloniae*, see Provost, 1993, 219–237.

48 See Scheidel, 2010 for his calculation of variations in real wages based on basic and respectable consumption baskets of commodities. For his reliance primarily on Allen's calculations (Allen, 2009), based on Diocletian's price edict, and Egyptian wages, see Scheidel, 2014, 210–211.

49 See Schachner, 1999.

50 Data taken from Kemp, 1977.

51 Thompson, 1988, 168.

52 Van Minnen, 1994, 234–237.

53 Thompson, 1979.

54 See Papathomas, 2006.

55 See Grilletto, 1981; Billy, 1992.

56 See Prominska, 1981; Hussein et al., 2006, 18, Table 2.

57 Molto, 2001.

58 See, for example, Masali, 1981, 225; Strouhal, 1986, 215; Zakrzewski, 2003, 224, Table 3; Raxter et al., 2008, 149, fig. 1.

59 See Bowman and Rathbone, 1992, 123–127.

60 Sharp, 2007, 223–230 offers references to the distribution of bread by the eutheniarchs at Oxyrhynchus. The practice starts with municipal officials baking bread for subsidized sale, beginning no later than 199 AD, for approximately 3,600 consumers. Eventually, up to 4,000 recipients are documented, for AD 268–272.

61 See Rathbone, 1991.

62 For the very different Roman land tenure system, and the much larger proportion of the agricultural land farmed by Roman smallholders, rather than aristocratic landowners working vast estates with landless labourers, as in England, see Kron, 2008a, 87–97.

63 See Cuvigny, 1996.

64 Cuvigny, 1996, 139.

65 Cuvigny, 1996, 141 citing Foxhall and Forbes, 1982. This practice of providing significant supplies of food in kind, particularly wheat, is reflected in Diocletian's price edict and in descriptions of pay for legionaries and other salaried workers, which generally included a significant amount in basic staples, much of it presumably for sale or trade by the recipient.

66 Cuvigny, 1996, 142.

67 Wages for labourers in the Nile valley seem to have been significantly lower in the second century AD, with an average of 25 dr. per month, according to Drexhage, 1990b, 425–429, but as Cuvigny, 1996, 141 notes, it is unclear if these wages include payment in kind, as they clearly did at Mons Claudianus.

68 Scheidel, 2010, 452–453, cited by Scheidel, 2014, 211.
69 See Van der Veen, 1998a; 1998b; 2001; Hamilton-Dyer, 2001. Archaeobotanical investigations of individual houses in Pompeii by Ciaraldi also provide clear evidence for a wide range of fruits, vegetables, nuts and spices or condiments being consumed by individuals of very different social statuses. See, for example, Ciaraldi, 2007, 114–115, 145–146.
70 See Hamilton-Dyer, 2001.
71 The spices included black pepper, capers, chicory, coriander, cumin, fennel, rue, mint, mustard, fenugreek, lotus, and basil. (Van der Veen, 1998a).
72 Kron, 2014c, 126–128.
73 See Duncan-Jones, 1974, 12, cited by Kron, 2014c, 128 n. 35, with further discussion.
74 See Davies, 1971 for an excellent discussion.
75 See Kron, 2014c, 126–128. Both Roman legionaries and British soldiers had money deducted from their pay to cover certain living expenses, but these stoppages, as they were called, generally absorbed most of the low base pay of the British, whereas Roman legionaries had significant surplus funds after living expenses, funds which were often kept on account and invested, accumulating interest, in banks controlling the funds of each legion.
76 I offer an overview of some of the evidence for high Roman agricultural productivity, with references to recent literature, in Kron, 2000; 2002; 2004a; 2008a, 73–79; 2012a; 2012b; 2014b; Forthcoming [b]. Many important monographs or studies can be cited, but note, in particular, Rinkewitz, 1984; Tchernia, 1986; Pleket, 1990; 1993; Marcone, 1997; Farrar, 1998; Peters, 1998; Brun, 2004a; 2004b; Bartoldus, 2012; Marzano, 2013c. These improved methods of intensive farming seem to have become dominant not only in Greece, Sicily, western Turkey, Carthaginian and Greek North Africa, and Italy, but also throughout much of Spain and southern France, gradually influencing, but not necessarily becoming universal in, northern France, the Balkans, Germany, and Egypt.
77 For the case for higher ancient meat consumption, see especially Kron, 2008a, 73–79. For evidence of technical innovation and large-scale investments in, and the productivity of, Roman animal husbandry and meat production as compared to medieval and Early Modern Europe, and the evidence of greater integration of animal husbandry with arable agriculture through convertible husbandry, see, for example, Lauwerier, 1988; Lepetz, 1996; Peters, 1998; Kron, 2000; 2002; 2004a; 2008b; MacKinnon, 2010b; 2014a; Gaastra, 2014. The importance of game farming, discussed further below, also testifies to the healthy market demand for meat among the Romans, including newer luxury varieties. See Rinkewitz, 1984; Peters, 1998; Kron, 2008b; 2014a; Forthcoming [b]. Meat production, however, is only one aspect of the significantly increased demand for a range of luxury foods among the Greeks and Romans, which is evident from their intensive and sophisticated agricultural practices and production of a wide range of fruits, vegetables, nuts, wine and other products, as I survey in Kron, 2012a.
78 For the predominance of pork over beef and mutton or lamb in Romanized sites, see King, 1998.
79 See Kron, 2008a, 79–86; 2012a.
80 See Rinkewitz, 1984; Kron, 2008b; 2014a; Bartoldus, 2012, 181–213; for some of the game species raised using *pastio villatica*, and the methods used, as well as the range of types of game found in Roman archaeozoological assemblages.
81 See Kron, 2000; and note subsequent investigations of possible archaeobotanical evidence of convertible husbandry, based on the identification of the presence of weeds associated with cereal cultivation in a significant new discovery of carbonized meadow hay at Pompeii (Ciaraldi, 2007, 84–85, 158–159). For other investigations suggesting convertible husbandry or intensive farming, based on the analysis of archaeobotanical and palynological evidence from archaeological soil strata, see Fraser et al., 2011; Bowes et al., 2015; Aguilera et al., 2016; Marchesini and Marvelli, Forthcoming.
82 See Kron, 2004a; 2008b, 80–83; Ciaraldi, 2007, 84–85; 158–159; Marchesini and Marvelli, Forthcoming.
83 See Lauwerier, 1988; Lepetz, 1996; Peters, 1998; Kron, 2002; 2008a, 73–79; 2008b, 176–185; 2014; MacKinnon, 2010b; Gaastra, 2014.
84 See Bartoldus, 2012, 218.
85 See Kron, 2008b, 181 for references. The great care taken to produce pork meat is reflected in the practice of feeding pigs with figs to enhance the flavour of their flesh (Cappers, 2006, 165).
86 See Bartoldus, 2012, 223–224, for example, on goat milk production.

87 See Kron, 2017b for a detailed discussion and further references to the importance of game farming in Roman agriculture, its effect in reducing the cost, and the consequent increase in consumption by ordinary people. Game, the most expensive, luxurious and socially exclusive type of specialty meat, is very well represented archaeologically, not only in luxury villas, where game was presumably consumed by the wealthy and privileged, but in much less socially exclusive contexts, including *villa rusticae*, villages, towns and cities. Moreover, alongside evidence for declining prices and expanding game farming, our literary sources describe the growing importance of a range of game meats in banquets for *collegia*, and the consequent democratization of the taste for wild game.

88 See Lauwerier, 1993a.

89 See Olive and Deschler-Erb, 1999.

90 See Bartoldus, 2012, 210–213.

91 Tchernia, 1986, 172–179.

92 See Kron, 2014b, 167, for further discussion and references.

93 Kron, 2008a, 86. Note, of course, that other sources of olive oil, are not included in Hesnard's figure, and that olive oil was used for non-food uses, although presumably not the better grades of oil that were part of the organized state trade imported from Spain and deposited at Monte Testaccio.

94 As noted by Bartoldus, 2012, 115 n. 667.

95 See Bakels and Jacomet 2003; Livarda and Van der Veen, 2008. Papyrological (Papathomas, 2006) and archaeobotanical (Van der Veen, 1998a; 1998b; 2001; Cappers, 2006) studies in Egypt show an equally extensive range of fruits, vegetables and spices in the Roman period.

96 Sadori et al. 2009; Marchesini and Marvelli, Forthcoming.

97 Sadori et al., 2009, 49–53.

98 See Paap, 1983, 317–318, fig 14:1.

99 See Kron, 2012a, 164–165; 2014b, 168–169; Bartoldus, 2012, 123–124; Marchesini and Marvelli, Forthcoming. There were also new hybrid fruits, whose exact nature is unclear, such as the apple-pumpkin, perhaps a cross of the melon and quince, the apple-plum and almond-plum.

100 See Bartoldus, 2012, 126–127.

101 See Bartoldus 2012, 128–133 for the demonstration that the Romans grew the lemon, and not just the citron, and may even have introduced the orange. For the discovery of archaeobotanical remains of the lemon and citron at Roman sites, primarily Pompeii, see Pagnoux et al., 2013.

102 Van der Veen and Wasylikowa, 2004.

103 Kron, 2012a, 164 n. 44.

104 See Jashemski, 1979; Farrar, 1998; Garcia Soler, 2001, 43–72; Bowe, 2004; Frass, 2006; Bartoldus, 2012, 113–123. For a comparison with nineteenth-century London and specific references and analysis, see Kron, 2014b, 168–171.

105 See Miller, 1969; Thüry and Walter, 1997; Garcia Soler, 2001, 341–367. For important archaeobotanical evidence of spices, see, for example, Cappers, 2006; Ciaraldi, 2007, 114, 145–146, and the many references in Bakels and Jacomet, 2003.

106 For wild asparagus, see Bartoldus, 2012, 122–123.

22

SKELETONS IN THE CUPBOARD?

Femurs and food regimes in the Roman world

Miko Flohr

The study of (mal)nutrition in the ancient world long was, as Peter Garnsey (1999, 43) called it, an 'undernourished plant', but since the turn of the millennium there has been a proliferation of studies discussing the quality of Roman food regimes. While Roman diets are being approached from a variety of angles and by a range of specialists, it is the study of skeletal remains that has, in the last decade, had the most impact on the terms of the debate. Progress in our understanding of the skeletal record has been spectacular. Scholars have begun to study evidence for stature on a larger scale, enhancing the statistical and historical significance of their work, and making it possible to assess changes in average human body length over the very long term. Well-known is the work by Koepke and Baten (2005) on the biological standard of living in Europe during the last two millennia. For Italy, Giannecchini and Moggi-Cecchi (2008) have analysed the chronological development of stature between the early Iron Age and the early Middle Ages. Unfortunately, work on a very large and promising dataset of all published skeletal remains from the Roman period by Klein Goldewijk has thus far remained unpublished except for one chart published by Jongman (2007b, 194) and a very short methodological article by Klein Goldewijk and Jacobs (2013). At the same time, scholars have begun to systematically analyse them for indications of ill health that can be associated with structural malnutrition, such as porotic hyperostosis, and dental enamel hypoplasia. While studies like those of Lazer (2009; 2017) at Pompeii, and those of Killgrove (this volume, with references) in the region around Rome highlight the possibilities of such approaches, most of this work is still more-or-less limited to the micro-scale, partially for problems of compatibility and transparency outlined by Killgrove in this volume, partially because this work is labour-intensive and requires specialist skills not common among archaeologists. However, both developments have significantly increased the amount of historical information that can be extracted from the skeletal record.

Not unexpectedly, however, scholars have not yet come to a broadly shared consensus on what the skeletal record has to say about Roman food regimes. As happens more often in the study of issues related to ancient economic history, there is a more optimistic camp, and a more pessimistic camp – the former highlighting Roman dietary achievement, the latter highlighting Roman dietary shortcomings. Two of the most thorough and detailed general explorations of the relation between malnutrition and skeletal evidence come from scholars that have a less optimistic take on Roman food regimes. Peter Garnsey's broad discussion of skeletal evidence in his book on food and society in the Ancient world leaves no doubt that the author believes earlier accounts on the topic to have been overly optimistic about the quality of ancient diets (Garnsey 1999, 43–61). More recently, Walter Scheidel spread a similar message in his chapter on physical well-being in the *Cambridge Companion to the Roman Economy* (2012b), incorporating the more recent literature. Particularly focusing on the issue of stature, more optimistic sounds have been made by Willem Jongman (2007b) in a chapter on the historical development of the Roman Economy in the imperial period, and by Geoffrey Kron, in a lengthy article on ancient health, nutrition and living standards in *Historia* (Kron, 2005a) and in the preceding chapter in this volume. As they appear, the two positions cannot be reconciled, and their very frontal opposition begs the question of how solid conclusions derived from skeletal remains at this point actually are, and to what extent skeletal remains actually can be used in methodologically satisfying ways – either one is right, and the other is wrong, or the skeletal evidence is simply less ready to contribute to robust historical scenarios than one may want it to be, and it will have to be approached with more caution until we have a better understanding of it.

Bones and biases

It certainly is not hard to find challenges involved in bringing together skeletons and economic historians. The most crucial problem perhaps is that it is almost impossible for individual scholars to completely master the theoretical and methodological complexities of the scholarly fields involved, which bears the risk of Roman historians handling the osteological evidence too superficially, and of osteoarchaeologists not asking the questions of their material that matter most to Roman historians. Additionally, there also is a vast difference in publication culture: whereas osteoarchaeologists tend to come from a rigidly analytical scientific tradition that highly values explicit methodological precision, Roman historians have strong roots in the more rhetorical classical tradition, where the reconstruction of palatable historical scenarios often is more highly valued than detailed discussion of all the methodological complexities involved. Furthermore, as Killgrove rightly emphasizes elsewhere in this volume, raw osteoarchaeological data are often extremely inaccessible, and key arguments in the debate rest, essentially, on evidence that remains partially unpublished and is not easily accessible (the repeated references in recent literature to Klein Goldewijk's unpublished work are a case in point). Moreover, predictably, the evidence that is published is not necessarily published in a way that allows it to be used by others too. This relative lack of conventions is probably typical for a fast-developing field, and it will undoubtedly get better in the future, but this will be a slow process.

Yet even without these practical difficulties in bringing together the relevant data and in discussing them in a way that successfully integrates both research cultures involved, the relationship between the excavated skeletal record and historical reality is extremely complex. First of all, it is impossible to ignore the extent to which the composition of the skeletal record has been influenced by excavation practice: bones have been found only at places that have been excavated, and it has only very rarely been the case that these places were selected for osteoarchaeological purposes only – the study of skeletal evidence is an epiphenomenon of excavation practice dictated by other agendas. For instance, the Casal Bertone excavation discussed by Killgrove essentially was a rescue excavation necessitated by the construction of a high-speed rail line (Musco et al., 2008); the same is true for the excavation at Castellaccio Europarco, which preceded the construction of a major extra-urban shopping mall (Buccellato, 2007, esp. fig. 4). In general, certain parts of the Roman world are much better known than others, and the evidence at our disposal is biased in several important ways. It is heavily skewed towards Italy and temperate Europe at the expense of the rest of the Roman world, including densely populated regions in North Africa, along the Nile, and in Asia Minor. More importantly, the known skeletal record privileges centralized necropolises over isolated graves and thus city and settlement over countryside: especially for the late Republic and for the imperial period, the large majority of excavated skeletal remains comes from contexts associated with cities or other large settlements. People who spent their lives on farmsteads on the countryside are, by consequence, structurally underrepresented in our evidence, as are classes of people that for some reason or another were buried outside necropolises – or not at all. Thus, while Killgrove rightly stresses that the osteoarchaeological record reaches social layers far below the strata that had access to epigraphy, it still does not necessarily include all groups in society, and we do not know precisely who is lacking: it is true that the Casal Bertone excavation included a lot of people who had been inhumated without any formal tomb or gravestone to indicate their burial place, but this does not mean that we have all relevant social layers. Moreover, even if we are optimistic about the urbanization rate, a large majority of the ancient population remains almost completely invisible, and it is very hard to find a way to make up for that.

Short Romans, tall Romans

As far as stature is concerned, it should be emphasized that both the 'optimistic' and the 'pessimistic' position have their weaknesses. Kron has argued that adult males in Roman Italy, on average, must have been around 168.3 cm tall, a figure that he uses to confirm that Romans (and Greeks) were 'significantly taller than the nineteenth century working class populations' (Kron 2007, 72–79; in this volume). He believes that this picture is corroborated by the fact that minimum recruitment heights for the Roman army as reported by Vegetius (*De Re Militari* 1.5) were much taller than those of nineteenth-century European armies. There are several methodological problems with this. First of all, there is no reason to suppose that Roman recruitment heights are directly comparable to those of the nineteenth century: as the technological context of warfare is completely different, so are the physical demands on soldiers in the battlefield. Moreover, as Kron himself indicates, the figures mentioned by Vegetius only applied to the cavalry and the *first* cohort of the legions, rather than to the army as a whole – indeed, when referring to them, Vegetius leaves no doubt that such heights even among Romans were exceptional rather than the norm: they date, he says, from a period when the flower of the nation sought military, rather than civil careers, and when the total amount of recruits was much higher ('*sed tunc erat amplior multitudo*', 1.5), suggesting that in his day, when recruitment was more problematic, it was often necessary to compromise on stature. More problematic still is that essentially, the difference between Kron and more conservative estimates of body heights depends on the fact that they use different formulae to calculate stature from long bones: Kron (this volume) uses the Trotter and Gleser formula for 'whites' and the method of Olivier; others have used Pearson's formula, or the Trotter and Gleser formula for 'blacks'. Significantly, Klein Goldewijk and Jacobs (2013, 11) have recently argued that the methods to reconstruct stature from long bones are essentially all unreliable, and that one should compare bones, not reconstructed heights (cf. Killgrove, this volume). However, underneath these methodological issues lies a more fundamental problem with Kron's approach: even if he was right in his assertion that Greeks and Romans were taller than the nineteenth-century working classes in northern Europe, then what does it *mean*? For all the achievements of the Greeks and Romans compared to medieval and Early Modern Europe, to fully appreciate the development of stature in the Greco-Roman world, it needs to be judged in its own historical context, both geographically *and* chronologically: a key question is how Greco-Roman food economies relate to Mediterranean food economies of the late Bronze Age and early Iron Age, and to those of late antiquity and the medieval period. Early industrial Europe does not constitute a valid direct historical comparison.

Those with a more pessimistic view on Roman stature have put more emphasis on differences between Roman, pre-Roman and post-Roman body lengths in the Mediterranean. Giannecchini and Moggi-Cecchi (2008) have argued that the Roman imperial period saw a marked decrease in stature, followed by a marked increase of bodily height in late antiquity; similarly Koepke and Baten (2005) have advocated a pan-European increase in bodily height between the fourth and sixth century AD – coinciding with the collapse of the western half of the Roman Empire. However, although both studies incorporate a lot of evidence, on closer inspection, their argument is not unproblematic. A crucial problem with the work of Giannecchini and Moggi-Cecchi is that the evidence used to assess the Roman imperial period to a considerable extent comes from one place, which, in turn, is barely represented in the datasets used to make sense of preceding and subsequent periods. More worryingly still, that place happens to be the city of Rome, where living conditions and the food economy were fundamentally different from anywhere else in the Roman world: of the 284 bodies analysed by Giannecchini and Moggi-Cecchi for the imperial period, 159 (56%) came from cemeteries in the direct environment of Rome (see Figure 22.1); in other periods, the balance is completely inversed: in the pre-Roman period, the skeletons come from all over Italy, but not from closer to Rome than Gabii (Osteria dell'Osa); in the post-Roman period, 73% of all skeletons come from Tuscany, and only 2% come from Rome (Giannecchini and Moggi-Cecchi 2008, 285–286). No statistical technique can make up for such a bias, and their analysis mainly suggests that people in the

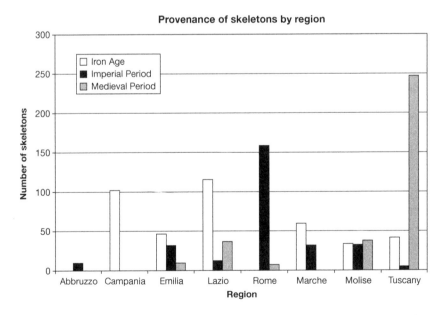

Figure 22.1 Provenance of evidence used by Giannecchini and Moggi-Cecchi (2008), by period.

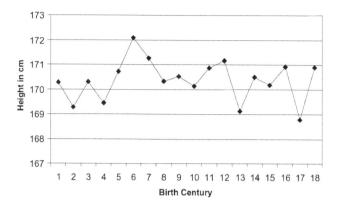

Figure 22.2 Height development, first to eighteenth centuries. From Koepke and Baten, (2005, 76, fig. 2).

Roman metropolis in the imperial period were shorter than people elsewhere in Italy in the Republican and late antique periods. This does not, of course, imply that there was a significant decline in body height in the Roman world at large. Moreover, even if the evidence from Rome suggested that the living conditions in the metropolis were worse than elsewhere in the Roman world (which it does not unequivocally do), it still would not follow that this was related to malnourishment – as is well known, stature has many determinants, and specifically in the case of the Roman metropolis, it is essential to point to the epigraphically attested seasonality of mortality patterns, which several scholars have linked to endemic malaria, and from which Scheidel (2013, with references) sketched a picture of a population that, from young age, suffered from bad health. While others have been more sceptical about the extent

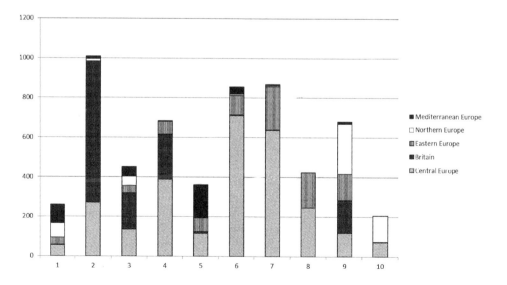

Figure 22.3 Regional provenance of the data used by Koepke and Baten, first to tenth centuries. Chart: Miko Flohr.

of malaria in and around the Roman metropolis (especially Lo Cascio, 2006), the point is that there is a range of credible possibilities for bad health, related to, for instance, the structural overpopulation in the metropolis, bad hygiene (classic, if overly dramatic, is Scobie, 1986), the water-rich nature of key zones in Rome's urban landscape, or, possibly, by structural shortage of food. It is unknowable which factor contributed what to the overall picture.

The analysis of Koepke and Baten (see Figures 22.2 and 22.3) operates on a much higher level of abstraction, but it uses a similar dataset and struggles with similar biases – for instance, it has only 11 Mediterranean skeletons for the second century, and only four for the fourth; this casts doubts about the validity of their claims for body length in the Roman Mediterranean, and while it is true that their data for Europe do suggest an increase in body length following the fall of the western Roman Empire, it should be noted that the peak coincides with the period in which the largest number of skeletons comes from southern Germany and the Rhine Region and when skeletons from Britain disappear from the equation (Koepke and Baten, 2005, 64). This is a typical bias that is not repeated in later periods, and which does not appear in their analysis as they have merged Britain, Germany and the Rhine region into one broad data category.

Rome and the Malthusian ceiling

Perhaps, one should reluctantly conclude that at this point, skeletal evidence remains essentially inconclusive as far as the historical development of stature is concerned. Theoretically, one possible way forward would be to reconstruct local developments in the long term in several specific places and compare these developments, but there are virtually no large necropolises that continue for more than three or four centuries, and there is no city or settlement where we can reliably follow local stature trends from the pre-Roman period until late antiquity. The only possible exception is the city of Rome, but Killgrove's analysis of skeletons from the city and the *suburbium* provides a clear example of the problems faced even here: while analysing chronological developments in bone-length within the context of one city is theoretically very promising, the results appear contradictory in themselves, with males and females going into different directions, and have a very weak statistical significance.

This is a sobering, but nonetheless important, result. While it is very well possible that, in the future, our knowledge of Roman skeletal remains will allow us to nuance and modify the models we use to make sense of living conditions in the Roman world, it is likely to remain essentially the other way around for considerable time to come: scholars will interpret excavated skeletal remains in the light of their preferred models of the nutritional status of Romans, and these models have been developed on the basis of other data. The big question at this point is whether those models should be optimistic, pessimistic or neutral in nature: is there reason to expect that undernourishment in the Roman world at large was bigger than, smaller than or comparable to that of pre- and post-Roman phases? In the end, most scholars seem to agree that this remains in the first place an issue of population pressure: it depends on the extent to which Rome's imperial food economies operated at a level close to their maximum capacity, so that further population growth would lead to food scarcity. To be sure, the ancient Mediterranean has a long history of communities sending out surplus population to places outside their political territory, and the consistency of this pattern suggests that, especially in the first millennium BC, many communities in the Ancient Mediterranean had to find ways to accommodate population growth above the carrying capacity of their hinterland – overpopulation was a familiar issue, but there was a ready solution, too: migration to places where there was still room for population growth. Is there any evidence that, in the Roman period, there were no places left to go to?

Scheidel (2009, 70) has argued that, by the early imperial period, the Mediterranean was operating close to its maximum carrying capacity, but it is worth emphasizing that there is no direct evidence unequivocally supporting this claim. Particularly, there is no reason why the Romans could not have lessened the pressure on their imperial ecosystem by founding more cities in fertile regions in the margins of their imperial network, and simply filling them with colonists and veterans. Several emperors, of course, did precisely this. Augustus founded a large number of towns throughout the empire, and he was able to emphasize (although probably not without exaggeration) that many of these places had become populous and famous already during his lifetime (*Res Gestae*, 28: '*quae vivo me celeberrimae et frequentissimae fuerunt*'). A century later, Trajan founded a series of cities a bit more beyond the immediate surroundings of the Mediterranean, such as Timgad in Numidia, Nicopolis in Moesia, and Xanten on the lower Rhine (Bennett, 1997, 315–316). Most of these cities also seem to have transformed into flourishing, independent communities, suggesting that by AD 100 there still was enough under-explored land available in the empire to resort to the strategy of colonization if population pressure became too high. As a demographic instrument, however, colonization does not really seem to have been used in the imperial period.

Indeed, on the whole, it should be noted that the Roman Empire, outside the direct environment of the central Mediterranean, does not appear to have been very densely populated. While our knowledge of Roman period settlements is not unbiased, plotting the settlements included in the Pleiades database on a map gives a relatively reliable indication of broad settlement trends (see Figure 22.4): settlements are very unequally divided over the Roman

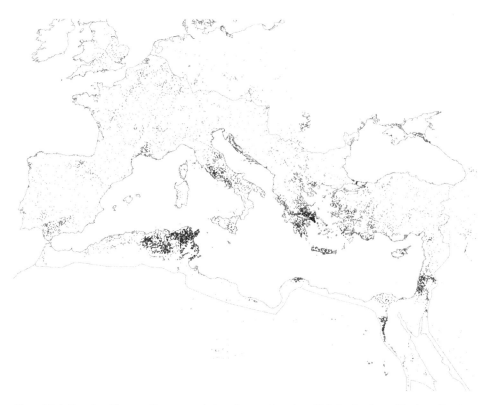

Figure 22.4 Density of known Roman-period settlements based on Pleiades Database (Version: October 21, 2015). Map: Miko Flohr.

world, and there are entire regions that appear rather empty. This is true for all river valleys in Gaul and Spain that flow towards the Atlantic, and for the very fertile Gharb region in what is now Morocco. It also seems true for large parts of the Ebro basin, which seems to have been rather thinly populated, particularly between the river and the Pyrenees. Some of these 'empty' regions were too cold for olives, but in others it is very well possible to cultivate the complete Mediterranean triad (Garnsey 1999, 12–20). In other words: there is no evidence suggesting that population pressure was getting the better of the Roman food economy on an empire-wide level – quite the contrary.

This does not mean that there was no undernourishment in the Roman world. Rather, it would suggest that this undernourishment was not necessarily directly related to the sheer quantity of people living in the Mediterranean. It is possible, and perhaps likely, that in some larger urban communities, and particularly (as already suggested above) in the Roman metropolis, there was, on a structural basis, friction undernourishment due to the malfunctioning of local and regional food markets. Well-attested institutions like the *annona* in Rome (and occasionally elsewhere in the Latin-speaking West), the grain distributions by wealthy benefactors, and the municipal grain funds (*sitonia*) in the Greek East, suggest that access to grain was not self-evident for all urban inhabitants (Erdkamp, 2005, 237–257; 2008; Zuiderhoek, 2008; Holleran, this volume): even if grain-distributions did not target those in need, they come from an ideology that assigns heavy weight to food security, highlighting the potential for malnutrition in urban contexts. These social and cultural echoes of food insecurity, in turn, suggest that those who grew up in bigger urban centres had higher chances of suffering from undernourishment during childhood, and of being shorter for that reason. If this means that the overall average stature is inversely related to the proportion of people living in large cities – the larger the number of urban inhabitants, the shorter the stature – then we may expect Romans *on average* to be a little bit shorter than their predecessors and their successors, and we may expect those on the pessimistic side of the debate to have a slightly stronger case. Yet given the biases in the dataset of, particularly, Giannecchini and Moggi-Cecchi one should be cautious not to overestimate these differences. After all, as the evidence collected by both Wilson (2011) and De Ligt (2012) highlights, many Roman cities were rather small, and rather unlike the Roman metropolis.

PART 5

Food on the market and in politics

23

MARKET REGULATION AND INTERVENTION IN THE URBAN FOOD SUPPLY

Claire Holleran

The vast majority of people in the Roman world lived in rural areas, but a notable minority lived in towns and cities and were dependent on the market for their food supply.[1] Most of the food that they consumed was produced locally, but the demand of some urban centres, most notably Rome, far outstripped the capacity of their immediate hinterlands. Such places were routinely reliant on food transported from further afield, while other towns and cities relied on the importation of external food supplies in times of poor local harvest. Markets could, however, be unstable, causing the price of food to fluctuate. On occasion then, it was deemed necessary to intervene and regulate the market; the aim of this chapter is to consider both the nature and extent of this regulation and intervention, and the motivation behind it. Was it driven by a genuine desire to ensure an adequate food supply for all and to protect the poor from the vicissitudes of the market, or was it only ever intended to assist a privileged few? The bulk of the discussion is related to Rome, since this was the largest food market in the Roman world, but the urban food supply outside Rome is also considered.[2] The focus is on the grain supply, because cereals formed the majority of the calorific intake in the Roman diet (see Heinrich in this volume). It is divided into two parts: the first considers direct food assistance through grain distributions, alimentary schemes, and public banquets, while the second explores both direct and indirect interventions in the market.

Direct assistance

Grain distributions

One of the most direct ways in which the Roman authorities intervened in the urban food supply was through the distribution of subsidised or free grain to urban populations, most famously in the city of Rome itself. Monthly sales of grain at a reduced price were first introduced as a permanent institution in Rome by Gaius Gracchus in 123 BC, although such measures had already been employed on an ad hoc basis by the aediles from the late third century BC.[3] These earlier distributions took place not in times of shortage, but rather in times of plenty, when the Roman state found itself with large amounts of tribute grain at its disposal. Similarly, Gracchus' law was not necessarily a reaction to poverty and food crisis in Rome. It was more likely motivated by a desire to reduce the power of individual politicians by removing the food supply from their gift and making it a structural issue for the Roman state; the acquisition of more tribute grain than was required to feed the Roman armies made this development possible (Erdkamp, 2000; 2005, 241). Laws were passed modifying Gracchus' measure in the 90s BC (*Lex Octavia*), in 73 BC (*Lex Terentia Cassia*), and in 62 BC (*Lex Porcia*), but the most important development took place in 58 BC when Clodius instituted a monthly distribution of free grain in Rome, a practice that continued into late antiquity.[4] The continued political importance of the distributions is made clear by Suetonius' comment that Augustus wanted to end the practice but could not take the risk that it would be revived by a political rival (Suet. *Aug.* 42.3).

However, not everybody in Rome was eligible to receive the free grain. Access was based on status rather than need, and while some recipients (known as the *plebs frumentaria*) may have been poor, it should be stressed that the grain distributions were a privilege rather than poor relief. Membership of the *plebs frumentaria* conveyed a certain status, something indicated by the fact that some recipients of the grain-dole at Rome advertised this distinction on their tombstones (*ILS* 2049, 6063–6065, 6067–6070, 9275; Woolf, 1990, 215). Membership was restricted to male citizens, probably over the age of ten (Suet. *Aug.* 41.2). The number of recipients was reduced from 320,000 to 150,000 by Julius Caesar in 46 BC, who registered those eligible *vicus* by *vicus* and instituted a lottery to be held by the praetor each year for the places of the deceased (Suet. *Iul.* 41.3; Dio Cass. 43.21.4). This system cannot have been effective for very long because the number of recipients increased in the following years until it was fixed again at just over 200,000 by Augustus in 2 BC (Aug. *RG* 15; Suet. *Aug.* 40.2; Dio Cass. 55.10.1). It is then highly unlikely that even all the male citizens in Rome were part of the *plebs frumentaria* in the imperial period. Membership was denoted by possession of a *tessera*, and by the early third century at least, if not earlier, *tesserae* could be bequeathed (*Dig.* 31.49.1; SHA *Aurel.* 35.1), gifted, or sold (*Dig.* 5.1.52.1, 31.87.pr), although since there is no evidence of extensive buying and selling, or any 'black market' in *tesserae* developing, Rickman (1980a, 244–249) argues that this process was probably somehow under the supervision of the state.

Five *modii* of grain were distributed to each recipient monthly, which works out at around 400 kg annually per person (Mattingly and Aldrete, 2000, 146). Garnsey (1983, 118) estimated the annual grain requirement per person at 200 kg, so the amount distributed would be sufficient to feed both the recipient and another person, although it would be insufficient to feed a family.[5] Assuming 200,000 recipients, as many as 400,000 people in Rome were fed at the expense of the Roman state. This amounts to well over a third of the population, which probably numbered around 1,000,000 by the first century BC. The market for grain in the city was therefore significantly reduced by the grain distributions, but demand no doubt remained considerable. Furthermore, the provision of free grain probably increased the demand for additional food items, as well as other consumer goods, since it freed up income that would ordinarily be spent on cereals. The situation may have changed somewhat in the later empire, since Septimius Severus added a ration of olive oil to the dole in the third century AD, and Aurelian later added pork and wine (SHA *Sev.* 18.3; *Aur.* 35.2, 48.1).

The grain was unmilled, which meant that it lasted longer but would have to be processed further before it could be consumed, either as some form of coarsely ground porridge, or bread. The ability to produce home-baked bread was a mark of status (Cic. *Pis.* 67), and most of the recipients probably lacked the means to produce bread at home, relying on local bakers to store, mill, and transform the grain into bread (Holleran, 2012, 134–135). The profits to be made are attested by the grand tomb of Eurysaces just outside the Porta Maggiore in Rome, a *pistor redemptoris* or bread contractor of the late first century BC. The continued importance of bakers in the process is indicated by the attention that Trajan paid to the bakers in the city (Gaius *Inst.* 1.34; Aur. Victor 13.5; Sirks, 1991, 311–322). Again the situation was somewhat different in late antiquity, since by the time of Aurelius, probably under Severus Alexander, the monthly grain ration had been replaced with a daily distribution of bread (SHA *Aurel.* 35.1, 48.1; Zosimus 1.61.3).[6] Grain was then supplied direct to bakers, a change that perhaps encouraged the development of state-sponsored watermills and the centralisation of milling in Rome (Tengström, 1974, 71–72; Wilson, 2000, 237).

The grain distributed was drawn principally from Sicily, Sardinia, North Africa, and (following its annexation by Augustus in 30 BC) Egypt. There is some debate over the relative extent of taxation in kind and the purchase of grain from landowners and merchants by the state, particularly in the imperial period, but it is probable that a considerable proportion of the grain distributed in Rome, if not all of it, was exacted directly from the provinces in the form of tribute.[7] Certainly this was the case in Egypt, although it should be noted that this did not preclude a market in Alexandrian wheat, since this was stored and used as collateral for a loan by merchants in Puteoli in the early empire (Casson, 1980, 26–29, 33). Some grain also came from imperial estates, which increased in number over the course of the empire (Erdkamp, 2005, 221–223).

Much of this can be classed as state redistribution of grain, but there was a good deal of private involvement in the process of collection and shipping of grain (Garnsey, 1983, 121–126). In the Republic, the state sold contracts to *publicani* for the collection of tax and rent grain and its transport to Rome (and to the army), offering the potential for huge profits to be made. By the second century AD – and probably much earlier in most areas – the system of *publicani* had been replaced by one in which grain was collected through the cities, with the process overseen by imperial officials. Seneca (*Ep.* 77.1–2) famously referred to the appearance of the Alexandrian grain fleet (*classis*) at Puteoli, and inscriptions indicate that by the time of Septimius Severus, this was under the supervision of an imperial procurator (*IG Italiae* 918, 919). An African grain fleet is also attested in the time of Commodus (SHA *Comm.* 17.7), but the precise meaning of *classis* (or *stolos* in our Greek sources) here is not entirely clear and is perhaps best understood as referring to a complex of vessels dedicated to this type of activity (Geraci, 2018). In any case, these do not appear to have been state merchant fleets, but consisted of private shippers (Rickman, 1980a, 129–130), and the actual transportation of the grain to Rome remained largely in the hands of private shippers.[8]

Grain distributions took place in cities other than Rome, but they were not commonplace. In Egypt, for example, Alexandria appears to have had a distribution (Eusebius *HE* 7.21.9), as did Hermopolis (*P. Lond.* 955, Vol. iii, 127–128), but the best documented is that of Oxyrhynchus in the third century, which modelled its monthly distribution on that of Rome.[9] They are also known of in other large cities by the late empire, such as Antioch, Constantinople, and possible Carthage (Woolf, 1990, 213).

Alimenta

Alimenta schemes were somewhat different to the grain distributions in that they provided funds specifically intended for the maintenance of children. These schemes are commonly associated with Trajan, who commemorated them with images on his coinage (e.g., *RIC* II 93, with the legend *ALIM. ITAL*), and on the carved stone balustrades of the Plutei Traiani in Rome.[10] The evidence indicates that more than 50 towns in Italy certainly benefited.[11] It was administered by a *quaestor alimentorum* (e.g., *ILS* 6620 from Assisi), and a well-known inscription from Veleia, dating to the early first century AD, sets out the details of the imperial scheme (*CIL* XI 1147).[12] The emperor provided a fund to the town, which was then invested in land through a system whereby local landowners were provided with a loan averaging 8% of the total value of their land, on which they paid 5% interest. The money that was given to the children came from the interest generated by the loans, which provided a stable and predictable return.

A number of private schemes are also documented, many of which predate the imperial schemes, such as those at Atina (*CIL* X 5056) and Florence (*CIL* XI 1602). Pliny also set up a scheme in his hometown of Como (*CIL* V 5262; Plin. *Ep.* 1.8, 7.18), and some are also known of outside of Italy, for example, in Sicca in Numidia in the second century AD (*CIL* VIII 1641).

In both the imperial and the private schemes, girls typically received less than boys, and for a shorter period of time. Furthermore, the round numbers of recipients of the funds, together with discrepancies between the sexes, indicates that eligibility was not based on need, and not all children from a town were necessarily included.[13] The Veleia inscription, for example, gives the details of both the imperial scheme and a much smaller pilot scheme set up by one Gallicus, which together provided funds for 300 children, comprising of 264 boys and 36 girls. Similarly, in the private scheme set up in Sicca in Numidia, 300 boys and 200 girls were to be supported, and those selected for inclusion were chosen by the duovirs (*CIL* VIII 1641).[14] Thus while a late fourth-century source, Pseudo-Aurelius Victor (12.4), claimed that Nerva set up the alimentary schemes in order that the boys and girls of needy (*egestas*) parents be supported at public expense throughout the towns of Italy, his attribution of a charitable motivation is almost certainly anachronistic, reflecting later Christian ideas of charity (Woolf, 1990, 204–205). The motivations that Pliny ascribes to Trajan for including children in donations in Rome are probably more pertinent (*Pan.* 26–28). Pliny presents this as a political measure, portraying Trajan as acting in his role as imperial benefactor and paternal figure. He also places an emphasis on the raising of loyal citizen children to serve in the army, although this need not imply any demographic crisis as such.[15]

Both the imperial and the private schemes are, therefore, to be seen within the wider context of imperial largesse and local euergetism. As with the grain distributions, some of those who received these donations may well have been in need, but by no means all the recipients were destitute; at Assisi, for example, the recipients used at least a proportion of the money that they obtained to set up an inscription to C. Alfius Clemens Maximus who administered the scheme on behalf of the emperor (*ILS* 6620). Nevertheless, these schemes must have had an impact on the local market for grain, since they increased the purchasing power of the urban population, albeit only modestly. At Veleia, for example, legitimate boys received 16 sesterces per month, enough to buy 4 *modii* of grain, assuming a price of 4 sesterces per *modius* (Duncan-Jones, 1982, 50–51).

Occasionally, food was also distributed by means of a public banquet (*epulum*), often connected with a religious festival or a public occasion, such as the dedication of a new public building. Pliny, for example, commemorated the dedication of his temple at Tifernum Tiberinum with a public banquet (*Ep.* 4.1.5–6), and Petronius talks of two municipal banquets at rates of 8 sesterces per head (45, 71).[16] However, such occasional banquets can hardly have had any long-lasting impact on urban diets, and in any case, only those of a certain social status would have been eligible to attend.

Market regulation and intervention

These measures were surely all well-received by the beneficiaries but they were far from poor relief and by no means all urban inhabitants were eligible. Many must have continued to rely on the market for their food supply, and the number of documented protests over the high prices of food surely indicates this, particularly in the early empire. During a period of prolonged drought and consequent high prices in Rome, for example, Claudius was apparently confronted in the forum and pelted with abuse and pieces of bread (Suet. *Claud.* 18.1–2; Tac. *Ann.* 12.43).[17] Outside of Rome, a speech of Dio Chrysostom relates to riots over high food prices that took place in his native Prusa around AD 100 (*Or.* 46).[18] The unpredictability and seasonality of ancient agriculture, coupled with the imperfect nature of ancient markets, meant that the market alone could not always be relied upon to provide a consistent supply of food at stable prices; the question is to what extent did the authorities intervene to regulate or influence this market?

Rome

The authorities had several options open to them to ensure that there was a supply of affordable grain on the market in Rome. They could, for instance, purchase or requisition additional grain directly; stockpile public grain to release on to the market; provide incentives to shippers and merchants to encourage them to supply grain to Rome; improve the administrative arrangements related to the grain supply; introduce rationing; invest in infrastructure; and/or fix the price of grain. This is not an exhaustive list of possible measures, nor are these measures mutually exclusive, but there is evidence to suggest that they were all employed at Rome at some point. Some were clearly short-term emergency measures introduced to deal with an immediate crisis in the grain supply, while others were more structural measures intended to stabilise the supply in the longer term. As will become apparent, the relative role of public and private grain and the extent of Roman intervention in the market remains something of an open question.[19]

Administration and infrastructure

From at least the mid-Republic, the grain supply of Rome was the concern of the aediles, although their focus appears to have been more on the distribution of grain than on its procurement (Rickman, 1980a, 34–36). They were also involved in its storage; Cicero writes that Caelius, the curule aedile in 50 BC, was in control of the Porta Flumentana, presumably referring to the granaries in that region (Cic. *Att.* 7.3.9). As the organisation of the grain supply became increasingly complex, Julius Caesar created two new aedileships, the *aediles cereales*, whose sole focus was the grain supply (Cass. Dio 43.51; *Dig.* 1.2.2.32). Prior to this development, however, in 57 BC, Pompey was granted command over the grain supply throughout the entire Roman world (*toto orbe terrarium*) for five years in the face of demonstrations over high prices in Rome, although this should of course be seen in the context of the politics of the late Republic and was far from a permanent solution to fluctuating prices (Cic. *Att.* 4.1.6–7; see also Plut. *Pomp.* 49–50).

With the emergence of a system of imperial government centred on the person of the emperor after the civil wars of the first century BC, it was both possible and expedient to turn to longer-term solutions for securing the grain supply of Rome. It took some time, however, for this to happen, and for much of his reign, Augustus continued to rely on *ad hoc* organisational measures and his own personal donations and interventions in times of shortage (see, for example, *RG* 5.1–2, 15.1, 18). Nevertheless, we can trace a gradual evolution in the administrative bureaucracy under Augustus (Rickman, 1980a, 62–65). In 22 BC, he took charge of the grain supply and instituted a commission run by two ex-praetors appointed annually, which later became known as the *praefecti frumenti dandi* (Suet. *Aug.* 37; Cass. Dio 54.1.4). This was concerned with the grain distributions, although the aediles still appear to have had oversight of the grain supply more generally. In 18 BC, the number of officials in the commission was raised to four (Cass. Dio 54.17.1). Following shortages in AD 6, Augustus appointed two ex-consuls to oversee the supply, a measure that he repeated in AD 7 (Cass. Dio 55.26.2–3, 55.31.4). Finally, at some point between AD 8 and AD 14, he instituted the office of the *praefectus annonae* (Tac. *Ann.* 1.7). This equestrian official was to have overall control of the grain supply of Rome and was answerable to the emperor personally.[20] A whole range of subordinates associated with the office developed over the first century AD (Robinson, 1992, 157). His chief assistant was called an *adiutor* but by the end of the second century was known as the *sub-praefectus annonae*; he was appointed directly by the emperor and commanded a substantial salary of 100,000 sesterces (Rickman, 1980a, 221–222).

There was also a proliferation of subsidiary posts in Rome, Ostia, and across the empire, especially in important grain-producing regions such as Egypt.[21] Already by the end of the second century BC, the main duties of the *quaestor Ostiensis* were linked to the grain supply, a role which continued into the early empire, although the full details of his involvement are unclear. In any case, with the development of the new harbour at Ostia under Claudius, he was replaced by the *procurator annonae Ostis* and the *procurator portus* (Suet. *Claud.* 24.2; Rickman, 1980a, 47–48; Robinson, 1992, 150).

This increasing bureaucracy was primarily concerned with the collection, transportation, and distribution of public grain, but its remit was much broader, encompassing the sale of grain by private merchants, as well as overseeing the distribution of other commodities, such as olive oil. An honorific dedication made in the reign of Hadrian to the *praefectus annonae* by the grain and olive oil dealers of Africa (*mercatores frumentarii et olearii Afrari*: *CIL* VI 1620), for example, suggests that the two groups had a similar relationship with the *praefectus annonae*. M. Petronius Honoratus, the *praefectus annonae* from 144-146/7 was even hailed as a patron by the olive oil dealers from Baetica (*CIL* VI 1625b; Potter and Mattingly, 1999, 191). Other officials were also involved in the supply of olive oil to Rome. A certain C. Pomponius Turpilianus, for instance, a procurator for oil in the warehouse of Galba, at Ostia, and at Portus in AD 175 (*proc(urator) ad oleum in Galbae Ostiae Portus utriusque*: *CIL* XIV 20), was presumably in charge of overseeing the movement of oil through the Horrea Galbana, which was probably closely associated with the nearby Monte Testaccio, an ancient rubbish dump composed of discarded olive oil amphorae from Baetica and North Africa (Holleran, 2012, 76–78; see also Rowan in this volume). An inscription from Hispalis in AD 166 (*CIL* II 1180) also honours one Sextus Julius Possessor, an assistant to the *praefectus annonae*, Ulpius Saturninus, who was in charge of overseeing the importation and transportation of Spanish and African oil, and may well have visited these regions in order to secure the supply of oil (Potter and Mattingly, 1999, 192).

The increasingly stable administration was likely to have had a positive effect on the market. The *praefectus annonae* headed a court, for instance, that dealt with disputes between parties involved in the food supply and those working for the *annona*, which may have reduced the risks and costs for contractors and merchants (e.g., *CIL* III 14165/8 for the case of the shippers from Arles in AD 201). The administration also ensured that the shipping lanes to Rome were kept free from piracy, that the Tiber was dredged (Suet. *Aug.* 30.1; SHA *Aurel.* 47.2–3), and the tow-paths maintained (Robinson, 1992, 91–93). Furthermore, capital investment was made in harbours, ports, and storage facilities, which can only have benefited private merchants.

By the early second century BC, the docks in the area of the Forum Boarium were becoming inadequate for the growing city, and the Aventine area began to be developed as an alternative river port. Notably it was the aediles M. Aemilius Lepidus and M. Aemilius Paulus who started this development in 193 BC, erecting a porticus outside the Porta Trigemina, together with an *emporium* stretching down to the Tiber (Livy 35.10.12).[22] Gaius Gracchus' grain law was apparently accompanied by the provision of additional granaries in Rome (Plut. *G. Gracc.* 6.3). These were presumably intended primarily for public grain, but their construction may have freed up space in existing granaries for private merchants. Further private storage facilities were also built over the course of the first century BC, such as the Horrea Lolliana and the Horrea Sulpicia, both of which came into imperial ownership over the course of the first century AD, with the latter becoming known as the Horrea Galbana (Holleran, 2012, 72–73). This reflects a general trend of increasing state involvement in the imperial period. Dock facilities were also constructed on both sides of the Tiber south of Tiber Island (Castagnoli, 1980).

There was no good natural harbour at Ostia, and in the Republic and early empire, large sea-going ships either had to unload onto smaller boats while riding at anchor offshore, or dock at Puteoli on the Bay of Naples and tranship their cargo to Rome. In AD 42 Claudius demonstrated a long-term interest in safeguarding the food supply of Rome by investing in the construction of a huge harbour basin 4 km to the north of Ostia. This had two curving breakwaters to provide shelter from the sea, a lighthouse, and was connected to the Tiber by canals (Suet. *Claud.* 20; Cass. Dio 60.11.1–5). This harbour, known as Portus, was not entirely successful, since ships within it were still vulnerable to storms (Tac. *Ann.* 15.18), but this problem was solved by Trajan's construction of a hexagonal inner harbour basin. Such measures can be classed as indirect, rather than direct, intervention in the market, but must have made the transportation and sale of grain and a range of other commodities much easier for traders.

Alongside the increasing administrative superstructure relating to the grain supply, the aediles continued to play a role in supervising the sale of both grain and other food in Rome. They oversaw sales in the *macella* ('luxury' food markets dedicated to the sale of meat and fish), enforced restrictions on the sale of food in cookshops, and regulated weights and measures (Robinson, 1992, 131–137; Holleran, 2012, 143, 175); at some point in the later empire, most of these roles passed into the hands of the urban prefect, although the date of the change is not known.

Stock piling, purchase, and requisition

If the state were to stockpile grain in the city, this could be released onto the market as necessary, thus manipulating prices by engineering a natural decrease. There are certainly some hints of state stockpiling in our ancient sources, although it is less clear how commonly this grain was released on the market.[23] In response to a famine in Rome in AD 6, for example, Augustus apparently doubled the amount of grain given to the recipients of the free distributions (Cass. Dio. 55.26.3); this was not market grain, but does suggest that large amounts were stored in the city. More than 200 years later, Septimius Severus is said to have managed the grain supply so well that on his death he left a surplus equivalent to seven years' tribute (*canon*; SHA *Sev.* 8.5–6, 23.2); the author(s) of the Historia Augusta claims that this was enough to distribute 75,000 *modii* of grain per day, although it is not clear if any such distributions actually took place or to whom the grain was given.[24]

Under Nero, grain was apparently stored in the city for so long that it went bad, and the emperor had it thrown into the Tiber in a very public demonstration that the grain supply was not a matter for concern (Tac. *Ann.* 15.18; Casson, 1980, 25). That this was grain intended for the market is indicated by Tacitus' follow-up remark that the price of grain was not raised, despite the additional accidental destruction of 300 grain ships in storm and fire. This is also implied by a further comment in Tacitus (*Ann.* 14.51) about Nero's appointment of Faenius Rufus as one of the commanders of the Praetorian Guard. He apparently chose Rufus for the role because of his popularity with the people, since he oversaw the provision of the capital without profit to himself, probably referring to his lack of profiteering in the sale of public grain. In his panegyric to Trajan (29), Pliny comments that harvests are no longer snatched from allies to perish in Rome's granaries, perhaps referring to the incident under Nero, or other unknown instances of spoiled grain under Trajan's predecessors. This passage also implies that such grain had in the past been requisitioned, whereas under Trajan, Pliny claims that grain was purchased at what appears to be a market price, as agreed between buyer and seller.

However, as Casson notes (1980, 25, 31 n.25), the importance placed on the arrival of grain ships in the city rather suggests that such stockpiles were not the norm. In AD 70, for example, after the apparent surplus of Nero's reign, the ships from Africa were delayed due to the harsh winter, and a rumour spread that Africa had revolted and the ports had been closed, causing fear among the people in the city (Tac. *Hist.* 4.38). Again, this does not appear to relate to grain intended for free distribution, since Tacitus notes that the people were accustomed to buy their food on a daily basis and therefore had no concerns other than the stability of the grain supply. If stockpiles of grain were the norm, the food supply would surely not be a matter of such perennial concern, nor would delay cause such anxiety in the city.

What this does indicate is that the authorities had an interest in the grain supply of Rome beyond the free distributions, and in fact they shipped far more grain to the city than was required annually for the dole (Erdkamp, 2005, 244). Much of this was grain exacted as tribute in kind and rent from the imperial estates, but as Pliny demonstrates (*Pan.* 29), grain could also be requisitioned or purchased by the state. However, on the basis of our sources, it is difficult to know the full extent of this practice. Neither is it clear exactly what happened to this additional public grain. It was probably not routinely stockpiled, but was most likely sold, and in normal circumstances at market price. Whether this was direct to consumers, to private merchants who acted as intermediaries, or even to bakers in the city is not certain.[25]

Rationing and price fixing

On only one occasion do we hear of grain being rationed in Rome, when this was introduced by Augustus in AD 6 as part of a range of measures intended to cope with a serious food shortage (Cass. Dio. 55.26.2–3), although as already noted above, there was apparently enough grain available for Augustus to double the amount given to the *plebs frumentaria*. The population was reduced through the banishment of gladiators and slaves for sale, the cutting of official retinues, a recess of the courts, and by official encouragement to senators to leave the city, while ex-consuls were appointed to oversee the supply of both grain and bread, ensuring that only a fixed quantity was sold to each person that remained.

Another option open to the authorities was to fix the price of grain and/or bread, but this does not seem to have been routine practice. As with rationing, this appears to have been largely an emergency measure introduced in times of shortage.[26] There are three instances known of in Rome. In AD 19, Tiberius fixed the price of grain after the people protested about high prices. This measure must have related to grain that was in the hands of private merchants, since Tiberius compensated them with a subsidy of 2 sesterces per *modius* (Tac. *Ann.*

2.87). In AD 64, Nero imposed a grain price of 3 sesterces per *modius* in the face of shortages caused by the great fire (Tac. *Ann*. 15.39.3). Finally in AD 189, Commodus ordered a general reduction in the price of grain, following shortages that appear to be primarily down to the political machinations of Cleander and Papirius Dionysius, the *praefectus annonae* (SHA *Comm*. 14.3; Herod. 1.12.3–4; Cass. Dio. 72.13.2).

Tiberius apparently proposed that the prices in the *macellum* should be regulated annually by the senate, but there is no evidence that this was actually implemented (Suet. *Tib*. 34.1). Furthermore, Suetonius presents this as a direct response to the sale of three mullets in the *macellum* for 30,000 sesterces, and it is part of a raft of measures intended to curb elite expenditure rather than stabilise food prices in general.[27]

The danger with price fixing is that merchants simply remove their grain from the market when it becomes unprofitable to sell, and the Romans were well aware of this problem.[28] The result of Commodus' reduction in prices was to make grain even rarer (SHA *Comm*. 14.3), and when discussing Julian's desire to reduce prices in Antioch, Ammianus Marcellinus (22.14.1) remarks that fixed prices tend to cause scarcity and famine if not properly regulated.[29] Price fixing would only really be a viable option in the long term if there was a fully public market for grain, or if other measures were taken to compensate private merchants, as with Tiberius' subsidy. Suetonius (*Aug*. 42) recognises that emperors had to achieve a delicate balance between the needs of the people and those of the farmers (*aratores*) and the grain dealers (*negotiantes*). In itself, this indicates that public grain only fulfilled a certain proportion of the demand for grain in Rome; the rest must have been supplied by the private market and it was therefore essential that the authorities did not alienate merchants. The availability of public grain on the market may also have been an issue here, since although it may have helped to stabilise prices, it may have made Rome an unattractive prospect for private traders. This of course largely depends on the amount of public grain available on the market, which is a matter of some debate. Erdkamp (2005, 257), for example, argues that two-thirds or more of the grain in Rome was public grain, while others see private merchants as the principal suppliers of the city.[30] Certainly the measures put in place to encourage merchants to bring grain indicate their importance, but what this actually means for their role in the food supply is less clear.

Encouragement to shippers

One of the major logistical problems of feeding Rome was ensuring that sufficient amounts of grain were shipped to the city. Claudius therefore offered incentives to merchants to bring grain to Rome even in the winter season (Suet. *Claud*. 18–19). He assumed the expense of any loss that might be suffered from storms, thus guaranteeing a profit. He also offered different inducements to merchants who built large ships, according to their status: citizens were exempted from the *Lex Papia Poppaea*; Latins were given the rights of Roman citizenship; and women were given the privileges allowed to those who had three or more children.[31] These were long-lasting measures that were apparently still in place in Suetonius' day. Nero also instituted tax breaks for merchants, since cargo-boats were not to be included in the assessment of a merchant's property nor were they to be treated as taxable (Tac. *Ann*. 13.51). By the second century, *negotiatores* and *navicularii* who were involved with the grain supply of Rome were granted immunity from public *munera* (*Dig*. 50.6.6.3–6; also 50.5.3). Notably, membership of a *corpus naviculariorum* was not in itself sufficient, but actual possession of ships had to be demonstrated, implying some fraud (see also *Dig*. 50.6.6.9). The organisation of those concerned with the grain supply, including shippers, boatmen, and porters, into such *corpora* and *collegia* at Ostia and Rome simplified the process on both sides.[32]

It is has been generally assumed that these incentives were intended to stimulate the market supply of grain, but it is equally likely, if not more so, that these measures relate to the shipping of public grain.[33] Certainly this is implied by Gaius' description of Claudius' measures, which includes the detail that Latins could acquire citizenship if they built a seagoing vessel with a capacity of at least 10,000 *modii* of grain and carried grain to Rome for six years (Gaius, *Inst.* 1.32c). The threshold was raised to 50,000 *modii* of grain in the second century AD (*Dig.* 50.5.3). The volume and regularity of supply almost certainly indicates a contract to ship public grain. If such incentives do indeed relate only to the shipment of public grain – and it should be noted that Rome never owned or controlled a grain fleet – then we can only assume that the sheer size of the market was enough to induce private merchants to supply the additional grain that was needed to feed the city, despite state intervention in the market.

Outside Rome

Rome was the largest and (at least from a political point of view) most important food market in the Roman world. However, the food supply was equally important for those living in other urban centres, and some similar measures were taken by local authorities to ensure the stability of supply and prices.

Price fixing

There is some evidence that officials were concerned with the regulation of prices in local markets, a role undertaken by aediles and *agoranomoi*. Pythias, the aedile that Lucius encounters in the market place in Hypata in Apuleius' novel *Metamorphoses*, for example, appears to be overseeing both quality and price, since he berates a fish seller for selling goods of inferior quality at a high price (1.24–25). Moreover, the *agoronamoi* at Roman Pergamum seem to be routinely fixing the price of small fish (*OGI* 484; Macro, 1976), although price fixing in general appears to be related either to shortages (and consequent high prices) or an anticipated period of high demand, such as a festival.[34] In Pisidian Antioch, for example, the provincial governor L. Antistius Rusticus ordered by edict the sale of stored grain at a fixed maximum price of four sesterces per *modius* during a time of high prices in AD 93 (*AE* 1925, 126; Erdkamp, 2005, 286–288). Notably this edict included the stipulation that all the citizens and inhabitants of Antioch must make any grain not needed for seed or for family use available to buyers, preventing merchants from simply withdrawing grain from the market.[35] In any case, the maximum price was still double what it had been before the shortage. This was a reactive measure, with the governor responding to a request for help from the local town councillors. Although not in force in this period, it is worth noting that a rescript of the emperors Marcus Aurelius and Lucius Verus in the later second century AD prohibited the local ordo from fixing prices for grain, stating also that were unable to force any decurion to sell grain below market price (*Dig.* 48.12.3, 50.1.8, 50.8.7(5)).

Known examples of price fixing are rare before late antiquity, when a number of instances are documented in Syrian Antioch in particular. These took place in AD 354, 362, and 384, and are perhaps reflective of a more general trend of increasing state interference in prices, although it is equally true that these may simply be exceptional examples or a coincidence of the availability of sources on the affairs of Antioch in this period (Erdkamp, 2005, 291–292). The lack of appetite for price fixing among local elites is hardly surprising. First, the local elites were very often landowners with an active interest in maximising grain prices (Lib. *Or.* 18.195–197), and second, price fixing blocked avenues for euergetism on their part during times of shortage. Furthermore, it alienated merchants from outside the local area since it made exporting grain to a city with a fixed price less attractive.

There is some evidence to suggest that the focus of local authorities was more on fixing the price of bread than the price of grain, with the weight and size of bread varying but the price of bread remaining roughly the same (Garnsey and Van Nijf, 1998, 312; Erdkamp, 2005, 298–302). The bulk of the evidence for this practice comes from Ephesus and relates to the food supply during a festival, but this was an approach common in early modern European cities, and a comment from a character in Petronius (*Sat.* 44) about the magistrates being in league with the bakers and the changing size of bread suggests that the practice was more widespread.[36]

Municipal grain funds

There were other means by which local authorities could regulate prices and ensure a consistent urban food supply. In the Greek East, municipal grain funds seem to be fairly common, especially in the second and early third century AD when numerous inscriptions, concentrated particularly but not exclusively in Asia Minor, testify to the presence of *sitonia* and their associated officials, *sitonai*.[37] Ulpian in fact seems to view grain funds (*frumentaria pecunia*) as essential for the survival of a community (*Dig.* 50.8.2.3; see also Herodian 7.3.5), although there is less evidence for such funds in the western provinces (and none at all in Egypt). Inscriptions testify to private donations to the grain funds, which may well have been the main source of their funds (e.g., *CIL* III 6998), making it difficult to separate grain funds out from the wider practice of *euergetism*, although Zuiderhoek (2008) argues for significant support from civic public finances also. Quite how these funds were used is not entirely clear. It is possible that they were used as a financial reserve to cushion against the worst effects of unforeseen shortages, but since grain would obviously be less available at such times, it would be more effective to purchase grain regularly and keep it in storage. Whether this was sold on the market or distributed, and whether it was made available to urban inhabitants regularly or just in times of shortage, is not known, but these funds must surely have had some impact on the workings of the private market.

The authorities also sometimes intervened to ensure that there was an adequate supply of olive oil on the market. Hadrian, for example, issued a decree regulating the sale of olive oil produced in Attica, with local producers obligated to sell one third of their olive oil to the 'oil buyers' (*elaionai*) in Athens and the details of exports recorded.[38] A passage in the *Digest* (50.4.18.5) attributed to the Diocletianic lawyer Arcadius Charisius, implies that *elaionai* were similar to *sitonai*, with both being regularly appointed officials charged with overseeing the purchase of oil and grain respectively, suggesting that the measures put in place by Hadrian were not unique to Athens.

The obligation on local producers to ensure that the local market was supplied before any agricultural produce was exported is also indicated by Ulpian's comment (*Dig.* 7.1.27.3) that it was typical practice for landowners to sell a fixed proportion of their produce to municipal authorities at a low price (although compare *Dig.* 48.12.3, 50.1.8, 50.8.7(5), discussed above). Furthermore, Arcadius Charisius (50.4.18.25) claims that some communities had the right to demand that those who held property in their territory provide a quantity of grain annually, according to the extent of their land. Political coercion, perhaps with additional social pressure, was then another means by which local authorities could ensure a stable food supply for urban centres, particularly in the staples of grain and olive oil.

RIC II = Mattingly, H. and Sydenham, E.A. 1926. *Roman Imperial Coinage. Volume 2, Vespasian to Hadrian.* London.

Notes

1 On urbanisation rates see, for example, Erdkamp, 2012b, 245–247.
2 At the very least, Rome required a minimum of 150,000 tonnes of grain per year to survive, assuming 200 kg of grain per person per year on the basis of a population of one million (Garnsey, 1983, 118); in reality, it must have needed much more, given the higher standard of living enjoyed by some and the probable rates of wastage (on which, see Geraci, 2018). See also Mattingly and Aldrete, 2000, 154 for higher subsistence requirements.
3 Grain from Spain and Africa was apparently distributed by the aediles at a low price of 4 asses per modius in 203 and 201 BC (Livy 30.26, 31.4), and 2 asses in 200 BC (Livy 31.50). See also Livy 33.42 for Sicilian grain distributed at 2 asses in 196 BC. For G. Gracchus' measure, see Cic. *Sest.* 25.55, 48.103; Vell. Pat. 2.6.3; Plut. *C. Gracch.* 5; Rickman, 1980a, 158–161.
4 For more details on these interim measures, see Rickman, 1980a, 161–172; also briefly Robinson, 1992, 151.
5 Other estimates range as high as 270 kg per person per annum; see Mattingly and Aldrete, 2000, 142; 158 n.8, with further references.
6 For Severus Alexander, see, for example, Wilson, 2000, 237; Erdkamp, 2005, 254.
7 See in particular Erdkamp, 2005, 206–237, also Garnsey, 1983, 120-21, *contra* Rickman, 1980a, 72.
8 See also pp. 291–292.
9 See Rea, 1972, for an archive of papyri documenting the details of this distribution (*P.Oxy.* XL 2892–2940).
10 See also Cass. Dio, 68.5.4. Interestingly, Pliny makes no mention of these schemes in his Panegyricus, but he does praise Trajan for including children in his donations in Rome (26–28). For later emperors and their involvement in these schemes, see SHA *Hadr.* 7.8; *Ant. Pius* 8.1; *Marc. Aur.* 7.8, 26.4-9; *Pert.* 9.3; *Alex. Sev.* 57.4-7; Woolf, 1990, 221–222.
11 Duncan-Jones (1982, 337–341, Appendix 5) gives a figure of 49 towns, to which two more can now be added, at Ticinum and Bovianum (Carlsen, 2013, 48).
12 A similar but less detailed inscription also survives from Ligures Baebiani (*CIL* IX 1455)
13 For an overview of historiography relating to the *alimenta* schemes and the debate over whether or not they reflect a genuine concern with providing economic aid to families, see Carlsen, 2013, 40–44.
14 A private scheme from Tarracina in Italy, recorded in an inscription dating to the second century AD, also included a limited number of recipients, although there was an even balance between the sexes, with 100 boys and 100 girls supported (*CIL* X 6328). Girls, however, only received three *denarii* a month up to the age of 14, while boys received five *denarii* up to the age of 16.
15 See Duncan-Jones, 1964, 127 for the argument that the primary aim of the scheme was to augment the birth rate.
16 For further discussion and references, see Duncan-Jones, 1982, 139–140.
17 See also Tac. *Ann.* 2.87; 6.13 for protests under Tiberius (also 4.6 for high food prices in Rome). Under Nero, see Suet. *Nero* 45.
18 See also Philostratus' account of a food riot in Aspendus (*VA* 1.15), although its fictional nature has been emphasised (Raeymaekers, 2000). Also Philostr. *VS* 23; Lib. *Or.* 1.205-9. On food riots in the Roman world, see Erdkamp, 2002.
19 On the one hand see, for example, Casson, 1980, who argues that aside from the grain distributions and the feeding of government personnel, the grain trade was largely in the hands of private traders. On the other hand, see, for example, Erdkamp, 2005, 237–257, who argues that public channels contributed more than private enterprise to the city of Rome. In general, see also Garnsey, 1983, 127–128.
20 For some example careers of the *praefectus annonae*, see Rickman, 1980a, 218–221.
21 On which see, for example, Mattingly and Aldrete, 2000, 151–153; Rickman, 1980a, 222–225.
22 See also Livy 40.51, 41.27.8–9 for further development of this area in 179 and 174 BC. Holleran, 2012, 65–67. In general, see Rickman, 1980a, 45–48.
23 See Geraci, 2018, who describes the fear of running out of food and resultant stockpiling as Rome's 'grain psychosis'.
24 He also apparently left such a surplus of oil that there was enough for five years' use not only in Rome, but in Italy as a whole (SHA *Sev.* 23.2).
25 See Erdkamp, 2005, 251–255 for both suggestions.
26 On price fixing of grain, see in particular Garnsey and Van Nijf, 1998.

27 Holleran, 2012, 175. See also 160–181 for the *macellum* as a luxury food market in Rome, 177–179 for high prices. Garnsey and Van Nijf, 1998, 304–305 link Tiberius' measure to demonstrations about the price of grain in the theatre in AD 32, but there is no evidence that grain was sold in the *macellum* and the two incidents are unlikely to be related. Certainly Tacitus (*Ann.* 6.13) makes no mention of this response to the demonstrations.

28 A similar argument is made by Garnsey and Van Nijf, 1998, 305.

29 See also Lib. *Or.* 15.21. Also Lactantius, *De Mort. Pers.* 7.6 for the market in goods drying up in response to Diocletian's Edict of Maximum Prices.

30 See note 19.

31 The *Lex Papia Poppaea* restricted the rights of the unmarried and childless to inherit. Women who had given birth to three children (and freedwomen to four) did not require a guardian.

32 Rickman, 1980b, 271; Garnsey, 1983, 125, 127–128; Mattingly and Aldrete, 2000, 148–149; Sirks, 2007, 177–78. See also the detailed study of Sirks, 1991, *passim.*

33 For these as measures intended to stimulate the market, see for example Casson, 1980, 25; Rickman, 1980a, 72; 1980b, 269. As related to the shipment of state grain, see Erdkamp, 2005, 245–249; Garnsey and Saller, 2014, 113.

34 See also Steinhauer, 1994, for maximum prices in first century BC Piraeus; Vatin, 1966 for price setting of fish at Delphi. For the link between festivals and fixed prices, see Garnsey and Van Nijf, 1998.

35 Similar measures are recorded in Oxyrhynchus in AD 246 (P. Oxy. 42.3048; Erdkamp, 2005, 288).

36 See also SHA *Aurel.* 47.1–2 for Aurelian adding an ounce to the bread for free distribution.

37 On municipal grain funds, see in particular Erdkamp, 2005, 268–283, on which the following is based. See also Zuiderhoek, 2008.

38 Erdkamp, 2005, 273.

24

FAMINE AND HUNGER
IN THE ROMAN WORLD

Paul Erdkamp

[The personification of Hunger is found in] a stubborn stony field,
Grubbing with nails and teeth the scanty weeds.
Her hair was coarse, her face sallow, her eyes sunken;
Her lips crusted and white; her throat scaly with scurf.
Her parchment skin revealed the bowels within;
Beneath her hollow loins jutted her withered hips;
Her sagging breasts seemed hardly fastened to her ribs;
Her stomach only a void; her joints wasted and huge,
Her knees like balls, her ankles grossly swollen.

(Ovid, Metamorphoses *799–808)*

Introduction

Ovid's description of the personification of Hunger as an emaciated woman finds a parallel in the painting of 'Famine' in the Temple of Chalkioikos, a pale and starved woman, with hands tied at her back. Hunger and the fear of starvation were omnipresent in the Roman world (as in most premodern societies) and most people had probably witnessed – if not experienced themselves – the ravages of deprivation. The fate of starving – or dying of its side-effects – undoubtedly affected only a small minority of the individuals that ever lived in the Roman world, but that does not mean that famine and starvation were marginal and of little concern to most people. Of course, not every disruption of the food supply caused real famine. Peter Garnsey defined famine as "a critical shortage of essential foodstuffs leading through hunger to starvation and a substantially increased mortality rate in a community or region". On most occasions the consequences of a subsistence crisis were less disastrous, merely leading to "a short-term reduction in the amount of available foodstuffs, as indicated by rising prices, popular discontent, hunger, in the worst cases bordering on starvation".[1] The differentiation between famine and shortage is important, but it also is an artificial distinction, and there is no clear dividing line between them. During famines people succumbed *en masse* to the lack of food or the diseases that went with it, but among the poorest classes of society individuals died of hunger and deprivation-related diseases at all times. In normal years, when harvests reached expected levels and no plundering armies roamed the land, the sustenance of most people was at least sufficient, even if the calories largely came from the kinds of grains and pulses that were scorned by the more privileged. There was a continuous fluctuation with the seasons between times of relative scarcity and times of relative abundance. In times of dearth, more households had to turn to food that they would otherwise have rejected as only fit for animals, and more individuals faced the threat of hunger and fatal disease. In other words, as times were hard or kind, the consumption of inferior foods and the threat of death ascended or descended the social ladder, but there is no clear boundary between famine and normality.

The literary sources

Famine and hunger are relatively invisible in our sources. Almost all literary texts were written by members of the elite – or people who socially, culturally and politically stood close to the elite – and these writers had little interest in the affairs of the poor and marginal people, a segment of society that includes many inhabitants of the countryside. A similar social blindness affects the epigraphic sources. Numerous inscriptions survive that honour benefactors and magistrates for their deeds when market prices were high and the food supply of their particular town was under pressure, but it is not in the nature of these commemorative texts to shed light on whether the shortage that occasioned the benefactor's or magistrate's intervention caused hunger and starvation among the common people.

We have several relatively detailed accounts of famines in the surviving texts. The Jewish historian Flavius Josephus (AD 37–c. 100), for example, mentions serious food shortages and severe famine several times in his works. His most detailed account describes events in 25/24 BC in Palestine. The bishop and church historian Eusebius (AD c. 260–340) describes a famine that struck Palestine in AD 312/313. In the so-called Chronicle of Joshua the Stylite (early sixth century AD) a graphic and detailed chronological account is given of the famine and pestilence that struck Edessa in AD 500/501,[2] while the early-Byzantine historian Procopius (AD c. 500–560) describes the severe scarcity that struck northern Italy during the wars against the Goths.[3] These detailed accounts bring together crucial aspects, such as weather conditions, harvests and emergency crops, seasonal developments, geographical scale, food prices, migration and disease, and sometimes even an estimate of the number of deaths, and thereby shed some light on causality and severity of these mortality crises. However, such narratives are rare, and their impressionistic nature, in particular the lack of quantitative data – or the lack of specificity of these data – rules out the kind of analysis that is possible for famines occurring in Europe from the fourteenth century onwards. Relatively numerous are brief mentions of shortages of the following kind: in AD 46/47 Jerusalem "was struck by a severe famine (*limos*) and many died because they lacked the money to buy what they needed" (Flavius Josephus, *AJ* 20.51). How many died and how widespread the dearth was beyond Jerusalem is impossible to say on the basis of this passing note.

Even more problematic is that the written sources remain silent on much of the Roman world for most of the time. Symptomatic is that Flavius Josephus merely mentions in passing that the dearth causing famine in Judea in 25/24 BC also affected the neighbouring lands, but no existing source sheds any light on how people there were affected by this shortage. Our sources are fairly good on political and cultural centres such as Rome, Alexandria and Constantinople, and we may safely assume that severe famines causing mass starvation in these cities would be known to us if they had occurred. However, less severe shortages that increased mortality to a lesser extent or mainly among the poor may still go under the radar. Most importantly, many regions – such as Spain, Gaul, Britain and Central Europe – remain in the dark, with at best occasional glimpses on local affairs if something happened that was deemed interesting from the perspective of the political and cultural centre. It is simply an effect of the surviving sources that we hear more about food shortages in Asia Minor or Palestine than in Spain or Britain. Moreover, the sixth century AD is represented well, because many texts from this period have survived and because Christian authors of that era became interested in apocalyptic events.[4] This is no indication at all that famine was rare at other times or in other regions – it only shows that none of the sparse surviving texts picked up the shortages that undoubtedly occurred in these regions and periods.

Natural causes and prevention strategies

Until the 1980s, explanations of famines focussed on the production side of the food supply, such as weather-induced harvest failures. With the works of Robert Fogel and Amartya Sen, attention shifted to the distribution-side of things. Interpreting the price-data for Early Modern England, Fogel concluded that in all years that subsistence crises occurred, the harvest had been sufficient to feed the entire populace and therefore argued that famines were caused by "dramatic redistributions of entitlements to grain" (Fogel, 1992; cf. Vanhaute, 2011, 50–51). Recent research has reaffirmed the importance of fluctuations in harvest size as causes of variations in mortality (Persson, 1999; Ó Gráda, 2007, 10; Campbell and Ó Gráda, 2011). The causality of subsistence crises is complex, but it is safe to say that natural causes are equally as important as the failure of commercial and governmental institutions and households to ensure equal access to available food.[5]

The success of crops depends on the right amount of precipitation at the right time of year. Many parts of the Mediterranean are especially vulnerable to unfavourable weather conditions, as summers tend to be dry or periods of heavy rainfall may cause flooding or damage to standing crops. In central Spain, southern Italy, southern Greece and parts of the Near East, average levels of precipitation are quite low for most types of cereals and legumes, thereby increasing the susceptibility to variations in the timing of precipitation within the year. If the drought set in before the crop was ready to ripen or if the field was flooded, yields were low or the crop entirely lost (Stathakopoulos, 2004, 36–39). Although our literary sources mainly tell us about the practice on the farms of prosperous landowners, comparative ethnographic research confirms that smallholders knew several strategies to cope with these dangers.[6] First, farmers diversified their crops, as for instance barley and millet are more drought resistant than most types of wheat, and also several kinds of legumes withstood dry and hot conditions well (e.g. Pliny, *Epist.* 1.20.16–17). Moreover, the growth cycle of some cereals and legumes was sufficiently short as to allow an emergency sowing in the spring if the autumn-sown crop had failed (e.g., Columella, *R.R.* 2.6.2). Second, farmers preferred to spread their land across the landscape, giving each farmer a share in different soil types and susceptibilities to weather conditions (e.g., Pliny, *Epist.* 3.19.4). Both strategies lowered the average volatility of the crops and spread the risks each farmer bore, but could not avoid local dearth when yields were disastrously low in some years. Whether yields failed did not only depend on the meteorological conditions, but also on the expectations of the farmers, who obviously knew the uncertainty of the weather. Comparison with more recent premodern farming in the Mediterranean shows that peasants aimed to produce more than needed. Average yields tended to produce a surplus, which peasants did not always sell, but often used to fatten an additional pig or increase next year's sowing. Storing reserves for future meagre times was also part of the coping strategies of smallholders, but the role of long-term storage beyond a year's needs should not be overrated. The general depiction of the winter and early spring as a period of scarcity, during which some country-dwellers even had to fall back on acorns and fodder, shows that many households lacked the reserves to alleviate the impact of bad harvests through inter-annual storage.

Finally, smallholders approached relatives and neighbours for assistance in times of need. For example, in a fictional account of rustic life, a peasant woman says: "Last year we borrowed some wheat just for seed, but we repaid them as soon as harvest time was come" (Dio Chrysostom, *Orat.* 7.68). This passage illustrates the seasonal constraints on smallholders' resources, but also the fact that many poor people had social ties with more prosperous members of the smallholding class. During minor crises, assistance from relatives and neighbours undoubtedly helped to ward off starvation. When rural communities were hit hard, however, one needed recourse to the help of wealthy landowners. The latter, however, weighed the advantages of social standing against the opportunities to make large profits by selling their crops for cash or on credit. Indebtedness of smallholders, in part resulting from the need to acquire food and seed, was a recurring issue in ancient politics and historiography. Moralist writers also lament the unwelcome side-effects of increased absentee landownership on the circumstances of the rural population.

In the end, none of the coping strategies was sufficient to evade the disastrous effects of major crises, which, as we shall see, pushed a large share of households into starvation or flight.

Man-made causes and coping strategies

Subsistence crises were partly a question of entitlement, which depended on economic status, political status, and on social status within the household and wider society. The state took control of a significant percentage of total available food in the form of taxation in kind, with armies adding requisitions, plunder and devastation in times of war. In a period when the average army was several times as large as most towns, warfare generally had an even more devastating impact on the food supply of local communities than bad weather (Erdkamp, 1998). The Romans soon realized that regular taxes in kind were the most effective way of feeding their armies, so from the third century BC onwards taxes were introduced that siphoned off a fixed percentage of the harvest (20% in the case of Sicily and Sardinia, 10% in Spain). Taxes in kind, in particular of Egypt (grain), Africa (grain and olive oil) and Spain (olive oil) remained important in imperial times, when the food supply of the city of Rome largely depended on it. Occasionally, when other sources failed, provincial cities profited from the imperial control of grain and their magistrates were allowed to buy Roman tax-grain. The distribution of tax-grain was solely governed by political status, as it were primarily the inhabitants of the capital city of Rome (and from about AD 330 the populace of Constantinople) and the Roman armies that had access to it, and only secondarily the inhabitants of those cities that had close political ties with the Roman imperial authorities, such as Athens and Ephesus.[7] Pliny the Younger (*Pan.* 30–31) boasts that even Egypt had to turn to the emperor for help when the harvests there had failed due to drought. Until the fourth century, Rome's control of foodstuffs had sufficient capacity to ward off severe food shortages in all major cities, but the majority of its subjects in smaller towns and in the countryside did not benefit from the imperial granaries.

During crises, the common people benefitted occasionally from the intervention of local and central authorities, for instance when the latter forced landowners to sell their stocks and imposed maximum prices on the market (Erdkamp, 2005, 265–268; cf. Holleran in the previous chapter). The authorities, who in normal times supervised, but not fixed market prices, resorted to market intervention in times of crisis in order to ensure local stability. In one famous case, the Roman governor was invited by the council of the relatively small town of Antioch in Pisidia to compel landowners to sell all their stocks beyond their personal need for the immediate future. For the measure to work, he also imposed a maximum price, which was still much higher than normal prices (Erdkamp, 2005, 286–288). Emperors failed when they imposed badly conceived measures on the urban market, as the historian Ammianus Marcellinus (22.14.1) observed regarding imperial intervention in fourth-century Antioch in Syria.[8]

Landowners and grain merchants are often blamed in our sources for causing shortages by withholding stocks from the market, but the scope for local estate-owners and local businessmen to drive up prices should not be overestimated (Erdkamp, 2005, 264–265; cf. Ó Gráda, 2007, 14). Businessmen undoubtedly profited from shortages to drive up their profits, but most traders were too small to corner the market. In general, authorities had every reason to ensure an adequate food supply and stable prices on the urban markets, and usually succeeded in doing so, but this has been dealt with in the previous chapter. The point is, that only a particular segment of society, in particular those living in cities and larger towns, profited from official market intervention.

Before Christianity dominated the Roman Empire, say, before the fourth century AD, authorities and benefactors did not aim their measures at the poor and destitute, but rather at those citizens that were deemed worthy of their attention. There are no known distributions or schemes that were particularly, let alone exclusively, aimed at those in desperate need. Lack of interest in our sources makes it impossible to assess the impact of the official measures on the situation of the poorest members of society in times of crisis. In his account of the famine that struck Palestine in the early fourth century AD, bishop Eusebius (*Hist. Eccl.* 9.8.14) underlines the respect and popularity that the Christians earned by their good deeds towards those in need in the absence of any official institution. Despite the obvious Christian bias, there may be much truth in his point.

Finally, we should not overestimate the role of commercial channels in alleviating local dearth. The drivers of trade were not hunger and local demand, but profit and buying power, while transaction costs acted as a brake on the activities of traders to connect supply and demand. Few people could afford to pay excessively high prices for a prolonged period, despite the threat of starvation, while the countryside lacked the necessary contacts, networks, and infrastructure to attract traders. The rural market, moreover, was dispersed over a wide region, adding costs to sellers. Cities, which were constantly bringing in outside supplies, were the preferred destinations of traders, as they offered a concentrated market, the necessary infrastructure, networks and communication channels to grain dealers (Erdkamp, 2005, 175–205). But even large cities could fail to attract sufficient commercial shipments, despite their advantages, as, for example, happened in Antioch in AD 362/3, when the emperor Julian had to bring in supplies from Egypt (Julian, *Misop.* 369b). In addition, high transportation costs over land soon made exporting trade to inland regions unprofitable, as illustrated by a famous passage in the works of Gregory of Nazianzus (*In laudem Basilii* 34–35):

> There was a food crisis, the most terrible in the memory of man. The city languished but there was no help from any part, no remedy for the calamity. Cities on the seacoast easily endure a shortage of this kind, importing by sea the things of which they are short. But we who live far from the sea profit nothing from our surplus, nor can we produce what we are short of, since we are able neither to export what we have nor import what we lack.

Food riots

A combination of an internalized mentality of social obligation, paternalist attitudes, and the endeavour to increase one's social status probably motivated many of the benefactions and market interventions by civilians and magistrates in the towns and cities of the Roman world, but in much of the Mediterranean world the urban populace did not hesitate to remind them of their duties when the market was under pressure and prices became high.[9] "A hungry people neither listens to reason, nor is appeased by justice, nor is bent by any entreaty," Seneca (*De brevitate vitae* 18.5) observes, lamenting furthermore that the emperor Gaius' foolish actions had nearly led to "the city's destruction and famine and the general revolution that follows famine". Food riots are often seen as a symptom of food shortage, but there is no linear connection between the threat of starvation and the willingness to riot. As E. P. Thompson famously said, people who are starving do not riot.

The satirical novel of Petronius (AD 27–66) provides an interesting, although fictional example of how dearth could lead to rumours and urban unrest. One of the characters, Ganymedes, is made to exclaim:

> You go talking about things which are neither in heaven nor earth, and none of you care all the time how the price of food pinches. I swear I cannot get hold of a mouthful of bread to-day. And how the drought goes on. There has been a famine for a whole year now. Damn the magistrates, who play "Scratch my back, and I'll scratch yours" in league with the bakers. So the little people come off badly; for the jaws of the upper classes are always keeping carnival. I do wish we had the fellows I found here when I first came out of Asia. [. . .] I remember Rafinius [. . .] You could trust him [. . .] So at that time food was dirt-cheap. Buying a loaf of bread for an as, it took more than two to eat it. One sees an ox's eye bigger now!
>
> (Petronius, *Sat. 44*)

During his tirade, Ganymedes makes the following remark: "If we had any spunk in us he [the magistrate] would not be so pleased with himself. Nowadays people are lions in their own houses and foxes out of doors" (*Sat.* 44). This is clearly a reflection of how rumours and dissatisfaction with public officials led to unrest and rioting.

Our examples of riots outside Rome are mostly limited to the towns of the Greek East. In a fictional account of a riot in the town of Aspendus, we are told that the outraged populace threatened to burn the local governor alive, because the local landowners had withdrawn their stocks of grain from the market (Philostratus, *Vit. Apoll.* 15; cf. Raeymaekers, 2000). Similarly, the orator Dio Chrysostom tells us in one of his orations that he was threatened by the town's populace, together with an unnamed neighbour, to be "stoned or burned to death", as he was held responsible for the city's food supply (Dio Chrysostom, *Orat.* 46,4–11).

Rioters aimed their demonstrations, often resorting to violence, against the people who they thought were responsible for taking the necessary measures, whether these were consuls, leading officials or emperors in Rome. At one time, the protesters threw pieces of stale bread at the emperor Claudius to express their discontent. In the fourth century AD, rioters burned down the house of the urban prefect because they were dissatisfied with the price of wine (Ammianus Marcellinus 27.3,4).[10] Rioters were sometimes more direct than resorting to loud and occasionally violent forms of communication. A not historic but nevertheless noteworthy account of the strained relations between the wealthy and the poor in Rome during the legendary first years of the Republic sheds light on this kind of mob violence:

> Their hatred did not lead to any irreparable mischief as often happens in like disorders. For on the one hand the poor did not attack the houses of the rich, where they suspected they should find stores of provisions laid up, nor attempt to raid the public stores.
>
> (Dionysius of Halicarnassus 7.18,3)

The author would not have deemed it necessary to note what he thought had not happened in early Rome, if it had not provided a striking contrast to the unrestrained violence of his own time, i.e., the late first century BC. In late Republican Rome, it seems, dearth and high prices were sufficient to legitimise the plundering of civilian and public stores. Nevertheless, a shortage of wine does not cause hunger, and starving people do not use bread to throw at the emperor. One final example: in first-century BC Rome, a riot was violently ended by soldiers, who afterwards plundered the nice clothes of the more affluent victims (Appian, *B.C.* 5.68). Real famine did not occur in ancient Rome, and hence the more prosperous citizens, who could afford better clothes, did not have to fear starvation. While we cannot rule out that the subsistence crises in these cases threatened the survival of at least part of the urban community, it was primarily the urban populace's sense of outrage that determined the violent nature of food riots in ancient cities.

Famine in Palestine, Edessa and Italy

We have several relatively detailed narratives of disastrous famines in the Roman world, which offer sufficient detail to give us an impression of the severity of the shortage. In addition we have numerous brief glimpses of similar phenomena, which may indicate widespread starvation, but do not allow a real understanding of the magnitude of the crisis. In view of my previous argument, we may be sure that the relatively few instances in the written sources seriously underrepresent the occurrence of famine in the Roman world.

Flavius Josephus (*AJ* 15.299ff) ascribes the famine that occurred in Palestine in 25/24 BC to severe drought. As all the stores were soon consumed, there was no seed for next year. Starvation was followed by epidemic, because – so Josephus tells us – the lack of food meant that eating habits changed and there was no nourishment for the diseased. Country-dwellers lost their livestock to the drought or slaughtered the animals for food. Also the neighbouring countries were hit hard, which made it difficult to alleviate the crisis through imports. King Herod, however, managed to acquire permission from the Roman governor of Egypt to buy grain there for food and seed, and thereby ended the shortage. The story is very impressionistic, lacking any figures, except for the quantity of grain that Herod acquired in Egypt.

Unlike Josephus, Eusebius (in AD 314 appointed bishop of Caesarea) was a contemporary of the famine in Palestine in AD 312/313. Again, the famine is said (*Hist. Eccl.* 9.8.1–15) to have been caused by drought and to have been followed by an epidemic disease that killed or blinded many people. Prices rose dramatically: a measure of wheat was sold for 2,500 Attic drachmae. People had to sell all their possessions to raise money to buy food and resorted to eating fodder and harmful plants. In the city, women of high birth begged in the streets; the destitute dropped dead while begging. Well-to-do citizens stopped handing out food to the needy as they saw no end coming to the famine and feared for their own fate. Eusebius observes that many died in the cities, but even more in the countryside and villages, referring to empty registers of peasants to substantiate his point. The crisis spared no one, he observed: those who had sufficient means to survive the famine – the rich, the magistrates and officials – succumbed to the epidemic. The Christians were the only ones who showed mercy, Eusebius underlines, handing out bread to the starving.

The town of Edessa was located on the upper Euphrates, about 200 km east of the Mediterranean. The famine of AD 500/501 is narrated in one of the most detailed accounts of the ancient world. The writer, conventionally known as Ps.-Joshua or Joshhua the Stylite (*Chron.* 39–46), pays much attention to the prices of foodstuffs such as wheat, barley, chickpeas, beans, lentils, wine and raisins, noting that at first meat was not dear, although prices of meat, fowl and eggs soared later. "Everything that was not edible was cheap, such as clothes and household utensils and furniture, for these things were sold for a half or a third of their value and did not suffice for the maintenance of their owners, because of the great dearth of bread" (39). Grain from the public granaries did not solve the crisis, because the poor lacked the money to buy bread. Instead, they bought turnips and cabbage, which they ate raw, but also vegetables became scarce. The villagers were eating bitter-vetch and – after the vintage – fallen, withered grapes; those in the city consumed stalks and leaves of vegetables. Even cannibalism occurred, the chronicler assures his readers. Distributions of money and bread did not suffice to end the famine. In February of the second year, there was a dearth of everything. The harvest did not succeed in alleviating the shortage and wheat prices remained high, although the harvest of dried grapes "amply supplied the poor". During the crisis Edessa was full of country-dwellers who had fled to the town and people died in the streets. The pestilence became worse in November and December. The infirmaries set up by the state and private benefactors attracted refugees from far and wide, as famine and pestilence struck the region as far as Antioch and Nisibis. In the second year, it is observed, the rich who had survived the famine died of disease. Finally, the new harvest succeeded in lowering the prices.

Procopius (*Bell. Goth.* 2.20-15-33) blames the harvest failure in northern Italy in approx. AD 530 on the disruption of agriculture caused by the war against the Goths. The people of Aemilia fled to Picenum in the expectation that the problems would be less severe closer to the sea. There was dearth also in Tuscany, where people processed acorns into bread. At least 50,000 peasants died in Picenum, Procopius writes, but even more in the regions that were further from the sea. People succumbed, he adds, while gathering grasses to satisfy their hunger.

Fames et pestilentia

All the themes of these famine narratives, such as the consumption of fodder and grass, recur in more fragmentary mentions of food shortages. The eating of grass, hay and even human flesh in such texts are dramatic elements accentuating the gravity of the crisis, but it seems likely that fodder and such plants that also play a role at normal times were more important emergency foodstuffs. A recent study of the famine striking Greece during World War II notes that people mainly resorted to foodstuffs that were eaten under normal conditions as well, although then more rarely and/or by a smaller – poorer – segment of society. The author argues that generally most famine foods were part of the diet in normal times (Hionidou, 2011; cf. Stathakopoulos, 2004, 81–87). Also the Roman agricultural writers mention such crops as vetch, lupins, rape and cabbage as eaten by the poor and in times of dearth.[11] Even acorns supplemented the diet of many households in normal years as well as during famine (Galen 6.522–523, 620). Because stocks of such crops were insufficient to feed entire communities and for many people these foods were part of their diet anyway, fodder and similar foodstuffs undoubtedly kept many individuals alive, but could not entirely ward off the effects of starvation in the worst of crises.

One element of subsistence crises that on the basis of documentary evidence is well-studied regarding Early Modern Europe, but that is nearly invisible in the literary texts of antiquity, is the economic malaise that was the result of inflated food prices, which meant that the demand for all other goods and services collapsed. Only the chronicler of Edessa noticed that non-edible goods were cheap, but such attention by the ancient writers is rare. People who offered goods and services for sale and depended on the market for their food were doubly hit, as they lost their livelihood at a time when food prices skyrocketed.[12]

Mobility and mass migration are invariably connected to serious food shortages in modern and premodern times, as people confronted with the lack of food at prices they could afford saw no other option than to seek better conditions elsewhere, where more food might be available or where public or private institutions were expected to offer some form of help, as in the case of Edessa. Country-dwellers fled to the city and from places inland to coastal regions. Public or state granaries were a feature of the urban world, as was the infrastructure of the grain trade, and smallholders and tenants were accustomed that their taxes and rents were brought to the town or city, so it was quite rational for them to expect that food was easier to come by in the nearest city. However, the refugees died in great numbers due to starvation and disease. The fourth-century orator Libanius remarked about the city of Antioch that the desperate position of the refugees constituted more of a problem than the absolute lack of food: "There is famine in the midst of plenty because of the crowds of squatters everywhere. The governors resent the migrations, but in the uncertainty about the future, they cannot stop them" (*Orat.* 19.59).

Mass mobility was one of the main reasons that food shortages were indissolubly connected to epidemics, and hence the phrase *fames et pestilentia* occurs frequently in the literary sources. The causal link between epidemic diseases on the one hand and food prices and starvation on the other has been studied in detail for early-modern Europe and modern famines (Mokyr and Ó Gráda, 2002; Ó Gráda, 2007, 20–23; Kelly and Ó Gráda, 2014, 359–360), but the sources attest this relationship in the ancient world as well.[13] Apart from the weakening of the undernourished individuals, which made them susceptible to many diseases, the movement of people from the countryside to an urban environment, in which infectious diseases to which they were rarely exposed in their isolated villages were endemic, caused an upsurge of diseases, which was intensified by the unsanitary living conditions of the refugees.[14] Most infectious diseases did not limit themselves to the starving, so that also those whose nourishment had been sufficient succumbed in large numbers. Josephus, Eusebius and the chronicler of Edessa all emphasize the latter point. Another causal link between famine and pestilence is illustrated by a subsistence crisis leading to political strife in Rome in 22 BC, a year during which the city of Rome also experienced a flooding of the Tiber:

> The pestilence raged throughout all Italy so that no one tilled the land, and I suppose that the same was the case in foreign parts. The Romans, therefore, reduced to dire straits by the disease and by the consequent famine . . .
>
> *(Cassius Dio 54.1.2; cf. 53.33.5)*

Although the authors do not make this point regarding the famines in Palestine, Edessa and Italy that we have just seen, the fleeing of farmers and the numerous deaths among them must have hampered the tilling of the land and thereby prolonged the crisis.

Population and demography

Although municipal and central authorities in the Roman world kept various kinds of records of their subjects, only occasionally do our literary sources offer concrete figures. The relationship between official registrations of people or burials and the figures we find in our sources is usually uncertain. "Thousands of people died in the cities", Eusebius (9.8.5) writes, referring also to empty registers of country-dwellers, but he does not give us any precise figures. Interesting is the following note of Orosius of the number of dead as a result of a plague of locusts[15] and subsequent epidemic in northern Africa in 125/124 BC:

In Numidia, where at that time Micipsa was king it is handed down that eight hundred thousand men perished, and along the maritime coast which lies especially close to Carthage and Utica, more than two hundred thousand, and at the city of Utica itself thirty thousand soldiers, who had been stationed there for the protection of all Africa, were destroyed and wiped out. This calamity was so sudden and so violent that at Utica at that time, in one day through one gate, more than one thousand five hundred bodies of the youth are said to have been carried out for burial.

(Orosius 5.11.1–7)

In view of the high number of deaths in nineteenth- and twentieth-century crises, a figure of about one million dead is certainly plausible.[16] The Late Ancient Christian writer Orosius, however, continues his account by observing that such calamities had not occurred in Christian times. He therefore had a possible motive to exaggerate the number of dead or to at least pick the highest estimate he could find in his sources. Livy mentioned the plague of locusts and epidemic too, but only a summary of his account survives, which gives no figures of casualties. On the one hand, the total figures are connected to various political units or – in case of the burials – to a particular register, which supports their credibility, on the other hand the numbers seem too round to be the result of registration. Casualties are often given in the number of burials, which may go back to registrations of burials at certain graveyards or records of certain gates. In the Chronicle of Joshua the Stylite (43), we are informed that between November and March every day more than 100 bodies – some days 120 or even 130 – were taken to the graveyard, in other words more than 15,000 in all. It is problematic to estimate a mortality rate on the basis of the Chronicle's figures, as a large proportion of victims were refugees coming from a very uncertain range beyond Edessa.

The census registrations and official registers once contained the data for an analysis of mortality crises in the Roman world, but unfortunately the data are lost, apart from a few glimpses in our literary sources. Hence, it is futile to attempt calculating even the basic demographic variables of ancient mortality crises. What we can do is see whether the much better-documented cases of later times provide insights that fit the conditions that we can reconstruct on the basis of the literary narratives. This will not replace the statistics that we seek, but allows a better understanding of the demography and population impact of famines in the Roman world.

Even though the circumstances in medieval England differed considerably from those in the ancient Mediterranean world – I would even say, precisely because of the difference – two recent studies of famines in medieval England provide additional insights. Famine, defined by increased mortality and lower marriage and birth rates, recurred in England until the mid-eighteenth century (Walter and Schofield, 1989; Campbell and Ó Gráda, 2011). Based on price data, Campbell and Ó Gráda calculated the harvest shortfalls in England in the thirteenth to fifteenth century. Kelly and Ó Gráda make the remarkable observation that in the Middle Ages the mortality rate among nobles responded to the same degree to harvest shocks as that of tenants, albeit lagging behind about a year.[17] "Wealth was no armour against death from epidemic disease that had incubated among hungry peasants" (2014, 369). There is no reason to assume that most parts of the Roman world – outside maybe the leading metropoles and their direct hinterland – performed significantly better concerning harvest shocks and their impact on living standards than medieval England. During famines, most individuals did not die directly of the physical consequences of starvation, but of the infectious diseases that soared as a result of famine conditions. As the famine narratives that we have seen above confirm, the impact of severe food shortages on the mortality rate of all socioeconomic levels consisted largely of the epidemic rise of diseases in the wake of famines that were endemic in normal times. In short, famines had a serious impact on population, even though actual starvation may have been limited largely to the poorer layers of society.

Mortality crises also caused a decline in fertility rates for the duration of the crisis. To begin with, undernourishment reduced the fertility of women (Le Roy Ladurie, 1975), but more importantly, marriages were disrupted by the high number of adult deaths and by the disruption of normal life (e.g., Sella, 1991). The admittedly impressionistic literary and juridical sources indicate that more children were exposed or killed during severe food shortages. Ovid (*Metam.* 8.849) tells of a father who sells his daughter during a famine – a fictional case, but one that refers to reality. The Codex Theodosianus (a compilation of earlier laws published in AD 438) contains a ruling (dated to the early fourth century AD) against the observed phenomenon of families not raising their children due to poverty (*Cod. Theod.* 11.27.1). The Chronicle of Joshua the Stylite (42) says that mothers abandoned their children as they could not feed them. In a contract from Oxyrhynchus (Egypt) dated to AD 554, a widow legally surrenders her nine year old daughter because, she says, she does not have the means to feed her (*P.Oxy.* 1895). The sale or surrender of children may have ensured their survival, but in extremely uncertain times the exposure and infanticide of new-born children increased the levels of mortality among infants, which were high at the best of times.

Modern research has shown the long-term effects on the physical and mental health of infants and children raised in conditions of deprivation, the signs of which may be visible in the skeletal and dental remains (Ó Gráda, 2007, 23–25). However, it is very difficult – if not impossible – for osteoarchaeologists to distinguish the effects of illnesses on the intake of nutrients among children from the effects of starvation. Studying the detrimental long-term effects of famines in antiquity is currently beyond the means of our sources.

Comparison with later times also shows that demographic trends were reversed in the wake of mortality crises. The death rate invariably fell below pre-crisis figures when conditions improved, because in particular the elderly, the physically weak and economically marginal had succumbed in large numbers during the crisis. In contrast, the marriage and birth rate increased, as the survivors profited from improved socioeconomic conditions, such as the increased availability of land, which they may have inherited, and the relative shortage of labour, while new marriages were formed among survivors (Ó Gráda, 2007, 23). Again, a similar demographic scenario seems very likely for the Roman world too, but cannot be proven on the basis of the currently available evidence.

Notes

1 Both definitions from Garnsey, 1988, 6. Cf. Stathakopoulos, 2004, 4-5; Ó Gráda, 2007, 5; Vanhaute, 2011, 49.
2 Cf. the detailed commentary in Stathakopoulos, 2004, 250–255.
3 Flavius Josephus, *Jud. Arch.* 15.299ff; Eusebius, Hist. Eccl. 9.8.1–15; Ps.-Joshua the Stylite, Chron. 39–46; Procopius, Bell. Goth. 2.20.15–33.
4 Stathakopoulos, 2004, 25. See this work also for its invaluable overview of sources.
5 See also D'Alessandro, 2011 on the role of the economic structure on the impact of harvest shocks.
6 On ethnography, see in particular Halstead, 2014b. See also Jameson, 1983; Garnsey, 1988, 43–86; Gallant, 1991.
7 Regarding the Later Roman Empire, see Stathakopoulos, 2004, 62–65.
8 Ammianus Marcellinus 14.7.2–6, 22.12-14; Libanius, *Orat.* 1.102, 126, 11.177–178, 15.20, 18.195; Julian, *Misop.* 368–370. Erdkamp, 2005, 291–294.
9 On food riots in the Roman world in general, Erdkamp, 2002. See also Kelly, 2007, and Holleran in the previous chapter.

10 See Chronicon Paschale 571 for similar events in Constantinople in AD 409. Stathakopoulos, 2004, 223.

11 Pliny, *Nat. Hist.* 18.127; Columella 2.6.2, 2.9.14, 2.10.1–3. See also Sperber, 1977, 404 on lupins as "normal" food in Palestine.

12 The economic malaise resulting from subsistence crises is discussed in detail by Abel, 1974.

13 The relationship between famine and epidemic is so clear, that one wonders how many visible epidemics in the ancient world were caused by invisible famines!

14 On diseases endemic in cities, Sallares, 1991, 221–293; Scheidel, 2003.

15 See for a detailed analysis of locusts in our sources, Stathakopoulos, 2004, 41–45.

16 Cf. about 20 million deaths in India in the second half of the nineteenth century. D'Alessandro, 2011.

17 Kelly and Ó Gráda, 2014, 365: "Rich and poor are succumbing at similar rates to the same infectious diseases." Cf. p. 368: "Nobles appear slightly less affected by falls in living standards than tenants."

BIBLIOGRAPHY

Abd El-Moniem, G.M. 1999. 'Sensory evaluation and *in vitro* protein digestibility of mung bean as affected by cooking time', *Journal of the Science of Food and Agriculture* 79, pp. 2025–2028.

Abel, W. 1974. *Massenarmut und Hungerkrisen im vorindustriellen Europa*. Hamburg: Parey.

Agache, R. and Bréart, B. 1975. *Atlas d'archéologie aérienne de Picardie: le Basin de la Somme et ses Abords à l'Époque protohistorique et romaine*. Amiens: Société des antiquaires de Picardie.

Agarwal, S. and B. Glencross, eds. 2011. *Social Bioarchaeology*. Oxford: Wiley-Blackwell.

Aguilera, M., Lepetz, S., Balasse, M. and Zech-Materne, V. 2016. 'Fertilisation des sols de culture par les fumiers et rôle potentiel des céréales dans l'affouragement du bétail: l'éclairage des analyses isotopiques sur restes carpologiques et archéozoologiques', in *Méthodes d'Analyse des différents Paysages ruraux dans le nord-est de la Gaule romaine: Études comparées*, ed. M. Reddé. Paris: École pratique des Hautes Études, pp. 41–47.

Ahmed, M., 2010. *Rural Settlement and Economic Activity: Olive Oil and Amphorae Production on the Tarhuna Plateau during the Roman Period*. PhD dissertation, University of Leicester.

Ahmad, W., Watts, M.J., Imtiaz, M., Ahmed, I. and Zia, M.H. 2012. 'Zinc deficiency in soils, crops and humans: A review', *Agrochimica* 51(2), pp. 65–97.

Akroyd, W.R. and Doughty, J. 1970. *Wheat in Human Nutrition*. Rome: FAO.

Akroyd, W.R., Doughty, J., and Walker, A., 1982. *Legumes in Human Nutrition*, 2nd revised edition. FAO Food and Nutrition Paper 20. Rome: FAO.

Alajaji, S.A. and El-Adawy. T.A. 2006. 'Nutritional composition of chickpea (*Cicer arietinum L.*) as affected by microwave cooking and other traditional cooking methods', *Journal of Food Composition and Analysis* 19, pp. 806–812.

Albarella, U. 2007. 'The end of the Sheep Age: people and animals in the Late Iron Age', in *The Later Iron Age in Britain and Beyond*, ed. C. Haselgrove and T. Moore. Oxford: Oxbow, pp. 389–402.

Albarella, U., Johnstone, C. and Vickers, K. 2008. 'The development of animal husbandry from the Late Iron Age to the end of the Roman period: a case study from south-east Britain', *Journal of Archaeological Science* 23, pp. 1828–1848.

Alberione Dos Reis, J. 2005. 'What conditions of existence sustain a tension found in the use of written and material documents in archaeology', in *Global Archaeological Theory: Contextual Voices and Contemporary Thoughts*, ed. P.P. Funari, A. Zarankin and E. Stovel. New York: Kluwer Academic, pp. 43–58.

Alcock, J. 2001. *Food in Roman Britain*. Stroud: Tempus.

Alcock, J.P. 2006. *Food in the Ancient World*. Westport, CT: Greenwood Press.

Aldrete, G.S. 2004. *Daily Life in the Roman City: Rome, Pompeii and Ostia*. Westport, CT: University of Oklahoma Press.

Aldrete, G.S. 2014. 'Hammers, axes, bulls, and blood: some practical aspects of Roman animal sacrifice', *Journal of Roman Studies* 104, pp. 28–50.

Aldrete, G.S. and Mattingly, D.S. 1999. 'Feeding the city: the organisation, operation, and scale of the supply system for Rome', in *Life, Death, and Entertainment in the Roman Empire*, ed. D.S. Potter and D.J. Mattingly. Ann Arbor: University of Michigan Press, pp. 171–204.

Bibliography

Alföldy, G. 1988. *The Social History of Rome*, trans. D. Braund and F. Pollock. Baltimore: Johns Hopkins University Press.

Allen, R.C. 2009. 'How prosperous were the Romans? Evidence from Diocletian's Price Edict (AD 301)', in *Quantifying the Roman Economy. Methods and Problems*, ed. A. Bowman and A.I. Wilson. Oxford, Oxford University Press, pp. 327–345.

Alston, R. and Van Nijf, O., eds. 2008. *Feeding the Ancient Greek City*, Leuven: Peeters.

Amberger, G. 1982. 'Tierknochenfunde aus eisenzeitlichen Siedlungsstellen der Göttinger Gegend', *Neue Ausgrabungen und Forschungen in Niedersachsen* 15, pp. 327–338.

Amouretti, M-C. 1986. *Le Pain et l'Huile dans la Grèce antique*. Paris: Belles Lettres.

André, J. 1961. *L'Alimentation et la cuisine à Rome*. Paris: C. Klincksieck.

André, J. 1981. *L'Alimentation et la Cuisine à Rome*, 2nd edition. Paris: Klincksieck.

André, J. 1985. *Les Noms des Plantes dans Rome Antique*. Paris: Belles lettres.

André, J. 1998. *Essen und Trinken im alten Rom*. Stuttgart: Reclam Verlag.

Angel, J.L. 1966. 'Porotic hyperostosis, anemias, malarias and marshes in the prehistoric Mediterranean', *Science* 153, pp. 760–763.

Angel, J.L. 1977. 'Anemias of Antiquity: Eastern Mediterranean', in *Porotic Hyperostosis: An Enquiry*, ed. E. Cockburn and A. Cockburn. Detroit: Paleopathology Association Monograph 2, pp. 1–5.

Anjum, F.M., Ahmad, I., Butt, M.S., Sheikh, M.A. and Pasha. I. 2005. 'Amino acid composition of spring wheats and losses of lysine during chapati baking', *Journal of Food Composition and Analysis* 18, pp. 523–532.

Antolín, F. and Buxó, R. 2011. 'Proposal for the systematic description and taphonomic study of carbonized cereal grain assemblages: a case study of an early Neolithic funerary context in the cave of Can Sadurní (Begues, Barcelona province, Spain)', *Vegetation History and Archaeobotany* 20, pp. 53–66.

Antolín, F., Steiner, B.L., Vach, W. and Jacomet, S. 2015. 'What is a litre of sediment? Testing volume measurement techniques for wet sediment and their implications in archaeobotanical analyses at the Late Neolithic lake-dwelling site of Parkhaus Opéra (Zürich, Switzerland)', *Journal of Archaeological Science* 61, pp. 36–44.

Apicius. *De Re Coquinaria*, trans. W.M. Hill 1936.

Arcini, C., Torbjörn, A. and Tagesson, G. 2014. 'Variation in diet and stature: are they linked? Bioarchaeology and paleodietary Bayesian mixing models from Linköping, Sweden', *International Journal of Osteoarchaeology* 24, pp. 543–556.

Arese, P. 2006. 'How genetics and biology helped humanity to survive falciparum malaria', *Parassitologia* 48, pp. 523–525.

Arese, P., Turrini, F., and Schwarzer, E. 2005. 'Band 3/complement-mediated recognition and removal of normally senescent and pathological human erythrocytes', *Cellular Physiology and Biochemistry* 16, pp. 133–146.

Arobba, D., Caramiello, R. and Martino, G.P. 2014. 'Il contributo delle analisi archeobotaniche per la storia del paesaggio agrario della città romana di Albintimilium (Ventimiglia)', *Rivista di studi liguri* 70, pp. 283–306.

Ascough, R. 2008. 'Forms of commensality in Greco-Roman associations', *Classical World* 102, pp. 33–45.

Ast, R. and Azzarello G. 2013. 'New perspectives on the Gemellus archive: Sabinus and his correpondence', in *Das Fayum in Hellenismus und Kaiserzeit. Fallstudien zu multikulturellem Leben in der Antike*, ed. C. Arlt and M. Stadler. Wiesbaden: Harassowitz, pp. 19–28.

Audouze, F. and Büchsenschütz, O. 1992. *Towns, Villages, and Countryside of Celtic Europe: From the Beginning of the Second Millennium to the End of the First Century BC*. London: B.T. Batsford.

Australian Government Department of Health and Ageing Office of the Gene Technology Regulator. 2013. *The Biology of Lupinus L.* Canberra: Office of the Gene Technology Regulator. Available at www.ogtr.gov.au/internet/ogtr/publishing.nsf/Content/biologylupin2013-toc/$FILE/biologylupin 2013-2.pdf (accessed 15 February 2015).

Baadsgaard, A., Boutin, A.T. and Buikstra, J. E., eds. 2011. *Breathing New Life into the Evidence of Death Contemporary Approaches to Bioarchaeology*. Santa Fe: School for Advanced Research Press.

Baatz, D. 1977. 'Reibschale und Romanisierung', *Acta RCRF* 17/18, pp. 147–158.

Backe-Dahmen, A. 2006. *Innocentissima Aetas. Römische Kindheit im Spiegel literarischer, rechtlicher und archäologischer Quellen des 1. bis 4. Jhs. n.Chr.* Mainz am Rhein: Philip von Zabern.

Badham, K. and Jones, G., 1985. 'An experiment in manual processing of soil samples for plant remains', *Circaea* 3(1), pp. 15–26.

Bagnall, R.S. 1993. *Egypt in Late Antiquity*. Princeton: Princeton University Press.

Bagnall, R. 2013. *Eine Wüstenstadt. Leben und Kultur in einer ägyptischen Oase im 4. Jahrhundert n. Chr.* Stuttgart; Steiner Verlag.

Bahl, P.N. 1990. 'The role of food legumes in the diets of populations of Mediterranean areas and associated nutritional factors', in *The Role of Legumes in the Farming Systems of the Mediterranean Areas*, ed. A.E. Osman, M.H. Ibrahim and M.A. Jones. Dordrecht, Boston, and London: Kluwer Academic Publishers, pp. 143–149.

Bakels, C. and Jacomet, S. 2003. 'Access to luxury foods in Central Europe during the Roman period: the archaeobotanical evidence', *World Archaeology* 34(3), pp. 542–557.

Balasse, M. and Tresset, A. 2002. 'Early weaning of Neolithic domestic cattle (Bercy, France) revealed by intra-tooth variation in Nitrogen isotope ratios', *Journal of Archaeological Science* 29, pp. 853–859.

Banducci, L.M. 2014a. 'Function and use of Roman pottery: a quantitative method for assessing use wear', *Journal of Mediterranean Archaeology* 27, pp. 187–210.

Banducci, L.M. 2014b. 'Ceramics: Roman Republican and Early Principate', in *Encyclopedia of Global Archaeology*, ed. Claire Smith. New York: Springer, pp. 1325–1331.

Banducci, L.M. 2015. 'Fuel, cuisine and food preparation in Etruria and Latium: cooking stands as evidence for change', in *Ceramics, Cuisine and Culture: The Archaeology and Science of Kitchen Pottery in the Ancient Mediterranean World*, ed. M. Spataro and A. Villing. Oxford: Oxbow Books, pp. 157–169.

Banducci, L.M. Forthcoming. 'Using fire damage on Roman cooking pots to address cooking technology', in *Fuel and Fire in the Ancient World*, ed. R. Veal and V. Leitch. McDonald Institute monographs. Cambridge: Cambridge University Press.

Barker, G. 1996. *Farming the Desert*, 2 Vols. London: UNESCO Publishing, Department of Antiquities (Tripoli) and Society for Libyan Studies.

Bartoldus, M.J. 2012. *Palladius Rutilius Taurus Aemilianus. Welt und Wert spätrömischer Landwirtschaft.* Augsburg: Wissner Verlag.

Baschet, J. 2000. 'Âme et corps dans l'occident médiéval: une dualité dynamique, entre pluralité et dualisme', *Archives de Sciences sociales des Religions* 112, pp. 5–30.

Bats, M. 1988. *Vaisselle et alimentation à Olbia de Provence (v. 350-v. 50 av. J.-C.): modèles culturels et catégories céramiques*. Revue archéologique de Narbonnaise. Paris: Centre National de la Recherche Scientifique.

Battaglia, E. 1989. *Artos. Il lessico della panificazione nei papiri greci*. Biblioteca di Aevum Antiquum 2. Milan: Vita e pensiero.

Baudrillart, A.1900. 'Lac', in *Dictionnaire des antiquités grecques et romaines. Vol. 6*, ed. C. Daremberg, E. Saglio, and E. Pottier. Paris, pp. 883–886.

Beard, M. 2010. *The Fires of Vesuvius: Pompeii Lost and Found*. Cambridge, MA: Harvard University Press.

Beard, M., North, J. and Price, S. 1998. *Religions of Rome*, 2 vols. Cambridge: Cambridge University Press.

Beauchamp, G.K., Keast R., Morel D., Lin, J., Pika, J., Han, Q., Lee, C-H., Smith, A.B. and P. Breslin. 2005. 'Phytochemistry: ibuprofen-like activity in extra-virgin olive oil', *Nature* 437, pp. 45–46.

Becker, M.J. 1999. 'Calculating stature from in situ measurements of skeletons and from long bone lengths: an historical perspective leading to a test of Formica's hypothesis at 5th century BCE Satricum, Lazio, Italy', *Rivista di Antropologia* 77, pp. 225–247.

Becker, M.J. 2000. 'Skeletal studies of the people of Sicily: An update on research on human remains from archaeological contexts', *International Journal of Anthropology* 15, pp. 191–239.

Becker, M.J. 2003. 'Review of *I Fuggiaschi di Ercolano: Paleobiologia delle vittime dell'eruzione Vesuviana del 79 D.C.* by L. Capasso', *The Journal of Roman Studies* 93, pp. 404–406.

Becker, T. 2007. 'Viehwirtschaft bei Kelten, Römern und Germanen im Rheinland', in *Krieg und Frieden. Kelten – Römer – Germanen*, ed. G. Uelsberg. Darmstadt: Primus Verlag, pp. 133–143.

Becker, T. 2012. 'Archäozoologische Untersuchungen an Tierknochenfunden von Wachttürmen und Kleinkastellen am Limes', in *Der Limes vom Niederrhein bis an die Donau. 6. Kolloquium der deutschen Limeskommission*, ed. P. Henrich. Beiträge zum Welterbe Limes 6. Stuttgart: Konrad Theiss Verlag, pp. 157–175.

Beer, M. 2010. *Taste or Taboo: Dietary Choices in Antiquity*. Totnes: Prospect Books.

Belayche, N. 2007. 'Religion et consommation de la viande dans le monde romain: des réalités voilées', *Food and History* 5, pp. 29–43.

Belcastro, G., Rastelli, E., Mariotti, V., Consiglio, C., Facchini, F. and Bonfiglioli, B. 2007. 'Continuity or discontinuity of the life-style in Central Italy during the Roman imperial age–early Middle Ages. Transition: diet, health, and behavior', *American Journal of Physical Anthropology* 132, pp. 381–394.

Beltrán Lloris, M. 2000. 'Mulsum betico. Nuevo contenido de las ánforas Haltern 70', in *Actas do III Congresso de Arqueologia Peninsular*. Porto, Adecap, pp. 323–345.

Bendini, A., Lorenzo C., Alegria C-P., Gómez-Caravaca, A.M., Segura-Carretero, A., Fernández-Gutiérrez, A. and G. Lercker. 2007. 'Phenolic molecules in virgin olive oils: a survey of their sensory properties, health effects, antioxidant activity and analytical methods. An overview of the last decade', *Molecules* 12, pp. 1679–1719.

Bennett, J. 1997. *Trajan, Optimus Princeps: A Life and Times*. Bloomington: Indiana University Press.

Bennion, E. 1986. *Antique Dental Instruments*. London: Sotheby's Philip Wilson Publishers Ltd.

Berger, E. 1982. *Antike Kunstwerke aus der Sammlung Ludwig II: Terrakotten und Bronzen*. Basel: Mainz am Rhein, Philipp von Zabern.

Bergmann, B. 1995. 'Greek masterpieces and Roman recreative fictions', *Harvard Studies in Classical Philology*, pp. 79–120.

Bernal, D. 2011. 'Arqueología de la acuicultura en Hispania. Problemas y reflexiones', in *Las Factorías de Salazones de Traducta: Primeros Resultados de las Excavaciones arqueológicas en la c/San Nicolás de Algeciras (2001–2006)*, ed. D. Bernal. Cádiz: Universidad de Cádiz, pp. 189–214.

Bernal Casasola, D. and Arévalo Gonzales, A. 2008. 'Baelo Claudia y sus industrias halieuticas: Sintesis de las ultimas actuaciones arqueologicas (2000–2004)', in *Ressources et Activités maritimes des Peuples de l'Antiquité: Actes du Colloque international de Boulogne-sur-Mer, 12, 13 et 14 mai 2005 organisé par le Centre de recherche en histoire atlantique et littorale, CRAHEL* (Les Cahiers du Littoral, série 2.6), ed. J. Napoli. Boulogne-sur-mer: Les cahiers du littoral, pp. 9–30.

Bertoldi, T. 2011. *Ceramiche Comuni Dal Suburbio Di Roma*. Studi di archeologia 1. Rome: Aracne.

Bhatty, R.S. 1988. 'Composition and quality of lentil (*Lens culinaris Medik*): a review', *Canadian Institute of Food Science and Technology Journal* 21(2), pp. 144–160.

Biddulph, E. 2008. 'Form and function: the experimental use of Roman samian ware cups', *Oxford Journal of Archaeology* 27(1), pp. 91–100.

Bilde, P. 2001. 'The common meal in the Qumran-Essene communities', in *Meals in a Social Context. Aspects of the Communal Meal in the Hellenistic and Roman World*, ed. I. Nielsen and H.S. Nielsen. Aarhus: Aarhus University Press, pp. 145–166.

Billy, G. 1992. 'La population de Douch (Oasis de Kharga), Égypte à l'époque romaine', *Bulletins et Mémoires de la Société d'Anthropologie de Paris*, N.S. tome 4, pp. 111–126.

Binford, L.R. 1962. 'Archaeology as anthropology', *American Antiquity* 28(2), 217–225.

Bintliff, J., Howard, P. and Snodgrass, A. 2007. *Testing the Hinterland: The Work of the Boeotia Survey (1989–1991) in the Southern Approaches to the City of Thespiai*. Oxford: MacDonald Institute of Archaeological Research.

Birkenhagen, B. 2013. 'Ein Spargelmesser aus dem Archäologiepark Römische Villa Borg', *Funde und Ausgrabungen im Bezirk Trier* 45, pp. 14–15.

Birley, A. 1997. 'Supplying the Batavians at Vindolanda', in *Roman Frontier Studies 1995: Proceedings of the XVIth International Congress of Roman Frontier Studies*, ed. W. Groenman-Van Waaterringe, B.L. Van Beek, W.J.H. Willems and S.L. Wyrria. Oxford: Oxbow, pp. 273–280.

Blake, S. H. 2016. 'The aesthetics of the everyday in Flavian art and literature', in *A Companion to the Flavian Age of Imperial Rome*, ed. A. Zissos. Chichester, UK, and Malden, MA: Wiley-Blackwell, pp. 344–360.

Blakely, J.A., Brinkmann, R. and Vitaliano, C.J. 1992. 'Roman mortaria and basins from a sequence at Caesarea: fabrics and sources', in *Caesarea Papers, Straton's Tower, Herod's Harbor, and Roman and Byzantine Caesarea*, ed. R.L. Vann. Ann Arbor, MI: Journal of Roman Archaeology, pp. 194–214.

Blandino, A., Al-Aseeri, M.E., Pandiella, S.S., Cantero, D. and Webb, C. 2003. 'Cereal-based fermented foods and beverages', *Food Research International* 36, pp. 527–543.

Blázquez, J.M. 1992. 'The latest work on the export of Baetican olive oil to Rome and the army', *Greece and Rome (Second Series)* 39, pp. 173–188.

Blázquez, J.M. et al. 1994–2013. *Estudios sobre el Monte Testaccio (Roma)* 1–6. Barcelona: Publicacions Universitat de Barcelona.

Boardman, S. and Jones, G. 1990. 'Experiments on the effects of charring on cereal plant components', *Journal of Archaeological Science* 17, pp. 1–11.

Boccone, S., Micheletti Cremasco, M., Bortoluzzi, S., Moggi-Cecchi, J. and Rabino Massa, E. 2010. 'Age estimation in subadult Egyptian remains', *Homo* 61, pp. 337–358.

Bocherens, H. and Drucker, D. 2003. 'Trophic level isotopic enrichment of carbon and nitrogen in bone collagen: case studies from recent and ancient terrestrial ecosystems', *International Journal of Osteoarchaeology* 13, pp. 46–53.

Bockius, R. 2008. 'Römische Kriegsschiffe auf der Mosel? Schiffarchäologisch-historische Betrachtungen zum Neumagener Weinschiff', *Funde und Ausgrabungen im Bezirk Trier* 40, pp. 37–49.

Bode, M. 1999. *Apicius: Anmerkungen zum römischen Kochbuch. Das Kochbuch des Apicius als Quelle zur Wirtschafts- und Sozialgeschichte.* St Katharinen: Scripta Mercaturae Verlag.

Bodel, J. 2001. 'Epigraphy and the ancient historian', in *Epigraphic Evidence: Ancient History from Inscriptions*, ed. J. Bodel. London: Routledge, pp. 1–56.

Bogaard, A., Heaton, T.H.E., Poulton, P. and Merbach, I. 2007. 'The impact of manuring on nitrogen isotope ratios in cereals: archaeological implications for reconstruction of diet and crop management practices', *Journal of Archaeological Science* 34(3), pp. 335–443.

Bogaard, A., Fraser, R.A., Heaton, T.H.E et al. 2013. 'Crop manuring and intensive land management by Europe's first farmers', *PNAS* 110(31), pp. 12589–12594.

Bokser, B. 1984. *The Origins of the Seder.* Berkeley: University of California Press.

Bolsden, J. 1984. 'Statistical evaluation of the basis for predicting stature from long bone lengths in European populations', *American Journal of Physical Anthropology* 65, pp. 305–311.

Bonfiglioli, B., Brasili, P. and Belcastro, M.G. 2003. 'Dento-alveolar lesions and nutritional habits of a Roman imperial age population (1st–4th c. AD): Quadrella (Molise, Italy)', *Homo* 54, pp. 36–56.

Bonsall, L. 2014. 'A comparison of female and male oral health in skeletal populations from late Roman Britain: implications for diet', *Archives of Oral Biology* 59, pp. 1279–1300.

Booth, A. 1991. 'The age for reclining and its attendant perils', in *Dining in a Classical Context*, ed. W. J. Slater. Ann Arbor: University of Michigan Press, pp. 105–120.

Boozer, A.L. 2015. A late Roman-Egyptian house in the Dakhla oasis: Amheida house B2. Available at http://dlib.nyu.edu/awdl/isaw/amheida-ii-house-b2/

Borgognini Tarli, S.M. and Mazzotta, F. 1986. 'Physical anthropology of Italy from the Bronze Age to the Barbaric Age', in *Ethnogenese europäischen Völker*, ed. B. Kandler Palsson. Stuttgart: Gustav Fischer Verlag, pp. 147–172.

Borhy, L. 2014. *Die Römer in Ungarn – mit einem Beitrag von M. Szabó.* Darmstadt: Verlag Philipp von Zabern.

Borhy, L. and E. Számadó, 2010. 'A III. számu épület figurális jeleneteinek ikonográfiai értelmezése. In Római kori falfestmények Brigetióból. A komáromi Klapka György Muzeum római kori falfestményeinek katalógusa', *Acta Archaeologica Brigetionensia Ser. I. Vol. 3.* Komárom: Komáromi Nyomda és Kiado Kft., pp. 103–106.

Bouby, L. and Marinval, P. 2004. 'Fruits and seeds from Roman cremations in Limagne (Massif Central) and the spatial variability of plant offerings in France', *Journal of Archaeological Science* 31, pp. 77–86.

Bouby, L., Bouchette, A. and Figueiral, I. 2011. 'Sebesten fruits (Cordia myxa L.) in Gallia Narbonensis (Southern France): a trade item from the Eastern Mediterranean?', *Vegetation History and Archaeobotany* 20(5), pp. 397–404.

Bourbou, C. 2005. 'Biological status in Hellenistic and Roman elites in Western Crete (Greece)', *Eres* 13, pp. 87–110.

Bourbou, C. and S. J. Garvie-Lok, 2009. 'Breastfeeding and weaning patterns in Byzantine times: evidence from human remains and written sources', in *Becoming Byzantine. Children and Childhood in Byzantium*, ed. A. Papaconstantinou and A.-M. Talbot. Dumbarton Oaks: Harvard University Press, pp. 65–83.

Bourbou, C. and Tsilipakou, A., 2009. 'Investigating the human past of Greece during the 6th and 7th centuries AD', in *New Directions in the Skeletal Biology of Greece*, ed. L.A. Schepartz, S.C. Fox, and C. Bourbou. Princeton: The American School of Classical Studies at Athens, pp. 121–136.

Bowe, P. 2004. *Gardens of the Roman World.* Los Angeles: Getty Museum.

Bowes, K., Mercuri, A.M., Rattighieri, E., Rinaldi, R., Arnoldus-Huyzendveld, A., Ghisleni, M., Grey, C., Mackinnon, M. and Vaccaro, E. 2015. 'Palaeoenvironment and land use of Roman peasant farmhouses in southern Tuscany', *Plant Biosystems* 149(1), pp. 174–184.

Bowie, E. 'Athenaeus [3]', in *Brill's New Pauly Online*. Accessed 1 March 2016.

Bowman, A.K. and Rathbone, D. 1992. 'Cities and administration in Roman Egypt', *The Journal of Roman Studies* 82, pp. 107–127.

Bowman, A.K. and Wilson, A.I., eds. 2011. *Settlement, Urbanization and Population.* Oxford: Oxford University Press.

Bowman, A.K. and Wilson, A.I. 2013. 'Introduction: quantifying Roman agriculture', in *The Roman Agricultural Economy: Organization, Investment, and Production*, ed. A. Bowman and A. Wilson. Oxford: Oxford University Press, pp. 1–32.

Braadbaart, F. and van Bergen, P.F. 2005. 'Digital imaging analysis of size and shape of wheat and pea upon heating under anoxic conditions as a function of the temperature', *Vegetation History and Archaeobotany* 14, pp. 67–75.

Braadbaart, F., Poole, I. and van Brussel, A.A. 2009. 'Preservation potential of charcoal in alkaline environments: an experimental approach and implications for the archaeological record', *Journal of Archaeological Science* 36, pp. 1672–1679.

Bradley, K. 1998. 'The Roman family at dinner', in *Meals in a Social Context. Aspects of the Communal meal in the Hellenistic and Roman World*, ed. I. Nielsen and H. Sigismund Nielsen. Aarhus: Aarhus University Press, pp. 36–55.

Bradley, K. 2000. 'Fictive families: family and household in the *Metamorphoses* of Apuleius', *Phoenix* 54, pp. 282–308.

Bradley, K. 2001. 'The Roman family at dinner', in *Meals in a Social Context: Aspects of the Communal Meal in the Hellenistic and Roman World*, ed. I. Nielsen and H.S. Nielsen. Aarhus: Aarhus University Press, pp. 36–55.

Brandtzaeg, B. 1979. *Nutrition and Technological Evaluation of Malted Flours from Ragi, Sorghum, and Green Gram for Flour Processing of Supplementary and Weaning Foods*. Oslo: Institute for Nutrition Research/FAO.

Braun, T. 1995. 'Barley cakes and emmer bread', in *Food in Antiquity*, ed. J. Wilkins, D. Harvey and M. Dobson. Exeter: University of Exeter Press, pp. 25–37.

Braund, D. 2000. 'Learning, luxury and empire: Athenaeus' Roman patron', in *Athenaeus and his World: Reading Greek Culture in the Roman Empire*, ed. D. Braund and J. Wilkins. Exeter: University of Exeter Press, pp. 3–22.

Braund, D. and Wilkins, J. 2000. 'Section II: Text, transmission and translation: Introductory remarks', in *Athenaeus and His World: Reading Greek Culture in the Roman Empire*, ed. D. Braund and J. Wilkins. Exeter: University of Exeter Press, pp. 39–40.

Breitinger, E. 1937. 'Ausgrabungen in Kerameikos', *Archäologischer Anzeiger* 1937, pp. 184–203.

Brickley, M. and Buckberry, J. 2015. 'Picking up the pieces: utilizing the diagnostic potential of poorly preserved remains', *International Journal of Paleopathology* 8, pp. 51–54.

Brickley, M. and Ives, R. 2008. *The Bioarchaeology of Metabolic Bone Disease*. Oxford: Academic Press.

Brickley, M. and McKinley, J.I. 2004. *Guidelines to the Standards for Recording Human Remains*. Southampton: BABAO, Department of Archaeology, University of Southampton.

Broekaert, W. 2016. 'The soldiers' kitchen along the limes: fish sauce consumption and economics', in *Food, Identity and Cross-Cultural Exchange in the Ancient World*, ed. W. Broekaert, R. Nadeau and J. Wilkins, Collection Latomus 354, 64-87.

Broekaert, W. and Zuiderhoek, A. 2012a. 'Food systems in classical antiquity', in *A Cultural History of Food in Antiquity*, ed. P. Erdkamp. London and New York: Berg, pp. 41–55.

Broekaert, W. and Zuiderhoek, A. 2012b. 'Food and politics in Classical Antiquity', in *A Cultural History of Food in Antiquity*, ed. P. Erdkamp. London: Bloomsbury, pp. 75–93.

Broshi, M, 2001. *Bread, Wine, Walls and Scrolls*. Sheffield: Sheffield Academic Press.

Brothwell, D. and Brothwell, P. 1969. *Food in Antiquity: A Survey of the Diet of Early Peoples*. London: Thames & Hudson.

Brown, P. 1988. *The Body and Society: Men, Women and Sexual Renunciation in Early Christianity*. New York: Columbia Classics.

Brüggler, M. 2012. 'Weeze-Vorselaer: eine einheimisch-römische Hofanlage im Umland von Xanten', in *Landleben im römischen Deutschland*, ed. V. Rupp and H. Birley. Stuttgart: Konrad Theiss Verlag, pp. 63–64.

Brüggler, M. 2016. 'Filling in the gaps – studying the Roman rural landscape on the German Lower Rhine', in *Méthodes d'analyse des différents paysages ruraux dans le nord-est de la Gaule romaine*, ed. M. Reddé, pp. 199–234. Available at https://hal.archives-ouvertes.fr/hal-01253470 (accessed 28 February 2016).

Brun, J.P. 2003. *Le vin et L'huile dans la Méditerranée antique: Viticulture, Olécultur et Procédés de Transformation*. Paris: Errance.

Brun, J.P. 2004a. *Archéologie du Vin et de l'Huile de la Préhistoire à l'Époque hellénistique*. Paris: Errance.

Brun, J.P. 2004b. *Archéologie du Vin et de l'Huile dans l'Empire romain*. Paris: Errance.

Brun, J.P. 2005. *Archéologie du Vin et de l'Huile en Gaule romaine*. Paris: Errance.

Brun, J.P., Rogers, G., Columeau, P., Thinon, M. and Gérard, M. 1989. 'La villa gallo-romaine de Saint-Michel à La Garde (Var). Un Domaine Oléicole au Haut-Empire', *Gallia* 46, pp. 103–162.

Bruun, C. 1991. *The Water Supply of Ancient Rome. A Study of Roman Imperial Administration*. Helsinki: Societas Scientarum Fennica.

Buccellato, A. 2007. 'L'antica via Laurentina: l'arteria e le infrastrutture', *Fasti OnLine Documents & Research* 88.

Buccellato, A., Catalano, P., Arrighetti, B., et al. 2003. 'Il comprensorio della necropoli di via Basiliano (Roma): un'indagine multidisciplinare', *Mélanges de l'École Française de Rome: Antiquité* 115, pp. 311–376.

Buccellato, A., Caldarini, C., Catalano, P., Musco, S., Pantano, W., Torri, C. and Zabotti, F. 2008. 'La nécropole de Collatina', *Les Dossiers d'Archéologie* 330, pp. 22–31.

Buckland, G. and Gonzáles, A.C. 2010. 'Trends in olive oil production, supply and consumption in Mediterranean countries from 1961 to the present day', in *Olives and Olive Oil in Health and Disease Prevention*, eds. V.R. Preedy and R.R. Watson. London: Academic Press, pp. 689–698.

Buikstra, J.E. 2006. 'Preface', in *Bioarchaeology: The Contextual Analysis of Human Remains*, ed. J.E. Buikstra and L.A. Beck. Amsterdam: Academic Press, pp. xvii–xx.

Buikstra, J.E. and Beck, L.A., eds. 2006. *Bioarchaeology: The Contextual Analysis of Human Remains*. Amsterdam: Academic Press.

Buikstra, J. and Ubelaker, D., eds. 1994. *Standards for Data Collection from Human Skeletal Remains: Proceedings of a Seminar at the Field Museum of Natural History*. Fayetteville: Arkansas Archeological Survey.

Bülow-Jacobsen, A. 2003. 'The traffic on the road and provisioning of the stations', in *La Route de Myos Hormos: L'Armée romaine dans le Désert oriental d'Egypte*, ed. H. Cuvigny. Cairo: Institut français d'archéologie orientale du Caire, pp. 399–426.

Burnett, J. 1979. *Plenty and Want*, 2nd edition. London: Scholars Press.

Cabouret, B. 2008. 'Rites d'hospitalité chez les élites de l'Antiquité Tardive', in *Pratiques et discours alimentaires en Méditerranée de l'Antiquité à la Renaissance*, ed. J. Leclant, A. Vauchez and M. Sartre, Paris: Belles Lettres, pp. 187–222.

Cagnazzi, L. De S. 1849. *Saggio sullo stato presente della popolazione del Regno di Puglia per servire da confronto allo stato antico*. Naples: Angelo Trani.

California and the World Olive Oil Statistics. 2004. Available from www.oleigest.com/international/california_and_world_trends.pdf (accessed 28 June 2015).

Camak, I., Ozkan, H., Braun, H.J., Welch, R.M. and Romheld, V. 2000. 'Zinc and iron concentrations in seeds of wild, primitive and modern wheats', *Food and Nutrition Bulletin* 21(4), pp. 401–403.

Campbell, B.M.S. and Ó Gráda, C. 2011. 'Harvest shortfalls, grain prices, and famines in preindustrial England', *Journal of Economic History* 71, pp. 859–886.

Campbell-Platt, G. 1994. 'Fermented foods: a world perspective', *Food Research International* 27, pp. 253–257.

Cao, I. 2010. *Alimenta: il racconto delle fonti*. Padua: Il Poligrafo.

Capasso, L. 2001. *I fuggiaschi di Ercolano: paleobiologia delle vittime dell'eruzione vesuviana del 79 d.C.* Rome: L'Erma di Bretschneider.

Cappers, R.T.J. 2006. *Roman Foodprints at Berenike: Archaeobotanical Evidence of Subsistence and Trade in the Eastern Desert of Egypt*. Los Angeles: Cotsen Institute of Archaeology, University of California.

Cappers, R.T.J. 2013. 'Modelling cereal selection in Neolithic Egypt: An evaluation of economic criteria', in *Neolithisation of Northeastern Africa*, ed. N. Shirai. Berlin: Ex Oriente, pp. 109–120.

Cappers, R.T.J. and Neef, R. 2012. *Handbook of Plant Palaeoecology*. Groningen: Barkhuis and University of Groningen Library.

Cappers, R.T.J., Heinrich, F.B.J., Kaaijk, S.R., Fantone, F., Darnell, J. and Manassa, C. 2014. 'Barley revisited: Production of barley bread in Umm Mawagir'. In *Current Research in Egyptology 2013. Proceedings of the Fourteenth Annual Symposium*, ed. K. Accetta, R. Fellinger, P.L. Concalves, S. Mussewhite and W.P. van Pelt. Oxford: Oxbow, pp. 49–63.

Carcopino, J. 1939. *La vie quotidienne à Rome à l'apogée de L'Empire*. Paris: Hachette.

Carcopino, J. 1941. *Daily Life in Ancient Rome: the People and the City at the Height of the Empire*. London: Routledge.

Cardauns, B. 2001. *Marcus Terentius Varro: Einführung in sein Werk*. Heidelberg: Universitätsverlag C. Winter.

Carlsen, J. 2013. *Land and Labour: Studies in Roman Social and Economic History*. Rome: L'Erma di Bretschneider.

Carruthers, W.J. 2000. 'The mineralised plant remains', in *Potterne 1982–5: Animal Husbandry in Later Prehistoric Wiltshire*, ed. A. Lawson and C. Gingell. Salisbury: Wessex Archaeology Report 17, pp. 72–84.

Casson, L. 1980. 'The role of the state in Rome's grain trade', in *The Seaborne Commerce of Ancient Rome: Studies in Archaeology and History*, ed. J. H. D'Arms and E. C. Kopff. Rome: American Academy in Rome, pp. 21–33.

Castagnoli, F. C. 1980. 'Installazioni portuali a Roma', in *The Seaborne Commerce of Ancient Rome: Studies in Archaeology and History*, ed. J. H. D'Arms and E. C. Kopff. Rome: American Academy in Rome, pp. 35–42.

Catalano, P. 2001. 'Bioarcheologia. Archivio antropologico', in *Archeologia e Giubileo. Gli Interventi a Roma e nel Lazio nel Piano del Grande Giubileo del 2000*, ed. F. Filippi. Rome: Ministero per i Beni e le Attività Culturali, Ufficio Centrale per i Beni Archeologici, Architettonici, Artistici e Storici.

Catalano, P. and Di Bernardini, M. 2001. 'Nota antropologica sull'intervento nell'area sub divo delle Catacombe di San Zotico', in *Archeologia e Giubileo. Gli Interventi a Roma e nel Lazio nel Piano del Grande Giubileo del 2000*, ed. F. Filippi. Rome: Ministero per i Beni e le Attività Culturali, Ufficio Centrale per i Beni Archeologici, Architettonici, Artistici e Storici, p. 269.

Catalano, P. and Nanni, A. 2001. 'Gabii. Nota antropologica', in *Archeologia e Giubileo. Gli Interventi a Roma e nel Lazio nel Piano del Grande Giubileo del 2000*, ed. F. Filippi. Rome: Ministero per i Beni e le Attività Culturali, Ufficio Centrale per i Beni Archeologici, Architettonici, Artistici e Storici, pp. 500–501.

Catalano, P., Egidi, R. and Minozzi, S. 2001a. 'Via Casal Ferranti. Ritrovamento dei resti della Via Latina e della necropoli', in *Archeologia e Giubileo. Gli Interventi a Roma e nel Lazio nel Piano del Grande Giubileo del 2000*, ed. F. Filippi. Rome: Ministero per i Beni e le Attività Culturali, Ufficio Centrale per i Beni Archeologici, Architettonici, Artistici e Storici, pp. 300–301.

Catalano, P., Arrighetti, B., Benedettini, et al. 2001b. 'Vivere e morire a Roma tra il primo ed il terzo secolo', *Mitteilungen des Deutschen Archäologischen Instituts, Römische Abteilung* 108, pp. 355–363.

Catalano, P., S. Minozzi, and W. Pantano. 2001c. 'Le necropoli romane di età Imperiale: un contributo all'interpretazione del popolamento e della qualità della vita nell'antica Roma', in *Urbanizzazione delle Campagne nell'Italia Antica.*, ed. L. Quilici and S. Quilici Gigli. Rome: L'Erma di Bretschneider, pp. 127–137.

Catalano, P., Minozzi, S., et al. 2001d. 'Le necropoli di Roma: Il contributo dell'antropologia.' *RM* 108, pp. 353–381.

Catalano, P., W. Pantano, C. Caldarini, F. De Angelis, A. Battistini, and A. Iorio. 2012. 'The contribution of the anthropological study to the analysis of ancient cemeteries: the demographic profile of six roman imperial age necropolis', *Journal of Biological Research – Bollettino della Società Italiana di Biologia Sperimentale* 85: 224-6.

Chandezon, C. 2004. 'Pratiques zootechniques dans l'antiquité grecque', *Revue des Études Grecques* 106, pp. 477–497.

Chandezon, C. 2015. 'Animals, meat, and alimentary by-products. Patterns of production and consumption', in *A Companion to Food in the Ancient World*, ed. J. Wilkins and R. Nadeau. Oxford: Wiley-Blackwell, pp. 135–146.

Chaniotis, A. 1988. 'Vinum Creticum Excellens: Zum Weinhandel Kretas', *Münstersche Beiträge zur Antiken Handelsgeschichte* 7(1), pp. 62–89.

Charles, M. 1998. 'Fodder from dung: the recognition and interpretation of dung-derived plant material from archaeological sites', *Environmental Archaeology* 1, pp. 111–122.

Chastagnol, A. 1950. 'Un scandale du vin à Rome sous le Bas-Empire. L'affaire du préfet Orfitus', *Annales* 5, pp. 166–183.

Chatterton, B.A. and Chatterton, L. 1984a. 'Medicago – its possible role in Romano-Libyan farming and its positive role in modern dry farming', *Libyan Studies* 14, pp. 157–160.

Chatterton, B.A. and Chatterton, L. 1984b. 'Alleviating land degradation and increasing cereal and livestock production in North Africa and the Middle East using annual medicago pasture', *Agriculture, Ecosystems and Environment* 11, pp. 117–129.

Chatterton, B.A. and Chatterton, L. 1985. 'A hypothetical answer to the decline of the granary of Rome', *Libyan Studies* 16, pp. 95–99.

Chavan, J.K. and Kadam, S.S. 1989. 'Critical reviews in food science and nutrition', *Food Science* 28, pp. 348–400.

Chenery, C., Müldner, G., Evans, J., Eckardt, H. and Lewis, M. 2010. 'Strontium and stable isotope evidence for diet and mobility in Roman Gloucester, UK', *Journal of Archaeological Science* 37, pp. 150–163.

Cheung, C., Schroeder, H. and Hedges, R.E.M. 2012. 'Diet, social differentiation and cultural change in Roman Britain: new isotopic evidence from Gloucestershire', *Archaeological and Anthropological Sciences* 4, pp. 61–73.

Chioffi, L. 1999. *Caro: il mercato della carne nell'Occidente romano*. Rome: L'Erma di Bretschneider.

Chouliara-Raïos, H. 1989. *L'abeille et le miel en Égypte d'après les papyrus grecs, Panepistemio Ioanninon Epistemonike Epeterida philosophikes Scholes "Dodone"'*. Parartema 30, Yanina: University of Yanina.

Ciaraldi, M. 2007. *People and Plants in Ancient Pompeii: A New Approach to Urbanism from the Microscope Room, the Use of Plant Resources at Pompeii and in the Pompeian Area from the 6th Century BC to AD 79*. London: Accordia Research Institute.

Cima, M., and Tomei, M.A., eds. 2012. *Vetri a Roma*. Milano: Electa.

Claflin, K.W. and Scholliers, P. 2012. 'Introduction: surveying global food historiograpy', in *Writing Food History: A Global Perspective*, ed. K. W. Claflin and P. Scholliers. London and New York: Berg, pp. 1–8.

Claridge, A. 2010. *Rome: An Oxford Archaeological Guide*. Oxford: Oxford University Press.

Clark, G. 2007. *A Farewell to Alms. A Brief Economic History of the World*. Princeton: Princeton University Press.

Clarke, J.R. 2003. *Art in the Lives of Ordinary Romans: Visual Representation and Non-Elite Viewers in Italy, 100 BC–AD 315*. Berkeley, University of California Press.

Clarysse, W. 1987. 'Greek loan-words in demotic', in *Aspects of Demotic Lexicography, Acts of the Second International Conference for Demotic Studies, Leiden*, ed. S.P. Vleeming. Leuven: Peeters, pp. 9–33.

Clarysse, W. 2001. 'Use and abuse of beer and wine in Graeco-Roman Egypt', in *Punica – Libyca – Ptolemaica. Festschrift für Werner Huss zum 65. Geburtstag dargebracht von Schülern, Freunden und Kollegen*, ed. K. Geus and K. Zimmermann. Studia Phoenicia 16, Orientalia Lovaniensia Periodica 104, Leuven: Peeters, pp. 159–166.

Clarysse, W. 2009. 'The archive of the toparch Leon once again', in *Faces of Hellenism. Studies in History of the Eastern Mediterranean (4th century BC–5th century AD)*, ed. P. Van Nuffelen. Studia Hellenistica 48. Leuven: Peeters, pp. 161–168.

Clarysse, W. 2013. 'Determinatives in Greek loan-words and proper names', in *Aspects of Demotic Orthography, Acts of an International Colloquium held in Trier*, ed. S.P. Vleeming. Leuven: Peeters, pp. 1–24.

Clarysse, W. and Thompson, D.J. 2006. *Counting the People in Hellenistic Egypt*. Cambridge: Cambridge University Press.

Clarysse, W. and Vandorpe, K. 1997. 'Viticulture and wine consumption in the Arsinoite Nome (P. Köln v 221)', *Ancient Society* 28, pp. 67–73.

Collingwood, R.G. and Wright, R.P. 1994. *The Roman Inscriptions of Britain: Volume II (Fascicule 6) Instrumentum Domesticum*. Avon: The Bath Press.

Colomer, R. and Menéndez, J.A. 2006. 'Mediterranean diet, olive oil and cancer', *Clinical and Translational Oncology* 8, pp. 15–21.

Colonnelli, G., Carpaneto, G.M., Cristaldi, M. 2000. 'Uso alimentare e allevamento del ghiro (Myoxus glis) presso gli antichi romani: materiale e documenti.' *Atti del 2 Convegno Nazionale di Archeozoologia. Asti, 14–16 Novembre 1997*. Forli, pp. 315–325.

Conedera, M., Krebs, P., Tinner, W., Pradella, M. and Torriani, D. 2004. 'The cultivation of *Castanea sativa* (Mill.) in Europe, from its origin to its diffusion on a continental scale', *Vegetation History and Archaeobotany* 13, pp. 161–179.

Cool, H. 2006. *Eating and Drinking in Roman Britain*. Cambridge: Cambridge University Press.

Cooley, A.E and Cooley, M.G.L. 2014. *Pompeii and Herculaneum: A Sourcebook*. London: Routledge.

Cooper, K. 1996. *The Virgin and the Bride: Idealized Womanhood in Late Antiquity*. Cambridge, MA: Harvard University Press.

Cooper, K. 2007. *The Fall of the Roman Household*. Cambridge and New York: Cambridge University Press.

Cooper, K. 2009. 'Gender and the fall of Rome', in *A Companion to Late Antiquity*, ed. P. Rousseau. Oxford: Wiley-Blackwell, pp. 187–200.

Copley, M.S., Berstan, R., Dudd, S.N., Straker, V., Payne, S. and Evershed, R.P. 2005. 'Dairying in antiquity. I. Evidence from absorbed lipid residues dating to the British Iron Age', *Journal of Archaeological Science* 32, pp. 485–503.

Corbier, M. 1989a. 'Le statut ambigu de la viande à Rome', *Dialogues d'histoire Ancienne* 15/2, pp. 107–158.

Corbier, M. 1989b. 'The ambiguous status of meat in ancient Rome', *Food and Foodways* 3, pp. 223–264.

Cordie-Hackenberg, R., Gerdes, C. and Wigg, A. 1992. 'Nahrungsreste aus römischen Gräbern und Aschengruben des Trierer Landes', *Archäologisches Korrespondenzblatt* 22, pp. 109–117.

Counihan, C. 2004. *Around the Tuscan Table. Food, Family and Gender in Twentieth-Century Florence.* London and New York: Routledge.

Courrier, C. 2014. *La plèbe de Rome et sa culture: (fin du IIe siècle av. J.C.-fin du Ier siècle ap. J.-C.).* Rome: École Française de Rome.

Cracco Ruggini, L. 1988. 'Roma e il vino nord-italico', in *La Mémoire perdue: à la Recherche des Archives oubliées, publiques et privées, de la Rome antique*, ed. S. Demougin. Paris: Publications de la Sorbonne, pp. 345–364.

Craig, O.E., Biazzo, M., O'Connell, T.C., et al. 2009. 'Stable isotopic evidence for diet at the Imperial Roman coastal site of Velia (1st and 2nd Centuries AD) in Southern Italy', *American Journal of Physical Anthropology* 139, pp. 572–583.

Craig, O.E., et al. 2013. 'Evaluating marine diets through radiocarbon dating and stable isotope analysis of victims of the AD 79 eruption of Vesuvius', *American Journal of Physical Anthropology* 152, pp. 345–352

Cramp, L.J.E., Evershed, R.P. and Eckardt, H. 2011. 'What was a mortarium used for? Organic residues and cultural change in Iron Age and Roman Britain', *Antiquity* 85(330), pp. 1339–1352.

Crandall, J.J, and Martin, D.L. 2012. 'On porotic hyperostosis and the interpretation of hominin diets. Comment on Manuel Domínguez-Rodrigo et al. 2010. Earliest porotic hyperostosis on a 1.5-million-year-old hominin, Olduvai Gorge, Tanzania', *PLOS ONE* 7, e46414.

Crawford, A. 2014. 'Ceramics, Roman Imperial', in *Encyclopedia of Global Archaeology*, ed. Claire Smith. New York: Springer, pp. 1303–1310.

Crawford, D. 1973. 'Garlic-growing and agricultural specialisation in Graeco-Roman Egypt', *Chronique d'Egypte* 48, pp. 350–363.

Crépon, K., Marget, P., Peyronnet, C., Carrouée, B., Arese, P., and Duc, G. 2010. 'Nutritional value of faba bean (*Vicia faba* L.) seeds for feed and food', *Field Crops Research* 115, pp. 329–339.

Cribellier, C. 2014. 'Jardins et habitats de l'agglomération de (Loiret, France)', in *Archéologie des jardins, analyse des espaces et méthodes d'approche*, ed. P. Van Ossel and A.-M. Guimier-Sorbets. Archéologie et histoire romaine 26. Montagnac: Editions Monique Mergoil, pp. 57–70.

Croisille, J.-M. 2015. *Natures Mortes dans la Rome antique.* Paris, Picard.

Crowe, F., Sperduti, A., O'Connell, T.C., Craig, O. E., Kirsanow, K., Germoni, P. Macchiarelli, R., Garnsey, P. and Bondioli, L. 2010. 'Water-related occupations and diet in two Roman coastal communities (Italy, first to third century AD): correlation between stable carbon and nitrogen isotope values and auricular exostosis prevalence', *American Journal of Physical Anthropology* 142, pp. 355–366.

Cruse A. 2004. *Roman Medicine.* Tempus: Stroud.

Cubberley, A. 1995. 'Bread-baking in ancient Italy', in *Food in antiquity*, ed. J.B. Wilkins, F.D. Harvey and M.J. Dobson. Exeter: University of Exeter Press.

Cubberley, A.L., Lloyd, J.A. and Roberts, P.C. 1988. 'Testa and Clibani: the baking covers of Classical Italy', *Papers of the British School at Rome* 56, pp. 98–119.

Cucina, A., Vargiu, R., Mancinelli, D., Ricci, R., Santandrea, E., Catalano, P. and Coppa, A. 2006. 'The necropolis of Vallerano (Rome, 2nd–3rd century AD): an anthropological perspective on the ancient Romans in the Suburbium', *International Journal of Osteoarchaeology* 16, pp. 104–117.

Cuomo di Caprio, N. 2007. *La ceramica in archeologia, 2: antiche tecniche di lavorazione e moderni metodi di indagine.* Studia archaeologica 144. Rome: L'Erma di Bretschneider.

Curiel, J.A., Coda, R., Centomani, I., Summo, C., Gobbetti, M. and Rizzello, C.J. 2015. 'Exploitation of the nutritional and functional characteristics of traditional Italian legume: the potential of sourdough fermentation', *International Journal of Food Microbiology* 196, pp. 51–61.

Curtis, R.I. 1979. 'The garum shop of Pompeii', *Cronache pompeiane* 5, pp. 5–23.

Curtis, R.I. 1984. 'A personalized floor mosaic from Pompeii'. *American Journal of Archaeology* 88(4), pp. 557–566.

Curtis, R.I. 1988. 'A. Umbricius Scaurus of Pompeii', in *Studia Pompeiana et Classica in Honor of Wilhelmina F. Jashemski*, ed. R. I. Curtis. New Rochelle, NY: A.D. Caratzas, pp. 19–50.

Curtis, R.I. 1991. *Garum and Salsamenta: Production and Commerce in Materia Medica.* New York: E.J. Brill.

Curtis, R.I. 2001. *Ancient Food Technology.* Leiden, Brill.

Curtis, R.I. 2008. 'Food processing and preparation', in *The Oxford Handbook of Engineering and Technology in the Classical World*, ed. J.P. Oleson. Oxford: Oxford University Press, pp. 369–392.

Curtis, R.I. 2012. 'Professional cooking, kitchens, and service work', in *A Cultural History of Food in Antiquity*, ed. P. Erdkamp. Oxford: Bloomsbury, pp. 95–112.

Cuvigny, H. 1996. 'The amount of wages paid to the quarry-workers at Mons Claudianus', *The Journal of Roman Studies* 86, pp. 139–145.

Cuvigny, H. 2003. *La route de Myos Hormos. L'armée romaine dans le désert oriental d'Egypte, Fouilles de l'IFAO 38.* Cairo: IFAO.

Cuvigny, H. 2007. 'Les noms du chou dans les ostraca grecs du désert oriental d'Egypte: κράμβη, κραμβίον, καυλίον', *BIFAO* 107, pp. 89–96.

Cuvigny, H. 2011. *Didymoi. Une garnison romaine dans le désert Oriental d'Egypte, I. Les fouilles et le matériel, Fouilles de l'IFAO 64.* Cairo: IFAO.

Cuvigny, H. 2014. 'La ration mensuelle d'un cavalier et de son cheval d'après un ostracon du praesidium de Dios (désert oriental d'Egypte)', in *De l'or pour les braves!*, Scripta antiqua 69. Bordeaux: Ausonius, pp. 71–90.

Dahiya, P.K., Linnemann, A.R., Nout, M.J.R., van Boekel, M.A.J.S. and Grewal, R.B. 2013. 'Nutrient composition of selected newly bred and established mung bean varieties', *Food Science and Technology* 54(1), pp. 249–256.

Dalby, A. 1996. *Siren Feasts: A History of Food and Gastronomy in Greece.* London: Routledge.

Dalby, A. 2003. *Food in the Ancient World from A–Z.* London: Routledge.

Dalby, A. and Grainger, S. 1996. *The Classical Cookbook.* London: British Museum Press.

D'Alessandro, S. 2011. 'Modernization, weather variability, and vulnerability to famine', *Oxford Economic Papers* 63, pp. 625–647.

D'Alessandro, W. 2006. 'Human fluorosis related to volcanic activity: a review', in *Environmental Toxicology*, ed. A. Kungolos, C. Brebbia, C. Samaras, and V. Popov. Southampton: WIT Press, pp. 21–30.

D'Alessandro, S. 2011. 'Modernization, weather variability, and vulnerability to famine', *Oxford Economic Papers* 63, pp. 625–647.

Daloz, J.-P. 2010. *The Sociology of Elite Distinction: From Theoretical to Comparative perspectives*, London: Palgrave Macmillan.

Dar, S. 1995. 'Food and archaeology in Romano-Byzantine Palestine', in *Food in Antiquity*, ed. J. Wilkins, D. Harvey and M. Dobson. Exeter: University of Exeter Press, pp. 326–335.

D'Arms, J. 1990. 'The Roman *convivium* and the ideal of equality', in *Sympotica: A Symposium on the Symposium*, ed. O. Murray. Oxford: Clarendon Press, pp. 308–320.

D'Arms, J. 1991. 'Slaves at Roman *convivia*', in *Dining in a Classical Context*, ed. W.J. Slater. Ann Arbor: University of Michigan Press, pp. 171–183.

D'Arms, J., 1995. 'Heavy drinking and drunkenness in the Roman world: four questions for historians', in *In Vino Veritas*, ed. O. Murray and M. Tecusan. London and Rome: British School at Rome, pp. 304–317.

Davidson, A., ed. 1999. *The Oxford Companion to Food.* Oxford: Oxford University Press.

Davies, D. 1795. *The Case of Labourers in Husbandry Considered.* Bath: R. Cruttwell.

Davies, R.W. 1971. 'The Roman military diet', *Britannia* 2, pp. 122–142.

Davies, R.W.1989. *Service in the Roman Army*, ed. D.J. Breeze and V.A. Maxfield. Edinburgh: Edinburgh University Press.

De Almeida Costa, G.E., da Silva Queiroz-Monici, K., Reis, S.M.P.M., and de Oliveira, A.C. 2006. 'Chemical composition, dietary fibre and resistant starch contents of raw and cooked pea, common bean, chickpea and lentil legumes', *Food Chemistry* 94, pp. 327–330.

De Boe, D., De Bie, M. and Van Impe, L. 1992. 'Neerharen-Rekem. Die komplexe Besiedlungsgeschichte einer von Kiesbaggern geretteten Fundstätte', in *Spurensicherung. Archäologische Denkmalpflege in der Euregio Maas-Rhein.* Kunst und Altertum am Rhein 136. Mainz: Verlag Philipp von Zabern, pp. 477–496.

De Caro, S. 2001. *La natura morta nelle pitture e nei mosaici delle città vesuviane.* Napoli: Electa Napoli, Soprintendenza archeologica di Napoli e Caserta.

De Cupere, B., Poblome, J., Hamilton-Dyer, S. and Van Haelst, S. 2015. 'Communal dining in the eastern suburbium of ancient Sagalassos: the evidence of animal remains and material culture', *HEROM. Journal on Hellenistic and Roman Material Culture* 4(2), pp. 173–197.

De Fillippo, C., Cavalieri, D., Di Paola, M., Ramazzotti, M., Poullet, J.B., Massart, S., Collini, S., Pieraccini, G. and Lionetti, P. 2010. 'Impact of diet in shaping gut microbiota revealed by a comparative study in children from Europe and rural Africa', *PNAS* 107(33), pp. 14691–14696.

De Haan, N. and Jansen, G. 1996. *Cura Aquarum in Campania. Proceedings of the Ninth International Congress on the History of Water Management and Hydraulic Engineering in the Mediterranean Region, Pompeii 1–8 October 1994*. Leiden: Peeters.

De Jong, F.M. 2010. *Ons Voedsel in Getallen*.'s-Gravenland: Fontaine Uitgevers.

De Ligt, L. 2012. *Peasants, Citizens, and Soldiers. Studies in the Demographic History of Roman Italy 225 BC–AD 100*. Cambridge: Cambridge University Press.

De Lorgeril, M., Salen, P., Martin, J-L., Monjaud, I., Delaye, J. and Mamelle, N. 1999. 'Mediterranean diet, traditional risk factors, and the rate of cardiovascular complications after myocardial infarction. Final report of the Lyon diet heart study', *Circulation* 99, pp. 779–785.

De Sena, E. C. 2005. 'An assessment of wine and oil production in Rome's hinterland: ceramic, literary, art, historical and modern evidence', in *Roman Villas around the Urbs: Interaction with Landscape and Environment. Proceedings of a Conference held at the Swedish Institute in Rome, September 17–18, 2004*, ed. B. Santillo Frizell and A. Klynne. Rome: Swedish Institute in Rome. Projects and Seminars, 2, pp. 135–149.

De Sena, E.C. and Ikäheimo, J.P. 2003. 'The supply of amphora-borne commodities and domestic pottery in Pompeii 150 BC-AD 79: preliminary evidence from the house of the vestals', *EJA* 6(3), pp. 301–321.

De Witte, S.N. and Stojanowski, C.M. 2015. 'The osteological paradox 20 years later: past perspectives, future directions', *Journal of Archaeological Research* 23, pp. 397–450.

Deines, P. 1980. 'The isotopic composition of reduced organic carbon. In *Handbook of Environmental Isotope Geochemistry*, ed. P. Fritz and J.C. Fontes.Amsterdam: Springer, pp. 329–406.

Deitch, R. 2003. *Hemp: American History Revisited: The Plant with a Divided History*. New York: Algora Publishing.

Delouis, O. and Mossakowska-Gaubert, M. (2015) *Le Vie quotidienne des Moines en Orient et en Occident (IVe–Xe sicèle), volume I. L'État des Sources*, Bibliothèque d'Etude 163, Cairo: IFAO.

DeNiro, M.J. and Epstein, S. 1981. 'Influence of diet on the distribution of nitrogen isotopes in animals,' *Geochimica et Cosmochimica Acta* 45, pp. 341–351.

Derreumaux, M., Lepetz. S., Jacques, A. and Prilaux, G. 2008. 'Food supply at two successive military settlements in Arras (France): An archaeobotanical and archaeozoological approach', in *Feeding the Roman Army. The Archaeology of Production and Supply in NW Europe*, ed. S. Stallibrass and R. Thomas. Oxford: Oxbow Books, pp. 52–68.

Deru, X. 2010. *Die Römer an Maas und Mosel*. Mainz: Verlag Philipp von Zabern.

Deschler-Erb, S. 2006. 'Leimsiederei- und Räuchereiwarenabfälle des 3. Jahrhunderts aus dem Bereich zwischen Frauenthermen und Theater von Augusta Raurica', *Jahresberichte aus Augst und Kaiseraugst* 27, pp. 323–346.

Deschler-Erb, S. 2013. 'Gallische Schinken und Würste neu aufgetischt', *Jahrbuch Archäologie Schweiz* 96, pp. 146–151.

Diederich, S. 2007. *Römische Agrarhandbücher zwischen Fachwissenschaft, Literatur und Ideologie*. Berlin: De Gruyter.

Dietler, M. and B. Hayden, eds. 2001. *Feasts: Archaeological and Ethnographical Perspectives on Food, Politics and Power*. Washington and London: Smithsonian Institution Press.

Dionisotti, A.C. 1982. 'From Ausonius' schooldays? A schoolbook and its relatives', *Journal of Roman Studies* 72, pp. 83–125.

Dixon, S. 1990. *The Roman Mother*. London: Routledge.

Dixon, S. 1992. *The Roman Family*. Baltimore: Johns Hopkins University Press.

Dixon, S., ed. 2001. *Childhood, Class and Kin in the Roman World*. London: Routledge.

Dobney, K. and Goodman, A.H. 1991. 'Epidemiological studies of dental enamel hypoplasias in Mexico and Bradford: their relevance to archaeological skeletal studies', in *Health in Past Societies: Biocultural interpretations of Human Skeletal Remains in Archaeological Contexts*, ed. H. Bush and M. Zvelebil. Oxford: BAR International Reports, pp. 81–100.

Dobney, K.M., Jaques, S.D. and Irving, B.G. 1996. *Of Butchers and Breeds. Report on Vertebrate Remains from various sites in the City of Lincoln*. Lincoln: City of Lincoln Archaeology Unit.

Dohm, H. 1964. *Mageiros: Die Rolle des Kochs in der Griechisch-Römishcen Komödie*. Munich: C.H. Beck.

Donahue, J.F. 2003. 'Towards a typology of Roman public feasting', *The American Journal of Philology* 124(3), Special Issue, Roman Dining, pp. 423–441.

Donahue, J.F. 2004a. *The Roman Community at Table during the Principate*. Ann Arbor: University of Michigan Press.

Donahue, J.F. 2004b. 'Iunia Rustica of Cartima: Female munificence in the Roman West', *Latomus* 63, pp. 873–891.

Donahue, J. F. 2015a. 'Roman dining' in *A Companion to Food in the Ancient World*, ed. J. Wilkins and R. Nadeau. Oxford: Wiley-Blackwell, pp. 253–264.

Donahue, J.F. 2015b. *Food and Drink in Antiquity: Readings from the Graeco-Roman World: a Sourcebook.* London: Bloomsbury.

Donahue, J.F. 2016. 'Nutrition', in *Blackwell Companion to Ancient Science, Medicine and Technology*, ed. G. Irby. Chichester, West Sussex and Malden, MA: Wiley-Blackwell, pp. 618–631.

Donnelly, A.J. 2015. 'Cooking pots in ancient and late antique cookbooks', in *Ceramics, Cuisine and Culture: The Archaeology and Science of Kitchen Pottery in the Ancient Mediterranean World*, ed. M. Spataro and A. Villing. Oxford: Oxbow Books, pp. 141–147.

D'Ortenzio, L., Brickley, M., Schwarcz, H. and Prowse, T. 2015. 'You are not what you eat during physiological stress: isotopic evaluation of human hair', *American Journal of Physical Anthropology* 157, pp. 374–388.

Doymaz, I., Gorel, O. and Akgun, N.A. 2004. 'Drying characteristics of the solid by-product of olive oil extraction', *Biosystems Engineering* 88, pp. 213–219.

Draguet, R. 1945. 'Le chapitre de l'Histoire Lausiaque sur les Tabennésiotes dérive-t-il d'une source copte?', *Le Muséon* 58, 15–95.

Drexhage, H.-J. 1990a. 'Λάχανον and λαχανοπώλης im römischen Aegypten (1.-3. Jh. n.Chr.)', *Münstersche Beiträge zur Antiken Handelsgeschichte* 9, pp. 103–108.

Drexhage, H.-J. 1990b. *Preise, Mieten/Pachten, Kosten und Lohne im romischen Aegypten bis zum Regierungsantritt Diokletians, Vorarbeiten zu einer Wirtschaftsgeschichte des romischen Aegypten I.* St. Katharinen: Scripta Mercatura Verlag.

Drexhage, H.-J. 1993. 'Garum und Garumhandel im römischen und spätantiken Ägypten', *Münstersche Beiträge zur Antiken Handelsgeschichte* 12, pp. 27–55.

Drexhage, H.J. 1996. 'Der Handel, die Produktion und der Verzehr von Käse nach den griechischen Papyri und Ostraka', *Münstersche Beiträge zur Antiken Handelsgeschichte* 15, pp. 33–41.

Drexhage, H.-J. 1997. 'Bierproduzenten und Bierhändler in der papyrologischen Überlieferung', *Münstersche Beiträge zur Antiken Handelsgeschichte* 16(2), pp. 32–39.

Drexhage, H.-J. 2012. 'Schweine und Schweinefleisch in den griechischen Papyri und Ostraka mit besonderem Blick auf die ersten drei Jahrhunderte n. Chr.', *Münstersche Beiträge zur Antiken Handelsgeschichte* 29, pp. 165–209.

Dubois-Pelerin, E. 2008. *Le luxe privée à Rome et en Italie au Ier siècle après J.-C.* Naples: Centre Jean Bérard.

Dunbabin, K. 1991. '*Triclinium* and *stibadium*', in *Dining in a Classical Context*, ed. W.J. Slater. Ann Arbor: University of Michigan Press, pp. 121–148.

Dunbabin, K. 1993. 'Wine and water at the Roman convivium', *Journal of Roman Archaeology* 6, pp. 116–141.

Dunbabin, K. 1999. *Mosaics of the Greek and Roman World.* Cambridge and New York: Cambridge University Press.

Dunbabin, K. 2003. *The Roman Banquet: Images of Conviviality.* Cambridge: Cambridge University Press.

Dunbabin, K., and Slater, W. 2011. 'Roman dining', in *The Oxford Handbook of Social Relations in the Roman World*, ed. M. Peachin. Oxford: Oxford University Press, pp. 438–466.

Duncan-Jones, R. 1964. 'The purpose and organization of the *alimenta*', *PBSR* 33, pp. 123–146.

Duncan-Jones, R. 1974. *The Economy of the Roman Empire: Quantitative Studies.* Cambridge: Cambridge University Press.

Duncan-Jones, R. 1982. *The Economy of the Roman Empire: Quantitative Studies*, 2nd edition. Cambridge: Cambridge University Press.

Dupont, F. 1977. *Le plaisir et la loi, du 'Banquet' de Platon au Satiricon.* Paris: F. Maspero.

Dupont, F. 1996. 'Grammaire de l'alimentation et des repas romains', in *Histoire de l'Alimentation*, ed. J-L. Flandrin and M. Montanari. Paris: Fayard, pp. 197–214

Dupont, F. 1999. 'De l'œuf à la pomme: la cena romaine', in *Table d'ici, Table d'ailleurs: Histoire et Ethnologie du Repas*, ed. J.-L. Flandrin and J. Cobi, Paris: Odile Jacob, pp. 59–85.

Dütting, M. K. and van Rijn, P. 2017. 'Wickerwork Fish Traps from the Roman period in the Netherlands', in *Wald und Holznutzung währen der römischen Antike. Akten der Rheinbacher Tagung 2014*, ed. T. Kaszab-Olschewski and I. Tamerl. Archäologische Berichte 27, pp. 37–59.

Dyson, S.L. 1995. 'Is there a text in this site?' in *Methods in the Mediterranean: Historical and Archaeological Views on Texts and Archaeology*, ed. D.B. Small. Leiden: Brill, pp. 25–44.

Dzierzbicka, D. 2018. *Oinos. Production and Import of Wine in Greco-Roman Egypt.* Warsaw: JJP Supplement, vol. 31.

Ebel-Zepezauer, W. 2009. 'Eine heile Welt? Alltag und Lebensgrundlage der Germanen in der älteren Römischen Kaiserzeit', in *2000 Jahre Varusschlacht Mythos*, ed. Landesverband Lippe. Stuttgart: Wissenschaftliche Buchgesellschaft, pp. 77–80.

Eck, W. 2004. *Köln in römischer Zeit. Geschichte einer Stadt im Rahmen des Imperium Romanum.* Geschichte der Stadt Köln 1. Köln: Greven Verlag.

Eckardt, H., ed. 2010. *Roman Diasporas: Archaeological Approaches to Mobility and Diversity in the Roman Empire.* Journal of Roman Archaeology Supplement 78.

Eden. Sir F.M. 1797. *The State of the Poor*, 3 vols. London: B&J White.

Effros, B. 2002. *Creating Community with Food and Drink in Merovingian Gaul.* New York: Palgrave.

Egidi, R., Catalano, P. and Spadoni, D. eds. 2003. *Aspetti di Vita Quotidiana dalle Necropoli della via Latina, Località Osteria del Curato.* Rome: Ministero per i Beni e le Attività Culturali, Soprintendenza Archeologica di Roma.

Ehmig, U. 2003. *Die römischen Amphoren aus Mainz.* Frankfurter Archäologische Schriften 4. Möhnsee: Reichert Verlag.

Ehmig, U. 2011/2012. 'Über alle Berge. Früheste Mediterrane Warenlieferungen in den römischen Ostalpenraum', *Römisches Österreich* 34/35, pp. 13–35.

Eideneier, H. 1971. 'Ghost-words in der griechischen Papyruslexicography', *Zeitschrift für Papyrologie und Epigraphik* 7, pp. 53–55.

Ekroth, G. 2007. 'Meat in ancient Greece: sacrificial, sacred or secular', *Food and History* 5, pp. 249–272

El-Mahdy, A.R. and El-Sebaiy, L.A. 1985. 'Proteolytic activity, amino acid composition and protein quality of germinating fenugreek seeds. (*Trigonella foenum graecum L.*)', *Food Chemistry* 18, pp. 19–33.

El Nasri, N.A. and El Tinay, A.H. 2007. 'Functional properties of fenugreek (Trigonella foenum graecum) protein concentrate', *Food Chemistry* 103, pp. 582–589.

Ellis, S.J.R. 2012. 'Eating and drinking out', in *A Cultural History of Food in Antiquity*, ed. P. Erdkamp. London: Bloomsbury, pp. 95–112.

Ellis, S.P. 1992. *Graeco-Roman Egypt.* Shire Egyptology. Haverfordwest: Shire Publications.

Elm, S. 1994. *Virgins of God: The Making of Asceticism in Late Antiquity.* Oxford and New York: Oxford University Press.

Erdkamp, P. 1998. *Hunger and the Sword: Warfare and Food Supply in Roman Republican Wars (264–30 BC).* Amsterdam: J.C. Gieben.

Erdkamp, P. 2000. 'Feeding Rome, or feeding Mars? A long-term approach to C. Gracchus' *lex frumentaria*', *Ancient Society* 30, pp. 53–70.

Erdkamp, P. 2002. 'A starving mob has no respect: urban markets and food riots in the Roman world, 100 BC–400 AD', in *The Transformations of Economic Life under the Roman Empire*, ed. L. de Blois and J. Rich. Amsterdam: J.C. Gieben, pp. 93–115.

Erdkamp, P. 2005. *The Grain Market in the Roman Empire: A Social, Political, and Economic Study.* Cambridge: Cambridge University Press.

Erdkamp, P. 2007. 'War and state formation in the Roman Republic', in *A Companion to the Roman Army*, ed. P. Erdkamp. Oxford: Blackwell, pp. 96–113.

Erdkamp, P. 2008. 'Grain funds and market intervention in the Roman world', in *Feeding the Ancient Greek City*, ed. R. Alston and O.M. van Nijf. Leuven: Peeters, pp. 109–126.

Erdkamp, P. 2011. 'Jews and Christians at the dinner table: a study in social and religious interaction', *Food and History* 9, pp. 71–107

Erdkamp, P., ed. 2012a. *A Cultural History of Food in Antiquity.* London and New York: Berg.

Erdkamp, P. 2012b. 'Urbanism', in *The Cambridge Companion to the Roman Economy*, ed. W. Scheidel. Cambridge: Cambridge University Press, pp. 241–265.

Erdkamp, P. 2012c. 'Food security, safety, and crises', in *A Cultural History of Food in Antiquity*, ed. P. Erdkamp. Oxford: Bloomsbury, pp. 57–74.

Eriksson, G., 2013. 'Stable isotope analysis of humans', in *The Oxford Handbook of the Archaeology of Death*, ed. S. Tarlow and L. Nilsson Stutz. Oxford: Oxford University Press, pp. 123–146.

Ervynck, A., Neer, W.V., Hüster-Plogmann, H. and Schibler, J. 2003. 'Beyond affluence: the zooarchaeology of luxury', *World Archaeology* 34(3), pp. 542–557.

Etienne, R. 1981. 'Les rations alimentaires des esclaves de la 'familia rustica' d'après Caton', *Index* 12, pp. 66–77.

Eveleth, P.B. and Tanner, J.M., 1990. *Worldwide Variation in Human Growth*. Cambridge: Cambridge University Press.

Evershed, R.P. 2008a. 'Experimental approaches to the interpretation of absorbed organic residues in archaeological ceramics', *World Archaeology* 40(1), pp. 26–47.

Evershed, R.P. 2008b. 'Organic residue analysis in archaeology: the archaeological biomarker revolution', *Archaeometry* 50(6), pp. 895–924.

Faas, P. 1994. *Around the Roman Table*. Chicago: University of Chicago Press.

Facchini, F., Rastelli, E., Brasili, P. 2004. 'Cribra orbitalia and cribra cranii in Roman skeletal remains from the Ravenna area and Rimini (I–IV Century AD)', *International Journal of Osteoarchaeology* 14, pp.126–136.

Facsády, A. R. 1996. 'Kaiserdarstellungen aus Terrakotta im Museum von Aquincum', in *Akten des 3. Internationalen Kolloquiums über Probleme des provinzialrömischen Kunstschaffens*, ed. G. Bauchhenß. Beihefte der Bonner Jahrbücher 51. Köln: Rheinland Verlag, pp. 21–25.

Fairclough, H.R. and Goold, G.P., eds. 2000. *Virgil, Volume II: Aeneid Books 7–12, Appendix Vergiliana*. Loeb Classical Library. Cambridge, MA: Harvard University Press.

Farrar, L. 1998. *Ancient Roman Gardens*. Phoenix Mill, Gloucestershire: Sutton.

Faust, S. and Schneider, F. 2013. 'Römische Spargelmesser im archäologischen Experiment. Zu antiken Messern mit Spargelgriff', *Funde und Ausgrabungen im Bezirk Trier* 45, pp. 7–13.

Fauve-Chamoux, A. 2001. 'Chestnuts', in *The Cambridge World History of Food* vol. I, ed. K.F. Kiple and K.C. Ornelas. Cambridge: Cambridge University Press, pp. 359–364.

FDA. 2004. 'Letter responding to health claim petition dated August 28, 2003: Monounsaturated fatty acids from olive oil and coronary heart disease (Docket No 2003Q-0559)', *Summary of Qualified Health Claims Subject to Enforcement Discretion*. Available at www.fda.gov/Food/IngredientsPackagingLabeling/LabelingNutrition/ucm072963.htm (accessed 3 July 2015).

FDA. 2014. 'Food labelling'. *Code of Federal Regulations 21*. Vol 2. Last updated April 1, 2014. Available at www.accessdata.fda.gov/scripts/cdrh/cfdocs/cfcfr/cfrsearch.cfm?fr=101.12 (accessed 27 June 2015).

Feely-Harnick, G. 1981. *The Lord's Table: The Meaning of Food in Early Judaism and Christianity*. Washington DC: Smithsonian Institute Press.

Fejerskov, O., Guldager Bilde, P., Bizzaro, M., Connelly, J.N., Skovhus Thomsen, J. and Nyvad, B. 2012. 'Dental caries in Rome, 50–100 AD', *Caries Research* 46, pp. 467–473.

Fentress, E. 2010. 'Cooking pots and cooking practice: an African bain-marie?' *Papers of the British School at Rome* 78, pp. 145–150.

Ferdière, A. 2011. *Gallia Lugdunensis. Eine römische Provinz im Herzen Frankreichs*. Mainz: Verlag Philipp von Zabern.

Fernández, A.G., Fernández Díez, M.J. and Adams, M.R. 1997. *Table Olives: Production and Processing*. London: Chapman & Hall.

Figueiral, I., Bouby, L., Buffat, L. Petitot, H. and Terral, J.-F. 2010. 'Archaeobotany, vine growing and wine producing in Roman Southern France: the site of Gasquinoy (Béziers, Hérault)', *Journal of Archaeological Science* 37, pp. 139–149.

Finn, R. 2009. *Asceticism in the Graeco-Roman World*. Key Themes in Ancient History. Cambridge and New York: Cambridge University Press.

Flandrin, J.-L. and M. Montanari, eds. 1996. *Histoire de l'Alimentation*, Paris: Fayard.

Flint-Hamilton, K.B. 1999. 'Legumes in ancient Greece and Rome: Food, medicine, or poison?', *Hesperia* 68(3), pp. 371–385.

Flohr, M., Marzano, A. and A.I. Wilson. 2013. 'Olive oil and wine presses database', *Oxford Roman Economy Project*. Available at http://oxrep.classics.ox.ac.uk/databases/olive_oil_and_wine_presses_database/ (accessed 15 June 2015).

Floud, R.W., Wachter, K. and Gregory, A. 1990. *Height, Health and History: Nutritional Status in the United Kingdom*. Cambridge: Cambridge University Press.

Flower, B. and Rosenbaum, E. 1958. *The Roman Cookery Book: A Critical Translation of The Art of Cooking by Apicius. For Use in the Study and the Kitchen*. London: George G. Harrap & Co.

Fogel, R. 1989/2012. 'Second thoughts on the European escape from hunger. Famines, chronic malnutrition, and mortality rates', *NBER Historical Working Paper* No. 1, issued in May 1989. Reprinted in *Explaining Long-Term Trends in Health and Longevity*. Cambridge: Cambridge University Press 2012, pp. 39–90.

Fogel, R.W. 1992. 'Second thoughts on the European escape from hunger: famines, chronic malnutrition, and mortality rates', in *Nutrition and Poverty*, ed. S.R. Osmani. Oxford: Oxford University Press, pp. 243–286. (Reprinted in *Explaining Long-Term Trends in Health and Longevity*, Cambridge: Cambridge University Press, pp. 39–90.)

Fogel, R.W. 2004. *The Escape from Hunger and Premature Death, 1700–2000: Europe, America, and the Third World*. Cambridge: Cambridge University Press.

Food and Agriculture Organization (FAO), 1994. *Definition and Classification of Commodities: 4. Pulses and Derived Products*. Available at www.fao.org/es/faodef/fdef04e.htm (accessed: 15 February 2015).

Food and Agriculture Organization (FAO), 2013. *FAO Statistical Yearbook 2013*. Geneva: FAO. Available at http://issuu.com/faooftheun/docs/syb2013issuu/281 (accessed 15 February 2015).

Food and Agriculture Organization, World Health Organization, and United Nations University. 1985. *Energy and Protein Requirements*. Technical report series No. 724. Geneva: FAO. Available at www.fao.org/docrep/003/aa040e/AA040E05.htm#ch5.6 (accessed 15 February 2015).

Food and Agriculture Organization, World Health Organization, and United Nations University. 2007. *Protein and Amino Acid Requirements in Human Nutrition*. Technical report series No. 935. Geneva: FAO. Available at http://whqlibdoc.who.int/trs/who_trs_935_eng.pdf (accessed 15 February 2015).

Formicola, V. 1983. 'Stature in Italian prehistoric samples, with particular reference to methodological problems', *Homo* 34, pp. 33–47.

Formicola, V. 1993. 'Stature reconstruction from long bones in ancient population samples: an approach to the problem of its reliability', *American Journal of Physical Anthropology* 90, pp. 351–358.

Foss, P.W. 1994. *Kitchens and Dining Rooms at Pompeii: The Spatial and Social Relationships of Cooking to Eating in the Roman Household*. PhD. Dissertation, Ann Arbor, MI: University of Michigan.

Fox, S. 2005. 'Health in Hellenistic and Roman times: the cases of Paphos, Cyprus and Corinth, Greece', in *Health in Antiquity*, ed. H. King. London: Routledge, pp. 59–82.

Fox, S. 2012. 'The bioarchaeology of children in Graeco-Roman Greece', in *L'Enfant et la Mort dans l'Antiquité II. Types de tombes et traitement du corps des enfants dans l'antiquité gréco-romaine*, ed. M.-D. Nenna. Alexandria: Centre d'Études Alexandrines, pp. 409–427.

Foxhall, L. 2007. *Olive Cultivation in Ancient Greece: Seeking the Ancient Economy*. Oxford: Oxford University Press.

Foxhall, L. and Forbes, H.A. 1982. 'Sitometreia: the role of grain as a staple food in classical antiquity', *Chiron* 12, pp. 41–90.

Frank, T. 1940. *An Economic Survey of Ancient Rome*. Baltimore: John Hopkins University Press.

Fraser, R., Bogaard, A., Heaton, T., et al. 2011. 'Manuring and stable nitrogen isotope ratios in cereals and pulses: towards a new archaeobotanical approach to the inference of land use and dietary practices', *Journal of Archaeological Science* 38, pp. 2790–2804.

Fraser, R.A., Bogaard, A., Heaton, T., et al. 2011. 'Manuring and stable nitrogen isotope ratios in cereals and pulses: towards a new archaeobotanical approach to the inference of land use and dietary practices', *Journal of Archaeological Science* 38, pp. 2780–2904.

Fraser, R.A., Bogaard, A., Schäfer, M., Arbogast, R.-M. and Heaton, T.H.E.H. 2013. 'Integrating botanical, faunal and human stable carbon and nitrogen isotope values to reconstruct land use and palaeodiet at LBK Vaihingen an der Enz, Baden-Württemberg', *World Archaeology* 45(3), pp. 492–517.

Frass, M. 2006. *Antike römische Gärten: soziale und wirtschaftliche Funktionen der Horti Romani*. Horn-Vienna: Burger und Söhne.

Frayn, J.M. 1979. *Subsistence Farming in Roman Italy*. London: Open Gate Press.

Freidenreich, D.M. 2011. *Foreigners and their Food: Constructing Otherness in Jewish, Christian, and Islamic Law*. Berkeley, CA: University of California Press.

Frémondeau, D., M.-P. Horard-Herbin, O. Buchsenschutz, J. Ughetto-Monfrin and M. Balasse 2015. 'Standardized pork production at the Celtic village of Levroux Les Arènes (France, 2nd c. BC): evidence from kill-off patterns and birth seasonality inferred from enamel δ18O analysis', *Journal of Archaeological Science: Reports* 2, pp. 215–226.

Friedländer, L. [1908]–1913. *Roman Life and Manners in the Early Empire*. London: Routledge.

Frier, B.W. 1983. 'Roman law and the wine trade: the problem of "vinegar sold as wine"', *Zeitschrift der Savigny-Stiftung für Rechtsgeschichte. Romanistische Abteilung* 100, pp. 257–295.

Froschauer, F. and Römer, C. 2006. *Mit den Griechen zu Tisch in Aegypten*. Nilus 12. Wien: Phoibos.

Fuller, B.T., Márquez-Grant, N. and Richards, M.P. 2010. 'Investigation of diachronic dietary patterns on the Islands of Ibiza and Formentera, Spain: Evidence from carbon and nitrogen stable isotope ratio analysis', *American Journal of Physical Anthropology* 143, pp. 512–522.

Fuller, B.T., Muldner, G., Van Neer, W., Ervynck, A. and Richards, M.P. 2012. 'Carbon and nitrogen stable isotope ratio analysis of freshwater, brackish and marine fish from Belgian archaeological sites (1st and 2nd millennium AD)', *Journal of Analytical Atomic Spectrometry* 27(5), pp. 807–820.

Fully, G. and Pineau, H. 1960. 'Détermination de la stature au moyen du squelette', *Annales de Médicine Légale* 40, pp. 145–153.

Funari, P.P.A. 1996. *Dressel 20 Inscriptions from Britain and the Consumption of Spanish Olive Oil*. Oxford: Tempus Reparatum.

Funari, P.P.A. 2001. 'Monte Testaccio and the Roman economy', *JRA* 14, pp. 585–588.

Funari, P.P.A. 2002. 'The consumption of olive oil in Roman Britain and the role of the army', in *The Roman Army and the Economy*, ed. P. Erdkamp. Amsterdam: Gieben, pp. 235–263.

Furger, A.R. 1994. 'Die urbanistische Entwicklung von Augusta Raurica vom 1. bis zum 3. Jahrhundert', *Jahresberichte aus Augst und Kaiseraugst* 15, pp. 29–38.

Gaastra, J.S. 2014. 'Shipping sheep or creating cattle: domesticate size changes with Greek colonisation in Magna Graecia', *Journal of Archaeological Science* 52, pp. 483–496.

Gabba, E. 1983. 'Literature', in *Sources for Ancient History*, ed. M. Crawford. Cambridge: Cambridge University Press, pp. 1–79.

Gaitzsch, W. 2010. 'Römische Siedlungsgrabungen im rheinischen Braunkohlenrevier. Forschungsschwer-punkte und Ergebnisse', in *Braunkohlenarchäologie im Rheinland. Entwicklung von Kultur, Umwelt und Landschaft*, ed. J. Kunow. Weilerswist: Verlag Ralf Liebe, pp. 76–86.

Galen. 2002. *Galen: On the Properties of Foodstuffs*, trans. O. W. Powell. New York: Cambridge University Press.

Gallant, T. 1991. *Risk and Survival in Ancient Greece: Reconstructing the Rural Domestic Economy*. Cambridge: Polity Press.

Garcia Soler, M.J. 2001. *El arte de comer en la antigua grecia*. Madrid: Biblioteca Nueva.

Gardner, J. 1998. *Family and Familia in Roman Law and Life*. Oxford: Clarendon Press.

Garnsey, P. 1983. 'Grain for Rome', in *Trade in the Ancient Economy*, ed. P. Garnsey, K. Hopkins and C. Whittaker. London: Chatto and Windus, pp. 118–130.

Garnsey, P. 1988. *Famine and Food Supply in the Graeco-Roman World: Responses to Risk and Crisis*. Cambridge: Cambridge University Press.

Garnsey, P. 1991. 'Mass diet and nutrition in the city of Rome', in *Nourrir le Plèbe*, ed. A. Giovanni. Basel: Friedrich Reinhardt Verlag, 67–101.

Garnsey, P. 1998. *Cities, Peasants, and Food in Classical Antiquity*. Cambridge: Cambridge University Press.

Garnsey, P. 1999. *Food and Society in Classical Antiquity*. Cambridge: Cambridge University Press.

Garnsey, P. and Saller, R. 2014. *The Roman Empire: Economy, Society, and Culture*, 2nd edition. London and New York: Bloomsbury.

Garnsey, P. and Van Nijf, O. 1998. 'Contrôle des prix du grain à Rome et dans les cités de l'Empire', in *La Mémoire perdue: Recherches sur l'Administration romaine*, ed. C Moatti. Rome: Ecole française de Rome, pp. 303–315.

Gasbarrini, G., Rickards, O., Martínez-Labarga, C., Pacciani, E., Chilleri, F., Laterza, L., Marangi, G., Scaldaferri, F., and Gasbarrini, A. 2012. 'Origin of celiac disease: how old are predisposing haplotypes?', *World Journal of Gastroenterology* 18, pp. 5300–5304.

George, M., ed. 2001. *The Roman Family in the Empire: Rome, Italy and Beyond*. Oxford: Oxford University Press.

Geraci, G. 2018. 'Feeding Rome: the grain supply', in *A Companion to the City of Rome*, ed. C.Holleran and A. Claridge. Malden, MA: Wiley-Blackwell, pp. 219–246.

Ghanbari, R., Farooq, A., Khalid, M.A., Anwarul-Hassan, G. and Nazamid, S. 2012. 'Valuable nutrients and functional bioactives in different parts of olive (*Olea europaea* L.): a review', *International Journal of Molecular Sciences* 13, pp. 3291–3340.

Giacosa, I. G. 1992. *A Taste of Ancient Rome*. Chicago: University of Chicago Press.

Giannecchini, M. and Moggi-Cecchi, J. 2008. 'Stature in archeological samples from central Italy: methodological issues and diachronic changes', *American Journal of Physical Anthropology* 135(3), pp. 284–292.

Gill, C., Whitmarsh, T. and Wilkins, J., eds. 2009. *Galen and the World of Knowledge*. Cambridge: Cambridge University Press.

Gilles, K.-J. 1999. *Bacchus und Sucellus. 2000 Jahre römische Weinkultur an Mosel und Rhein*. Briedel: Rhein-Mosel-Verlag.

Goffin, B. 2002. *Euergetismus in Oberitalien*. Bonn: Rudolf Habelt.

Gomes, T. Paradiso, V.M. and Delcuratolo, D. 2010. 'Non-conventional parameters for quality evaluation of refined olive oil and olive oil commercial classes', in *Olives and Olive Oil in Health and Disease Prevention*, ed. V.R. Preedy and R.R. Watson. Amsterdam: Academic Press, pp. 139–154

Goodman, A.H. and Rose, J.C. 1990. 'Assessment of systemic physiological perturbations from dental enamel hypoplasias and associated histological structures', *American Journal of Physical Anthropology* 33, pp. 59–110.

Goodman, A.H. and Martin, D.L. 2002. 'Reconstructing health profiles from skeletal remains', in *The Backbone of History: Health and Nutrition in the Western Hemisphere*, ed. R. Steckel and J. Rose. Cambridge: Cambridge University Press, pp. 11–60.

Goodrich, R.J. 2007. *Contextualising Cassian: Aristocrats, Asceticism, and Reformation in Fifth-Century Gaul.* Oxford: Oxford Early Christian Studies.

Goody, J. 1982. *Cooking, Cuisine and Class. A Study in Comparative Sociology.* Cambridge: Cambridge University Press.

Gottschalk, R. 2014. *Römer und Franken in Hürth.* Hürther Beiträge zur Geschichte, Kultur und Regional-kunde 93. Bonn: Habelt Verlag.

Gowers, E. 1993. *The Loaded Table: Representations of Food in Roman Literature.* Oxford: Clarendon Press.

Gowland, R.L. and Garnsey, P. 2010. 'Skeletal evidence for health, nutritional status, and malaria in Rome and the Empire and implications for mobility', in *Roman Diasporas: Archaeological Approaches to Mobility and Diversity in the Roman Empire*, ed. H. Eckardt Portsmouth, RI: Journal of Roman Archaeology, Supplement 78, pp. 131–156.

Graham, E.J. 2005. 'Dining *al fresco* with the living and the dead in Roman Italy', in *Consuming Passions. Dining from Antiquity to the Eighteenth Century*, ed. M. Carroll, D.M. Hadley and H. Willmott. Stroud: Tempus, pp. 49–66.

Grainger, S. 2006. *Cooking Apicius: Roman Recipes for Today.* Totnes: Prospect Books.

Grant, M. 1999. *Roman Cookery: Ancient Recipes for Modern Kitchens.* London: Serif.

Grant, M. 2000. *Galen on Food and Diet.* London: Routledge.

Greene, L.S. 1993. 'G6PD deficiency as protection against *falciparum* malaria: an epidemiologic critique of population and experimental studies', *American Journal of Physical Anthropology* 36(17), pp. 153–178.

Grewe, K. 1986. *Atlas der römischen Wasserleitungen nach Köln.* Rheinische Ausgrabungen 26. Köln: Rheinland-Verlag.

Grewe, K. 2010. *Meisterwerke antiker Technik.* Mainz: Verlag Philipp von Zabern.

Grewe, K. and Knauff, M. 2012. *Die lange Leitung der Römer. Der Römerkanal-Wanderweg Nettersheim-Köln.* Düren: Verlag Eifelverein.

Griffiths, D.M. 1978. 'Use-marks on historic ceramics: a preliminary study', *Historical Archaeology* 12, pp. 68–81.

Grilletto, R. 1981. 'Premiers resultats anthropologiques des fouilles de la necropole d'Antinoe en Egypte', *Bulletins et Mémoires de la Société d'anthropologie de Paris*, XIIIe S., 8, pp. 281–287.

Grimm, V. 1996. *From Feasting to Fasting, the Evolution of a Sin: Attitudes to Food in Late Antiquity.* London and New York: Routledge.

Grocock, C. and S. Grainger, eds. 2006. *Apicius: A Critical Edition with an Introduction and English Translation.* Totnes: Prospect Books.

Grottanelli, C. 1996. 'La viande et ses rites', in *Histoire de l'Alimentation*, ed. J.-L. Flandrin and M. Montanari. Paris: Fayard, pp. 117–132.

Haard, N.F., Odunfa, S.A., Lee, C.H., Quitero-Ramirez R., Lorence-Quinones, A. and Wacher-Radarte, C. 1999. *Fermented Cereals: A Global Perspective.* Rome: FAO.

Hackworth-Peterson, L. 2003. 'The baker, his tomb, his wife, and her breadbasket: the monument of Eurysaces in Rome', *The Art Bulletin*, pp. 230–257.

Hallbäck, G. 2001. 'Sacred meal and social meeting: Paul's argument in 1. Cor. 11.17–34', in *Meals in a Social Context. Aspects of the Communal Meal in the Hellenistic and Roman World*, ed. I. Nielsen and H.S. Nielsen. Aarhus: Aarhus University Press, pp. 167–176.

Halstead, P. 1998. 'Mortality models and milking: problems of uniformitarianism, optimality and equifinality reconsidered', *Anthropozoologica* 27, pp. 3–20.

Halstead, P. 2014a. 'Archaeological science and the Neolithic: the power and perils of proxy measures', in *Early Farmers: The View from Archaeology and Science* (Proceedings of the British Academy 198), ed. A. Whittle and P. Bickle. London: Oxford University Press for the British Academy, pp. 419–433.

Halstead, P. 2014b. *Two Oxen Ahead: Pre-Mechanized Farming in the Mediterranean*, Chichester: Wiley Blackwell.

Hamad, A.M. and Fields, M.L. 1979. 'Evaluation of the protein quality and available lysine of germinated and fermented cereals', *Journal of Food Science* 44(2), pp. 456–459.

Hamilton-Dyer, S. 1990. 'Quatrième campagne de fouille au Mons Claudianus: Rapport préliminaire. Annexe II – The Animals Remains', *BIAO* 90, pp. 65–81.

Hamilton-Dyer, S. 2001. 'Ch. 9 The faunal remains', in *Mons Claudianus, Survey and Excavation: Vol 2 Excavations part 1*, ed. D.P.S. Peacock and V.A. Maxfield. Cairo: Institut français d'archéologie orientale, pp. 249–310.

Hanbury, C.D., White, C.L., Mullan, B.P. and Siddique, K.H.M. 2000. 'A review of the potential of *Lathyrus sativus* L. and L. *cicera* L. grain for use as animal feed', *Animal Feed Science and Technology* 87, pp. 1–27.

Hankinson, R.J., ed. 2008. *The Cambridge Companion to Galen*. Cambridge: Cambridge University Press.

Hansen, A.M., Walker, B.J. and Heinrich F.B.J., 2017. 'Impressions of the Mamluk agricultural economy. Archaeobotanical evidence from clay ovens ṭābūn at Tall Ḥisbān (Jordan)', *Tijdschrift voor Mediterrane Archeologie* 56, pp. 58–67.

Hansen, M.H. 2006. *The Shotgun Method: The Demography of the Ancient Greek City-State Culture*. Columbia: University of Missouri Press.

Hansen, M.H. 2008. 'An update on the shotgun method', *GRBS* 48, pp. 259–286.

Harcum, C.G. 1921. 'Roman cooking utensils in the Royal Ontario Museum of Archaeology', *American Journal of Archaeology* 25(1), 37–54.

Hardy, K., Blakeney, T., Copeland, L., Kirkham J., Wrangham, R. and Collins, M. 2009. 'Starch granules, dental calculus and new perspectives on ancient diet', *Journal of Archaeological Science* 36, pp. 248–255.

Harland, P. 2012. 'Banqueting values in the associations: rhetoric and reality', in *Meals in the Early Christian World: Social Formation, Experimentation, and Conflict at the Table*, ed. D.E. Smith and H. Taussig. New York: Palgrave Macmillan, pp. 73–85.

Harris, M. 1985. *Good to Eat*. New York; Simon and Schuster.

Harris, W.V. 2007. 'The late republic', in *The Cambridge Economic History of the Greco-Roman World*, eds. W. Scheidel, I. Morris and R. Saller. Cambridge: Cambridge University Press, pp. 511–540.

Hartley, K.F. 1973. 'The marketing and distribution of mortaria', in *Current Research in Romano-British Coarse Pottery*, ed. A.P. Detsicas. London: Council for British Archaeology, pp. 39–51.

Harwood, J.L. and Yaqoob, P. 2002. 'Nutritional and health aspects of olive oil', *European Journal of Lipid Science and Technology* 104, pp. 685–697.

Hasbach, W. 1908. *A History of the English Agricultural Labourer*. London: P.S. King and Son.

Hashmi, M.A., Afsar K., Hanif, M., Farooq U. and P. Shagufta. 2015. 'Traditional uses, phytochemistry, and pharmacology of *Olea europaea* (olive)', *Evidence-Based Complementary and Alternative Medicine* 2015, pp. 1–29.

Hather, J. G. 1993. *An Archaebotanical Guide to Root and Tuber Identification: Europe and South Asia*. Oxbow Monograph 28. Oxford: Oxbow.

Hather, J. G. 2000. *Archaeological Parenchyma*. London: Archetype.

Hatton, T.J. and Bray, B.E. 2010. 'Long run trends in the heights of European men, 19th–20th centuries', *Economics and Human Biology* 8, pp. 405–413.

Heaton, T.H.E., Jones, J., Halstead, P. and Tsipropoulos, T. 2009. 'Variations in the 13C/12C ratios of modern wheat grain, and implications for interpreting data from Bronze Age Assiros Toumba, Greece', *Journal of Archaeological Science* 36, 2224–2233.

Hedges, R. 2009. 'Studying human diet', in *The Oxford Handbook of Archaeology*, ed. B. Cunliffe, C. Gosden, and R. A. Joyce. Oxford: Oxford University Press, pp. 484–516.

Hedrick Jr., C.W. 1995. 'Thucydides and the beginnings of archaeology', in *Methods in the Mediterranean: Historical and Archaeological Views on Texts and Archaeology*, ed. D.B. Small. Leiden: Brill, pp. 45–88.

Hefnawy, T.H. 2011. 'Effect of processing methods on nutritional composition and anti-nutritional factors in lentils (Lens culinaris)', *Annals of Agricultural Science* 56(2), pp. 57–61.

Heimberg, U. 2002/2003. 'Römische Villen an Rhein und Maas', *Bonner Jahrbücher* 202/203, pp. 57–148.

Hein, A., Müller, N.S., Day, P.M. and Kilikoglou, V. 2008. 'Thermal conductivity of archaeological ceramics: The effect of inclusions, porosity and firing temperature', *Thermochimica Acta* 480(1–2), pp. 35–42.

Heinrich, F.B.J. 2012. *Nitrogen and Carbon Stable Isotope Analysis and Manuring: Agricultural Practices in the Upper Thames Valley during the Iron Age and Roman Period: The Case of Gravelly Guy*. Unpublished MSc dissertation. University of Oxford.

Heinrich, F.B.J. 2017. 'Modelling crop-selection in Roman Italy. The economics of agricultural decision making in a globalizing economy', in *The Economic Integration of Roman Italy: Rural Communities in a Globalizing World*, ed. Tymon de Haas and Gijs Tol. Leiden/Boston: Brill, pp. 136–164.

Heinrich, F.B.J. and Hansen, A.M. Forthcoming. 'Mudbricks, cereals and the agricultural economy. Archaeobotanical investigations at the New Kingdom town', in *AcrossBorders 2: Living in New Kingdom Sai*, ed. J. Budka.

Heinrich, F.B.J. and Erdkamp, P. 2018. 'The role of modern malnutrition in modelling Roman malnutrition: aid or anachronism?', *Journal of Archaeological Science: Reports*, 19 pp. 1016–1022.

Heinrich, F.B.J. and Erdkamp, P. forthcoming. 'Stable isotopes and the Roman economy: a review'.

Heinrich, F.B.J. and van Pelt, W.P. 2017a. 'Graantransport en graanprijzen in Ramessidisch Egypte. Het recto van P. Amiens en P. Baldwin gekwantificeerd', *Tijdschrift voor Mediterrane Archeologie* 57, pp. 1–12.

Heinrich, F.B.J. and van Pelt, W.P. 2017b. 'Ramessidische graantransporten, landerijen en landbelastingen botanisch gekwantificeerd: Het verso van Papyrus Amiens + Baldwin', in *Paleo-Palfenier*, ed. M. Schepers and G. Aalbersberg. Groningen: Barkhuis, pp. 31–42.

Heinrich, F.B.J. and Wilkins, D.A. 2014. 'Beans, boats and archaeobotany: A new translation of Phasolus or why the Romans ate neither kidney beans nor cowpeas', *Palaeohistoria* 55/56, pp. 149–176.

Heiss, A.G. and Kreuz, A. 2007. 'Brot für die Salinenarbeiter-das Keltenbrot von Bad Nauheim aus archäobotanischer Sicht', *hessenARCHÄOLOGIE 2006*. Stuttgart: Konrad Theiss Verlag, pp. 70–73.

Henrich, P. 2010. *Die römische Nekropole und Villenanlage von Duppach-Weiermühle, Vulkaneinfel*. Trierer Zeitschrift Beiheft 33. Trier: Verlag des Rheinisches Landesmuseums.

Herchenbach M. and Meurers-Balke, J. Forthcoming. 'Stadt, Land, Fluss . . . und Baum – archäobotanische Betrachtungen zur Romanisierung des Niederrheingebietes', in *Wald und Holznutzung währen der römischen Antike. Akten der Rheinbacher Tagung 2014*, eds. T. Kaszab-Olschewski and I. Tamerl. Archäologische Berichte.

Heron, C. and Evershed, R.P. 1993. 'The analysis of organic residues and the study of pottery use', *Archaeological Method and Theory* 5, pp. 247–284.

Herter, H. 1964. 'Amme oder Saugflasche', in *Mullus. Festschrift Theodor Klauser*. Münster: Aschendorff, pp. 168–172.

Heslin, K. 2011. 'Dolia shipwrecks and the wine trade in the Roman Mediterranean'. In *Maritime Archaeology and ancient Trade in the Mediterranean*, ed. D. Robinson and A.I. Wilson. Oxford, Oxbow, pp. 157–168.

Hickey, T.M. 2012. *Wine, Wealth and the State in Late Antique Egypt: The House of Apion at Oxyrhynchus*. Ann Arbor: University of Michigan Press.

Higginbotham, J. 1997. *Piscinae. Artificial Fishponds in Roman Italy*. Chapel Hill: University of North Carolina Press.

Hill, S. and Bryer, H. 1995. 'Byzantine Porridge: tracta, trachanás and tarhana', in J. Wilkins, D. Harvey and M. Dobson, eds. *Food in Antiquity*. Exeter: University of Exeter Press, pp. 44–54.

Hillman, G. 1981. 'Reconstructing crop husbandry practices from charred remains of crops', in *Farming Practice in British Prehistory*, ed. R. Mercer. Edinburgh: Edinburgh University Press, pp. 123–163.

Hillson, S. 2001. 'Recording dental caries in archaeological human remains', *International Journal of Osteoarchaeology* 11, pp. 249–289.

Hin, S. 2012. *The Demography of Roman Italy: Population Dynamics in an Ancient Conquest Society (201 BCE–14 CE)*. Cambridge: Cambridge University Press.

Hingley, R. 2005. *Globalizing Roman Culture: Unity, Diversity and Empire*. London and New York: Routledge.

Hionidou, V. 2011. 'What do starving people eat? The case of Greece through oral history', *Continuity and Change* 26, pp. 113–134.

Hitchner, R. B. 1999. 'More Italy than province? Archaeology, texts, and culture change in Roman Provence', *Transactions of the American Philological Association* 129, pp. 375–379.

Hitchner, R.B. 2002. 'Olive production and the Roman economy: the case for intensive growth in the Roman Empire', in *The Ancient Economy*, ed. W. Scheidel and S. von Reden. Edinburgh: Edinburgh University Press, pp. 71–86.

Hobbs, R. 2010. 'Platters in the Mildenhall treasure', *Britannia* 4, pp. 324–333.

Hodge, A.T. 1992. *Roman Aqueducts and Water Supply*. London, Duckworth.

Højte, J. M. 2005. 'Archaeological evidence for fish processing in the Black Sea Region', in *Ancient Fishing and Fish Processing in the Black Sea Region*, ed. T. Bekker-Nielsen. Aarhus: Aarhus University Press, pp. 133–160.

Höpken, C. 2015. 'Cervesia für Bonn?' In *non solum . . . sed etiam. Festschrift für Thomas Fischer zum 65. Geburtstag*, ed. P. Henrich, C. Miks, J. Obmann and M. Wieland. Rahden: Verlag Marie Leidorf, pp. 195–198.

Höpken, C. 2016. 'Entscheidende Wandfragmente: Untersuchungen zum Inhalt von Amphoren aus Köln und Bonn', *Archäologisches Korrespondenzblatt* 46, pp. 101–112.

Hörter, F. 2000. 'Vom Reibstein zur römischen Kraftmühle', in *Steinbruch und Bergwerk. Denkmäler römischer Technikgeschichte zwischen Eifel und Rhein*. Vulkanpark-Forschungen 2. Mainz: Verlag des Römisch-Germanischen Zentralmuseums, pp. 58–70.

Hohlwein, N. 1939. 'Palmiers et palmeraies dans l'Egypte romaine', *Etudes de Papyrologie* 5, pp. 1–74.

Holleran, C. 2011. 'The street life of Ancient Rome', in *Rome, Ostia, Pompeii: Movement and Space*, eds. R. Laurence and D. Newsome. Oxford: Oxford University Press, pp. 245–261.

Holleran, C. 2012. *Shopping in Ancient Rome: The Retail Trade in the Late Republic and Principate*. Oxford: Oxford University Press.

Holtmeyer-Wild, V. 2012. 'Reib- und Mühlsteingewinnung am Vulkan "Ruderbüsch" bei Oberbettingen, Landkreis Vulkaneifel. Archäologische Untersuchungen zur Eisenzeit und zum Mittelalter', *Funde und Ausgrabungen im Bezirk Trier* 44, pp. 19–27.

Hopkins, K. 2002. 'Rome, taxes, rents and trade', in *The Ancient Economy*, ed. W. Scheidel and S. Von Reden. New York, Routledge, pp. 190–230.

Horden, P. and Purcell, N. 2000. *The Corrupting Sea: A Study of Mediterranean History*. London: Wiley-Blackwell.

Hosch, S. and Zibulski, P. 2003. 'The influence of inconsistent wet-sieving procedures on the macroremain concentration in waterlogged sediments', *Journal of Archaeological Science* 30, pp. 849–857.

Hubbard, R.N.L.B. and al Azm, A. 1990. 'Carbonized seeds; and investigating the history of *Friké* production', *Journal of Archaeological Science* 17, pp. 103–106.

Hudson, N. 1989. 'Food in Roman satire', in *Satire and Society in Ancient Rome*, ed. S. Braund. Exeter: Exeter University Press, pp. 69–87.

Hudson, N. 2010. 'The archaeology of the Roman "convivium"', *American Journal of Archaeology* 114, pp. 663–695.

Humer, F. 2014. 'Wie sahen die Carnuntiner Privathäuser innen aus?' in *Carnuntum – Wiedergeborene Stadt der Kaiser*, ed. F. Humer. Darmstadt: Verlag Philipp von Zabern, pp. 102–107.

Hummel, C. 1999. *Das Kind und seine Krankheiten in der griechischen Medizin. Von Aretaios bis Johannes Aktuarios (1. Bis 14. Jahrhundert)*. Frankfurt am Main: Peter Lang.

Huskinson, J. 2011. 'Picturing the Roman family', in *A Companion to Families in the Greek and Roman Worlds*, ed. B. Rawson. Chichester, West Sussex and Malden, MA: Wiley-Blackwell, pp. 521–541.

Hussein, F.H., Al Banna, R., Sarry, El. and Din, A.M. 2006. 'Non-specific stress indicators in ancient Egyptians from Giza and Bahriyah Oasis', *Journal of the Arab Society for Medical Research* 1, pp. 13–27.

Ikäheimo, J.P. 2003. *Late Roman African Cookware of the Palatine East Excavations, Rome: A Holistic Approach*. BAR international series 1143. Oxford: Archaeopress.

Jackes, M. 2011. 'Representativeness and bias in archaeological skeletal samples', in *Social Bioarchaeology*, eds. S.C. Agarwal and B.A. Glencross. Malden: Wiley-Blackwell, pp. 107–146.

Jackson, R. 1988. *Doctors and Diseases in the Roman Empire*. London: British Museum Publications.

Jacob, C. 2013. *The Web of Athenaeus*. Washington, DC: Center for Hellenic Studies at Harvard University.

Jacomet, S. 2006. *Identification of Cereal Remains from Archaeological Sites*, 2nd edition. Basel: IPAS, Basel University.

Jacomet, S. 2012. 'Archaeobotany: analyses of plant remains from waterlogged archaeological sites', in *The Oxford Handbook of Wetland Archaeology*, ed. F. Menotti and A. O'Sullivan. Oxford: Oxford University Press, pp. 497–514.

Jacomet, S. and Kreuz, A. 1999. *Archäobotanik. Aufgaben, Methoden und Ergebnisse vegetations- und agrargeschichtlicher Forschung*. Stuttgart: Verlag Eugen Ulmer.

Jacomet, S., Kučan, D., Ritter, A., Suter, G. and Hagendorn, A. 2002. '*Punica granatum* L. (pomegranates) from early Roman contexts in Vindonissa (Switzerland)', *Vegetation History and Archaeobotany* 11, pp. 79–92.

Jaeggi, S. Forthcoming. 'Un biberon sur une fontaine d'époque augustéenne à Palestrina?', *Latomus* 77.

Jameson, M. 1983. 'Famine in the Greek world', in *Trade and Famine in Classical Antiquity* ed. P. Garnsey and C.R. Whittaker. Cambridge: Cambridge University Press, pp. 6–16.

Janssen, A.M. 1992. *Obelisk and Katepwa Wheat Gluten: A Study of Factors Determining Bread Making Performance*. PhD thesis. University of Groningen Press.

Jashemski, W.F. 1979. *The Gardens of Pompeii*, 2 vols. New Rochelle, NY: Caratzas Brothers.

Jashemski, W. F. and Meyer, F.G. 2002. *The Natural History of Pompeii*. Cambridge and New York: Cambridge University Press.

Jasny, N. 1941–1942. 'Competition among grains in Classical Antiquity', *American Historical Review* 47(4), 747–764.

Jasny, N. 1944a. *The Wheats of Classical Antiquity*. Baltimore: John Hopkins Press.

Jasny, N. 1944b. 'Wheat prices and milling costs in classical Rome', *Wheat Studies of the Food Research Institute* 20(4), pp. 137–170.

Jasny, N. 1950. 'The daily bread of the ancient Greeks and Romans', *Osiris* 9, pp. 227–253.

Joachim, H.-E. 2002. *Porz-Lind. Ein mittel- bis spätlatènezeitlicher Siedlungsplatz im Linder Bruch (Stadt Köln)*. Rheinische Ausgrabungen 47. Mainz: Verlag Philipp von Zabern.

Johns, C. 2010. *The Hoxne Late Roman Treasure: Gold Jewellery and Silver Plate*. London: British Museum Press.

Johnson, L. A. 2010. 'Lilies do not spin: a challenge to female social norms', *New Testament Studies* 56(4), pp. 475–490.

Jones, A.H.M. 1964. *The Later Roman Empire 284–602*. Oxford: Blackwell.

Jones, G. 1984. 'Interpretation of archaeological plant remains: ethnographic models from Greece', in *Plants and ancient Man: Studies in Palaeoethnobotany*, ed. W. van Zeist and W.A. Casperie. Rotterdam: A.A. Balkema, pp. 43–61.

Jones, G. 1987. 'A statistical approach to the archaeological identification of crop processing', *Journal of Archaeological Science* 14, pp. 311–323.

Jones, G. 1991. 'Numerical analysis in archaeobotany', in *Progress in Old World Palaeoethnobotany*, ed. W. van Zeist, K. Wasylikowa and K.-E. Behre. Rotterdam: A. A. Balkema, pp. 63–80.

Jones, G. 1998. 'Distinguishing food from fodder in the archaeobotanical record', *Environmental Archaeology* 1, pp. 95–98.

Jones, G. 2002. 'Weed ecology as a method for the archaeobotanical recognition of crop husbandry practices', *Acta Palaeobotanica* 42, pp. 185–193.

Jones, G. 2006. 'Tooth eruption and wear observed in live sheep from Butser Hill, the Cotswold Farm Park and five farms in the Pentland Hills, UK', in *Recent Advances in Ageing and Sexing Animal Bones*, ed. D. Ruscillo. Oxford: Oxbow Books, pp. 155–178.

Jones, G. and Halstead, P. 1995. 'Maslins, mixtures and monocrops: on the interpretation of archaeological crop samples of heterogenous composition', *Journal of Archaeological Science* 22: 103-14.

Jones, G., Charles, M., Bogaard, A. and Hodgson, J. 2010. 'Crops and weeds: the role of weed functional ecology in the identification of crop husbandry methods', *Journal of Archaeological Science* 37, pp. 70–77.

Jones, M.J. 1990. 'The role of forage legumes in rotation with cereals in Mediterranean areas', in *The Role of Legumes in the Farming Systems of the Mediterranean Areas*, ed. A.E. Osman, M.H. Ibrahim and M.A. Jones. Dordrecht: Kluwer Academic Publishers, pp. 143–149.

Jongman, W. 1988. *The Economy and Society of Pompeii*. Amsterdam, Gieben.

Jongman, W. 2002. 'Beneficial symbols. Alimenta and the infantilization of the Roman citizen', in *After the Past. Essays in Ancient History in Honour of H. W. Pleket*, ed. W. Jongman and M. Kleijwegt. Leiden: Brill, pp. 47–80.

Jongman, W. 2007a. 'The early Roman Empire: consumption', in *The Cambridge Economic History of the Greco-Roman World*, ed. W. Scheidel, I. Morris and R. Saller. Cambridge: Cambridge University Press, pp. 592–618.

Jongman, W. M. 2007b. 'Gibbon was right: the decline and fall of the Roman Empire', in *Crises and the Roman Empire*, ed. O. Hekster, G. de Kleijn and D. Slootjes. Leiden: Brill, pp. 183–199.

Jongman, W. 2014. 'Re-constructing the Roman economy', in *The Cambridge History of Capitalism, vol. 1*, ed. L. Neal and J. Williamson. Cambridge: Cambridge University Press, pp. 75–100.

Jung, C., Odiot, T., et al. 2001. 'La viticulture antique dans le Tricastin (moyenne vallée du Rhône)', *Gallia* 58, pp. 113–128.

Junkelmann, M. 1997. *Panis militaris. Die Ernährung des römsichen Soldaten oder der Grundstoff der Macht*, Kulturgeschichte der alten Welt 75. Mainz am Rhein: von Zabern.

Junkelmann, M. 2006. *Panis militaris. Die Ernährung des römsichen Soldaten oder der Grundstoff der Macht*, 3rd edition. Kulturgeschichte der alten Welt 75. Mainz am Rhein: von Zabern.

Kalis, A. J. and Meurers-Balke, J. 2007. 'Landnutzung im Niederrheingebiet zwischen Krieg und Frieden', in *Krieg und Frieden. Kelten – Römer – Germanen*, ed. G. Uelsberg, Darmstadt: Primus Verlag, pp. 144–153.

Kalogeropoulos, N. and A. Chiou. 2010. 'Recovery and distribution of macro- and selected microconstituents after pan-frying of Mediterranean fish in virgin olive oil', in *Olives and Olive Oil in Health and Disease Prevention*, eds. V.R. Preedy and R.R. Watson. Amsterdam: Academic Press, pp. 755–765.

Kaszab-Olschewski, T. 2015. 'Mit den Göttern speisen – Keramikgefäße bei rituellen Handlungen. In *Keramik im Spannungsfeld zwischen Handwerk und Kunst*, ed. S. Glaser, Wissenschaftliche Beibände zum Anzeiger des Germanischen Nationalmuseums 40. Nürnberg: Verlag des Germanischen Nationalmuseums, pp. 31–38.

Kaszab-Olschewski, T. and Meurers-Balke, J. 2014. 'Die Römische Küche in der CCAA', in *Küche und Keller in Antike und Früh mittelalter*, ed. J. Drauschke, R. Prien and A. Reis. SAFM 6. Hamburg: Verlag Dr. Kovač, pp. 133–154.

Katzenberg, M.A. 2008. 'Stable isotope analysis: a tool for studying past diet, demography, and life history', in *Biological Anthropology of the Human Skeleton*, ed. M.A. Katzenberg and S. Saunders. Hoboken, NJ: Wiley-Liss, pp. 413–442.

Katzenberg, M.A. 2012. 'The ecological approach: understanding past diet and the relationship between diet and disease', in *A Companion to Paleopathology*, ed. A.L. Grauer. Chichester: Wiley-Blackwell, pp. 97–113.

Katzenberg, M.A. and Saunders, S.R., eds. 2011. *Biological Anthropology of the Human Skeleton*, 2nd edition. Hoboken, NJ: John Wiley & Sons.

Keenleyside, A., Schwarcz, H., Stirling, L. and Ben Lazreg, N. 2009. 'Stable isotopic evidence for diet in a Roman and Late Roman population from Leptiminus, Tunisia', *Journal of Archaeological Science* 36, pp. 51–63.

Kehne, P. 2011. 'War- and peacetime logistics: supplying imperial armies in East and West', in *A Companion to the Roman Army*, ed. P. Erdkamp. Oxford: Wiley-Blackwell, pp. 321–338.

Kellner, C.M. and Schoeninger, M.J. 2007. 'A simple carbon isotope model for reconstructing prehistoric human diet', *American Journal of Physical Anthropology* 133, pp. 1112–1127.

Kelly, B. 2007. 'Riot control and imperial ideology in the Roman empire', *Phoenix* 61, pp. 150–176.

Kelly, M., and Ó Gráda, C. 2014. 'Living standards and mortality since the Middle Ages', *Economic History Review* 67, pp. 358–381.

Kemp, B.J. 1977. 'The city of El-Amarna as a source for the study of urban society in Ancient Egypt', *World Archaeology* 9, pp. 123–139.

Kenward, H.K., Hall, A.R. and Jones, A.K.G. 1980. 'A tested set of techniques for the extraction of plant and animal macrofossils from waterlogged archaeological deposits', *Science and Archaeology* 22, pp. 3–15.

Kern, A., Kowarik, K., Rausch, A.W. and Reschreiter, H., eds. 2008. *Salz-Reich. 7000 Jahre Hallstatt*. Veröffentlichungen der Prähistorischen Abteilung 2. Wien: Verlag des Naturhistorischen Museums.

Kertzer, D. and Saller, R., eds. 1991. *The Family in Italy: From Antiquity to the Present*. New Haven: Yale University Press.

Khattab, R.Y. and Arntfield, S.D. 2009. 'Nutritional quality of legume seeds as affected by some physical treatments 2. Antinutritional factors', *Food Science and Technology* 42, pp. 1113–1118.

Khokhar, S. and Owusu Apenten, R.K. 2009. 'Antinutritional factors in food legumes and effects of processing', in *The Role of Food, Agriculture, Forestry and Fisheries in Human Nutrition* Vol. IV, ed. V.R. Squires. Paris: UNESCO-EOLSS. Available at: www.eolss.net/sample-chapters/c10/e5-01a-06-05.pdf (accessed 5 February 2015).

Killgrove, K. 2010a. *Migration and Mobility in imperial Rome*. Unpublished PhD Thesis. University of North Carolina at Chapel Hill.

Killgrove, K. 2010b. 'Identifying immigrants to Imperial Rome using strontium isotope analysis', in *Roman Diasporas: Archaeological Approaches to Mobility and Diversity in the Roman Empire*, ed. H. Eckardt, Journal of Roman Archaeology Supplement 78, pp. 157–174.

Killgrove, K. 2013. 'Biohistory of the Roman Republic: the potential of isotope analysis of human skeletal remains', *Post-Classical Archaeologies* 3, pp. 41–62.

Killgrove, K. 2014. 'Bioarchaeology in the Roman Empire', in *Encyclopedia of Global Archaeology*, ed. C. Smith. New York: Springer, pp. 876–882.

Killgrove, K. 2015. *Roman Osteology Database: Two Cemeteries from Imperial Rome*. Available at http://figshare.com/articles/Roman_Osteology_Database_Two_Cemeteries_from_Imperial_Rome/1468571.

Killgrove, K. 2017. 'Imperialism and physiological stress in Rome (1st–3rd centuries AD)', in *The Bioarchaeology of Contact, Colonialism, and Imperialism*, ed. M. Murphy and H. Klaus. Gainesville: University Press of Florida.

Killgrove, K. Forthcoming. 'Using biological distance techniques to investigate the heterogeneous population of Imperial Rome'. Under review in *The Archaeology of Circulation, Exchange, and Human Migration*, ed. D. Peterson, J. Dudgeon, and C. Freiwald. Equinox.

Killgrove, K. and Montgomery, J., 2016. 'All roads lead to Rome: Exploring human migration to the Eternal City through biochemistry of skeletons from two Imperial-era cemeteries (1st–3rd c AD)', *PLOS ONE* 11(2), e0147585.

Killgrove, K., and Tykot, R.H. 2013. 'Food for Rome: a stable isotope investigation of diet in the Imperial period (1st–3rd centuries AD)', *Journal of Anthropological Archaeology* 32, pp. 28–38.

Killgrove, K., and Tykot, R.H. 2018. 'Diet and collapse: a stable isotope study of Imperial-era Gabii (1st–3rd centuries AD)' *Journal of Archaeological Science: Reports*, pp. 1041–1049.

King, A. 1978. 'A comparative survey of bone assemblages from Roman sites in Britain', *Bulletin of the Institute of Archaeology London* 15, pp. 207–232.

King, A. 1998. 'Diet in the Roman Empire: a regional inter-site comparison of the mammal bones', *Journal of Roman Archaeology* 12, pp. 168–202.

King, A. 1999. 'Diet in the Roman world: a regional inter-site comparison of the mammal bones', *Journal of Roman Archaeology* 12, pp. 160–202.

King, A. 2002. 'Mammals: evidence from wall paintings, sculpture, mosaics, faunal remains, and ancient literary sources', in *The Natural History of Pompeii*, ed. W. F. Jashemski and F.G. Meyer. Cambridge; Cambridge University Press, pp. 401–450.

King, A. 2005. 'Animal remains from temples in Roman Britain', *Britannia* 36, pp. 329–369.

King, H., ed. 2005. *Health in Antiquity*. London: Routledge.

Kiple, K. and K. Ornelas, eds. 2000. *The Cambridge World History of Food*. Cambridge: Cambridge University Press.

Kislev, M. 1989. 'Origins of the cultivation of *Lathyrus sativus* and *L. cicera* (Fabaceae)', *Economic Botany* 43(2), pp. 262–270.

Klein Goldewijk, G., and Jacobs, J. 2013. 'The relation between stature and long bone length in the Roman Empire', *SOM Research Reports*, vol. 13002-EEF, University of Groningen.

Kleiner, D.E.E. 1992. *Roman Sculpture*. New Haven: Yale University Press.

Kneissl, P. 1981. 'Die utricularii. Ihr Rolle im gallo-römischen Transportwesen und Weinhandel', *Bonner Jahrbücher* 181, pp. 169–204.

Knörzer, K.-H. 1970. *Römerzeitliche Pflanzenfunde aus Neuss*. Limesforschungen 10. Berlin: Gebr. Mann Verlag.

Knörzer, K.-H. 2007. *Geschichte der synanthropen Flora im Niederrheingebiet. Pflanzenfunde aus archäologischen Ausgrabungen*. Rheinische Ausgrabungen 61. Mainz: Verlag Philipp von Zabern.

König, J. 2012. *Saints and Symposiasts: The Literature of Food and the Symposium in Greco-Roman and Early Christian Culture*. Cambridge: Cambridge University Press.

Koepke, N. and Baten, J. 2005. 'The biological standard of living in Europe during the last two millennia', *European Review of Economic History* 9, pp. 61–95.

Koepke, N. and Baten, J. 2008. 'Agricultural specialization and height in ancient and medieval Europe', *Explorations in Economic History* 45(2), pp. 127–146.

Konen, H. 1995. 'Die Kürbisgewächse (Cucurbitaceen) als Kulturpflanzen im römischen Aegypten (1.–3 Jh. n. Chr.)', *Münstersche Beiträge zur Antiken Handelsgeschichte* 14, pp. 43–81.

Konen. H. 2013. 'Bierhandel im römischen Kaiserreich. Einige Überlegungen zu Volumen, Reichweite und Bedeutung', in *Salutationes – Beiträge zur Alten Geschichte und ihrer Diskussion. Festschrift für Peter Herz zum 65. Geburtstag*, ed. B. Edelmann-Singer and H. Konen. Region im Umbruch 8. Berlin: Frank & Timme, pp. 187–205.

Kooistra, L. 2009. 'The provenance of cereals for the Roman Army in the Rhine Delta', in *Kelten am Rhein. Akten des dreizehnten Internationalen Keltologiekongresses 1. Archäologie. Ethnizität und Romanisierung*. Beihefte der Bonner Jahrbücher 58. Mainz: Verlag Philipp von Zabern, pp. 219–237.

Körber-Grohne, U. 1995. *Nutzpflanzen in Deutschland von der Vorgeschichte bis heute*. Hamburg: Nikol Verlag.

Kosso, P. 1995. 'Epistemic independence between textual and material evidence', in *Methods in the Mediterranean: Historical and Archaeological Views on Texts and Archaeology*, ed. D.B. Small. Leiden: Brill, pp. 177–186.

Kraemer, D. C. 2009. *Jewish Eating and Identity through the Ages*. London: Routledge.

Kramer, J. (1990), 'Die Bedeutung von σπανέλαιον', *Zeitschrift für Papyrologie und Epigraphik* 81, pp. 261–264.

Krause, O. 2009. *Der Arzt und sein Instrumentarium in der römischen Legion*. Remshalden: Verlag Bernhard Albert Greiner.

Krauss, S. 1910. *Talmudische Archäologie*, vol. 1. Leipzig: Fock.

Krausse, D. 2007. 'Das Phänomen Romanisierung. Antiker Vorläufer der Globalisierung?' in *Krieg und Frieden. Kelten – Römer – Germanen*, ed. G. Uelsberg, Darmstadt: Primus Verlag, pp. 14–27.

Kreuz, A. 2000. 'Functional and conceptual archaeobotanical data from Roman cremations', in *Burial, Society and Context in the Roman World*, ed. J. Pearce, M. Millett and M. Struck. Oxford: Oxbow, pp. 45–51.

Kreuz, A. 2004. 'Landwirtschaft im Umbruch? Archäobotanische Untersuchungen zu den Jahrhunderten um Christi Geburt in Hessen und Mainfranken', *Bericht der Römisch Germanischen Kommission* 85, pp. 97–292.

Kreuz, A. 2010. 'Nüsse und Südfrüchte. Pflanzenfunde aus spätaugusteischen Brunnen von Waldgirmes im Lahntal', *hessenARCHÄOLOGIE 2009*. Stuttgart: Konrad Theiss Verlag, pp. 82–84.

Kreuz, A. 2012a. 'Archäobotanische Forschungsergebnisse zu Landwirtschaft und Ernährung im kulturhistorischen Kontext', in *Neustart – Hessische Landesarchäologie 2001–2011. Konzeption – Themen – Perspektiven*, ed. Schallmayer, E. 2. Sonderband Jahrbuch hessenARCHÄOLOGIE. Stuttgart: Konrad Theiss Verlag, pp. 153–159.

Kreuz, A 2012b. 'Ackerbau im römischen Deutschland', in *Landleben im römischen Deutschland*, ed. V. Rupp and H. Birley. Stuttgart: Konrad Theiss Verlag, pp. 35–37.

Kron, G. 2000. 'Roman ley-farming', *Journal of Roman Archaeology* 13, pp. 277–287.

Kron, G. 2002. 'Archaeozoology and the productivity of Roman livestock farming', *Münstersche Beiträge zur Antiken Handelsgeschichte* 21(2), pp. 53–73.

Kron, G. 2004a. 'A deposit of carbonized hay from Oplontis and Roman fodder quality', *Mouseion Series III* 4, pp. 275–331.

Kron, G. 2004b. 'Roman livestock farming in Southern Italy: The case against environmental determinism', in *Espaces intégrés et gestion des ressources naturelles dans l'Empire romain*, ed. M. Clavel-Léveque and E. Hermon. Franche-Comté: Presses universitaires de Franche-Comté, pp. 119–134.

Kron, G. 2005a. 'Anthropometry, physical anthropology, and the reconstruction of ancient health, nutrition, and living standards', *Historia: Zeitschrift für Alte Geschichte* 54, pp. 68–83.

Kron, G. 2005b. 'The Augustan census and the population of Italy', *Athenaeum* 92, pp. 441–495.

Kron, G. 2005c. 'Sustainable Roman intensive mixed farming methods: water conservation and erosion control', in *Concepts, Pratiques et Enjeux environnementaux dans l'Empire romain, Caesarodunum*, ed. R. Bedon and E. Hermon, pp. 285–308. Limoges: Pulim.

Kron, G. 2008a. 'The much maligned peasant: comparative perspectives on the productivity of the small farmer in classical antiquity', in *People, Land, and Politics: Demographic Developments and the Transformation of Roman Italy 300 BC–AD 14*, ed. L. de Ligt and S. Northwood. Leiden: Brill, pp. 71–119.

Kron, G. 2008b. 'Animal husbandry, hunting, fishing and pisciculture', in *The Oxford Handbook of Engineering and Technology in the Classical World*, ed. J.P. Oleson. New York: Oxford University Press, pp. 176–222.

Kron, G. 2011. 'The distribution of wealth at Athens in comparative perspective', *Zeitschrift für Papyrologie und Epigraphik* 179, pp. 129–138.

Kron, G. 2012a. 'Food production', in *The Cambridge Companion to the Economic History of the Roman World*, ed. W. Scheidel. Cambridge: Cambridge University Press, pp. 156–174.

Kron, G. 2012b. 'Agriculture, Roman Empire', in *The Encyclopedia of Ancient History*, ed. R. Bagnall, K. Broderson, A. Erskine and S. Heubner. Oxford: Wiley Blackwell, pp. 217–222.

Kron, G. 2012c. 'Nutrition, hygiene, and mortality. Setting parameters for Roman health and life expectancy consistent with our comparative evidence', in *L'Impatto della 'Peste Antonina'*, ed. E. Lo Cascio. Bari: Edipuglia, pp. 193–252.

Kron, G. 2013. 'Fleshing out the demography of Etruria', *The Etruscan World*, ed. J.M. Turfa. London: Routledge, pp. 56–78.

Kron, G. 2014a. 'Animal husbandry', in *The Oxford Handbook of Animals in Classical Thought and Life*, ed. G. Campbell. Oxford; Oxford University Press, pp. 109–135.

Kron, G. 2014b. 'Agriculture', in *A Companion to Food in the Ancient World*, ed. J. Wilkins and R. Nadeau. Oxford: Wiley Blackwell, pp. 160–172.

Kron, G. 2014c. 'Comparative evidence and the reconstruction of the ancient economy: Greco-Roman housing and the level and distribution of wealth and income', in *Quantifying the Greco-Roman Economy and Beyond*, ed. F. de Callataÿ. Bari: Edipuglia, pp. 123–146.

Kron, G. 2017a. 'The population of Northern Italy and the debate over the Augustan census figures: weighing the documentary, literary, and archaeological evidence', *Popolazione e risorse nell'Italia del nord dalla romanizzazione ai Longobardi*, ed. E. Lo Cascio and M. P. Balbo. Bari: Edipuglia, pp. 49–98.

Kron, G. 2017b. 'The diversification and intensification of Italian agriculture: the complementary roles of the small and wealthy farmer', *Rural Communities in a Globalizing Economy: New Perspectives on the Economic Integration of Roman Italy*, ed. T. de Haas and G. Tol. Leiden: E.J. Brill, pp. 112–140.

Krueger, H. and Sullivan, C. 1984. 'Models for carbon isotope fractionation between diet and bone', *Stable Isotopes in Nutrition, ACS Symposium Series* 258, pp. 205–220.

Kruit, N. 1992. 'The meaning of various words related to wine', *Zeitschrift für Papyrologie und Epigraphik* 90, pp. 265–276.

Kučan, D. 1992. 'Die Pflanzenfunde aus dem römischen Militärlager Oberaden', in *Das Römerlager in Oberaden 3. Die Ausgrabungen im nordwestlichen Lagerbereich und weitere Baustellenuntersuchungen der Jahre 1962–1988*, ed. J.-S. Kühlborn. Bodenaltertümer Westfalens 27. Münster: Aschendorff Verlag, pp. 237–265.

Künzl, E. 2002. *Medizin in der Antike. Aus eine Welt ohne Narkose und Aspirin.* Stuttgart: Konrad Theiss Verlag.

Küster, H. 1995. 'Weizen, Pfeffer, Tannenholz. Botanische Untersuchungen zur Verbreitung von Handelsgütern in römischer Zeit', *Münstersche Beiträge zur Antiken Handelsgeschichte* XIV(2), pp. 1–26.

Kurien, P.P., Desikachar, H.S.R. and Parpia, H.A.B. 1972. *Processing and Utilization of Grain-Legumes in India.* Tropical Agricultural Research Series no. 6. Tokyo: Ministry of Agriculture and Forestry.

Kurlovich, B.S. 2002. 'This history of lupin development', in *Lupins: Geography, Classification, Genetic Resources and Breeding*, ed. B.S. Kurlovich. St. Petersburg: INTAN, pp. 147–164.

Lachiche, C. and Deschler-Erb, S. 2007. 'De la viande pour les hommes et pour les dieux – sa gestion dans deux villes de la Suisse romaine', *Food and History* 5(1), pp. 107–131.

Laes, C. 2011. *Children in the Roman Empire: Outsiders Within.* Cambridge: Cambridge University Press.

Laes, C. 2015. 'Children and their occupations in the city of Rome (300–700 CE)', in *Children and Family in Late Antiquity. Life, Death and Interaction*, ed. C. Laes, K. Mustakallio and V. Vuolanto. Leuven: Peeters, pp. 79–109.

Laes, C. and Strubbe, J. 2014. *Youth in the Roman Empire: The Young and the Restless Years?* Cambridge: Cambridge University Press.

Lagia, A. 1999. 'Στοιχεία καθημερινού βίου. Το ανθρωπολογικό υλικό από την ανασκαφή του ρωμαϊκού ταφικού κτίσματος αρ. 1. στο νεκροταφείο του Κεραμεικού', *Athenische Mitteilungen* 114, pp. 291–303.

Lagia, A. 2000. 'Kerameikos Grabung 1999: preliminary analysis of the human remains', *Archäologisher Anzeiger* 3, pp. 481–493.

Lahelma, E., et al. 2015. 'Social class inequalities in health among occupational cohorts from Finland, Britain and Japan: a follow-up study', *Health & Place* 31, pp. 173–179.

Lalueza Fox, C., Juan, J. and Albert, R.M. 1996. 'Phytolith analysis on dental calculus, enamel surface, and burial soil: information about diet and paleoenvironment', *American Journal of Physical Anthropology* 101, pp. 101–113.

Larsen, C.S. 2002. 'Bioarchaeology: the lives and lifestyles of past people', *Journal of Archaeological Research* 10, pp. 119–166.

Larsen, C.S. 2015. *Bioarchaeology: Interpreting Behavior from the Human Skeleton*, 2nd edition. Cambridge: Cambridge University Press.

Laubenheimer, F., Ouzoulias, P., et al. 2003. 'La bière en Gaule. Sa fabrication, les mots pour le dire, les vestiges archéologiques: première approche', *Revue archéologique de Picardie* 1–2, pp. 47–63.

Laudani, G. 2004. *Moretum.* Naples: Loffredo Editore.

Laurence, R. 2005. 'Health and the life course at Herculaneum and Pompeii', in *Health in Antiquity*, ed. H. King. London, New York: Routledge, pp. 83–96.

Laurence, R. 2007. *Roman Pompeii: Space and Society.* London: Routledge.

Laurence, R. 2017. 'Children and the urban environment: agency in Pompeii', in *Children and Everyday Life in the Roman and Late Antique World*, ed. C. Laes and V. Vuolanto. London and New York: Routledge, pp. 27–42.

Lauwerier, R.C.G.M. 1988. *Animals in Roman Times in the Dutch Eastern River Area.* Amersfoort: ROB.

Lauwerier, R.C.G.M. 1993a. 'Twenty-eight bird briskets in a pot; Roman preserved food from Nijmegen', *Archaeofauna* 2, pp. 15–19.

Lauwerier, R.C.G.M. 1993b. 'Bird remains in Roman graves', *Archaeofauna* 2, pp. 75–82.

Lauwerier, R.C.G.M. 1999. 'Eating horsemeat: the evidence in Roman Netherlands', *Archaeofauna* 8, pp. 101–113.

Lauwerier, R.C.G.M. and Robeerst, J.M.M. 2001. 'Horses in Roman times in the Netherlands', in *Animals and Man in the Past. Essays in Honour of Dr. A.T. Clason*, ed. H. Buitenhuis and W. Prummel. Groningen: ARC-Publicaties, pp. 275–290.

Layton, B. 2002. 'Social structure and food consumption in an early Christian monastery: the evidence of Senoute's canons and the White Monastery federation AD 385–465', *Le Muséon* 115, pp. 25–55.

Lazer, E. 2009. *Resurrecting Pompeii*. New York: Routledge.

Lazer, E. 2017. 'Skeletal remains and the health of the population at Pompeii', in *The Economy of Pompeii*, ed. M. Flohr and A. Wilson. Oxford: Oxford University Press, pp. 135–159.

Le Bohec, Y. 2015. *The Encyclopedia of the Roman Army*. Chichester: Wiley Blackwell.

Le Roux, P. 1995. 'Le ravitaillement des armées romaines sous l'Empire', in *Du latifundium au latifondo. Un héritage de Rome, une création médiévale ou moderne? (Actes 363 de la Table ronde internationale du CNRS Université Michel de Montaigne-Bordeaux III 17- 19 décembre 1992)*, Paris: Diffusion, De Boccard, pp. 395–416.

Le Roy Ladurie, E. 1975. 'Famine amenorrhoea (seventeenth-twentieth centuries)', in R. Forster and O. Ranum (eds.), *The Biology of Man in History*, Baltimore: Johns Hopkins University Press, pp. 163–178.

Lee-Thorp, J.A. 2008. 'On isotopes and old bones', *Archaeometry* 50, pp. 925–950.

Lefort, H.-T. 1933. *S. Pachomii vitae sahidice scriptae*, CSCO 99, SC 9, Paris.

Lefort, H.-T. 1943. *Les Vies Coptes de Saint Pachôme et de ses premiers Successeurs*. Louvain: Bibliothèque du Muséon.

Legge, A.J. 1981. 'The agricultural economy', in *Grimes Graves Excavations 1971–72*, ed. R. J. Mercer. London: Her Majesty's Stationery Office, pp. 79–103.

Legge, A.J., Williams, J. and Williams, P. 1991. 'The determination of season of death from the mandibles and bones of the domestic sheep (*Ovis aries*)', *Rivista di Studi Liguri* 57, pp. 49–65.

Legge, A.J., Williams, J. and Williams, P. 2000. 'Lambs to the slaughter: sacrifice at two Roman temples in southern England', in *Animal Bones, Human Societies*, ed. P. Rowley-Conwy. Oxford: Oxbow Books, pp. 152–157.

Leguilloux, M. 2003. 'Les animaux et l'alimentation d'après la faune: les restes de l'alimentation carnée des fortins de Krokodilô et Maximianon', in *La route de Myos Hormos. L'armée romaine dans le désert oriental d'Egypte, Fouilles de l'IFAO 38*, ed. H. Cuvigney. Cairo: IFAO, pp. 550–588.

Leguilloux, M. 2011. Les animaux à Didymoi d'après les restes fauniques du dépotoir extérieur', in *Didymoi. Une garnison romaine dans le désert Oriental d'Egypte, I. Les fouilles et le matériel, Fouilles de l'IFAO 64*, ed. H. Cuvigney. Cairo: IFAO, pp. 167–204.

Leguilloux, M. 2018. 'L'exploitation des animaux dans les praesidia des routes de Myos Hormos et de Bérénice: alimentation, transports et matières premières artisanales', in *Le désert oriental d'Egypte durant la période gréco-romaine: bilans archéologiques*, ed. J.P. Brun, T. Faucher, B. Redon et al. Paris: Collège de France. DOI: 10.4000/books.cdf.5175.

Leigh, M. 2015. 'Food in Latin literature', in *A Companion to Food in the Ancient World*, ed. J. Wilkins and R. Nadeau. Oxford: Wiley-Blackwell, pp. 43–52.

Leighty, C.E. 1933. 'Botanical and zoological reports', in *Karanis: The Temples, Coin Hoards, Botanical and Zoological Reports, Seasons 1924–31*, ed. A.E.R. Boak. Ann Arbor: Michigan University Press, pp. 87–93.

Lemaître, S. 1998. 'Note sur les importations de vins de Méditerranée orientale à Lyon sous le Haut Empire', in *El Vi a l'Antiguitat: Economia, Producció i Comerç al Mediterrani occidental: II Col·loqui Internacional d'Arqueologia Romana*. Badalona, Museu de Badalona, pp. 163–167.

Lepetz, S. 1996. *L'animal dans la Société gallo-romaine de la France du Nord*. Amiens: Revue archéologique de Picardie.

Lepetz, S. 2007. 'Boucherie, sacrifice et marché à la viande en Gaule romaine septentrionale: l'apport de l'archéozoologie', *Food and History* 5(1), pp. 73–105.

Lequément, R. 1980. 'Le vin africain à l'époque impériale', *Antiquités Africaines* 16: 185-193.

Lev-Tov, J. 2003. ' "Upon what meat doth this our Caesar feed . . . ?" A dietary perspective on Hellenistic and Roman influence in Palestine', in *Zeichen aus Text und Stein: Studien auf dem Weg zu einer Archäologie des Neuen Testaments*, ed. S. Alkier and J.K. Zangenberg. Tübingen, Basle: A. Francke, 420–446.

Lewit, T. 2011. 'Dynamics of fineware production and trade: the puzzle of supra-regional exporters', *JRA* 24, pp. 313–332.

Leyerle, B. 1995. 'Clement of Alexandria on the importance of table etiquette', *Journal of Early Christian Studies* 3(2), pp. 123–141.

Leyser, C. 2000. *Authority and Asceticism from Augustine to Gregory the Great*. Oxford: Clarendon Press.

Lieberman, S. 1955. *Tosefta Ki-fshuṭah*, v. 1. New York: Jewish Theological Seminary of America

Lieverse, A.R. 1999. 'Diet and the aetiology of dental calculus', *International Journal of Osteoarchaeology* 9, pp. 219–232.

Lightfoot, E., Šlaus, M. and O'Connell, T.C. 2012. 'Changing cultures, changing cuisines: cultural transitions and dietary change in Iron Age, Roman, and early medieval Croatia', *American Journal of Physical Anthropology* 148, pp. 543–556.

Lignereux, Y. and Peters, J. 1996. 'Techniques de boucherie et rejets osseux en Gaule Romaine', *Anthropozoologica* 24, pp. 45–98.

Lindsay, H. 1997. 'Who was Apicius?' *Symbolae Osloenses* 72, pp. 144–154.

Lindsay, H, 2001. 'Eating with the dead: the Roman funerary banquet', in *Meals in a Social Context: Aspects of the Communal Meal in the Hellenistic and Roman World*, ed. I. Nielsen and H.S. Nielsen. Aarhus: Aarhus University Press, pp. 67–80.

Lintott, A. 1999. *Violence in Republican Rome*. Oxford: Oxford University Press.

Liu, J. 2008. 'The economy of endowments: The case of the Roman *Collegia*', in *Pistoi dia tèn technèn: Bankers, Loans and Archives in the Ancient World*, ed. V. Chankowski, K. Vandorpe and K. Verboven. Leuven: Peeters, pp. 231–256.

Livarda, A. 2008a. *Introduction and Dispersal of Exotic Food Plants into Europe During the Roman and Medieval Periods*. Doctoral thesis, Department of Archaeology. University of Leicester.

Livarda, A. 2008b. 'New temptations? Olive, cherry and mulberry in Roman and medieval Europe', in *Food and Drink in Archaeology I*, ed. S. Baker, M. Allen, S. Middle and K. Poole. Blackawton: Prospect Books, pp. 73–83.

Livarda, A. 2011. 'Spicing up life in northwestern Europe: exotic food plant imports in the Roman and medieval world', *Vegetation History and Archaeobotany* 20, pp. 143–164.

Livarda, A. 2013. 'Date, rituals and socio-cultural identity in the northwestern Roman provinces', *Oxford Journal of Archaeology* 32(1), 101–117.

Livarda, A. 2017. 'Tastes in the Roman provinces: an archaeobotanical approach to socio-cultural change', in *Taste and the Ancient Senses*, ed. K. Rudolph. London: Routledge, pp. 179–196.

Livarda, A. and Kotzamani, G. 2014. 'The archaeobotany of Neolithic and Bronze Age Crete: synthesis and prospects', *The Annual of the British School at Athens* 108, pp. 1–29.

Livarda, A. and Orengo, H.A. 2015. 'Reconstructing the Roman London flavourscape: new insights into the exotic food plant trade using network and spatial analyses', *Journal of Archaeological Science* 55, pp. 244–252.

Livarda, A. and Van der Veen, M. 2008. 'Social access and dispersal of condiments in North-West Europe from the Roman to the medieval period', *Vegetation History and Archaeobotany* 17, pp. 201–209.

Lo Cascio, E. 1999. 'Canon frumentarius, suarius, vinarius: stato e privati nell'approvvigionamento dell'Urbs', in *The transformations of Urbs Roma in late Antiquity*, ed. W. V. Harris. Portsmouth, JRA suppl. 33, pp. 163–182.

Lo Cascio, E. 2006. 'Did the population of imperial Rome reproduce itself?', in *Urbanism in the Preindustrial World: Cross-Cultural Approaches*, ed. G. Storey. Tuscaloosa: University of Alabama Press, pp. 52–68

Lo Cascio, E. 2007. 'The early Roman Empire: the state and the economy', in *The Cambridge Economic History of the Greco-Roman World*, ed. W. Scheidel, I. Morris and R. Saller. Cambridge: Cambridge University Press, pp. 619–650.

Lo Cascio, E. 2009. 'Urbanisation as an index of demographic and economic growth', in *Quantifying the Roman Economy: Methods and Problems*, ed. A. Bowman and A.I. Wilson. Oxford: Oxford University Press, pp. 87–106.

Lo Cascio, E. and Malanima, P. 2009. 'GDP in Premodern Agrarian Economies (1–1820 AD)', *Rivista di Storia Economica* 25, pp. 391–420.

Lo Cascio, E. and Malanima, P. 2014. 'Ancient and premodern economies: GDP in the Roman Empire and early modern Europe', in *Quantifying the Greco-Roman Economy and Beyond*, ed. F. de Callataÿ. Bari: Edipuglia, pp. 229–251.

Locker, A. 2007. '*In piscibus diversis*: the bone evidence for fish consumption in Roman Britain', *Britannia* 38, pp. 141–180.

Lodwick, L. 2014. 'Condiments before Claudius: new plant foods at the Late Iron Age oppidum at Silchester, UK', *Vegetarian History and Archaeobotany* 53, pp. 543–549.

Lösch, S., Moghaddam, N., Grossschmidt, K., Risser, D.U. and Kanz, F. 2014. 'Stable isotope and trace element studies on gladiators and contemporary Romans from Ephesus (Turkey, 2nd and 3rd Ct. AD) – implications for differences in diet', *PLoS ONE* 9(10), e110489.

Lombardo, M. 1995. 'Food and "frontier" in the Greek colonies of South Italy', in *Food in Antiquity*, ed. J. Wilkins, D. Harvey and M. Dobson. Exeter: Exeter University Press, pp. 256–272.

López-López, A., Montaño, A. and Garrido-Fernández, A. 2010. 'Nutrient profiles of commercial table olives: proteins and vitamins', in *Olives and Olive Oil in Health and Disease Prevention*, ed. V.R. Preedy and R.R. Watson. Amsterdam: Academic Press, pp. 705–714.

Los, A. 1997. 'Qui exportait le vin crétois en Campanie à l'époque julio-claudienne?', *Antiquitas* 22, pp. 63–76.

Lukacs, J.R. 1989. 'Dental palaeopathology: methods for reconstructing dietary patterns', in *Reconstruction of Life from the Skeleton*, ed. M.Y. İşcan and K.A.R. Kennedy. New York: Alan R. Liss, Inc., pp. 261–286.

Lukacs, J.R. 2012. 'Oral health in past populations: context, concepts and controversies', in *A Companion to Paleopathology*, ed. A.L. Grauer. Chichester: Wiley-Blackwell, pp. 553–581.

Lukinovich, A. 1990. 'The play of reflections between literary form and sympotic theme in the *Deipnosophistae* of Athenaeus', in *Sympotica: a Symposium on the Symposion*, ed. O. Murray. Oxford: Clarendon Press, pp. 263–271.

Luley, B.P. and Piquès, G.L. 2016. 'Communal eating and drinking in early Roman Mediterranean France: a possible tavern at Lattara, c. 125–75 BC', *Antiquity* 90(349), pp. 126–142.

Lytle, E. 2010. 'Fish lists in the wilderness: the social and economic history of a Boiotian price decree', *Hesperia*, 79, pp. 253–303.

McCobb, L.M.E. and Briggs, D.E.G. 2001. 'Preservation of fossil seeds from a 10th century AD cess pit at Coppergate, York', *Journal of Archaeological Science* 28, pp. 929–940.

McCobb, L.M.E., Briggs, D.E.G., Carruthers, W.J. and Evershed, R.P. 2003. 'Phosphatisation of seeds and roots in a Late Bronze Age deposit at Potterne, Wiltshire, UK', *Journal of Archaeological Science* 30, pp. 1269–1281.

MacDonald, N. 2008. *What Did the Ancient Israelites Eat?* Grand Rapids, Michigan, and Cambridge: William B. Eerdmans Publishing Company.

McGowan, A. 1999. *Ascetic Eucharist: Food and Drink in Early Christian Ritual Meals*. Oxford: Clarendon Press.

McGowan, A. 2005. 'Food, ritual, and power', in *A People's History of Christianity, Vol. 2: Late Antique Christianity*, ed. V. Burrus, Minneapolis: Fortress, pp. 145–164.

McKay L.L. and Baldwin, K.A. 1990. 'Applications for biotechnology: present and future improvements in lactic acid bacteria', *FEMS Microbiology Reviews* 87, pp. 3–14.

MacKinnon, M. 2001. 'High on the hog: linking zooarchaeological, literary and artistic data for pig breeds in Roman Italy', *American Journal of Archaeology* 105, pp. 649–673.

MacKinnon, M. 2004. *Production and Consumption of Animals in Roman Italy: Integrating the Zooarchaeological and Textual Evidence*. Portsmouth, RI: Journal of Roman Archaeology, Suppl. Series 54.

MacKinnon, M. 2007. 'State of the discipline: osteological research in classical archaeology', *American Journal of Archaeology* 111, pp. 473–504.

MacKinnon, M. 2010a. '"Romanizing" ancient Carthage: evidence from zooarchaeological remains', in *Anthropological Approaches to Zooarchaeology: Complexity, Colonialism and Animal Transformations*, ed. D. Campana, P. Crabtree, S.D. deFrance, J. Lev-Tov and A. Choyke. Oxford: Oxbow, pp. 168–177.

MacKinnon, M. 2010b. 'Cattle "breed" variation and improvement in Roman Italy: connecting the zooarchaeological and ancient textual evidence', *World Archaeology* 42, pp. 55–73.

MacKinnon, M. 2014a. 'Animals, economics and culture in the Athenian Agora: comparative zooarchaeological investigations', *Hesperia* 83, pp. 189–255.

MacKinnon, M. 2014b. 'Crying fowl: re-evaluating the role poultry in Roman dietary and funeral contexts', Poster presented at the Archaeological Institute of America Conference, Chicago.

MacMahon, A. 2005. 'The *taberna* counters of Pompeii and Herculaneum', in *Roman Working Lives and Urban Living*, ed. A. MacMahon and J. Price. Oxford: Oxbow Books, pp. 70–87.

MacMullen, R. 1974. *Roman Social Relations, 50 BC to AD 284*. New Haven: Yale University Press.

Macro, A.D. 1976. 'Imperial provisions for Permanum: OGIS 484', *GRBS* 17, pp. 169–179.

Magyar-Hárshegyi, P. 2016. 'Supplying the Roman army on the Pannonian Limes. Amphorae on the territory of Budapest, Hungary (Aquincum and Albertfalva)', in *Rei Cretaria Romana Fautorum Acta* 44, pp. 619–632.

Makarewicz, C.A. and Sealy, J. 2015. 'Dietary reconstruction, mobility, and the analysis of ancient skeletal tissues: expanding the prospects of stable isotope research in archaeology', *Journal of Archaeological Science* 56, pp. 146–158.

Malama, P. and Triantaphyllou, S. 2002. 'Ανθρωπολογικές πληροφορίες από το ανατολικό νεκροταφείο της Αμφίπολης', *Το Αρχαιολογικό Έργο στη Μακεδονία και Θράκη*, 16, pp. 127–136.

Maltby, M. 1985. 'Patterns in faunal assemblage variability', in *Beyond Domestication in Prehistoric Europe*, ed. G. Barker and C. Gamble. New York: Academic Press, pp. 33–74.

Maltby, M. 2006. 'Salt and animal products: linking production and use in Iron Age Britain', in *Integrating Zooarchaeology*, ed. M. Maltby. Oxford: Oxbow, pp. 117–122.

Maltby, M. 2007. 'Chop and change: specialist cattle carcass processing in Roman Britain', in *TRAC 2006: Proceedings of the 16th Annual Theoretical Roman Archaeology Conference*, ed. B. Croxford, N. Ray and R. Roth. Oxford: Oxbow, pp. 59–76.

Manzi, G., Sperduti, A. and Passarello, P. 1991. 'Behavior-induced auditory exostoses in imperial Roman society: evidence from coeval urban and rural communities near Rome', *American Journal of Physical Anthropology* 85, pp. 253–260.

Manzi, G., Salvadei, L., Vienna, A. and Passarello, P. 1999. 'Discontinuity of life conditions at the transition from the Roman Imperial age to the early Middle Ages: example from central Italy evaluated by pathological dento-alveolar lesions', *American Journal of Physical Anthropology* 11, pp. 327–341.

Maravela-Solbakk, A. 2009. 'Byzantine inventory lists of food provisions and utensils', *Zeitschrift für Papyrologie und Epigraphik* 170, pp. 127–146.

Marchesini, M. and Marvelli, S. Forthcoming. 'Paesaggio vegetale e agricoltura nella pianura padana in età romana', *Popolazione e Risorse nell'Italia settentrionale dall'Età preromana ai Longobardi*, ed. E. Lo Cascio and M. Maiuro. Bari: Edipuglia.

Marchesini, M., Marvelli, S., Gobbo I. and Accorsi, C.A. 2008. 'Alla ricerca di paesaggi carpigiani perduti. Il paesaggio vegetale, l'ambiente e l'economia ricostruiti attraverso le indagini polliniche', in *Storia di Carpi – La città e il territorio dalle origini all'affermazione dei Pio*, ed. P. Bonacini and A.M. Ori. Modena: Mucchi, pp. 51–76.

Marchesini, M., Marvelli, S., Gobbo, I. and Rizzoli, E. 2010. 'Paesaggio, ambiente e attività antropica dalla Bologna villanoviana (VII–VI sec. a.C.) alla Bononia romana (I sec. d.C.) attraverso le analisi archeobotaniche', in *Alla ricerca di Bologna antica e medievale. Da Felsina a Bononia negli scavi di Via d'Aazeglio*, ed. L. Malnati, R. Curina, C.Negrelli and L. Pini. Florence: All'Insegna del Giglio, pp. 145–162.

Marcone, A. 1997. *Storia dell'Agricoltura romana. Dal Mondo arcaico all'Età imperiale*. Rome: Carocci.

Marinova, E., van der Valk, J.M.A., Valamoti, S.M. and Bretschneider, J. 2011. 'An experimental approach for tracing olive processing residues in the archaeobotanical record, with preliminary examples from Tell Tweini, Syria', *Vegetation History and Archaeobotany* 20, pp. 471–478.

Markus, R. 1990. *The End of Ancient Christianity*, Cambridge and New York: Cambridge University Press.

Marlière, E. 2002. *L'outre et le tonneau dans L'Occident romain*. Montagnac: Editions Monique Mergoil.

Marlière, E. and Torres Costa, J. 2005. 'Tonneaux et amphores à Vindolanda: contribution à la connaissance de l approvisionnement des troupes stationnées sur le mur d Hadrien (II)', in *Vindolanda Excavations 2003–2004*, ed. A. Birley and J. Blake. Bardon Mill, Hexham: Vindolanda Trust, pp. 214–236.

Márquez-Grant, N. and Fibiger, L., eds. 2011. *The Routledge Handbook of Archaeological Human Remains and Legislation: An International Guide to Laws and Practice in the Excavation and Treatment of Archaeological Human Remains*. New York: Taylor & Francis.

Marshall, C.W. 2017. 'Breastfeeding in Greek literature and thought', *Illinois Classical Studies* 42, pp. 185–201.

Martin, A. 2008. 'Imports at Ostia in the imperial period and late antiquity: the amphora evidence from the DAI-AAR excavations', in *The Maritime World of Ancient Rome. Proceedings of 'The Maritime World of Ancient Rome' Conference held at the American Academy in Rome 27–29 March 2003*, ed. R.L. Hohlfelder. Ann Arbor, pp. 105–118.

Martin, D.L., Harrod, R.P. and Pérez, V.R. 2014. *Bioarchaeology: An Integrated Approach to Working with Human Remains*. New York: Springer.

Martin-Kilcher, S. 1987. Die römischen Amphoren aus Augst und Kaiseraugst Ein Beitragzur römischen Handels – und Kulturgeschichte I: Die südspanischen Ölamphoren (Gruppe I). Augst: Römermuseum Augst. Blázquez

Martínez-González, M.A., Salas-Salvadó, J., Estruch, R., Corella, D., Fitó, M. and E. Ros. 2015. 'Benefits of the Mediterranean diet: insights from the PREDIMED study', *Progress in Cardiovascular Diseases* 58, pp. 50–60.

Marzano, A. 2007. *Roman Villas in Central Italy. A Social and Economic History*. Leiden-Boston: Brill.

Marzano, A. 2013a. 'Agricultural production in the hinterland of Rome: wine and olive oil', in *The Roman Agricultural Economy: Organisation, Investment and Production*, ed. A.K. Bowman and A.I. Wilson. Oxford, Oxford University Press, pp. 85–106.

Marzano, A. 2013b. *Harvesting the Sea: The Exploitation of Maritime Resources in the Roman Mediterranean*. Oxford: Oxford University Press.

Marzano, A. 2013c. 'Capital investment and agriculture: multi-press facilities from Gaul, the Iberian Peninsula, and the Black Sea region', in *The Roman Agricultural Economy: Organization, Investment, and Production*, ed. A. Bowman and A. Wilson. Oxford: Oxford University Press, pp. 107–141.

Marzano, A. and Brizzi, G. 2009. 'Costly display or economic investment? A quantitative approach to the study of marine aquaculture', *Journal of Roman Archaeology* 22, pp. 215–230.

Masali, M. 1981. 'Les prédynastiques de Gebelen (Haute Egypte)', *Bulletins et Mémoires de la Société d'anthropologie de Paris*, XIII Série, tome 8 fascicule 3, pp. 253–263.

Mason, S.L.R. 1996. 'Acornutopia? Determining the role of acorns in past human subsistence', in *Food in Antiquity*, ed. J. Wilkins, D. Harvey and M. Dobson. Exeter: University of Exeter Press, pp. 12–24.

Matterne, V. and Derreumaux, M. 2008. 'A Franco-Italian investigation of funerary rituals in the Roman world, "les rites et la mort à Pompéi", the plant part: a preliminary report', *Vegetation History and Archaeobotany* 17(1), pp. 105–112.

Matthews, J. 2006. *The Journey of Theophanes: Travel, Business and Daily Life in the Roman East*. New Haven and London: Yale University Press.

Mattingly, D.J. 1988a. 'Megalithic madness and measurement. Or how many olives could an olive press press?', *OJA* 7, pp. 177–195.

Mattingly, D.J. 1988b. 'The olive boom: oil surpluses, wealth and power in Roman Tripolitania', *LibSt* 19, pp. 21–42.

Mattingly, D.J. 1988c. 'Oil for export? A comparison of Libyan, Spanish and Tunisian olive oil production in the Roman Empire', *JRA* 1, pp. 33–56.

Mattingly, D.J. 1993. 'Maximum figures and maximizing strategies of oil production? Further thoughts on the processing capacity of Roman olive presses', *La Production du Vin et de l'Huile en Méditerrannée de l'Age du Bronze à la Fin du XVIème Siècle*, ed. M.C. Amouretti and J.-P. Brun. Athens-Paris: École Française d'Athènes, pp. 483–498.

Mattingly, D. and Aldrete, G. 2000. 'The feeding of imperial Rome: the mechanics of the food supply system', in *Ancient Rome: the Archaeology of the Eternal City*, ed. J. Coulston and H. Dodge. Oxford: Oxford University School of Archaeology, pp. 142–165.

Mattson, M.P. and Calabrese, E.J., eds. 2009. *Hormesis: A Revolution in Biology, Toxicology and Medicine*. New York: Humana Press.

Mau, A. 1899. *Pompeii: Its Life and Art*. London: Macmillan & Co.

Maxfield, V.A and Peacock D.P.S. 2001. *Survey and Excavation Mons Claudianus 1987–1993, II.1*. Cairo: IFAO.

Mayer, E. E. 2012. *The Ancient Middle Classes Urban Life and Aesthetics in the Roman Empire, 100 BCE–250 CE*. Cambridge, MA: Harvard University Press.

Mayer, E. Forthcoming. 'Was there a culture of the Roman plebs?' *Journal of Roman Archaeology*.

Mayerson, P. 2001. 'Radish oil: a phenomenon in Roman Egypt', *BASP* 38, pp. 109–117.

Mayerson, P. 2002. 'Qualitative distinctions for ἔλαιον (oil) and ψωμίον (bread)', *BASP* 39, pp. 101–109.

Mays, S. 1995. 'The relationship between Harris lines and other aspects of skeletal development in adults and juveniles', *Journal of Archaeological Science* 22, pp. 511–520.

Mazzini, I. 1999. 'Diet and medicine in the ancient world', in *Food: A Culinary History from Antiquity to the Present*, ed. A. Sonnenfeld. New York and Chichester: Columbia University Press, pp. 141–152.

Meadows, K. 1997. 'Much ado about nothing: the social context of eating and drinking in early Roman Britain', in *Not so Much a Pot, More a Way of Life*, ed. C.G. Cumberpatch and P.W. Blinkhorn. Oxford: Oxbow, pp. 17–27.

Meadows, K. 1999. 'The appetites of households in early Roman Britain', in *The Archaeology of Household Activities*, ed. P. Allison. London: Routledge, pp. 101–120.

Meier, C. 1997. *Caesar: A Biography*, trans. D. McLintock. New York: Perseus Book Group.

Méniel, P. 2014. 'Une *favissa* dans le sanctuaire de Mercure au sommet du puy de Dôme', in *Transalpinare. Mélanges offerts à Anne-Marie Adam*, ed. G. Alberti, C. Féliu and G. Pierrevelcin. Bordeaux: Ausonius, pp. 235–245.

Merlo, M. 2005. 'Distribution of impasto chiaro sabbioso pottery in ancient Italy', in *Papers in Italian Archaeology VI: Communities and Settlements from the Neolithic to the Early Medieval Period*, ed. P.A.J. Attema, A Nijboer and A. Zifferero. BAR international series 1452, Oxford: Archaeopress, pp. 417–425.

Metzler, J. and Gaeng, C. 2005. 'Protohistoire', in *Préhistoire et Protohistoire au Luxemburg*. Les collections du Musée national d histoire et d art. Luxemburg: Saint-Paul Luxembourg, pp. 125–221.

Meurers-Balke, J. and Kaszab-Olschewski, T., eds. 2010. *Grenzenlose Gaumenfreuden. Römische Küche in einer germanischen Provinz*. Mainz: Verlag Philipp von Zabern.

Meyer, F.G. 1980. 'Carbonized food plants of Pompeii, Herculaneum, and the Villa at Torre Annunziata', *Economic Botany* 34, pp. 401–437.

Mielsch, H. 2001. *Römische Wandmalerei*. Stuttgart: Theiss.

Milanovic, B., Lindert, P.H. and Williamson, J.G. 2007. *Measuring Ancient Inequality*. Policy Research Working Paper 4412. The World Bank Development Research Group Poverty Team (www.world bank.org).

Millar, F. 1983. 'Epigraphy', in *Sources for Ancient History*, ed. M. Crawford. Cambridge: Cambridge University Press, pp. 80–136.

Miller, J.I. 1969. *The Spice Trade of the Roman Empire, 29 BC to AD 641*. Oxford: Clarendon Press.

Miller, N.F. 1988. 'Ratios in paleoethnobotanical analysis', in *Current Paleoethnobotany: Analytical Methods and Cultural Interpretations of Archaeological Plant Remains*, ed. C.A. Hastorf and V.S. Popper. Chicago and London: University of Chicago Press, pp. 72–85.

Milne, G. 1985. *The Port of Roman London*. London: B.T. Batsford.

Minniti, C., Valenzuela-Lamas, S., Evans, J. and Albarella, U. 2014. 'Widening the market. Strontium isotope analysis on cattle teeth from Owslebury (Hampshire, UK) highlights changes in livestock supply between the Iron Age and the Roman period', *Journal of Archaeological Science* 42, pp. 305–314.

Minozzi, S., Catalano, P., di Giannantonio, S. and Fornaciari, G. 2013. 'Salute e malattia nella roma imperiale attraverso le evidenze scheletriche', *Medicina nei Secoli Arte e Scienza* 25, pp. 119–138.

Mirti, P. and Davit, P. 2001. 'Technological characterization of Campanian pottery of Type A, B and C and of regional products from ancient Calabria (Southern Italy)', *Archaeometry* 43(1), pp. 19–33.

Mitthof, F. 2001. *Annona militaris. Die Heeresversorgung im spätantiken Ägypten*, Florence: Gonnelli.

Moffett, L. 1996. 'Charred plant remains', in *Roman Alcester: Defences and Defended Area, Vol. 1, Gateway Supermarket and Gas House Lane*, ed. S. Cracknell. York: CBA Research Report 106, pp. 112–114.

Mokyr, J. and Ó Gráda, C. 2002. 'What do people die of during famines: the Great Irish Famine in comparative perspective', *European Review of Economic History* 6, pp. 339–363.

Molto, J.E. 2001. 'The comparative skeletal biology and paleoepidemiology of the people from Ein Tirghi and Kellis, Dakhleh Oasis, Egypt', in *The Oasis Papers I: The Proceedings of the First Conference of the Dakhleh Oasis Project*, ed. C.A. Marlow and A.J. Mills. Oxford: Oxbow, pp. 81–100.

Mols, S. and Moorman, E.M. 1993–1994. 'Ex parvo crevit: Proposta per una lettura iconografica della Tomba di Vestorius Priscus fuori Porta Vesuvio a Pompei', *Rivista di studi pompeiani* 6, pp. 15–52.

Monasterio, I. and Graham, R.D. 2000. 'Breeding for trace minerals in wheat', *Food and Nutrition Bulletin* 21(4), pp. 392–396.

Montanari, M., ed. 2012. *A Cultural History of Food in the Medieval Age*. London and New York: Berg.

Monteix, N. 2007. 'Du couteau au boucher: remarques préliminaires sur la préparation et le commerce de la viande à Pompéi', *Food and History* 5(1), pp. 169–195.

Monfort, C.C. 2002. 'The Roman military supply during the Principate: transportation and staples', in *The Roman Army and the Economy*, ed. P. Erdkamp. Amsterdam: Gieben, pp. 70–87.

Monson, A. 2006. 'The ethics and economics of Ptolemaic religious associations', *Ancient Society* 36, pp. 221–238.

Montgomery, J., Evans, J.A., Chenery, S., Pashley, V. and Killgrove, K. 2010. ' "Gleaming, white and deadly": lead exposure and geographic origins in the Roman period', in *Roman Diasporas: Archaeological Approaches to Mobility and Diversity in the Roman Empire*, ed. H. Eckardt. Portsmouth, RI: Journal of Roman Archaeology, Supplement 78, pp. 199–226.

Moore, M.K. and Ross, A.H. 2013. 'Stature estimation', in *Research Methods in Human Skeletal Biology*, ed. E.A. Di Gangi and M.K. Moore. London: Elsevier, pp. 151–180.

Moore-Jansen, P.H., Jantz, R.L. and Ousley, S.D. 1994. *Data Collection Procedures for Forensic Skeletal Material*. University of Tennessee at Knoxville Forensic Anthropology Center.

Morelli, F. 1996. *Olio e retribuzioni nell'Egitto tardo (V-VIII d.C.)*. Florence: Istituto Papirologico Vitelli.

Morelli, F. 2004. 'Il λαχανόσπερμον, il ῥαφανέλαιον, e il sesamo: olii e oleaginose fantasma', *Zeitschrift für Papyrologie und Epigraphik* 149, pp. 138–142.

Moritz, L.A. 1958. *Grain Mills and Flour in Classical Antiquity*. Oxford: Clarendon Press.

Morley, N. 1996. *Metropolis and Hinterland: The City of Rome and the Italian Economy, 200BC–AD200*. Cambridge, Cambridge University Press.

Morley, N. 2007. *Trade in Classical Antiquity*. Cambridge: Cambridge University Press.

Morra, V., De Bonis, A., Grifa, C., Langella, A., Cavassa, L. and Piovesan, R. 2013. 'Minero-petrographic study of cooking ware and Pompeian Red Ware (rosso Pompeiano) from Cuma (southern Italy)', *Archaeometry* 55(5), pp. 852–879.

Morris, I. 1992. *Death-Ritual and Social Structure in Classical Antiquity*. Cambridge: Cambridge University Press.

Mossakowska-Gaubert, M. 2015. 'Alimentation, hygiène, vêtements et sommeil chez les moines égyptiens (IVe-VIIIe siècle): l'état des sources archéologiques et écrites', in *Le Vie quotidienne des Moines en Orient et en Occident (IVe–Xe sicèle), volume I. L'État des Sources*, ed. O. Delouis and M. Mossakowska-Gaubert. Bibliothèque d'Etude 163, Cairo: IFAO, pp. 23–56.

Mossman, J. 1997. 'Plutarch's dinner of the seven wise men and its place in symposion literature', in *Plutarch and his Intellectual Word: Essays on Plutarch*, ed. J. Mossman. London: Duckworth, pp. 119–140.

Mould, Q. 2011. 'Domestic life', in *Artefacts in Roman Britain: Their Purpose and Use*, ed. L. Allason-Jones. New York: Cambridge University Press, pp. 153–179.

Müldner, G. 2013. 'Stable isotopes and diet: their contribution to Romano-British research', *Antiquity* 87(335), pp. 137–149.

Müldner, G. and Richards, M.P. 2007. 'Stable isotope evidence for 1500 years of human diet at the city of York, UK', *American Journal of Physical Anthropology* 133, pp. 682–697.

Müldner, G., Chenery, C. and Eckardt, H. 2011. 'The "headless Romans": multi-isotope investigations of an unusual burial ground from Roman Britain', *Journal of Archaeological Science* 38, pp. 280–290.

Müller, N.S., Kilikoglou, V. and Day, P.M. 2015. 'Home-made recipes: tradition and innovation in Bronze Age cooking pots from Akrotiri, Thera', in *Ceramics, Cuisine and Culture: The Archaeology and Science of Kitchen Pottery in the ancient mediterranean world*, ed. M. Spataro and A. Villing. Oxford: Oxbow Books, pp. 37–48.

Murphy, C., Thompson, G. and Fuller, D.Q. 2013. 'Roman food refuse: urban archaeobotany in Pompeii, Regio VI, Insula 1', *Vegetation History and Archaeobotany* 22(5), pp. 409–419.

Murray, O., ed. 1990. *Sympotika: A Symposium on the Symposium*. Oxford: Clarendon Press.

Musco, S., Catalano, P., Caspio, A., Pantano, W. and Killgrove, K. 2008. Le complexe archéologique de Casal Bertone. *Les Dossiers d'Archéologie* 330, pp. 32–39.

Musselman, L.J. and al-Mouslem, A.B. 2001. 'Triticum Durum in northern Syria: parched corn (Frikeh) of the Bible?', *Economic Botany* 55(2), pp. 187–189.

Mylona, D. 2008. *Fish-Eating in Greece from the Fifth Century BC to the Seventh Century AD: A Story of Impoverished Fishermen or Luxurious Fish Banquets?* BAR Int. Series 1754. Oxford: Archaeopress.

Mylona, D. 2015. 'Fish', in *A Companion to Food in the Ancient World*, ed. J. Wilkins and R. Nadeau. Oxford: Wiley-Blackwell, pp. 147–159.

Myrdal, G. 1944. *An American Dilemma: The Negro Problem and Modern Democracy*. New York: Harper and Brothers.

Nadeau, R. 2010. *Les Manières de Table dans le Monde gréco-romain. Table des Hommes*. Rennes/Tours: Presses universitaires François-Rabelais.

Nadeau, R. 2012. 'Body and soul', in *A Cultural History of Food in Antiquity*, ed. P. Erdkamp. London: Bloomsbury, pp. 145–162.

Nadeau, R. 2015. 'Cookery books', in *A Companion to Food in the Ancient World*, ed. J. Wilkins and R. Nadeau. Oxford: Wiley-Blackwell, pp. 53–58.

Nanni, A. and Maffei, L. 2004. *Nodo di Roma. Penetrazione Urbana A V – Linea FM2. Italferr/TAV. Relazione Antropologica. Area AI (E). Casal Bertone. Necropoli e Mausoleo*. Soprintendenza Archeologica di Roma, Servizio di Antropologia.

Naumann-Steckner, F. 1991. 'Depictions of glass in Roman wall paintings', in *Roman Glass: Two Centuries of Art and Invention*, ed. M. Newby and K.S. Painter. London: Society of Antiquaries of London, pp. 86–98.

Nehren, R. and Strauch, F. 2012. 'Austern, andere Muscheln und Schnecken – Leckereien auf der römischen Speisetafel', in *ZeitTunnel. 2000 Jahre Köln im Spiegel der U-Bahn-Archäologie*, ed. M. Trier and F. Naumann-Steckner. Köln: Wienand Verlag, pp. 56–57.

Nelsestuen, G.A. 2015. *Varro the Agronomist: Political Philosophy, Satire and Agriculture in the Late Republic.* Columbus: Ohio State Press.

Nelson, M. 2003. 'The cultural construction of beer among Greeks and Romans', *Syllecta Classica* 14, pp. 101–120.

Nielsen, H.S. 2001. 'Roman children at mealtimes', in *Meals in a Social Context. Aspects of the Communal Meal in the Hellenistic and Roman World*, ed. I. Nielsen and H.S. Nielsen. Aarhus: Aarhus University Press, pp. 67–80.

Nielsen, I. and Nielsen, H.S., eds. 2001. *Meals in a Social Context: Aspects of the Communal Meal in the Hellenistic and Roman World.* Aarhus: Aarhus University Press.

Nippel, W. 1995. *Public Order in Ancient Rome.* Cambridge: Cambridge University Press.

Nobis, G. 1973. 'Tierreste aus einer Siedlung der vorrömischen Eisenzeit bei Sünninghausen (Kr. Beckum-Westfalen)', *Bodenaltertümer Westfalens* 13, pp. 143–173.

Noddle, B.A. 1983. 'Size and shape, time and place: skeletal variations in cattle and sheep', in *Integrating the Subsistence Economy*, ed. M. Jones. Oxford: BAR, pp. 211–238.

Noethlichs, K.L. 'Edictum [3] Edictum Diocletiani', in *Brill's New Pauly Online.* Accessed 1 March 2016.

Nour, A.A.M. and Magboul, B.I. 1986. 'Chemical and amino acid composition of fenugreek seeds grown in Sudan', *Food Chemistry* 22, pp. 1–5.

Noy, D. 2001. 'The sixth hour is the mealtime for scholars: Jewish meals in the Roman world', in *Meals in a Social Context: Aspects of the Communal Meal in the Hellenistic and Roman World*, ed. I. Nielsen and H.S. Nielsen. Aarhus: Aarhus University Press, pp. 134–144.

Nutton, V. 1995. 'Galen and the traveller's fare', in *Food in Antiquity*, ed. J. Wilkins, D. Harvey and M. Dobson. Exeter: University of Exeter Press, pp. 359–370.

O'Connell, S. 2015. *Surface, Suggestion, and Seeing Through: Visual Perception and The Significance of Objects Depicted in Roman Wall Painting.* PhD Dissertation. Johns Hopkins University.

O'Connor, T. 1988. *Bones from the General Accident Site, Tanner Row.* London: Council for British Archaeology.

O'Connor, T.P. 1993. 'Process and terminology in mammal carcass reduction', *International Journal of Osteoarchaeology* 3, pp. 63–67.

Ó Gráda, C. 2007. 'Making famine history', *Journal of Economic Literature* 45, pp. 5–38.

Olcese, G. 2003. *Ceramiche comuni a Roma e in Area romana: Produzione, Circolazione e Tecnologia: tarda Età repubblicana-prima Età imperiale.* Mantua: SAP.

Olive, C. and Deschler-Erb, S. 1999. 'Poulets de grain et rôtis du cerf. Produits de luxe pour les villes Romaines.' *Archäologie der Schweiz* 22, pp. 35–38.

Olsen, K.C., White, C.D., Longstaffe, F. J., von Heyking, K., George McGlynn, G., Grupe, G. and Rühli, F.J. 2014. 'Intraskeletal isotopic compositions ($\delta^{13}C$, $\delta^{15}N$) of bone collagen: Nonpathological and pathological variation', *American Journal of Physical Anthropology* 153, pp. 598–604.

Orme, N. 2001. *Medieval Children.* New Haven and London: Yale University Press.

Ørsted, P. 1998. 'Salt, fish, and the sea in the Roman Empire', in *Meals in a Social Context: Aspects of the Communal Meal in the Hellenistic and Roman World*, ed. I. Nielsen and H.S. Nielsen. Aarhus: Aarhus University Press, pp. 13–35.

Ortiz-Monasterio, J.I., Palacios-Rojas, N., Meng, E., Pixley, K., Trethowan, R. and Peña, R.J. 2007. 'Enhancing the mineral and vitamin content of wheat and maize through plant breeding', *Journal of Cereal Science* 46, pp. 293–307.

Ortner, D. 2003. *Identification of Pathological Conditions in Human Skeletal Remains.* San Diego: Academic Press.

Ortner, D. 2012. 'Differential diagnosis and issues in disease classification', in *A Companion to Paleopathology*, ed. A.L. Grauer. Chichester: Wiley-Blackwell, pp. 250–267.

Osgood, J. 2011. 'Making Romans in the family', in *The Oxford Handbook of Social Relations in the Roman World*, ed. M. Peachin. Oxford: Oxford University Press, pp. 69–83.

Osman, A.E., Pagnotta, M., Russi, L., Cocks, P.S. and M. Falcinelli. 1990. 'The role of legumes in improving marginal lands', in *The Role of Legumes in the Farming Systems of the Mediterranean Areas*, ed. A.E. Osman, M.H. Ibrahim and M.A. Jones. Dordrecht, Boston and London: Kluwer Academic Publishers, pp. 143–149.

Ottini, L., Ricci, R., Angeletti, L., Costantini, R., and Catalano, P. 2001. 'Le condizioni di vita nella popolazione di età imperiale', *Mitteilungen des Deutschen Archäologischen Instituts, Römische Abteilung* 108, 364–366.

Oxenham, M.F. and Cavill, I. 2010. 'Porotic hyperostosis and cribra orbitalia: the erythropoietic response to iron-deficiency anaemia', *Anthropological Science* 118, pp. 199–200.

Paap, N. 1983. 'Economic plants in Amsterdam: qualitative and quantitative analysis', in *Integrating the Subsistence Economy*, ed. M. Jones. Oxford: BAR, pp. 315–325.

Päffgen, B. 2014. 'Küche und Keller – Produktion, Vorratshaltung und Konsum in römischer Antike und Frühmittelalter. Einleitende Bemerkungen zum Tagungsthema', in *Küche und Keller in Antike und Früh mittelalter*, ed. J. Drauschke, R. Prien and A. Reis. SAFM 6. Hamburg: Verlag Dr. Kovač, pp. 3–57.

Pagnoux, C. et al. 2013. 'The introduction of citrus to Italy, with reference to the identification problems of seed remains', *Vegetation History and Archaeobotany* 22, pp. 421–438.

Panel on Macronutrients, Subcommittees on Upper Reference Levels of Nutrients and Interpretation and Uses of Dietary Reference Intakes, and the Standing Committee on the Scientific Evaluation of Dietary Reference Intakes. 2005. 'Introduction to dietary reference intakes', in *Dietary Reference Intakes for Energy, Carbohydrate, Fiber, Fat, Fatty Acids, Cholesterol, Protein, and Amino Acids*. Washington: The National Academies Press, pp. 21–36. Available at www.nal.usda.gov/fnic/DRI/DRI_Water/21-36.pdf (accessed 1 July 2015).

Papathanasiou, A., Richards, M.P. and Fox, S.C., ed. 2015. Archaeodiet in the Greek World: Dietary Reconstruction from Stable Isotope Analysis. Princeton: American School of Classical Studies at Athens.

Papathomas, A. 2006. 'Zu den Luxusspeisen und -getränken in griechischen Papyri', *Zeitschrift für Papyrologie und Epigraphik* 158, pp. 193–200.

Parasescoli, P. and P. Scholliers, eds. 2012. *A Cultural History of Food, Volumes 1–6*. London: Bloomsbury.

Parkin, T. 2012. 'Life cycle', in *A Cultural History of Childhood and Family in Antiquity*, ed. M. Harlow and R. Laurence. Oxford: Berg, pp. 97–114.

Parlasca, K. and Seemann, H. 1999. *Augenblicke. Mumienporträts und ägyptische Grabkunst aus römischer Zeit, Eine Ausstellung der Schirn Kunsthalle Frankfurt*. Frankfurt: Schirn Kunsthalle.

Parsons, P. 1977. 'The oyster', *Zeitschrift für Papyrologie und Epigraphik* 24, pp. 1–12.

Pasqui, A. 1906. 'Region I. (Latium et Campania) IV. Ostia – Nuove scoperte presso il Casone', *Notizie degli scavi di antichità*, pp. 357–373.

Pastor-Cavada, E., Juan, R., Pastor, J.E., Alaiz, M., and Vioque, J. 2011. 'Nutritional characteristics of seed proteins in 15 *Lathyrus* species (fabaceae) from Southern Spain', *Food Science and Technology* 44, pp. 1059–1064.

Pastor-Cavada, E., Juan, R., Pastor, J.E., Aliaz, M. and Vioque, J. 2014. 'Protein and amino-acid composition of select wild legume species of tribe Fabeae', *Food Chemistry* 163, pp. 97–102.

Patterson, J.R. 2006. *Landscapes and Cities: Rural Settlement and Civic Transformation in Early Imperial Italy*. Oxford: Oxford University Press.

Paulas, J. 2012. 'How to read Athenaeus' Deipnosophists', *American Journal of Philology* 133, pp. 403–439.

Payne, S. 1973. 'Kill-off patterns in sheep and goats: the mandibles from Aşvan Kalé', *Anatolian Studies* 23, pp. 281–303.

Peacock, D.P.S. and Williams, D.F. 1986. *Amphorae and the Roman Economy: An Introductory Guide*. London: Longman.

Peacock, D., Blue, L. et al. 2011. *Myos Hormos – Quseir al-Qadim. Roman and Islamic ports on the Red Sea, Volume 2: Finds from the Excavations 1999–2003*, BAE International series 2286. Oxford: Oxbow books.

Pearsall, D.M. 2000. *Paleoethnobotany: A Handbook of Procedures*, 2nd edition. San Diego: Academic Press.

Pearson, K.L. 1997. 'Nutrition and early-medieval diet', *Speculum* 72, pp. 1–32.

Pearson, S. 2015. 'Bodies of meaning: figural repetition in Pompeian painting', in *Beyond Iconography: Materials, Methods, and Meaning in Ancient Surface Decoration*, ed. S. Lepinski and S. McFadden. Boston: Archaeological Institute of America, pp. 149–166.

Pellegrini, N., Serafini, M., Colombi, B., Del Rio, D., Salvatore, S., Bianchi, M. and Brighenti, F. 2003. 'Total antioxidant capacity of plant foods, beverages and oils consumed in Italy assessed by three different in vitro assays', *The Journal of Nutrition* 133, pp. 2812–2819.

Pelling, C. 2000. 'Fun with fragments: Athenaeus and the historians'. In *Athenaeus and his World: Reading Greek Culture in the Roman Empire*, ed. D. Braund and J. Wilkins. Exeter: University of Exeter Press, pp. 171–190.

Pelling, R., Campbell, G., Carruthers, W., Hunter, K. and Marshall, P. 2015. 'Exploring contamination (intrusion and residuality) in the archaeobotanical record: case studies from central and southern England', *Vegetation History and Archaeobotany* 24(1), pp. 85–99.

Peña, J.T. 1990. 'Internal red-slip cookware (Pompeian red ware) from Cetamura del Chianti, Italy: mineralogical composition and provenience', *American Journal of Archaeology* 94, pp. 647–661.

Peña, J.T. 2007. *Roman pottery in the archaeological record*. Cambridge: Cambridge University Press.

Pena, M.J. and Barreda, A. 1997. 'Productores de vino del nordeste de la Tarraconense. Estudio de algunos nomina sobre ánforas Laietana 1 (=Tarraconense 1)', *Faventia* 19(2), pp. 51–73.

Peña, J.T. and Gallimore, S.C. 2014. 'Black-gloss ware, North Etrurian red-slip ware, and Italian terra sigillata from Cetamura Del Chianti: composition, provenance, supply, and consumption', *HEROM* 3(1), pp. 71–244.

Peña-Chocarro, L. and Peña, L.Z. 1999. 'History and traditional cultivation of *Lathyrus sativus* L. and *Lathyrus cicero* L. in the Iberian Peninsula', *Vegetation History and Archaeobotany* 8, pp. 49–52.

Pepe, C., Giardini, M., Giraudi, C., Masi, A., Mazzini, I. and Sadori, L., 2013. 'Plant landscape and environmental changes recorded in marginal marine environments: the ancient Roman harbour of Portus (Rome, Italy)', *Quaternary International* 303, pp. 73–81.

Pereira, J.A., Pereira, A., Ferreira, I., Valentão, P., Andrade, P., Seabra, R., Estevinho, L. and Bento, A. 2006. 'Table olives from Portugal: Phenolic compounds, antioxidant potential, and antimicrobial activity', *Journal of Agricultural and Food Chemistry* 54, pp. 8425–8431.

Perpillou-Thomas, F. 1992. 'Une bouillie de céréales: l'athèra', *Aegyptus* 72, pp. 103–110.

Perpillou-Thomas, F. 1993. *Fêtes d'Egypte ptolémaïque et romaine d'après la Documentation papyrologique grecque*. Studia Hellenistica 31. Leuven: Peeters.

Perry, M. 2007. 'Is bioarchaeology a handmaiden to history?', *Journal of Anthropological Archaeology* 26, pp. 486–515.

Perry, J.S. 2011. 'Organized societies: *collegia*', in *The Oxford Handbook of Social Relations in the Roman World*, ed. M. Peachin. Oxford: Oxford University Press, pp. 499–515.

Persson, K.G. 1999. *Grain Markets in Europe, 1500–1900. Integration and Deregulation*, Cambridge: Cambridge University Press.

Peters, J. 1998. *Römische Tierhaltung und Tierzucht: eine Synthese aus archäozoologischer Untersuchung und schriftlich-bildlicher Überlieferung*. Rahden: Leidorf.

Pferdehirt, B. 2012. 'Die rechtlichen Auswirkungen', in *Bürgerrecht und Krise. Die Constitutio Antoniniana 212 n. Chr. und ihre innenpolitischen Folgen*, ed. B. Pferdehirt and M. Scholz. Forschungen am Römisch-Germanischen Zentralmuseum 9. Mainz: Verlag des Römisch-Germanischen Zentralmuseums, pp. 59–60.

Phang, S.E. 2008. *Roman Military Service: Ideologies of Discipline in the Late Republic and Early Principate*. Cambridge: Cambridge University Press.

Philonenko, Marc. 1968. *Joseph et Aséneth: Introduction, Texte critique, Traduction, et Notes*. Studia Post Biblica. Leiden: E. J. Brill.

Piccioli, A., Gazzaniga, V. and Catalano, P., eds. 2015. *Bones: Orthopaedic Pathologies in Roman Imperial Age*. New York: Springer.

Pieraccini, L. 2000. 'Families, feasting, and funerals: funerary ritual at ancient Caere', *Etruscan Studies* 7, pp. 35–49.

Pieroni, A. 1996. 'Gathered wild food plants in the Upper Valley of the Serchio River (Garfagnana), Central Italy', *Economic Botany* 53(3), pp. 327–341.

Piketty, T. 2005. 'Top income shares in the long run: an overview', *Journal of the European Economic Association* 3, pp. 382–392.

Piketty, T. 2014. *Capital in the Twenty-First Century*. Cambridge, MA: Harvard University Press.

Piketty, T. and Saez, E. 2004. 'Income inequality in the United States, 1913–2002', in *Top Incomes over the Twentieth Century: A Contrast between European and English-Speaking Countries*, ed. T. Piketty and A.B. Atkinson. Oxford: Oxford University Press.

Pilkington, N. 2013. 'Growing up Roman: infant mortality and reproductive development', *Journal of Interdisciplinary History* 44, pp. 1–36.

Pilon, F., Maames, K. and Jedrusiak, F. 2014. 'Approche archéologique et paléoenvironnementale des parcelles de l'agglomération gallo-romaine de Chäteaubleau', in *Archéologie des Jardins, Analyse des Espaces et Méthodes d'approche*, ed. P. Van Ossel and A.-M. Guimier-Sorbets. Archéologie et histoire romaine 26. Montagnac: Editions Monique Mergoil, pp. 95–112.

Pinhasi, R. and Bourbou, C. 2008. 'How representative are human skeletal assemblages for population analysis?', in *Advances in Human Palaeopathology*, ed. R. Pinhasi, S. Mays and S. Chichester: John Wiley & Sons Ltd, pp. 31–44.

Pisarikova, B., Zraly, Z., Bunka, F. and Trckova, M. 2008. 'Nutritional value of white lupine cultivar Butan in diets for fattening pigs', *Veterinarni Medicina* 53(3), pp. 123–134.

Pitts, M. 2015. 'The archaeology of food consumption', in *A Companion to Food in the Ancient World*, ed. J. Wilkins and R. Nadeau. Oxford: Wiley-Blackwell, pp. 95–104.

Pleket, H.W. 1990. 'Die Landwirtschaft in der römischen Kaiserzeit', in *Europäische Wirtschafts- und Sozialgeschichte in der Römischen Kaiserzeit*, ed. F. Wittinghoff. Stuttgart: Klett-Cotta.

Pleket, H.W. 1993. 'Agriculture in the Roman Empire in comparative perspective', in *De Agricultura. In Memoriam Pieter Willem de Neeve (1945–1990)*, ed. H. Sancisi-Weerdenburg. Amsterdam: J.C. Gieben, pp. 214–237.

Pollard, A.M., Ditchfield, P., McCullagh, J.S.O., et al. 2011. '"These boots were made for walking": the isotopic analysis of a C_4 Roman inhumation from Gravesend, Kent, UK', *American Journal of Physical Anthropology* 146, pp. 446–456.

Pollini, J. 2003. 'Slave boys for sexual and religious service: images of pleasure and devotion', in *Flavian Rome: Culture, Image, Text*, ed. A.J. Boyle and W.J. Dominik. Leiden: Brill, pp. 149–166.

Pontrandolfo, A., ed. 2002. *Pittura parietale in Macedonia e Magna Grecia:atti del Convegno internazionale di studi in ricordo di Mario Napoli, Salerno-Paestum, 21–23 novembre 1996*. Salerno: Pandemos.

Popper, V.S. 1988. 'Selecting quantitative measurements in paleoethnobotany', in *Current Paleoethnobotany: Analytical Methods and Cultural Interpretations of Archaeological Plant Remains*, ed. C.A. Hastorf and V.S. Popper. Chicago and London: University of Chicago Press, pp. 53–71.

Pösche, H. 2010. 'Der letzte Broiler – Hühnchen in römischen Gräbern', in *Grenzenlose Gaumenfreuden. Römische Küche in einer germanischen Provinz*, ed. J. Meurers-Balke and T. Kaszab-Olschewski. Mainz: Verlag Philipp von Zabern, pp. 115–116.

Potter, D.S. and Mattingly, D.J. 1999. *Life, Death, and Entertainment in the Roman Empire*. Ann Arbor: University of Michigan Press.

Pounds, N.J.G. 1969. 'The urbanization of the classical world', *Annals of the Association of American Geographers* 59, pp. 135–157.

Poupin, N., Bos, C., Mariotti, F., Huneau, J.F., Tome, D. and Fouillet, H. 2011. 'The nature of the dietary protein impacts the tissue-to-diet 15N discrimination factors in laboratory rats', *PloS One* 6(11), e28046.

Poupin, N., Mariotti, F., Huneau, J.F., Hermier, D. and Fouillet, H. 2014. 'Natural isotopic signatures of variations in body nitrogen fluxes: a compartmental model analysis', *PLoS Computational Biology* 10(10), e1003865.

Powell, L.A., et al. 2014. 'Infant feeding practices in Roman London: evidence from isotopic analyses', in *Infant Health and Death in Roman Italy and beyond*, ed. M. Carroll and E.-J.Graham. Portsmouth, RI: Journal of Roman Archaeology (Supplementary volume 96), pp. 89–110.

Preedy, V.R. and Watson, R.R. 2010. *Olives and Olive Oil in Health and Disease Prevention*. Amsterdam: Academic Press.

Prell, M. 1997. Sozialökonomische Untersuchungen zur Armut in Antiken Rom: Von den Gracchen bis Kaiser Diokletian. Stuttgart: Franz Steiner Verlag.

Preston, B. 2000. 'The functions of things: a philosophical perspective on material culture', in *Matter, Materiality and Modern Culture*, ed. P Graves-Brown. New York: Routledge, pp. 22–49.

Principal, J. 2006. 'Late Hellenistic black-gloss wares in the north-eastern Iberian Peninsula: production traditions and social practices', in *Old Pottery in a New Century: Innovating Perspectives on Roman Pottery Studies*, ed. D. Malfitana, J. Poblome, and J. Lund. Catania: Ibam, pp. 41–55.

Prominska, E. 1981. 'La stature des habitants de l'oasis de Dakhleh sous la XXVIe dynastie et à l'époque ptolémaique', *Bulletins et Mémoires de la Société d'anthropologie de Paris*, XIIIe S., 8, pp. 275–280.

Provost, M. 1993. *Le Val de Loire dans l'Antiquité*. Paris: CNRS éditions.

Prowse, T. 2001. *Isotopic and Dental Evidence for Diet from the Necropolis of Isola Sacra (1st–3rd Centuries AD), Italy*. PhD dissertation. McMaster University.

Prowse, T. 2011. 'Diet and dental health through the life course in Roman Italy', in *Social Bioarchaeology*, ed. S. Agarwal and B. Glencross. Oxford: Wiley-Blackwell, pp. 410–437.

Prowse, T.L., et al. 2004. 'Isotopic paleodiet studies of skeletons from the Imperial Roman-age cemetery of Isola Sacra, Rome, Italy', *Journal of Archaeological Science* 31, 259–272.

Prowse, T., Schwarcz, H. P., Saunders, S., Macchiarelli, R. and Bondioli, L. 2005. 'Isotopic evidence for age-related variation in diet from Isola Sacra, Italy', *American Journal of Physical Anthropology* 128, pp. 2–13.

Prowse, T.L., et al. 2007. 'Isotopic evidence for age-related immigration to imperial Rome', *American Journal of Physical Anthropology* 132, pp. 510–519.

Prowse, T., Saunders, S., Schwarcz, H., Garnsey, P., Macchiarelli, R., and Bondioli, L. 2008. 'Isotopic and dental evidence for infant and young child feeding practices in an imperial Roman skeletal sample', *American Journal of Physical Anthropology* 137, pp. 294–308.

Prowse, T., Barta, J., von Hunnius, T. and Small, A. 2010. 'Stable isotope and mtDNA evidence for geographic origins at Vagnari', in *Roman Diasporas: Archaeological Approaches to Mobility and Diversity in the Roman Empire*, ed. H. Eckardt. Journal of Roman Archaeology Supplement 78, pp. 175–197.

Pucci, G. 2001. 'Inscribed *instrumentum* and the ancient economy', in *Epigraphic Evidence: Ancient History from Inscriptions*, ed. J. Bodel. London: Routledge, pp. 137–152.

Pugliese Carratelli, G., ed. 1998. *Pompei: pitture e mosaici*. Roma: Istituto della Enciclopedia Italiana.

Pugsley, P. 2003. *Roman Domestic Wood*. Oxford: British Archaeological Reports.

Purcell, N. 1985. 'Wine and wealth in ancient Italy', *Journal of Roman Studies* 75, pp. 1–19.

Purcell, N. 2003. 'The way we used to eat', *American Journal of Philology* 124(3), pp. 329–358.

Raboy, V. 2000. 'Low-phytic-acid grains', *Food and Nutrition Bulletin* 21(4), pp. 423–427.

Raeymaekers, J. 2000. 'The grain hoarders of Aspendus: Philostratus on the intervention of Appollonius of Tyana (Vita Apollonii 1.15)', in *Politics, Administration, and Society in the Hellenistic and Roman World*, ed. L. Mooren. Leuven: Peeters, pp. 275–286.

Raga. E. 2009. 'Bon mangeur, mauvais mangeur. Pratiques alimentaires et critique sociale dans l'œuvre de Sidoine Apollinaire et de ses contemporains', *Revue Belge de Philologie et d'Histoire* 87(2), pp. 165–196.

Raga, E. 2016. 'Interdire la viande à la table monastique entre Antiquité tardive et haut Moyen âge en Occident. Un bricolage normatif autour de la problématique du plaisir', in *Religions et interdits alimentaires. Archéozoologie et Sources littéraires*, ed. B. Caseau and H. Monchot. Paris: PUPS.

Randic, M. 2001. 'Nutrition on the Adriatic islands: an ethnological view on nutrition of the Croatian Adriatic island population', *Sociologija sela* 39, pp. 319–341.

Rapp, C. 2013. *Holy Bishops in Late Antiquity: The Question of the Nature of Christian Leadership in an Age of Transition*, Berkley: University of California Press.

Rathbone, D. 1991. *Economic Rationalism and Rural Society in Third-Century Egypt: The Heroninos Archive and the Appianus Estate*. Cambridge: Cambridge University Press.

Rathbone, D. 2009. 'Earnings and costs: living standards and the Roman economy (first to third centuries AD)', in *Quantifying the Roman Economy. Methods and Problems, Oxford Studies on the Roman Economy*, ed. A. Bowman and A. Wilson. Oxford: Oxford University Press, pp. 299–326.

Rawson, B. 1986. *The Family in Ancient Rome: New Perspectives*. Ithaca, NY: Cornell University Press.

Rawson, B., ed. 1991. *Marriage, Divorce, and Children in Ancient Rome*. Oxford: Clarendon Press.

Rawson, B. 2003. *Children and Childhood in Roman Italy*. Oxford: Oxford University Press.

Rawson, B. 2010. 'Family and society', in *The Oxford Handbook of Roman Studies*, ed. A. Barchiesi and W. Scheidel. Oxford: Oxford University Press, pp. 610–623.

Rawson, B. and Weaver, P. 1999. *The Roman Family in Italy: Status, Sentiment, Space*. Oxford: Clarendon Press.

Raxter, M.H., et al. 2008. 'Stature estimation in ancient Egyptians: a new technique based on anatomical econstruction of atature', *American Journal of Physical Anthropology* 136, pp. 147–155.

Rea, J.R. 1972. *The Oxyrhynchus Papyri, Volume XL*. London: Egypt Exploration Society.

Reddé, M. 2016. 'Some critical thinking about large and small rural settlements in north-eastern Roman Gaul', in *Méthodes d'Analyse des Différentes Paysages ruraux dans le Nord-est de la Gaule romaine: Études comparées (Hiérarchisation des Exploitations; potentialités agronomiques des Sols; Systèmes de Production; Systèmes sociaux)*, ed. M. Reddé. Paris: École pratique des Hautes Études, pp. 7–40.

Redfern, R.C., Hamlin, C. and Athfield, N.B. 2010. 'Temporal changes in diet: a stable isotope analysis of Late Iron Age and Roman Dorset, Britain', *Journal of Archaeological Science* 37, pp. 1140–1160.

Redfern, R.C., et al. 2015. 'Urban-rural differences in Roman Dorset, England: a bioarchaeological perspective on Roman settlements', *American Journal of Physical Anthropology* 157, pp. 107–120.

Reekmans, T. 1996. *La Consommation dans les Archives de Zénon*. Papyrologica Bruxellensia 27. Brussels: Fondation égyptologique reine Elisabeth.

Reichmann, C. 2014. *Römer und Franken am Niederrhein*. Mainz: Nünnerich-Asmus Verlag.

Reiter, F. 2004. *Die Nomarchen des Arsinoites. Ein Beitrag zur Steuerwesen im römischen Ägypten*. Papyrologica Coloniensia 31. Cologne: Verlag Ferdinand Schöningh.

Reitsema, L.J. 2013. 'Beyond diet reconstruction: stable isotope applications to human physiology, health, and nutrition', *American Journal of Human Biology* 25, pp. 445–456.

Rejano, L., Montaño, A., Casado, F.J., Sánchez, A.H. and de Castro, A. 2010. 'Table olives: varieties and variations', in *Olives and Olive Oil in Health and Disease Prevention*, ed. V.R. Preedy and R.R.Watson. Amsterdam: Academic Press, pp. 5–15.

Remesal Rodríguez, J. 1986. *La Annona Militaris y el Commercio de aceite bético a Germania*. Madrid: Editorial de la Universidad Complutense.

Remesal Rodríguez, J. 2002. 'Baetica and Germania. Notes on concept of "provincial interdependence" in the Roman Empire'. In *The Roman Army and the Economy*, ed. P. Erdkamp. Amsterdam, pp. 293–308.

Renfrew, J.M. 1973. *Palaeoethnobotany. Prehistoric Food Plants of the Near East and Europe*. London: Methuen.

Renfrew, J.M. 2004. *Roman Cookery: Recipes and History*. London: English Heritage.

Reuter, M. 2005. 'Weinbau im römischen Südwestdeutschland? Von Genießern und Trunkenbolden', in *Imperium Romanum. Roms Provinzen an Neckar, Rhein und Donau*, ed. Archäologisches Landesmuseum Baden-Württemberg. Darmstadt: Wissenschaftliche Buchgesellschaft, pp. 301–305.

Ricci, R., Mancinelli, D., Vargiu, R., Cucina, A., Santandrea, E., Capelli, A., and Catalano, P. 1997. 'Pattern of porotic hyperostosis and quality of life in a II century AD farm near Rome', *Rivista di Antropologia* 75, 117–128.

Richard, J. 2012. *Water for the City, Fountains for the People: Monumental Fountains in the Roman East: An Archaeological Study of Water Management*. Turnhout, Brepols.

Richards, M.P., Hedges, R.E.M., Molleson, T.I. and Vogel, J.C. 1998. 'Stable isotope analysis reveals variations in human diet at the Poundbury Camp cemetery site', *Journal of Archaeological Science* 25, pp. 1247–1252.

Richardson, J., Thompson, G. and Genovese, A. 1997. 'New directions in economic and environmental research at Pompeii', in *Sequence and Space in Pompeii*, ed. S.E. Bon and R. Jones. Oxford: Oxbow, pp. 88–101.

Richardson-Hay, C. 2009. 'Dinner at Seneca's table: the philosophy of food', *Greece & Rome* 56, pp. 71–96.

Rickman, G. 1980a. *The Corn Supply of Rome*. Oxford: Clarendon Press.

Rickman, G. 1980b. 'The grain trade under the Roman Empire', in *The Seaborne Trade of Ancient Rome: Studies in Archaeology and History*, ed. J.H. D'Arms, and E.C. Kopff. Rome: American Academy in Rome, pp. 261–275.

Rinkewitz, W. 1984. *Pastio Villatica. Untersuchungen zur intensiven Tierhaltung in der römischen Landwirtschaft*. Frankfurt: P. Lang.

Ritter, St. 2002/2003. 'Zur Bildsprache römischer Alltagsszenen: Die Mahl- und Küchenreliefs am Pfeilergrabmal von Igel', *Bonner Jahrbücher* 202/203, pp. 149–170.

Riz, A.E. 1990. *Bronzegefässe in der römisch-pompeianischen Wandmalerei*. Mainz am Rhein: Philipp von Zabern.

Rizzello, C.J., Calasso, M., Campanella, D., De Angelis, M. and Gobbetti, M. 2014. 'Use of sourdough fermentation and mixture of wheat, chickpea, lentil and bean flours for enhancing the nutritional, texture and sensory characteristics of white bread', *International Journal of Food Microbiology* 180, pp. 78–87.

Roberts, C.A., 2013. 'The bioarchaeology of health and well-being: its contribution to understanding the past', in *The Oxford Handbook of the Archaeology of Death*, ed. S. Tarlow and L. Nilsson Stutz. Oxford: Oxford University Press, pp. 79–98.

Roberts, C.A. and Cox, M. 2003. *Health and Disease in Britain: From Prehistory to the Present Day*. Phoenix Mill: Sutton Publishing.

Robinson, M. 2002. 'Domestic burnt offerings and sacrifices at Roman and pre-Roman Pompeii, Italy', *Vegetation History and Archaeobotany* 11, pp. 93–99.

Robinson, M. and Rowan, E. 2015. 'Roman food remains in archaeology and the contents of a Roman sewer at Herculaneum', in *A Companion to Food in the Ancient World*, ed. J. Wilkins and R. Nadeau. Oxford: Wiley-Blackwell, pp. 105–115.

Robinson, O.F. 1992. *Ancient Rome: City Planning and Administration*. London: Routledge.

Rodríguez, J.R. 1998. 'Baetical olive oil and the Roman economy', in *The Archaeology of early Roman Baetica*, ed. S. Keay. Portsmouth: Journal of Roman Archaeology, 183–199.

Rodriguez-Almeida, E. 1972. 'Novedades de epigrafia anforaria del Monte Testaccio', *Publications de l'École française de Rome* 10(1), pp. 107–241.

Rösch, M. 2014. 'Direkte archäologische Belege für alkoholische Getränke von der vorrömischen Eisenzeit bis ins Mittelalter', in *Küche und Keller in Antike und Früh mittelalter*, ed. J. Drauschke, R. Prien and A. Reis. SAFM 6. Hamburg: Verlag Dr. Kovač, pp. 306–326.

Roller, N. 2003. 'Horizontal women: posture and sex in the Roman *convivium*', *The American Journal of Philology* 124(3), Special Issue, Roman Dining, pp. 377–422.

Roller, M. 2006. *Dining Posture in Ancient Rome: Bodies, Values, and Status.* Princeton: Princeton University Press.

Rollet, C. 2001. *Les enfants au XIXe siècle.* Paris: Hachette.

Romeri, L. 2002. *Philosophes entre mots et mets. Plutarque, Lucien et Athénée autour de la table de Platon.* Grenoble: Éditions Jérôme Million.

Ros, J., Evin A., Bouny, L. and Ruas, M-P. 2014. 'Geometric morphometric analysis of grain shape and the identification of two-rowed barley (*Hordeum vulgare* subsp. *distichum* L.) in southern France', *Journal of Archaeological Science* 41, pp. 568–575.

Rosenblum, J.D. 2010. *Food and Identity in Early Rabbinic Judaism.* Cambridge: Cambridge University Press.

Rosenfeld, B.-Z. and Menirav, J. 2005. *Markets and Marketing in Roman Palestine.* Leiden: Brill.

Rossiter, J.J. 1981. 'Wine and oil processing at Roman farms in Italy', *Phoenix* 35(4), 345–361.

Roth, J. 1999. *The Logistics of the Roman Army at War (264 BC–AD 235).* Leiden: Brill.

Rothenhöfer, P. 2005. *Die Wirtschaftsstrukturen im südlichen Niedergermanien. Untersuchungen zur Entwicklung eines Wirtschaftsraumes an der Peripherie des Imperium Romanum.* Kölner Studien zur Archäologie der Römischen Provinzen 7. Rahden/Westf: Verlag Marie Leidorf.

Rousselle, A. 1974. 'Abstinence et continence dans les monastères de Gaule méridionale à la fin de l'Antiquité et au début du Moyen Age. Étude d'un régime alimentaire et de sa fonction', in *Hommage à André Dupont*, Montpellier, pp. 239–254.

Rovira, N. and Chabal, L. 2008. 'A foundation offering at the Roman port of Lattara (Lattes, France): the plant remains', *Vegetation History and Archaeobotany* 17, pp. 191–200.

Rowan, E. 2014a. 'The fish remains from the Cardo V sewer: New insights into consumption and the fishing economy of Herculaneum', in *Fish and Ships. Production et commerce des* salsamenta *durant l'Antiquité*, ed. E. Botte and V. Leitch. Bibliothèque d'Archéologie Méditerranéenne et Africaine 17. Arles and Aix-en-Provence: Errance and Centre Camille Jullian, pp. 61–73.

Rowan, E. 2014b. *Roman Diet and Nutrition in the Vesuvian Region: A Study of the Bioarchaeological Remains from the Cardo V Sewer at Herculaneum.* Unpublished PhD thesis. University of Oxford.

Rowan, E. 2015. 'Olive oil pressing waste as a fuel source in antiquity', *AJA* 119(4), pp. 465–482.

Roy, J. 2007. 'The consumption of dog-meat in Classical Greece', in *Cooking up the Past: Food and Culinary Practices in the Neolithic and Bronze Age Aegean*, ed. C. Mee and J. Renard, Oxford: Oxbow, 342–353.

Ruffing, K. 1997. '. . . qui emere vina et vendere solet . . . Zum Berufsbild des Weinhändlers nebst einigen Bemerkungen zur Terminologie', in *Miscellanea oeconomica. Festschrift für Harald Winkel zum 65. Geburtstag*, ed. K. Ruffing and B. Tenger. St. Katharinen: Scripta Mercaturae Verlag, pp. 116–134.

Ruffing, K. 1998. 'Herstellung, Sorten, Qualitätsbezeichnungen von Wein im römischen Ägypten', *Münstersche Beiträge zur Antiken Handelsgeschichte* 17, pp. 11–31.

Ruffing, K. 2001. 'Einige Überlegungen zum Weinhandel im römischen Ägypten (1.-3. Jh. n. Chr.)', *Münstersche Beiträge zur Antiken Handelsgeschichte* 20(1), pp. 55–80.

Rutgers, L., van Strydonck, M., Boudin, M. and van der Linde, C. 2009. 'Stable isotope data from the early Christian catacombs of ancient Rome: new insights into the dietary habits of Rome's early Christians', *Journal of Archaeological Science* 36, pp. 1127–1134.

Sadeghi, G H., Pourreza, J., Samci, A., and H. Rahmani. 2009a. 'Chemical composition and some anti-nutrient content of raw and processed bitter vetch (*Vicia ervilia*) seed for use as feeding stuff in poultry diet', *Tropical Animal Health and Production* 41, pp. 85–93.

Sadeghi, G.H., Mohammadi, L., Ibrahim, S.A., and Gruber, K.J. 2009b. 'Use of bitter vetch (*Vicia ervillia*) as a feed ingredient for poultry', *World's Poultry Science Journal* 65(1), pp. 51–64.

Sadori, L., et al. 2009. 'The introduction and diffusion of the peach in ancient Italy', in *Plants and Culture: Seeds of the Cultural Heritage of Europe*, ed. J.-P. Morel. Bari: Edipuglia, pp. 45–61.

Sadori, L., Allevato, E., Bellini, C., et al. 2015. 'Archaeobotany in Italian ancient Roman harbours', *Review of Palaeobotany and Palynology* 218, pp. 217–230.

Sallares R. 1991. *The Ecology of the Ancient Greek World.* Ithaca: Cornell University Press.

Sallares, R. 1995. 'Molecular archaeology and ancient history', in J. Wilkins, D. Harvey and M. Dobson, eds. *Food in Antiquity.* Exeter: University of Exeter Press, pp. 87–100.

Sallares, R. 2002. *Malaria and Rome: A History of Malaria in Ancient Italy.* Oxford: Oxford University Press.

Saller, R. 2003. 'Women, slaves and the economy of the Roman household', in *Early Christian Families in Context. An Interdisciplinary Dialogue*, ed. D. Balch and C. Osiek. Michigan: Eerdmans, pp. 185–206.

Saller, R. 2012. 'Human capital and growth', in *The Cambridge Companion to the Roman Economy*, ed. W. Scheidel. Cambridge: Cambridge University Press, pp. 71–86.

Salvadei, L., Ricci, F. and Manzi, G. 2001. 'Porotic hyperostosis as a marker of health and nutritional conditions during childhood: studies at the transition between Imperial Rome and the early Middle Ages', *American Journal of Human Biology* 13, 709–717.

Salza Prina Ricotta, E. 1983. *L'Arte del Convito nella Roma antica. Con 90 ricette*. Rome: 'L'Erma' di Bretschneider.

Sandy, D.B. 1989. *The Production and Use of Vegetable Oils in Ptolemaic Egypt*. BASP Supplement 6. Atlanta: Scholars Press.

Sarpaki, A. and Jones, G. 1990. 'Ancient and modern cultivation of *Lathyrus clymenum* L. in the Greek islands', *The Annual of the British School at Athens* 85, pp. 363–368.

Sassi, A.B., Boularbah, A., Jaouad, A., Walker, G. and Boussaid, A. 2006. 'A comparison of the Olive oil Mill Wastewaters (OMW) from three different processes in Morocco', *Process Biochemistry* 41, pp. 74–78.

Schachner, A. 1999. *Von der Rundhütte zum Kaufmannshaus: kulturhistorische Untersuchungen zur Entwicklung prähistorischer Wohnhäuser in Zentral-Ost und Südostanatolien*. Oxford: Archaeopress.

Schallmayer, E. 2010. *Der Odenwaldlimes – entlang der römischen Grenze zwischen Main –und Neckar*. Stuttgart: Konrad Theiss Verlag.

Schamuhn, S. 2010. 'Brot für die Toten', in *Grenzenlose Gaumenfreuden. Römische Küche in einer germanischen Provinz*, ed. J. Meurers-Balke and T. Kaszab-Olschewski. Mainz: Verlag Philipp von Zabern, p. 60.

Schamuhn, S. and Zerl, T. 2009. 'Zur Landwirtschaft der Kelten und Germanen im Gebiet von Nordrhein-Westfalen', in *Kelten am Rhein. Akten des dreizehnten Internationalen Keltologiekongresses 1. Archäologie. Ethnizität und Romanisierung*. Beihefte der Bonner Jahrbücher 58. Mainz: Verlag Philipp von Zabern, pp. 239 –250.

Schatzmann, R. 2013. *Die Spätzeit der Oberstadt von Augusta Raurica. Untersuchungen zur Stadtentwicklung im 3. Jahrhundert*. Forschungen in Augst 48. Augst: Schwabe Verlag.

Scheffer, C. 1981. *Cooking and Cooking Stands in Italy, 1400–400 BC*. Skrifter utgivna av Svenska Institutet i Rom. 4°= Acta Instituti romani regni Sueciae. Series in 4°. Stockholm.

Scheid, J. 1990. *Romulus et ses Frères. Le Collège des Frères arvales, Modèle du Culte public dans la Rome des Empereurs*. Rome: École française de Rome.

Scheid, J. 2005. *Quand faire, c'est croire: les rites sacrificiels des Romains*. Paris: Aubier.

Scheid, J. 2007. 'Le statut de la viande à Rome', *Food and History* 5, pp. 19–28.

Scheid, J. 2012. 'Roman animal sacrifice and the system of being', in *Greek and Roman Animal Sacrifice: Ancient Victims, Modern Observers*, ed. C. Faraone and F.S. Naiden. Cambridge: Cambridge University Press, pp. 84–95.

Scheidel, W. 1995. 'The most silent women of Greece and Rome: Rural labour and women's life in the ancient world', *Greece and Rome* 42(2), pp. 202–217.

Scheidel, W. 2003. 'Germs for Rome', in *Rome the Cosmopolis*, ed. C. Edwards and G. Woolf. Cambridge: Cambridge University Press, pp. 158–176.

Scheidel, W. 2006. 'Stratification, deprivation and quality of life', in *Poverty in the Ancient World*, ed. M. Atkins and R. Osborne. Cambridge: Cambridge University Press, pp. 40–59.

Scheidel, W. 2007. 'Roman population size: the logic of the debate', *Princeton/Stanford Working Papers in Classics*. Available from www.princeton.edu/~pswpc/pdfs/scheidel/070706.pdf (accessed 17 April 2016).

Scheidel, W. 2009. 'In search of Roman economic growth', *Journal of Roman Archaeology* 22, pp. 46–70.

Scheidel, W. 2010. 'Real wages in early economies: evidence for living standards from 1800 BCE to 1300 CE', *Journal of the Economic and Social History of the Orient* 53(3), pp. 425–462.

Scheidel, W. 2012a. 'Roman well-being and the economic consequences of the Antonine plague', in *L'impatto della 'peste antonina'*, ed. E. Lo Cascio. Bari: Edipuglia, pp. 265–295.

Scheidel, W. 2012b. 'Physical wellbeing', in *Cambridge Companion to the Roman Economy*, ed. W. Scheidel. Cambridge: Cambridge University Press, pp. 321–333.

Scheidel, W. 2013. 'Disease and death', in *The Companion to Ancient Rome*, ed. P. Erdkamp. Cambridge: Cambridge University Press, pp. 45–59.

Scheidel, W. 2014. 'Roman real wages in context', in *Quantifying the Greco-Roman Economy and Beyond*, ed. F. de Callataÿ. Bari: Edipuglia, pp. 209–218.

Scheidel, W. and Friesen, S.J. 2009. 'The size of the economy and the distribution of income in the Roman Empire', *Journal of Roman Studies* 99, pp. 61–91.

Schepartz, L.A., Fox, S.C. and Bourbou, C., eds. 2009. *New Directions in the Skeletal Biology of Greece*. Athens: American School of Classical Studies at Athens.

Schibler, J. and Furger, A.R. 1988. *Die Tierknochenfunde aus Augusta Raurica (Grabungen 1955-1974)*. Augst: Amt für Museen und Archäologie des Kantons Basel-Landschaft.

Schiffer, M.B. 1992. *Technological Perspectives on Behavioral Change*. Tuscon: University of Arizona Press.

Schimmer, F. 2009. *Amphoren aus Cambodunum/Kempten. Ein Beitrag zur Handelsgeschichte der römischen Provinz Raetia*. Münchner Beiträge zur Provinzialrömischen Archäologie 1. Wiesbaden: Reichert Verlag.

Schmid, E. 1972. *Atlas of Animal Bones*. Amsterdam: Elsevier.

Schmitt-Pantel, P. 1992. *La Cité au Banquet: Histoire des Repas publics dans les Cités grecques*. Rome: Publications de l'Ecole Française de Rome.

Schmölder-Veit, A. 2009. *Brunnen in den Städten des westlichen Römischen Reichs*. Wiesbaden: Reichert Verlag.

Schnebel, M. 1925. *Die Landwirtschaft im hellenistischen Aegypten*. Münchener Beiträge 7. München: C.H.Beck'sche Verlagsbuchhandlung.

Schoeninger, M.J. and DeNiro, M.J. 1984. 'Nitrogen and carbon isotopic composition of bone collagen from marine and terrestrial animals', *Geochimica et Cosmochimica Acta* 48, pp. 625–639.

Schoeninger, M., DeNiro, M. and Tauber, H. 1983. 'Stable nitrogen isotope ratios of bone collagen reflect marine and terrestrial components of prehistoric human diet', *Science* 220, pp. 1381–1383.

Schofield, P.R. 2006. 'Medieval diet and demography', in *Food in Medieval England: Diet and Nutrition*, ed. M. Woolgar, D. Serjeantson and T. Waldron. Oxford: Oxford University Press, pp. 239–253.

Scholz, M. and C. Pause, 2010. 'Mit Dionysos zu Tisch: eine Gebäckform aus Neuss', in *Grenzenlose Gaumenfreuden. Römische Küche in einer germanischen Provinz*, ed. J. Meurers-Balke and T. Kaszab-Olschewski. Mainz: Verlag Philipp von Zabern, p. 47.

Schultz, M. 2001. 'Paleohistopathology of bone: a new approach to the study of ancient diseases', *Yearbook of Physical Anthropology* 44, pp. 106–147.

Schwarcz, H.P. and Schoeninger, M.J. 1991. 'Stable isotope analyses in human nutrition and ecology', *Yearbook of Physical Anthropology* 34, pp. 282–321.

Schwartz, S. 2001. *Imperialism and Jewish Society, 200 BCE to 640 CE*. Princeton, NJ, and Oxford: Princeton University Press.

Scobie, A. 1986. 'Slums, sanitation, and mortality in the Roman world', *Klio* 68, pp. 399–433.

Scorrano, G., Brilli, M., Martínez-Labarga, C., et al. 2014. 'Palaeodiet reconstruction in a woman with probable celiac disease: a stable isotope analysis of bone remains from the archaeological site of Cosa (Italy)', *American Journal of Physical Anthropology* 154, pp. 349–356.

Sealy, J., 2001. 'Body tissue chemistry and palaeodiet', in *Handbook of Archaeological Sciences*, ed. D.R. Brothwell and A.M. Pollard. Chichester: John Wiley and Sons Ltd, pp. 269–279.

Seetah, K. 2006. 'Multidisciplinary approach to Romano-British cattle butchery', in *Integrating Zooarchaeology*, ed. M. Maltby. Oxford: Oxbow, pp. 109–116.

Segan, F. 2004. *The Philosopher's Kitchen: Recipes from Ancient Greece and Rome for the Modern Cook*. New York: Random House.

Sella, D. 1991. 'Coping with famine: the changing demography of an Italian village in the 1590's', *Sixteenth Century Journal* 22, pp. 185–197.

Sen, A. 1981. *Poverty and Famines: An Essay on Entitlement and Deprivation*. Oxford: Clarendon Press.

Sen, A. 1990. 'More than 100 Million Women Are Missing', *The New York Review of Books*, December 20, 1990.

Shanzer, D. 2001. 'Bishops, letters, fast, food and feast in later Roman Gaul', in *Society and Culture in Late Roman Gaul: Revisiting the Sources*, ed. R.W. Mathisen and D. Shanzer. Liverpool: Liverpool University Press, pp. 217–236.

Sharp, M. 2007. '17. The food supply', in *Oxyrhynchus: A City and its Texts*, ed. A.K. Bowman. Oxford: Oxford University Press, pp. 218–230.

Shaw, B. 1982–1983. '"Eaters of flesh; drinkers of milk": the ancient Mediterranean ideology of the pastoral nomad', *Ancient Society* 13–14, pp. 5–31.

Shaw, T.M. 1998. *The Burden of the Flesh. Fasting and Sexuality in Early Christianity*, Minneapolis: Fortress Press.

Shelton, J. 1998. *As the Romans Did: A Sourcebook in Roman Social History*. Oxford: Oxford University Press.

Shelton, J. 2015. 'Creating a malaria test for ancient human remains', *Yale News*. http://news.yale.edu/2015/03/17/creating-malaria-test-ancient-human-remains (accessed 9 July 2015).

Shen, J., Wilmot, K., Ghasemzadeh, N., et al. 2015. 'Mediterranean dietary patterns and cardiovascular health', *Annual Review of Nutrition* 35.

Shewry, P.R. 2009. 'Darwin review wheat', *Journal of Experimental Botany*, pp. 1537–1553.

Shewry, P.R., Halford, N.G., Belton, P.S., and Tatham, A.S. 2002. 'The structure and properties of gluten: an elastic protein from wheat grain', *Philosophical Transaction of the Royal Society London: Biological Sciences* 357, pp. 133–142.

Shillito, L.M. and Almond, M.J. 2010. 'Comment on: Fruit and seed biomineralization and its effect on preservation by E. Messager et al.; in Archaeological and Anthropological Sciences 2:25–34', *Archaeological and Anthropological Sciences* 2, pp. 225–229.

Sidebotham S.E. 2011. *Berenike and the Ancient Maritime Spice Route*, Berkeley, CA: University of California Press.

Sigismund Nielsen, H. 1998. 'Roman children at mealtimes', in *Meals in a Social Context: Aspects of the Communal Meal in the Hellenistic and Roman World*, ed. I. Nielsen and H. Sigismund Nielsen. Aarhus: Aarhus University Press, pp. 56–67.

Sijpesteijn, P.J. 1987. *Customs Duties in Graeco-Roman Egypt, Studia Amstelodamensia ad epigraphicam, ius antiquum et papyrologicam pertinentia*. Amsterdam: Gieben.

Simons, A. 1989. *Bronze- und eisenzeitliche Besiedlung in den rheinischen Lößbörden. Archäologische Siedlungsmuster im Braunkohlengebiet*. BAR Internat. Ser. 467. Oxford: Archaeopress.

Sippel, D.V. 1989. 'Dietary deficiency among the lower classes of the Late Republican and Early Imperial Rome', *The Ancient World* 16, pp. 47–54.

Sirks, B. 1991. *Food for Rome*. Amsterdam: J.C. Gieben.

Sirks, B. 2007. 'Supplying Rome: safeguarding the system', in *Supplying Rome and the Empire*, ed. E. Papi. Portsmouth, RI: Journal of Roman Archaeology, pp. 173–178.

Slater, W., ed. 1991. *Dining in a Classical Context*. Ann Arbor: University of Michigan Press.

Slater, W. 2000. 'Handouts at dinner', *Phoenix* 54, pp. 107–122.

Šlaus, M., Pećina-Šlaus, N. and Brikć, H. 2004. 'Life stress on the Roman limes in continental Croatia', *Homo* 54, pp. 240–263.

Šlaus, M., Bedić, Z., Šikanjić, P.R., Vodanović, M. and Kunić, D. 2011. 'Dental health at the transition from the Late Antique to the early medieval period on Croatia's eastern Adriatic coast', *International Journal of Osteoarchaeology* 21, pp. 577–590.

Small, D.B. 1995. 'Introduction', in *Methods in the Mediterranean: Historical and Archaeological Views on Texts and Archaeology*, ed. D.B. Small. Leiden: Brill, pp. 1–22.

Smith, B.N. and Epstein, S. 1971. 'Two categories of $^{13}C/^{12}C$ ratios of higher plants', *Plant Physiology* 47, pp. 380–384.

Smith, D.E. 2003. *From Symposium to Eucharist: The Banquet in the Early Christian World*. Minneapolis: Fortress Press.

Smith, D.E. 2015. 'Food and dining in early Christianity', in *A Companion to Food in the Ancient World*, ed. J. Wilkins and R. Nadeau. Oxford: Wiley-Blackwell, pp. 357–364.

Smith, D.E. and Taussig, H., eds. 2012. *Meals in the Early Christian World: Social Formation, Experimentation, and Conflict at the Table*. New York: Palgrave Macmillan.

Smith, J.M. 2005. *Europe after Rome: A New Cultural History 500–1000*. Oxford: Oxford University Press.

Solomon, J. 1995. 'The Apician sauce: Ius apicianum', in *Food in Antiquity*, ed. J. Wilkins et al. Exeter: Exeter University Press, pp. 115–131.

Sõukand, R., Pieroni, A., Biró, M., et al. 2015. 'An ethnobotanical perspective on traditional fermented plant foods and beverages in Eastern Europe', *Journal of Ethnopharmacology* 170, pp. 284–296.

Soyer, A.B. 1853. *The Pantropheon or, History of Food, and its Preparation, from the Earliest Ages of the World*. London: Simpkin, Marshall.

Spanier, E. 2010. *The Good Farmer in Ancient Rome: War, Agriculture and the Elite from the Republic to Early Empire*. Unpublished PhD Thesis. University of Washington.

Sparkes, B. 1962. 'The Greek kitchen', *The Journal of Hellenic Studies* 82, pp. 121–137.

Sparks, H.F.D., ed. 1984. *The Apocryphal Old Testament*. Oxford: Oxford University Press.

Sperber, D. 1977. 'Aspects of agrarian life in Roman Palestine I. Agricultural decline in Palestine during the later principate', *Aufstieg under Niedergang der römischen Welt* 2(8), pp. 397–443.

Sperduti, A. 1997. 'Life conditions of a Roman Imperial age population: occupational stress markers and working activities in Lucus Feroniae (Rome, 1st–2nd cent. AD)', *Human Evolution* 12, pp. 253–267.

Spigelman, M., Hoon Shin, D. and Kahila, Bar Gal, G. 2012. 'The promise, the problems and the future of DNA analysis in paleopathology studies, in *A Companion to Paleopathology*, ed. A.L. Grauer. Chichester: Wiley-Blackwell, pp. 133–151.

Spivey, N. 1997. *Etruscan Art*. London: Thames & Hudson.

Spurr, M., 1983. 'The cultivation of millet in Roman Italy', *Papers of the British School at Rome* LI, pp. 1–15.

Spurr, M.S. 1986. *Arable Cultivation in Roman Italy c. 200 BC–AD 100*. Journal of Roman Studies Monograph III. London: Society for the Promotion of Roman Studies.

Squire, M. 2009. *Image and text in Graeco-Roman Antiquity*. New York: Cambridge University Press.

Stallibrass, S. 2000. 'Dead dogs, dead horses: site formation processes at Ribchester Roman fort', in *Animal Bones, Human Societies*, ed. P. Rowley-Conwy. Oxford: Oxbow Books, pp. 158–165.

Stark, A.H. and Madar, Z. 2002. 'Olive oil as a functional food: epidemiology and nutritional approaches', *Nutrition Reviews* 60, pp. 170–176.

Stathakopoulos, D.C. 2004. *Famine and Pestilence in the Late Roman and Early Byzantine Empire: A Systematic Survey of Subsistence Crises and Epidemics*. Farnham: Ashgate.

Steckel, R.H. 1995. 'Stature and the standard of living', *Journal of Economic Literature* 33, pp. 1903–1940.

Steckel, R.H. 2009. 'Heights and human welfare: recent developments and new directions', *Explorations in Economic History* 46, pp. 1–23.

Steckel, R.H. and Rose, J.C., eds. 2002. *The Backbone of History: Health and Nutrition in the Western Hemisphere*. Cambridge: Cambridge University Press.

Steckel, R.H., Larsen, C.S., Sciulli, P.W. and Walker, P.L., eds. 2005. *Data Collection Codebook*. The Global History of Health Project. Available at http://global.sbs.ohio-state.edu (accessed 9 July 2015).

Stefani, G., ed. 2005. *Cibi e Sapori a Pompei e Dintorni: Antiquarium di Boscoreale, 3 Febbraio–28 Maggio 2005*. Cava de' Tirreni: Grafica Metelliana.

Stegl, M. and Baten, J. 2009. 'Tall and shrinking Muslims, short and growing Europeans: the long-run welfare development of the Middle East, 1850–1980', *Explorations in Economic History* 46(1), pp. 132–148.

Steingräber, S. 2006. *Abundance of Life: Etruscan Wall Painting*. Translated by R. Stockman. Los Angeles: J. Paul Getty Museum.

Steidl, B. 2008. *Welterbe Limes: Roms Grenze am Main*. Obernburg: Logo Verlag.

Stein, A.J. 2010. 'Global impacts of human mineral nutrition', in *Potassium Role and Benefits in Improving Nutrient Management for Food Production, Quality and Reduced Environmental Damages Proceedings of the IPI-OUAT-IPNI International Symposium (2009). Vol I.*, ed. M.S. Brar and S.S. Mukhopadhyay. Horgen/Norcross: IPI/IPNI.

Stein-Hölkeskamp, E. 2005. *Das romische Gastmahl. Eine Kulturgeschichte*. Munich: Beck.

Steiner, B.L., Antolín, F. and Jacomet, S. 2015. 'Testing of the consistency of the sieving (wash-over) process of waterlogged sediments by multiple operators', *Journal of Archaeological Science Reports* 2, pp. 310–320.

Steinhauer, G. 1994. 'Inscription agoranomique du Pirée', *Bulletin de Correspondance hellénique* 118, pp. 51–68.

Steinkraus, K.H. 1994. 'Nutritional significance of fermented foods', *Food Research International* 27, pp. 259–267.

Stephan, E. 2005. 'Haus- und Wildtiere. Haltung und Zucht in den Provinzen nördlich der Alpen,' in *Imperium Romanum. Roms Provinzen an Neckar, Rhein und Donau*, ed. Archäologisches Landesmuseum Baden-Württemberg. Darmstadt: Wissenschaftliche Buchgesellschaft, pp. 294–300.

Stern, M. 1976. *Greek and Latin Authors on Jews and Judaism*, Vol. 1. Jerusalem: The Israel Academy of Sciences and Humanities.

Stern, M. 1980. *Greek and Latin Authors on Jews and Judaism*, Vol. 2. Jerusalem: The Israel Academy of Sciences and Humanities.

Sternberg, M. 1998. 'Les Produits de la pêche et la modification des structures halieutiques en Gaule Narbonnaise du IIIe siècle av. J.-C. au Ier siècle ap. J.-C.: Les Données de Lattes (Hérault), Marseille (Bouches-du-Rhône) et Olbia-de-Provence (Var)', *Mélanges d'archéologie et d'histoire de l'Ecole Française de Rome* 110/111, pp. 81–109.

Stika, H.-P. 2005. 'Cultura. Acker-, Garten- und Obstbau', in *Imperium Romanum. Roms Provinzen an Neckar, Rhein und Donau*, ed. Archäologisches Landesmuseum Baden-Württemberg. Darmstadt: Wissenschaftliche Buchgesellschaft, pp. 290–293.

Stöger, H. 2011. 'The spatial organization of the movement economy: the analysis of Ostia's *Scholae*', in *Rome, Ostia, Pompeii: Movement and Space*, ed. R. Laurence and D. Newsome. Oxford: Oxford University Press, pp. 215–242.

Stokes, P. 2000. 'A cut above the rest? Officers and men at South Shields Roman fort', in *Animal Bones, Human Societies*, ed. P. Rowley-Conwy. Oxford: Oxbow Books, pp. 145–151.

Strank, K.J. and Meurers-Balke, J., eds. 2008. *Obst, Gemüse und Kräuter Karls des Grossen. ". . . dass man im Garten alle Kräuter habe . . .".* Mainz: Verlag Philipp von Zabern.

Strouhal, E. 1986. 'Anthropology of the late period cemetery in the tomb of King Horemheb at Saqqara (Egypt) (Preliminary Report)', *International Journal of Anthropology* 1, pp. 215–224.

Stuart, P. 2013. *Nehalennia van Domburg. Geschiedenis van de stenen Monumenten*. Utrecht: Uitgeverij Matrijs.

Stuart, P. and Bogaers, J.E. 1971. *Deae Nehalenniae. Gids bij de tentoonstelling*. Middelburg: Koninklijk Zeeuwsch Genootschap der Wetenschappen.

Süntar, İ.P., Akkol, E.K. and Baykal, T. 2010. 'Assessment of anti-inflammatory and antinociceptive activities of *Olea europaea* L.', *Journal of Medicinal Food* 13, pp. 352–356.

Super, J.C. 2002. 'Review essay: food and history', *Journal of Social History* 36(1), pp. 165–178.

Swift, E. 2014. 'Design, function and use-wear in spoons: reconstructing everyday Roman social practice', *Journal of Roman Archaeology* 27, pp. 203–237.

Szirmai, K. 1997. 'Aquincum', in *Out of Rome Augusta Raurica, Aquincum. Das Leben in zwei römischen Provinzstädten*, ed. K. Kob. Basel: Schwabe Verlag, p. 273.

Tacoma, L.E. 2008. 'Urbanisation and access to land in Roman Egypt', in *Feeding the Ancient Greek City*, ed. R. Alston and O. Van Nijf. Leuven: Peeters, pp. 85–108.

Tafuri, M.A., Craig, O.E. and Canci, A. 2009. 'Stable isotope evidence for the consumption of millet and other plants in Bronze Age Italy', *American Journal of Physical Anthropology* 139, pp. 146–153.

Tamburino, R., Guida, V., Pacifico, S., Rocco, M., Zarelli, A., Parente, A., and Di Maro, A. 2012. 'Nutritional values and radical scavenging capacities of grass pea (*Lathyrus sativus* L.) seeds in Valle Agricola district, Italy', *Australian Journal of Crop Science* 6(1), pp. 149–156.

Tamerl, I. 2010. *Das Holzfass in der römischen Antike*. Innsbruck: StudienVerlag.

Tamm, J. 2005. 'Argentum potorium and the Campanian wall-painter', *Babesch Annual Papers on Mediterranean Archaeology*, pp. 73–89.

Tassinari, S. 1993. *Il Vasellame Bronzeo Di Pompei*. Rome: 'L'Erma' di Bretschneider.

Tchernia, A. 1986. *Le Vin de l'Italie romaine: Essai d'Histoire économique d'après les Amphores*. Rome: École française de Rome.

Tchernia, A. 1987. 'Modèles économiques et commerce du vin à la fin de la République et au début de l'Empire', in *El Vi a l'antiguitat: Economia, Producció i Comerç al Mediterrani occidental. Badalona, 28 Nov. 1985*. Badalona: Museu de Badalona, pp. 327–336.

Tchernia, A. 2000. 'La vente du vin', in *Mercati permanenti e Mercati periodici nel Mondo romano. Atti degli Incontri capresi di storia dell'economia antica (Capri 13–15 ottobre 1997)*, ed. E. Lo Cascio. Bari, Edipuglia, pp. 199–209.

Tchernia, A. 2008. 'Le convivium romain et la distinction sociale', in *Pratiques et Discours Alimentaires en Méditerranée de l'Antiquité à la Renaissance*, ed. J. Leclant, A. Vauchez and M. Sartre. Paris: Belles Lettres, pp. 147–156.

Tengström, E. 1974. *Bread for the People: Studies in the Corn-Supply of Rome During the Late Empire*. Stockholm: Svenska institutet i Rom.

Terzi, G., Celik T.H. and Nisbet, C. 2008. 'Determination of nenzo [a] pyrene in Turkish döner kebab samples cooked with charcoal or gas fire', *Irish Journal of Agricultural and Food Research* 47, pp. 187–193.

Thanheiser, U., Walter, J., and Hope, C.A. 2002. 'Roman agriculture and gardening in Egypt as seen from Kellis', in *Dakhleh Oasis Project: Monograph n. Preliminary reports on the 1994–1995 to 1998–1999 Field Seasons*, ed. C.A. Hope and G.E. Bowen. Oxford: Oxbow Books, pp. 299–307.

Thanheiser, U. and Heiss, A.G. 2014. 'Die pflanzliche Ernährung der Carnuntiner', in *Carnuntum – Wiedergeborene Stadt der Kaiser*, ed. F. Humer. Darmstadt: Verlag Philipp von Zabern, pp. 126–128.

Therios, I.N. 2009. *Olives*. Cambridge, MA: CABI.

Thissen, H.J. 1984. 'Der demotische Ammenvertrag aus Tebtynis', in *Grammata demotica. Festschrift für Erich Lüddeckens*, ed. H.-J. Thissen and K.T. Zauzich. Würzburg: Gisela Zauzich Verlag, pp. 235–244.

Thompson, D.J. 1979. 'Food: tradition and change in Hellenistic Egypt', *World Archaeology* 11, pp. 136–146.

Thompson, D.J. 1988. *Memphis Under the Ptolemies*. Princeton: Princeton University Press.

Thompson, D.J. 1995. 'Food for Ptolemaic temple workers', in *Food in Antiquity*, ed. J. Wilkins, D. Harvey and M. Dobson. Exeter: University of Exeter Press, pp. 316–325.

Thompson, D.J. 2012. *Memphis Under the Ptolemies*, 2nd edition. Princeton: Princeton University Press.

Thurmond, D.L. 2006. *A Handbook of Food Processing in Classical Rome: For Her Bounty No Winter*. Leiden/Boston: Brill.

Thüry, G.E. 2007. *Kulinarisches aus dem römischen Alpenvorland*. Linzer archäologische Forschungen Sonderheft 39. Linz: Stadtkommunikation Linz.

Thüry, G.E. 2010. 'Ein "Motor" der Ernährungsgeschichte: Die "Kulinarische Akkulturation"', in *Grenzenlose Gaumenfreuden. Römische Küche in einer germanischen Provinz*, ed. J. Meurers-Balke and T. Kaszab-Olschewski. Mainz: Verlag Philipp von Zabern, pp. 11–12.

Thüry, G.E. and Walter, J. 1997. *Condimenta: Gewürzpflanzen in Koch- und Backrezepten aus der römischen Antike: Begleitbuch zur Pflanzenschau 'Altrömische Gewürze'*. Vienna: Institut für Botanik und Botanischer Garten der Universität Wien.

Thüry, G.E. and Walter, J. 2001. *Condimenta. Gewürzpflanzen in Koch- und Backrezepten aus der römischen Antike*. Herrsching: Rudolf Spann Verlag.

Toedt, J., Koza, D. and van Cleef-Toedt, K. 2005. *The Chemical Composition of Everyday Products*. Westport: Greenwood Publishing Group.

Tolar, T., Jacomet, S., Velušček, A. and Čufar, K., 2009. 'Recovery techniques of waterlogged archaeological sediments – a comparison of different treatment methods of samples from Neolithic Lake shore settlements', *Vegetation History and Archaeobotany* 19(1), pp. 53–68.

Tomlinson, P.R. 1991. 'Vegetative plant remains from waterlogged deposits in York', in *New Light on early Farming*, ed. J. Renfrew. Edinburgh: Edinburgh University Press, pp. 109–119.

Torino, M., Rognini, M. and Fornaciari, G. 1995. 'Dental fluorosis in ancient Herculaneum', *Lancet* 345, p. 1306.

Touzeau, A., et al. 2014. 'Diet of ancient Egyptians inferred from stable isotope systematics', *Journal of Archaeological Science* 46, pp. 114–124.

Toynbee, J. 1971. *Death and Burial in the Roman World*. London: Thames & Hudson.

Toynbee, J. 1973. *Animals in Roman Life and Art*. London: Thames & Hudson.

Trotter, M. and Gleser, G. 1952. 'Estimation of stature from long bones of American whites and negroes', *American Journal of Physical Anthropology* 10, pp. 463–514.

Trotter, M. and Gleser, G. 1977. 'Corrigenda to "Estimation of stature from long limb bones of American whites and negroes, *American Journal Physical Anthropology* (1952)"', *American Journal of Physical Anthropology* 47, pp. 355–356.

Tykot, R.H. 2014. 'Bone chemistry and ancient diet', in *Encyclopedia of Global Archaeology*, ed. C. Smith. New York: Springer, pp. 931–941.

Ubelaker, D.H. and Rife, J.L. 2011. 'Skeletal analysis and mortuary practice in an early Roman chamber tomb at Kenchreai, Greece', *International Journal of Osteoarchaeology* 21, pp. 1–18.

Udayasekhara Rao, P. and Sharma, R.D. 1987. 'An evaluation of protein quality of fenugreek seeds (Trigonella foenumgraecum) and their supplementary effects', *Food Chemistry* 24, pp. 1–9.

Unwin, T. 1996. *Wine and the Vine: An Historical Geography of Viticulture and the Wine Trade*. London: Routledge.

Upex, S. 2008. *The Romans in the East of England: Settlement and Landscape in the Lower Nene Valley*. Stroud: Tempus.

Urso, C. 1997. 'L'alimentazione al tempo di Gregorio di Tours. *Consuetudines* e scelte culturali', *Quaderni medievali* 43, pp. 6–24.

US Department of Agriculture. 2011a. *USDA DRI Tables. Dietary Reference Intakes Homepage. Food and Nutrition Information Center*. Last updated 22 October 2015. Available at www.iom.edu/Activities/Nutrition/SummaryDRIs/~/media/Files/Activity%20Files/Nutrition/DRIs/5_Summary%20Table%20Tables%201-4.pdf) (accessed 27 June 2015).

US Department of Agriculture. 2011b. *USDA National Nutrient Database for Standard Reference*. Release 28. Nutrient Data Laboratory Home Page. Last updated Dec. 7, 2011. Available at http://ndb.nal.usda.gov/ (accessed June–July 2015).

US Department of Agriculture and US Department of Health and Human Services. 2010. *Dietary Guidelines for Americans, 2010*, 7th edition. Washington, DC: US Government Printing Office, December 2010. Available at www.cnpp.usda.gov/sites/default/files/dietary_guidelines_for_americans/PolicyDoc.pdf (accessed 20 October 2015).

Vaccaro, E. and MacKinnon, M. 2014. 'Pottery and animal consumption: new evidence from the "Excavating the Roman Peasant Project"', *HEROM. Journal on Hellenistic and Roman Material Culture* 3, pp. 225–257.

Vaccaro, E., Ghisleni, M., Arnoldus-Huyzendveld, A., Grey, C., Bowes, K., MacKinnon, M., Mercuri, A.M., Pecci, A., Ángel Cau Ontiveros, M., Rattigheri, E., and Rinaldi, R. 2013. 'Excavating the Roman peasant II: excavations at Case Nuove, Cinigiano (GR)', *Papers of the British School at Rome* 81, pp. 129–179.

Valamoti, S.M. 2013. 'Towards a distinction between digested and undigested glume bases in the archaeobotanical record from Neolithic northern Greece: a preliminary experimental investigation', *Environmental Archaeology* 18(1), 31–42.

Valamoti, S.M. and Charles, M. 2005. 'Distinguishing food from fodder through the study of charred plant remains: an experimental approach to dung-derived chaff', *Vegetation History and Archaeobotany* 14, pp. 528–533.

Valamoti, S.M., Moniaki, A., and Karathanou, A. 2011. 'An investigation of processing and consumption of pulses among prehistoric societies: archaeobotanical, experimental and ethnographic evidence from Greece', *Vegetation History and Archaeobotany* 20, pp. 381–396.

Van Pelt, W.P. and Heinrich, F.B.J., Forthcoming. 'Emmer wheat and barley prices in the Late New Kingdom: a Ramessid price paradox resolved', *Journal of Egyptian Archaeology*.

Van der Veen, M. 1998a. 'A life of luxury in the desert? The food and fodder supply to Mons Claudianus', *Journal of Roman Archaeology* 11, pp. 101–116.

Van der Veen, M. 1998b. 'Gardens in the desert', in *Life on the Fringe: Living in the Southern Egyptian Deserts During the Roman and Early-Byzantine Periods. Proceedings of a Colloquium Held in Cairo, 9–12 December 1996*. Leiden: E.J. Brill, pp. 221–242.

Van der Veen, M. 1999. 'The economic value of chaff and straw in arid and temperate zones', *Vegetation History and Archaeobotany*, 8, pp. 221–224.

Van der Veen, M. 2001. 'The botanical evidence', in *Survey and Excavations at Mons Claudianus 1987–1993. Volume 2: The Excavations: Part 1*, ed. V.A. Maxfield and D.P.S. Peacock. Cairo: Institut Français d'Archéologie Orientale du Caire: Documents de Fouilles 43, pp. 174–247.

Van der Veen, M. 2003. 'When is food a luxury?', *World Archaeology* 34(3), pp. 405–427.

Van der Veen, M. 2007. 'Formation processes of desiccated and carbonised plant remains – the identification of routine practice', *Journal of Archaeological Science* 34, pp. 968–990.

Van der Veen, M. 2018. 'Archaeobotany: the archaeology of human-plant interactions', in *The Science of Roman History: Biology, Climate, and the Future of the Past*, ed. W. Scheidel. Princeton: Princeton University Press. pp. 53–94.

Van der Veen, M. and Fieller, N.R.J. 1982. 'Sampling seeds', *Journal of Archaeologica Science* 9, pp. 287–298.

Van der Veen, M. and Tabinor, H. 2007. 'Food, fodder and fuel at Mons Porphyrites: the botanical evidence', in *The Roman Imperial Quarries. Survey and Excavation at Mons Porphyrites 1994–1998. Volume 2: The Excavations*, ed. D.P.S. Peacock and V.A. Maxfield. London: Egypt Exploration Society, pp. 83–142.

Van der Veen, M. and Wasylikowa, K. 2004. 'An archaeobotanical contribution to the history of watermelon: *Citrullus lanatus* (Thunb.)', *Vegetation History and Archaeobotany* 13, pp. 213–217.

Van der Veen, M., Livarda, A. and Hill, A. 2007. 'The archaeobotany of Roman Britain: current state and identification of research priorities', *Britannia* 38, pp. 181–210.

Van der Veen, M., et al. 2011. *Consumption, Trade and Innovation: Exploring the Botanical Remains from the Roman and Islamic Ports at Quseir al-Qadim, Egypt*. Frankfurt am Main: Africa Magna Verlag.

van Nijf, O. 1997. *The Civic World of Professional Associations in the Roman East*. Amsterdam: Brill.

van Minnen, P. 1994. 'House to house enquiries: an interdisciplinary approach to Roman Karanis', *Zeitschrift für Papyrologie und Epigraphik* 100, pp. 227–251.

van Minnen, P. 2001. 'Dietary hellenization or ecological transformation? Beer, wine and oil in later Roman Egypt', in *Atti del XXII Congresso internazionale di Papirologia*, ed. I. Andorlini, G. Bastianini, M. Manfredi and G. Menci. Florence: Istituto Papirologico Vitelli, pp. 1265–1280.

Van Neer, W., Lernau, O, Friedman, R., Mumford, G., Poblome, J., and Waelkens, M. 2004. 'Fish remains from archaeological sites as indicators of former trade connections in the Eastern Mediterranean', *Paléorient* 30(1), pp. 101–148.

Van Neer, W., Wouters, W., Ervynck, A. and Maes, J. 2005. 'New evidence from a Roman context in Belgium for fish sauce locally produced in Northern Gaul', *Archaeofauna* 14, pp. 171–182.

Van Neer, W., Hamilton-Dyer, S., Cappers, R., Desender, K. and Ervynck, A. 2007. 'The Roman trade in salted nilotic fish products: some examples from Egypt', *Documenta Archaeobiologiae* 4, pp. 173–188.

Van Neer, W., Wildekamp, R., Küçük, F., and Unlüsayin, M. 2008. 'The 1997–1999 surveys of the Anatolian fish fauna and their relevance to the interpretation of trade at Sagalassos', in *Sagalassos VI. Geo- and Bio-Archaeology at Sagalassos and in its Territory*, ed. P. Degryse and M. Waelkens. Leuven: Leuven University Press, pp. 299–323.

Van Neer, W., Ervynck, A. and Monsieur, P. 2010. 'Fish bones and amphorae: evidence for the production and consumption of salted fish products outside the Mediterranean region', *Journal of Roman Archaeology* 23, pp. 161–195.

Van Neer, W., et al. 2015. 'Découverte de deux salaisons de poissons à Oxyrynchus, el Bahnasa, Egypte', *Nova Studia Aegyptiaca* 9, pp. 567–578.

Vanhaute, E. 2011. 'From famine to food crisis: what history can teach us about local and global subsistence crises', *Journal of Peasant Studies* 38, pp. 47–65.

Vanna, V. 2007. 'Sex and gender related health status differences in ancient and contemporary skeletal populations', *Papers from the Institute of Archaeology* 18, pp. 114–147.

Vanpoucke, S., Mainland, I., de Cupere, B. and Waelkens, M. 2009. 'Dental microwear study of pigs from the classical site of Sagalassos (SW Turkey) as an aid for the reconstruction of husbandry practices in ancient times', *Environmental Archaeology* 14(2), pp. 137–154.

Vatin, C. 1966. 'Un tarif de poisons à Delphes', *Bulletin de Correspondance hellénique* 90, pp. 274–280.

Versluys, M.J. and Pitts, M., eds. 2014. *Globalisation and the Roman World: World History, Connectivity and Material Culture.* Cambridge: Cambridge University Press.

Vigne, J.-D. 1991. 'The meat and offal weight (MOW) method and the relative proportion of ovi caprines in some ancient meat diets of the north-western Mediterranean', *Rivista di Studi Liguri* 57, pp. 21–47.

Virlouvet, C. 1995. *Tessera frumentaria. Les Procédures de la Distribution du Blé public à Rome.* Rome: École francaise de Rome.

Virlouvet, C. 2009. *La Plèbe frumentaire dans les Témoignages épigraphiques. Essai d'Histoire sociale et administrative du Peuple de Rome antique.* Rome: École francaise de Rome.

Visioli, F., Poli A. and C. Gall. 2002. 'Antioxidant and other biological activities of phenols from olives and olive oil', *Medicinal Research Reviews* 22, pp. 65–75.

Vitruvius. 1999. *Ten Book of Architecture.* Translation and commentary by I. Rowland and T.N. Howe. Cambridge: Cambridge University Press.

Vleeming S.P., et al. 2005. *A Berichtigungsliste of Demotic Documents.* Leuven: Peeters.

Vogel, K.P., Johnson, V.A. and Mattern, P.J. 1978. 'Protein and lysine contents of endosperm and bran of the parents and progenies of crosses of common wheat', *Crop Science* 18, pp. 751–754.

Volpert, H.-P. 1997. 'Die römische Wassermühle einer villa rustica in München-Perlach', *Bayerische Vorgeschichtsblätter* 62, pp. 243–278.

von Reden, S. 2007. 'Classical Greece: consumption', in *The Cambridge Economic History of the Greco-Roman World*, ed. W. Scheidel, I. Morris and R. Saller. Cambridge, Cambridge University Press, pp. 385–406.

Vörös, I. 2000. 'Tierhaltung in römischen Ungarn', in *Von Augustus bis Attila. Leben am Ungarischen Donaulimes*, ed. Gesellschaft für Vor- und Frühgeschichte in Württemberg und Hohenzollern e.V. Schriften des Limesmuseums Aalen 53. Stuttgart: Konrad Theiss Verlag, pp. 68–72.

Vössing, K. 2004. *Mensa Regia. Das Bankett beim hellenistischen König und beim römischen Kaiser.* Munich: Saur.

Vössing, K. 2012. 'Family and domesticity', in *A Cultural History of Food in Antiquity*, ed. P. Erdkamp. London: Bloomsbury, pp. 133–143.

Vuolanto, V. 2005. 'Children and asceticism: strategies of continuity in the late fourth and early fifth centuries', in *Hoping for Continuity. Childhood, Education and Death in Antiquity and the Middle Ages*, ed. K. Mustakallio et al. Rome: Institutum Romanum Finlandiae, pp. 119–132.

Vuolanto, V. 2015. *Children and Asceticism in Late Antiquity. Continuity, Family Dynamics and the Rise of Christianity.* London: Ashgate.

Währen, M. 1983. 'Brot in einem römischen Brandgrab aus Saffig', *Pellenz Museum* 2, pp. 5–24.

Währen, M. 1990. 'Brot und Gebäck in keltischen Brandgräbern und römischen Aschengruben. Identifizierung von Brot- und Gebäckfunden aus dem Gräberfeld von Wederath-Belginum', *Trierer Zeitschrift* 53, pp. 195–224.

355

Währen, M. 2000. 'Neue Identifizierungen von seltenem Backwerk aus einem römischen Brandgrab mit Aschengruben im Saarland und der Zusammenhang mit anderem Bestattungs-brauchtum', in *Archäologische Untersuchungen im Trassenverlauf der Bundesautobahn A 8 im Landkreis Merzig-Wadern*, ed. A. Miron. Saarbrücken: Landesdenkmalamt im Ministerium für Umwelt, pp. 153–168.

Wahle, K., Caruso, D., Ochoa, J.J. and Quiles, J.L. 2004. 'Olive oil and modulation of cell signaling in disease prevention', *Lipids* 39, 1223–1231.

Waldron, T. 1994. *Counting the Dead: The Epidemiology of Skeletal Populations*. Chichester: John Wiley and Sons Ltd.

Waldron, T. 2006. 'Nutrition and the skeleton', in *Food in Medieval England: Diet and nutrition*, ed. C.M. Woolgar, D. Serjeantson and T. Waldron. Oxford: Oxford University Press, pp. 254–266

Waldron, T. 2009. *Palaeopathology*. Cambridge: Cambridge University Press.

Walker, P.L. and DeNiro, M.J. 1986. 'Stable nitrogen and carbon isotope ratios as indices of prehistoric dietary dependence on marine and terrestrial resources in Southern California', *American Journal of Physical Anthropology* 71, pp. 51–61.

Walker, P.L., Bathurst, R.R., Richman, R., Gjerdrum, T. and Andrushko, V.A. 2009. 'The causes of porotic hyperostosis and cribra orbitalia: a reappraisal of the iron-deficiency-anemia hypothesis', *American Journal of Physical Anthropology* 139, pp. 109–125.

Wallace, M. and Charles, M. 2013. 'What goes in does not always come out: the impact of the ruminant digestive system of sheep on plant material, and its importance for the interpretation of dung-derived archaeobotanical assemblages', *Environmental Archaeology* 18(1), pp. 18–30.

Wallace-Hadrill, A. 1994. *Houses and Society in Pompeii and Herculaneum*. Princeton: Princeton University Press.

Walter J. and Schofield, R. 1989. 'Famine, disease and crisis mortality in early modern society', in *Famine, Disease and the Social Order in Early Modern Society*, ed. J. Walter and R. Schofield. Cambridge: Cambridge University Press, pp. 1–73.

Wanek, J., Papageorgopoulou, C., Rühli, F. 2012. 'Fundamentals of paleoimaging techniques: bridging the gap between physicists and paleopathologists', in *A Companion to Paleopathology*, ed. A.L. Grauer. Chichester: Wiley-Blackwell, pp. 324–338.

Wang, N., Hatcher, D.W., Tyler, R.T., Toews, R. and Gawalko, E.J. 2010. 'Effect of cooking on the composition of beans (*Phaseolus vulgaris* L.) and chickpeas (*Cicer arietinum* L.)', *Food Research International* 43, pp. 589–594.

Warinner, C., Hendy, J., Speller, C., et al. 2014. 'Direct evidence of milk consumption from ancient human dental calculus', *Scientific Reports* 4(7104).

Warnock, P. 2007. *Identification of Ancient Olive Oil Processing Methods Based on Olive Remains*. Oxford: Archaeopress.

Waterlow, J.C. 1989. 'Diet of the classical period of Greece and Rome', *European Journal of Clinical Nutrition* 43(2), p. 3–12.

Wecowski, M. 2014. *The Rise of the Greek Aristocratic Banquet*. Oxford: Oxford University Press.

Wedenig, R. 2005. 'Tonmedaillon und Kuchenform aus Flavia Solva', in *Synergia. Festschrift für F. Krinzinger 2*, ed. B. Brandt, V. Gassner and S. Ladstätter. Wien: Phoibos Verlag, pp. 485–489.

Weeber, K.-W. 2013. *Wasser, Wein und Öl. Die Lebenssäfte der römischen Welt*. Darmstadt: Wissenschaftliche Buchgesellschaft.

Weinberger, K. 2003. 'The impact of micronutrients on labor productivity: evidence from rural India', *Annual Meeting 2003, August 16-22, International Association of Agricultural Economists, Durban*.

Weingarten, S. 'Food in Roman Palestine: ancient sources and modern research', in *Food and History* 5(2), pp. 41–67.

Welch, R.M. and Graham, R.D. 2000. 'A new paradigm for word agriculture: productive, sustainable, nutritious healthful food systems', *Food and Nutrition Bulletin* 21(4), pp. 361–366.

Wesenberg, B. 1993. 'Zum integrierten Stilleben in der Wanddekoration des zweiten pompejanischen Stils', in *Functional and Spatial Analysis of Wall Painting: Proceedings of the Fifth International Congress on Ancient Wall Painting, Amsterdam, September 1992*, ed. E.M. Moorman. Leiden: BABESCH, pp. 160–167.

White, K.D. 1970. *Roman Farming*. Ithaca: Cornell University Press.

White, K.D. 1976. 'Food requirements and food supplies in classical times in relation to the diet of the various classes', *Progress in Food and Nutrition Science* 2, pp. 143–191.

White, K.D. 1995. 'Cereals, bread and milling in the Roman world', in *Food in Antiquity*, ed. J. Wilkins, D. Harvey and M. Dobson. Exeter: University of Exeter Press, pp. 38–43.

White, L.M. 2001. 'Regulating fellowship in the communal meal: early Jewish and Christian evidence', in *Meals in a Social Context: Aspects of the Communal Meal in the Hellenistic and Roman World*, ed. I. Nielsen and H.S. Nielsen. Aarhus: Aarhus University Press, pp. 177–205.

Whittaker, C.R. 1985. 'Trade and the aristocracy in the roman empire', *Opus* 4, pp. 49–75.

Whittaker, H. 2003. 'Women and fasting in early Christianity', in *Gender, Cult, and Culture in the Ancient World from Mycenae to Byzantium. Proceeding of the Nordic Symposium on Gender and Women's History in Antiquity. Helsinki 20–22 October 2000*, ed. L. Larsson Lovén and A. Stromberg. Sävedalen: Paul Åströms Förlag, pp. 100–115.

Wickham, C. 2009. *The Inheritance of Rome: A History of Europe from 400 to 1000*. London, Allen Lane.

Wieland, G., ed. 1999. *Keltische Viereckschanzen. Einem Rätsel auf der Spur*. Stuttgart: Konrad Theiss Verlag.

Wies, E.W. 1992. *Capitulare de villis et Curtis imperialibus (Verordnung über die Krongüter und Reichshöfe) und die Geheimnisse des Kräutergartens Karls des Großen*. Aachen: Einhard Verlag.

Wieser, H. 2006. 'Chemistry of gluten proteins', *Food Microbiology* 24, pp. 115–119.

Wildman, R.E., ed. 2007. *Handbook of Nutraceuticals and Functional Foods*. Florida: CRC Press.

Wilkins, J. 2000. 'Dialogue and comedy: the structure of the *Deipnosophistae*', in *Athenaeus and his World: Reading Greek Culture in the Roman Empire*, ed. D. Braund and J. Wilkins. Exeter: University of Exeter Press, pp. 23–37.

Wilkins, J. 2003. 'Land and sea: Italy and the Mediterranean in the Roman discourse of dining', *The American Journal of Philology* 124(3), Special Issue: Roman Dining, pp. 359–375.

Wilkins, J. 2012. 'Food and drink in the ancient world', in *Writing Food History: A Global Perspective*, ed. K.W. Claflin and P. Scholliers. London and New York: Berg, pp. 11–23.

Wilkins, J.M. and Hill, S. 1996. 'The sources and sauces of Athenaeus', in *Food in Antiquity*, ed. J. Wilkins, D. Harvey and M. Dobson. Exeter: University of Exeter Press, pp. 429–438.

Wilkins, J. and Hill, S. 2006. *Food in the Ancient World*. Oxford: Blackwell.

Wilkins, J. and Nadeau, R., eds. 2015. *A Companion to Food in the Ancient World*. Oxford: Wiley-Blackwell.

Wilkins, J., Harvey, D. and Dobson, M. 1995. *Food in Antiquity*. Exeter: Liverpool University Press.

Wilkinson, K. 2015. *Women and Modesty in Late Antiquity*. Cambridge: Cambridge University Press.

Wilkinson, R. and Pickett, K., 2011. *The Spirit Level: Why Equality Makes Societies Stronger*. London: Bloomsbury Press.

Willerding, U. 1971. 'Methodische Probleme bei der Untersuchung und Auswertung von Pflanzenfunden in vor- und frühgeschichtlichen Siedlungen', *Nachrichten aus Niedersachsens Urgeschichte* 40, pp. 180–198.

Willerding, U. 1991. 'Präsenz, Erhaltung und Repräsentanz von Pflanzenresten in archäologischem Fundgut (Presence, preservation and representation of archaeological plant remains)', in *Progress in Old World Palaeoethnobotany: A Retrospective View on the Occasion of 20 Years of the International Work Group for Palaeoethnobotany*, ed. W. van Zeist, K. Wasylikowa and K-E. Behre. Rotterdam: A.A. Balkema, pp. 25–51.

Williamson, J.G. and Lindert, P.H. 1980. *American Inequality: A Macroeconomic History*. New York: Academic Press.

Wilson, A. 2000. 'The water-mills on the Janiculum', *Memoirs of the American Academy of Rome* 45, pp. 219–246.

Wilson, A. 2009. 'Indicators for Roman economic growth: a response to Walter Scheidel', *Journal of Roman Archaeology* 22, pp. 71–82.

Wilson, A. 2011. 'City sizes and urbanization in the Roman Empire', in *Settlement, Urbanization, and Population*, ed. A. Bowman and A. Wilson. Oxford: Oxford University Press, pp. 161–195.

Wittenburg, A. 1980. 'Zur Qualität des Olivenöls in der Antike', *Zeitschrift für Papyrologie und Epigraphik* 38, pp. 185–189.

Wittwer-Backofen, U. and Kiesewetter, U. 1997. 'Menschliche Überreste der Neuen Ausgrabungen in Troia – Funde der Kampagnen 1989–1995', *Studia Troia* 7, pp. 509–537.

Wood, J.W., Milner, G.R., Harpending, H.C. and Weiss, K.M. 1992. 'The osteological paradox: problems of inferring prehistoric health from skeletal samples', *Current Anthropology* 33, pp. 343–370.

Woolf, G. 1990. 'Food, poverty and patronage: the significance of the epigraphy of the Roman alimentary schemes in early Imperial Italy', *Papers of the British School at Rome* 58, pp. 197–228.

Woolf, G. 1998. *Becoming Roman: The Origins of Provincial Civilization in Gaul*. Cambridge: Cambridge University Press.

World Health Organization (WHO). 2004. 'Vitamin B_{12}', in *Vitamin and Mineral Requirements in Human Nutrition*, 2nd edition. Geneva: World Health Organization.

Worm, C. 1696. *Dissertatio: De faba Pythagorica*. Copenhagen: Hafniae.

Wright, L.E. and Yoder, C.J. 2003. Recent progress in bioarchaeology: approaches to the osteological paradox. *Journal of Archaeological Research* 11, pp. 43–70.

Wright, P. 2003. 'Preservation or destruction of plant remains by carbonization?', *Journal of Archaeological Science* 30, pp. 577–583.

Wright, P. 2005. 'Flotation samples and some paleoethnobotanical implications', *Journal of Archaeological Science* 32, pp. 9–26.

Wu, G., Jaeger, L.A., Bazer, F.W., and Marc Rhoads, J. 2004. 'Arginine deficiency in preterm infants: biochemical mechanisms and nutritional implications', *Journal of Nutritional Biochemistry* 15, pp. 442–551.

Youtie, H.C. 1978. 'ΚΟΡΥΜΒΑΣ', *Zeitschrift für Papyrologie und Epigraphik* 31, p. 107. Scriptiunculae posteriores 1. Bonn: Rudolf Habelt Verlag, pp. 482–483.

Zach, B. 2002. 'Vegetable offerings on the Roman sacrificial site in Mainz, Germany – short report on the first results', *Vegetation History and Archaeobotany* 11, 101–106.

Zakrzewski, S.R. 2003. 'Variation in ancient Egyptian stature and body proportions', *American Journal of Physical Anthropology* 121, pp. 219–229.

Zanda, E. 2011. *Fighting Hydra-like Luxury: Sumptuary Regulation in the Roman Republic*. London: Bloomsbury Publishing.

Zhernakova, A., Elbers, C.C., Ferwerda, B., Romanos, J., Trynka, G., Dubois, P.C., de Kovel, C.G.F., Franke, L., Oosting., M, Barisani., D., Bardella, M.T., Finnish Celiac Disease Study Group, Joosten, L.A.B., Saavalainen, P., van Heel, D.A., Catassi, C., Netea, M.G. and Wijmenga, C. 2010. 'Evolutionary and functional analysis of celiac risk loci reveals SH2B3 as a protective factor against bacterial infection', *American Journal of Human Genetics* 86(6), pp. 970–977.

Zifferero, A. 2004. 'Ceramica preromana e sistemi alimentari: elementi per una ricerca', in *Bridging the Tiber, Approaches to Regional Archaeology in the Middle Tiber Valley*, ed. H. Patterson. London: British School at Rome, pp. 255–268.

Zuiderhoek, A. 2008. 'Feeding the citizens: municipal grain funds and civic benefactors in the Roman East', in *Feeding the Ancient Greek City*, ed. O. van Nijf and R. Alston. Leuven: Peeters, pp. 159–180.

INDEX

References to diagrams, pictures, and tables are given in italics.

CPSIA information can be obtained
at www.ICGtesting.com
Printed in the USA
LVHW061732040223
738684LV00013B/857